Handbook of
STRESS, COPING,
and HEALTH

Handbook of STRESS, COPING, *and* HEALTH

Implications
for
Nursing
Research,
Theory,
and
Practice

Virginia Hill Rice
Editor

 Sage Publications, Inc.
International Educational and Professional Publisher
Thousand Oaks ▪ London ▪ New Delhi

For information:

Sage Publications, Inc.
2455 Teller Road
Thousand Oaks, California 91320
E-mail: order@sagepub.com

Sage Publications Ltd.
6 Bonhill Street
London EC2A 4PU
United Kingdom

Sage Publications India Pvt. Ltd.
M-32 Market
Greater Kailash I
New Delhi 110 048 India

Printed in the United States of America

Library of Congress Cataloging-in-Publication Data

Main entry under title:

Handbook of stress, coping, and health: Implications for nursing research, theory,
   and practice / edited by Virginia Hill Rice.
         p. cm.
      Includes bibliographical references and index.
      ISBN 0-7619-1820-5 (cloth: acid-free paper)
      ISBN 0-7619-1821-3 (paperback: acid-free paper)
   1. Stress (Physiology)—Handbooks, manuals, etc. 2. Stress (Psychology)—
   Handbooks, manuals, etc. 3. Stress management—Handbooks, manuals,
   etc. 4. Stress (Psychology)—Research—Methodology—Handbooks,
   manuals, etc. 5. Nursing—Research—Methodology—Handbooks, manuals,
   etc. I. Rice, Virginia Hill.
      QP82.2.S8 H357 2000
      158.7'2'024513—dc21   99-050741

      02   03   04   05   06   10   9   8   7   6   5   4   3   2

Acquiring Editor:	Jim Brace-Thompson
Editorial Assistant:	Anna Howland
Production Editor:	Astrid Virding
Editorial Assistant:	Nevair Kabakian
Typesetter/Designer:	Marion Warren
Indexer:	Teri Greenberg
Cover Designer:	Michelle Lee

This book is dedicated to my husband, Dr. Bill,
and to our sons, Grantland and Garrett,
for their loving support.

Contents

PART VI   FUTURE DIRECTIONS

Acknowledgments

I thank Dr. Brenda Lyon for her expertise and invaluable support in creating this text and the following people for serving as expert content reviewers of the chapters in this book. They provided essential feedback to me and to the chapter authors:

Kenneth R. Burns,
   Northern Illinois University

Stephen J. Cavanagh,
   Wayne State University

Carol A. Craft,
   St. Louis University

May T. Dobal,
   Wayne State University

Patricia R. Ebright,
   University of Cincinnati

Carol J. Farran,
   Rush University

Bonnie J. Garvin,
   Ohio State University

Margaret Grey,
   Yale University

Maureen W. Groer,
   University of Tennessee

Thomas L. Hardie,
   University of Delaware

Jean E. Johnson,
   University of Rochester

Brenda L. Lyon,
   Indiana University

Marilyn A. McCubbin,
   University of Wisconsin

Marilyn T. Oberst,
   Wayne State University

Rosalind Peters,
   Medical College of Ohio

Renee Twibell,
   Ball State University

April Hazard Vallerand,
   Wayne State University

Clarann Weinert,
   Montana State University

Felita Wilson,
   Wayne State University

Frances B. Wimbush,
   Wayne State University

Julie Johnson Zerwic,
   University of Illinois

Preface

nterest in the phenomena of
stress and coping and their relationship to health has reached an
all-time high not only in psychology and the
behavioral sciences but also in nursing. Stress,
coping, and health content have become an
integral part of nursing curricula, theory,
research, and practice at all educational and
practice levels. There are undergraduate programs whose structural underpinnings are
built on the relationships among these constructs; most, if not all, undergraduate textbooks include selected content in this area
(Craven & Hirnle, 1996; Porth, 1994).

At the master's level, stress and coping
are core content in most graduate programs
and are essential knowledge for certification
at the advanced practice level (American
Nurses Credentialling Center Commission on
Certification, 1999). At the doctoral level,
there are many schools of nursing that offer a
minor in this area of study (e.g., Wayne State
University). In many instances, stress, coping,
and their relationship to health are foundational to dissertation research.

The extensive attention given to these
phenomena is reflected in the periodical literature for nursing. The *Cumulative Index for
Nursing and Allied Health* lists more than
2,800 stress and coping articles published under these keywords since 1982. When stress
and coping topics are specified, such as hardiness or personal control, the literature volume
increases exponentially.

The stress, coping, and health field is a
broad one, developing across many disciplines, including nursing, psychology, medicine, sociology, and biology. This has resulted
in an unevenness and lack of systematic development. Nonetheless, I and the contributing authors believe there is much to be gained
through exploring a cross section of developments in the field. An attempt has been made
to synthesize stress, coping, and health findings of the past 30 years.

The book's content reflects the evolution
and testing of various theoretical models of
stress, coping, and health and their particular
relevance for the profession and the discipline
of nursing. Of necessity, choices of content

were made because of the extraordinary breath and depth of this field. Selected for inclusion in this book was content considered to be the most thoroughly developed and studied. Every attempt was made to present a balance between theoretical development, research, measurement, and implications for nursing practice and to critique the content within those contexts.

Part I, the Introduction, discusses the diverse conceptualizations of stress, coping, and health and the importance of these for nursing and other disciplines. It also addresses some of the major problems and issues surrounding the various conceptualizations. Part II presents the response-oriented theories of stress, beginning with the hallmark works of Cannon (1929) and Selye (1936). In these models, stress is considered to be within the person as a result of some internal or external stressor and is viewed as a nonspecific response to any demand on the organism. Studies of nursing investigators who have used the response conceptualization include Chavez and Faber's (1987) study of family members in the intensive care unit, Thomas and Friedman's (1990) work with cardiac patients, Toth's (1988) psychophysiological model for explaining the responses of acute myocardial infarction patients, and Fallon, Gould, and Wainwright's (1997) research with transplant patients.

Part III presents the stimulus-oriented theories of stress, in which stress is viewed as the spark or catalyst. Stress is considered to come from without, and the human organism responds both psychologically and physiologically. The assumption is that change is stressful, regardless of individual differences, and that there is inherent stress in events such as death, pain, and loss, regardless of the person experiencing them. The early life events work of psychologists Holmes and Rahe (1967) is relevant. Important for nursing is research by Volicer and Bohannon (1975) with their Hospital Stress Rating Scale, Bigbee's (1990) study of stressful life events and illness occurrence in rural versus urban women, and

Thoma, Hockenberry-Eaton, and Kemp's (1993) examination of life change events and coping in families of children with cancer.

In contrast to major life events, day-to-day irritating and joyous experiences called hassles and uplifts, respectively, are proposed to have a greater effect on psychological well-being and health than major life events (Kanner, Coyne, Schaefer, & Lazarus, 1981). Such daily happenings have been examined in rheumatoid arthritis patients (Crosby, 1988), adolescent girls (DeMaio-Esteves, 1990), and critical care nurses' job burnout (Stechmiller & Yarandi, 1993) and contrasted with life events by Klemm (1994).

Part IV examines theories proposed to describe, predict and/or explain the relationships among stress and coping and health outcomes. Theories developed in psychology that have proved useful for nursing include Salutogenesis and Sense of Coherence (Antonovsky, 1979) and the interactional (Lazarus, 1966) and transactional (Lazarus & Folkman, 1984) stress and coping models. Researchers using these theoretical approaches or modifications of them or both to study nursing phenomena include Scott, Oberst, and Dropkin (1980), Rice, Sieggreen, Mullin, and Williams (1988), and Mahat (1997).

Part V examines moderating factors found to affect the relationships among stress, coping, and health. These include antecedent variables such as age (Sharrer & Ryan-Wenger, 1995), family (Friedemann & Webb, 1995), and culture (Ani, 1993). Other factors are social support (Ducharme, Stevens, & Rowat, 1994; Northouse, 1988), hardiness (Post-White et al., 1996), sense of coherence (Nyamathi, 1993), Type A behavior pattern (Thomas & Friedmann, 1990), and self-regulation (Alonzo & Reynolds, 1997). Additional mediators include personal control (Rice, Beck, & Stevenson, 1997), hope (Farran, Herth, & Popovich, 1995), self-efficacy (Pohl, Martinelli, & Antonakos, 1998), and uncertainty (Mishel, 1991).

Part VI proposes a theoretical model that includes most of the concepts discussed in the book. Its purpose is to provide some direction for a more holistic view of stress, coping, and health and to point the way for future research and model building in nursing science.

The general format for most of the chapters is historical evolution and critical examination of prominent model, theories, and constructs within a "parent" discipline or in nursing or both. For example, Toth's (1988) cardiovascular recovery model was derived from Selye's (1936) general adaptation syndrome, Pollock's (1989) work was borrowed from Kobasa's (1979) hardiness model, and Norbeck's (1981) social support model was founded in the work of Cobb (1976). Scott et al.'s (1980) stress-coping and Mishel's (1991) uncertainty models were both derived from the work of Lazarus and Folkman (1984). Descriptions of the respective model, theory, or construct follow with a discussion of the level of theory development within nursing science and a schematic representation.

A critical examination of the empirical adequacy of the model, theory, or construct in nursing and related disciplines is followed by a detailed description of measures of the phenomenon. Intervention tables are included in some, but not all, of the chapters. Last, implications of the construct, concept, or theory for practice, theory development, and future research are discussed.

This book is intended as a primary source for graduate students in nursing and for other health care scientists and may serve as a secondary source for undergraduate students in nursing and for students of other health disciplines. The book has considerable utility as a reference work for researchers and scholars in a variety of health sciences.

For the clinician, it can be a guide to the most pertinent findings for the understanding, prevention, intervention, and treatment of stress-related disorders. Last, it has significant import for those in stress, coping, and health theory development and testing who wish to have foundational knowledge. This book is very important because no other comprehensive handbook was found that addresses specifically the state of the knowledge of stress, coping, and health for nursing.

➤ REFERENCES

Alonzo, A., & Reynolds, N. (1997). Responding to symptoms and signs of acute myocardial infarction: How do you educate the public? *Heart & Lung, 26,* 263-272.

American Nurses Credentialling Center Commission on Certification. (1999). *1999 board certification catalog.* Washington, DC: Author.

Ani, N. S. (1993). A comparison of American and Egyptian cancer patients' attitudes and unmet needs. *Cancer Nursing, 16,* 193-203.

Antonovsky, A. (1979). *Health, stress and coping.* San Francisco: Jossey-Bass.

Bigbee, J. (1990). Stressful life events and illness occurrence in rural versus urban women. *Journal of Community Health Nursing, 7,* 105-113.

Chavez, C. W., & Faber, L. (1987). Effect of an education-orientation program on family members who visit their significant other in the intensive care unit. *Heart & Lung: Journal of Critical Care, 16,* 92-99.

Cobb, S. (1976). Social support as a moderator of life stress. *Psychosomatic Medicine, 38,* 300-314.

Craven, R. F., & Hirnle, C. J. (1996). *Fundamentals of nursing: human health and function.* Philadelphia: Lippincott-Raven.

Crosby, L. J. (1988). Stress factors, emotional stress, and rheumatoid arthritis disease activity. *Journal of Advanced Nursing, 13,* 452-461.

DeMaio-Esteves, M. (1990). Mediators of daily stress and perceived health status in adolescent girls. *Nursing Research, 39,* 360-364.

Ducharme, F., Stevens, B., & Rowat, K. (1994). Social support: Conceptual and methodological issues for research in mental health nursing. *Issues in Mental Health Nursing, 15,* 373-392.

Fallon, M., Gould, D., & Wainwright, S. P. (1997). Stress and quality of life in the renal transplant patient: A preliminary investigation. *Journal of Advanced Nursing, 25,* 562-570.

Farran, C., Herth, K., & Popovich, J. (1995). *Hope and hopelessness: Critical clinical constructs.* Thousand Oaks, CA: Sage.

Friedemann, M. L., & Webb, A. (1995). Family health and mental health six years after economic stress and unemployment. *Issues in Mental Health Nursing, 16,* 51-66.

Holmes, T. H., & Rahe, R. (1967). The social readjustment rating scale. *Journal of Psychosomatic Research, 12,* 213-218.

Kanner, A. D., Coyne, J. C., Schaefer, C., & Lazarus, R. S. (1981). Comparison of two modes of stress measurement: Daily hassles and uplifts versus major life events. *Journal of Behavioral Medicine, 4*, 1-39.

Klemm, P. R. (1994). Variables influencing psychosocial adjustment to lung cancer: A preliminary study. *Oncology Nursing Forum, 21*, 1059-1062.

Kobasa, S. C. (1979). Stressful life events, personality, and health: An inquiry into hardiness. *Journal of Personality and Social Psychology, 37*, 1-11.

Lazarus, R. S. (1966). *Psychological stress and the coping process.* New York: McGraw-Hill.

Lazarus, R. S., & Folkman, S. (1984). *Stress, appraisal, and coping.* New York: Springer.

Mahat, G. (1997). Perceived stressors and coping strategies among individuals with rheumatoid arthritis. *Journal of Advanced Nursing, 25*, 1144-1150.

Mishel, M. (1991). The measurement of uncertainty. *Nursing Research, 30*, 258-263.

Norbeck, J. (1981). Social support: A model for clinical research and application. *Advances in Nursing Science, 3*, 43-59.

Northouse, L. L. (1988). Social support in patients' and husbands' adjustment to breast cancer. *Nursing Research, 37*, 91-95.

Nyamathi, A. M. (1993). A sense of coherence in minority women at risk for HIV infection. *Public Health Nursing, 10*, 151-158.

Pohl, J., Martinelli, A., & Antonakos, C. (1998). Predictors of participation in a smoking cessation intervention group among low-income women. *Addictive Behaviors, 23*, 699-704.

Pollock, S. E. (1989). The hardiness characteristic: A motivating factor in adaptation. *Advances in Nursing Science, 11*, 53-62.

Porth, C. (1994). *Pathophysiology: Concepts of altered health states* (5th ed.). Philadelphia: J. B. Lippincott.

Post-White, J., Ceronsky, C., Kreitzer, M., Nickelson, K., Drew, D., Mackey, K., Koopmeiners, L., & Gutknecht, S. (1996). Hope, spirituality, sense of coherence, and quality of life in patients with cancer. *Oncology Nursing Forum, 23*, 1571-1579.

Rice, V. H., Beck, C., & Stevenson, J. S. (1997). Ethical issues relative to autonomy and personal control in independent and cognitively impaired elders. *Nursing Outlook, 45*, 27-34.

Rice, V. H., Sieggreen, M., Mullin, M., & Williams, J. (1988). Development and testing of an arteriography information intervention for stress reduction. *Heart & Lung: Journal of Critical Care, 17*, 23-28.

Scott, D. W., Oberst, M., & Dropkin, M. (1980). A stress coping model. *Advances in Nursing Science, 3*(1), 9-23.

Selye, H. (1936). A syndrome produced by diverse noxious agents. *Nature, 138*, 132-135.

Sharrer, V., & Ryan-Wenger, N. (1995). A longitudinal study of age and gender differences in school-age children's stressors and coping strategies. *Journal of Pediatric Health Care, 9*, 123-130.

Stechmiller, J. K., & Yarandi, H. (1993). Predictors of burnout in critical care nurses. *Heart & Lung, 22*, 534-541.

Thoma, M., Hockenberry-Eaton, M., & Kemp, V. (1993). Life change events and coping behaviors in families of children with cancer. *Journal of Pediatric Oncology Nursing, 10*, 105-111.

Thomas, S., & Friedman, E. (1990). Type A behavior and cardiovascular responses during verbalization in cardiac patients. *Nursing Research, 39*, 48-53.

Toth, J. (1988). Measuring the stressful experience of hospital discharge following acute myocardial infarction. In C. Waltz & O. Strickland (Eds.), *Measurement of nursing outcomes* (pp. 3-23). New York: Springer.

Volicer, B. J., & Bohannon, M. W. (1975). A hospital stress rating scale. *Nursing Research, 24*(5), 352-359.

PART I

Introduction

CHAPTER 1

Stress, Coping, and Health

A Conceptual Overview

Brenda L. Lyon

lthough the term *stress* as it relates to the human experience has been in the scientific literature since the 1930s and in the nursing literature since the late 1950s, the word did not become popular vernacular until the late 1970s and early 1980s. Today, the term is used in everyday vocabulary to capture a variety of human experiences that are disturbing or disruptive in some manner: "You wouldn't believe how much stress I had today!" "I was really stressed out."

Subjective sensations commonly experienced in conjunction with "feeling stressed" are headache, shortness of breath, light-headedness or dizziness, nausea, muscle tension, fatigue, gnawing in the gut, palpitations, loss of appetite or hunger, and problems with sleep. Behavioral manifestations of stress commonly reported are crying, smoking, excessive eating, drinking alcohol, fast talking, and trembling. It is also commonplace for people to complain that stress negatively af-

fects their functioning. It impairs concentration ability, problem-solving ability, decision-making ability, and the ability to get work done (Goleman & Gurin, 1993; Ornstein & Sobel, 1988; Pelletier, 1992, 1995).

The word "stress" began appearing in nursing journals in 1956. Stress, as a construct, was not widely recognized by nurse researchers until the 1970s (Lyon & Werner, 1987). Stress gained recognition as a phenomenon of interest for nursing because anecdotal data from patients and empirical evidence from researchers suggested that stress and health were inextricably related concepts. Nursing, as a discipline, was not alone in recognizing the importance that stress played in health. Other health-related disciplines had already begun to contribute to both theory development and empirical testing of the phenomenon of stress and its connection with health.

Several different health-related disciplines (e.g., psychology, social psychology, nursing, and medicine) have identified stress and coping as important variables affecting health. Stress has been linked to the onset of diseases, such as cardiovascular conditions (Benschop et al., 1998; Dimsdale, Ruberman, & Carleton, 1987; Pashkow, 1999; Ornish, Scherwitz, & Doody, 1983), cancer (Cohen & Rabin, 1998; Siegel, 1986), and colds (Cohen et al., 1998; Cohen, Tyrrell, & Smith, 1991), as well as the exacerbation of symptoms such as asthma (Wright, Rodriquez, & Cohen, 1998), irritable bowel syndrome (Bennett, Tennant, Piesse, Badcock, & Kellow, 1998; Dancey, Taghavi, & Fox, 1998), ulcerative colitis (Whitehead & Schuster, 1985), arthritis (Crofford, Jacobson, & Young, 1999; Lorig et al., 1989), skin disorders (Lebwohl & Tan, 1998), and diabetes (Inui et al., 1998; Surwit, Schneider, & Feinglos, 1992). In addition, stress has been linked to symptomatic experiences such as headaches (Davis, Holm, Myers, & Suda, 1998; Fanciullacci, Alessandri, & Fanciullacci, 1998; Holm, Lokken, & Myers, 1997; Holroyd, Nash, Pingel, Cordingley, & Jerome, 1991), musculoskeletal pain (Dyrehag et al., 1998; Stacy, Kaplan, & Williams, 1992), gastrointestinal upset (Whitehead & Schuster, 1985), hyperventilation (Ringsberg & Akerlind, 1999), insomnia (Vgontzas et al., 1998), and fatigue (Glaser & Kiecolt-Glaser, 1998). Also, coping behaviors have been identified as mediating the effect of stress on blood sugar (Cox & Gonder-Frederick, 1992; Fukunishi, Akimoto, Horikawa, Shirasaka, & Yamazaki, 1998), heart rate (Fontana & McLaughlin, 1998; Suarez & Williams, 1989), blood pressure (Krantz, DeQuattro, & Blackburn, 1987; Schnall, Schwartz, Landsbergis, Warren, & Pickering, 1998; Syme, 1987), and 17- hydroxycorticosteriods (Oken, 1967).

The experience of stress, particularly chronic stress, takes a significant toll on the well-being of individuals in terms of emotional and physical discomforts as well as functional ability. Health care utilization research has repeatedly demonstrated that from 30% to 60% of all physician office visits are for illness experiences that are nondisease

based with stress as the common contributor (Cummings & Vandenbos, 1981; Sobel, 1995). As early as 1982, the United States Clearing House for Mental Health Information reported that industry had lost $17 billion in production capacity due primarily to stress-related problems. In addition, it was estimated in the late 1980s that $60 billion was lost annually by businesses because of stress-related physical illness (Matteson & Ivancevich, 1987). It has been estimated that businesses lose up to $150 billion per year due to stress-related absenteeism, lost productivity, retraining, and stress-related health care costs (deCarteret, 1994).

Although it is commonly accepted that stress affects health, all of the psychobiological connections are not understood. For example, why does a person who has had an unpleasant interaction with his or her supervisor develop a tension headache? Or why does a woman who is struggling to balance the demands of work and home develop stomach pains every Monday morning? Theoretical development in the area of stress, coping, and health has been hampered by confusion regarding each of the concepts.

The purpose of this chapter is to present an overview of theoretical approaches to explaining the concepts of stress, coping, and health and their interrelationships with some historical perspectives. Problems and issues regarding the conceptualizations of each of these constructs will be identified. Attention will be paid to reconciling some of the diverse conceptualizations of stress, coping, and health for nursing.

➤ THEORETICAL APPROACHES TO DEFINING STRESS, COPING, AND HEALTH

In this section, I present an overview of the conceptualizations of the stress and health connection. The content regarding coping will appear, as appropriate, in the presentation of each of the major theoretical orientations to stress. Discussion of each construct includes identification of conceptual and theoretical problems and measurement challenges. The theoretical orientations to explaining stress have been categorized into three types: response based, stimulus based, and transactional based.

Stress as a Response

The response-based orientation was initially developed and examined by Hans Selye and summarized in *The Stress of Life* (1956). Selye was a pioneer in the development and testing of theory pertinent to stress from a physiological and medical perspective. As a physician, he was intrigued by the common inflammatory responses he observed in patients regardless of their particular disease or exposure to medical procedures. Many of Selye's main concepts stemmed historically from Cannon's (1932) notion that sympathoadrenal changes were "emergency functions."

Selye viewed stress as a response to noxious stimuli or environmental stressors and defined it as the "nonspecific response of the body to noxious stimuli" (Selye, 1956, p. 12). He defined stress as a response, and it became the dependent variable in stress research. Selye's work focused on describing and explaining a physiological response pattern known as the general adaptation syndrome (GAS). The following are the basic ideas in Selye's theory: (a) The stress response (GAS) was a defensive response that did not depend on the nature of the stressor; (b) the GAS, as a defense reaction, progressed in three well-defined stages (alarm, resistance, and exhaustion); and (c) if the GAS was severe and prolonged, disease states could result (the so-called diseases of adaptation). Selye (1956) proposed that cognitive variables such as "perception" played no role in contributing to the initiation or moderation of the GAS. In his 1983 edition of *Stress of Life,* Selye extended his thinking to include both negatively and positively toned (eustress) experiences that could be contributed to and moderated by cognitive factors. It is important to note, how-

ever, that Selye's basic theoretical premise that stress was a physiological phenomenon was not altered. In the absence of a modification of his theory, it was not possible to explain "psychological stress." This could not be done in the context of a theory that was strictly limited to physiology and neglected cognitive-perceptual factors. In fact, problems inherent in a normative or generalized response theory were demonstrated when Mason (1971, 1975a, 1975b) disconfirmed the "nonspecificity" of physiological responses to noxious stimuli in rats and monkeys.

Although Selye did not specifically address the concept of coping in his work, his notions of "defense" and "adaptation" are conceptually similar to that of coping. The alarm reaction phase of the GAS is triggered when there is a noxious stimulus. This reaction is characterized by sympathetic nervous system stimulation. In the second phase, or stage of resistance, physiologic forces are mobilized to resist damage from the noxious stimulus. Often, the stage of resistance leads to adaptation or the improvement or disappearance of symptoms and does not progress to the third stage of exhaustion. The stage of resistance can also lead to diseases of adaptation, such as hypertension, arthritis, and cancer. Exhaustion occurs when the stressor is prolonged or sufficiently severe to use up all remaining adaptive energy. It is important to note that Selye conceptualized adaptive energy as limited by an individual's genetics. That is, each individual is proposed to have a certain amount of adaptive energy, similar to a bank account, from which he or she can withdraw but cannot deposit. When adaptive energy is depleted, death ensues (Selye, 1983).

Much of the response-based research on stress has used animal models with the intent of extrapolating results to humans. There have been many attempts to measure the stress response in humans using such indices as heart rate, blood pressure, plasma and urinary cortisol, and antibody production. As Lindsey (1993) correctly noted, however, it is not possible to capture the proposed "stress response" and the magnitude of the response by such variables alone.

There are several theoretical, measurement, and practice-related problems with defining stress as a nonspecific response to noxious stimuli or, as Selye (1983) stated, to any stress-inducing demand or stressor. First, the generality of the definition as the sum of all nonspecific reactions of the body obscures the more specific response patterns of psychophysiological responses. As early as 1957, Schachter demonstrated differential autonomic responses for anger and anxiety.

In 1967, Arnold summarized the empirical evidence of how the physiological correlates of anger and fear differed. Fear demonstrates primarily an adrenergic effect, whereas anger demonstrates primarily a cholinergic effect. By the mid-1970s, there was evidence that a single emotion such as anxiety could trigger different physiological responses depending on how a person coped with it (Schalling, 1976).

Second, Selye uses the term *stressor* to refer to the "noxious" condition that triggers the response and the term *stress* to refer to both the initial impact of the stressor (alarm reaction) on tissues and the adaptive mechanisms that are a reaction to the stressor. In addition, conceptual confusion about the meaning of the term stress was heightened because Selye sometimes defined stress as the wear and tear, damage, or disease consequences of prolonged GAS responses. Third, the absence of cognitive factors such as appraisal and meaning shortchanged what occurred in psychological stress. Fourth, the normative nature of the nonspecific physiological response pattern or GAS does not allow for individual differences in perception of a stimulus situation or how a person uniquely copes with a threatening situation.

In a classic study, Ursin, Baade, and Levine (1978) demonstrated that effective coping behavior produced a significant reduction in physiological activation. Their study of parachutist trainees found that general ability level, defense mechanisms, motivation, and role identification explained "considerable

portions" of the variance in stress response. Increased activation of the pituitary adrenocortical axis was positively correlated only with defense mechanisms and low performance, whereas cortisol levels returned to baseline as coping processes were established. In general, the Ursin et al. study supports the idea that an individual's perception of a threatening situation and his or her coping behavior are the primary determinants of the neuroendocrine response pattern. Fifth, the measurement of stress as a dependent variable must be operationalized by physiological variables. It has long been known that there is a disassociation between subjective experiences and objective signs of both the central and the autonomic nervous systems (Lacy, 1967). Sixth, in terms of adoption of the theory to guide nursing practice, the assumptions underlying the theory are not compatible with nursing's philosophical presuppositions, rendering its application to nursing practice awkward at best. Specifically, the presupposition that each individual is unique and that perception or meaning is central to personal experiences are not compatible with Selye's propositions.

In their critical review of nursing research on stress, Lyon and Werner (1987) noted that from 1974 to 1984 approximately 24% of the studies used a response framework to study stress. As noted earlier, the use of the response framework necessitated that stress be the dependent variable—it is the disruption caused by a noxious stimulus or stressor. Commonly, stress was operationalized in nursing research by both psychological and physiological measures. Physiological measures were typically vital signs (Guzetta & Forsyth, 1979), urinary Na:K ratio and 17-ketosteroids (Far, Keene, Samson, & Michael, 1984), cardiovascular complaints (Schwartz & Brenner, 1979), anxiety (Guzetta & Forsyth, 1979), or all these. Most of the research studies critically reviewed by Lyon and Werner used independent variables such as relaxation (Tamez, Moore, & Brown, 1978) or information (Toth, 1980) that were purported to mediate between the stressor (commonly assumed to be hospitalization, a threatening medical procedure, or unit transfer) and the stress response. Use of such mediating variables is inconsistent with Selye's theoretical propositions.

Contrary to Selye's GAS theory, studies of stress using the response-based orientation to stress in humans indicate that stress is stimulus- or situation-specific and subject to individual response. Although there is no empirical support for the "nonspecific and uniform response" to the noxious stimuli postulate in humans, there is abundant evidence that a person's perception of an event and his or her coping behaviors do vary in physiological correlates.

Stress as a Stimulus

In the 1960s, psychologists became interested in applying the concept of stress to psychological experiences. Masuda and Holmes (1967) and Holmes and Rahe (1967), stimulated by their interest in what happens when a person experiences "change" in life circumstances, proposed a stimulus-based theory of stress. The stimulus approach treats life changes or "life events" as the stressor to which a person responds. Therefore, unlike the response-based model, stress is the independent variable in research.

The work of the aforementioned researchers resulted in the development of tools known as the Social Readjustment Rating Scale (SRRS) and Schedule of Recent Experiences (Holmes & Rahe, 1967). Both tools were purported to measure stress defined and operationalized as the adjustment required by selected major life changes or events. The central proposition of the stimulus model is that too many life changes increase one's vulnerability to illness. The SRRS consisted of 42 life events (e.g., marriage, loss of a loved one, pregnancy, vacation, divorce, retirement, and change in residence) that were assigned a priori weights derived from the mean ratings of the estimated amount of adjustment the events would require (Holmes & Rahe, 1967). In their early research with Navy recruits, the

researchers demonstrated a small but significant relationship between adaptation scores (assigned to different events) and illness experiences during the subsequent year.

The stimulus-based model was built on assumptions that are inherently problematic in explaining human phenomenon. The primary theoretical proposition was based on the premise that (a) life changes are normative and that each life change results in the same readjustment demands for all persons, (b) change is stressful regardless of the desirability of the event to the person, and (c) there is a common threshold of readjustment or adaptation demands beyond which illness results. During their early work, Holmes and Rahe viewed the person as a passive recipient of stress. Furthermore, stress was conceptualized as an additive phenomenon that was measurable by researcher-selected life events that had preassigned normative weights. Later in their work, however, the researchers incorporated consideration of a person's interpretation of the life event as a negative or positive experience (Rahe, 1978).

During the 1970s, hundreds of studies were conducted on the ability of life event scores to predict illness. Illness was typically operationalized as morbidity or disease states. Collectively, these studies have consistently accounted for not more than 4% to 6% of the incidence of illness with low correlations of .20 to .30 (Johnson & Sarason, 1979a). One important explanation for why the low correlations reached statistical significance is that sample sizes in these studies were typically very large. The low correlations may also simply reflect the fact that people commonly experience stress that is not related to major life changes.

Sarason, Johnson, and Seigel (1979) developed a different measure, the Life Experiences Survey (LES), that not only incorporated the person's view of whether the life event was desirable or undesirable but also incorporated the degree of impact the event had on the individual's life. This 57-item self-report measure has been widely used in life stress studies. Despite the fact that development of the LES represented a theoretically useful step forward in the assessment of life stress, researcher-selected events do not have a uniform effect on individuals and there are many other variables influencing the stress-health outcome relationship (Johnson & Sarason, 1979b; Lazarus & Folkman, 1984). Despite the fact that LSE correlations with illness (operationalized as disease) are higher than those achieved by the SRRS, they are still very low. It is plausible that these low correlations were contributed to by researchers neglecting to assess factors such as social support, hardiness, and perceived control.

An important study, disconfirming the central postulate of the stimulus-based approach, was conducted by Kobasa in 1979. She introduced the notion of "hardiness" as an important moderator variable. Initially, hardiness was described as (a) a strong commitment to self, (b) a vigorous attitude toward the environment, (c) a sense of meaningfulness, and (d) an internal locus of control. Kobasa operationalized these elements by using several different extant surveys, including the Internal-External Locus of Control Scale, Alienation Test, and Achievement Scale of the Personality Research Form. In a study of 837 middle- and upper-level executives, the findings showed that those with higher hardiness had lower illness scores despite scoring higher on significant life events (SRRS). Executives who had higher SRRS scores and low hardiness scores, however, had significantly more illness. Kobasa demonstrated that hardiness was a powerful moderator between stress, measured by SRRS, and illness.

Although Kobasa (1979) found a mediating effect for hardiness on the relationship between life events and health outcomes, there have been inconsistent findings in other studies. Manning, Williams, and Wolfe (1988) found hardiness, rather than acting as a mediator between stress and health outcomes, to have direct effects on emotional and psychological factors thought to be related to well-being and work performance. These included a higher quality of life, more positive affect, and fewer somatic complaints.

A construct closely related to hardiness but different enough to be a more powerful mediator between life event stress and illness is sense of coherence (Antonovsky, 1987). Sense of coherence (SOC) is characterized by (a) comprehensibility—the degree to which a situation is predictable and explicable, (b) manageability—the availability of sufficient resources (internal and external) to meet the demands of the situation, and (c) meaningfulness—the degree to which life's demands are worth the investment of energy. A person with a high SOC has a tendency to view the world as ordered, predictable, and manageable. Importantly, Antonovsky (1982) argued that we often ask the wrong question—that is, "Why do people become ill?"—when perhaps we should be asking "Why do people stay healthy despite life stress?"

Notwithstanding the dominance of the stimulus approach to studying the relationship between life event stress and illness (disease) in the 1970s and early 1980s, the effectiveness of this paradigm in explaining the relationship between stress and illness was not confirmed. In an attempt to come to grips with the issues regarding a priori weighted measures of major life events, Kanner, Coyne, Schaefer, and Lazarus (1981) proposed a measure of chronic daily hassles and uplifts—the Hassles Scale consisting of 117 items and the Uplifts Scale containing 135 items. Hassles are "relatively minor" daily experiences and demands that are appraised as potentially threatening or harmful, and uplifts are favorable experiences and events. On the Hassles Scale, respondents indicate whether or not an occurrence of any of the items "hassled or bothered" them within the past week or month and, if so, whether the hassle was "somewhat," "moderately," or "extremely" severe. Similarly, on the Uplifts Scale, respondents indicate if they experienced an item as an uplift (a positive event) and, if so, to what extent was it strong ("somewhat," "moderate," or "extremely"). Using the Hassles Scale and a life events questionnaire, Delongis, Coyne, Dakof, Folkman, and Lazarus (1982) were able to demonstrate, through a multiple regression analysis, that the hassle scores were more strongly associated with somatic health than were life event scores. Interestingly, the uplift scores made very little contribution to health that was independent of hassles. Despite the stronger performance of hassles in predicting illness, the authors concluded that the experiences of daily hassles or uplifts are insufficient in predicting health outcomes.

In 1987, Lyon and Werner noted that approximately 30% of the nursing research on stress from 1974 to 1984 used a stimulus-based or life event approach. In fact, Volicer and Bohannon (1975) adapted the SRRS to stressful events of hospitalization and developed the Hospital Stress Rating Scale (HSRS). Consistent with findings from other disciplines, the correlations between life event or HSRS scores and physical or mental disruption were small in magnitude ($r = .20-.28$). By the late 1980s, the stimulus-based approach to defining and measuring stress without appraisal had fallen out of favor in nursing.

In 1993, Werner significantly modified and extended the notion that stress and health-related responses were triggered from events. She proposed a framework to examine trigger events or stimuli that result in the experience of stress or significant physical or psychosocial reaction. Werner labeled the trigger event a "stressor" and proposed that there are four types of stressors: event, situation, conditions, and cues. An *event* is something noteworthy that happens. A *situation* is composed of a combination of circumstances at any given moment. A *condition* is a state of being, and a *cue* is a feature indicating the nature of something perceived (Table 1.1). In addition to identifying types of stressors, Werner identified ways to categorize stressors with respect to locus (internal or external), duration and temporality (acute, time limited; chronic, intermittent; and chronic), forecasting (predictable or unpredictable), tone (positive or negative), and impact (normative or catastrophic). Integrating these elements, Werner proposed an organizing schema for stressor research in nursing. Although it is unlikely that specific responses to stressors in any of the categories

proposed by Werner would be the same across individuals, it might be possible to identify common themes within specified categories in similar cultures.

Stress as a Transaction

As a social-personality psychologist, Richard Lazarus became interested in explaining the dynamics of troublesome experiences. He developed and tested a transactional model of stress (Lazarus, 1966; Lazarus & Folkman, 1984). Lazarus believed that stress as a concept had heuristic value, but in and of itself was not measurable as a single variable. Lazarus (1967) contended that stress does not exist in the "event" but rather is a result of a transaction between a person and his or her environment. As such, stress encompasses a set of cognitive, affective, and coping variables.

Precursor models to Lazarus's transactional model of stress include those proposed by Basowitz, Persky, Korchin, and Grinker (1955), Mechanic (1962), and Janis (1954). Each of these models, although different in many ways, shared some commonalties. Basowitz et al. defined stress as feelings that typically occur when an organism is threatened. In Mechanic's model of stress, it is defined as "discomforting responses of persons in particular situations" (p. 7). The factors proposed to influence whether or not a situation is experienced as discomforting include the abilities or capacities of the person, skills and constraints produced by group practices and traditions, resources available to the person in the environment, and norms that define where and how the individual could be comfortable in using the means available. Behavior that a person uses to respond to demands is termed *coping behavior.* Janis (1954) proposed a model of disaster that included three major phases of stress: (a) the threat phase, in which persons perceive objective signs of danger; (b) the danger impact phase, in which the danger is proximal and the chance of the

TABLE 1.1 Organizing Schema for Stressor Research in Nursing

Stressor Category	Working Definition
Life-Related Normative (L-RN)	Events, situations, conditions, or cues which are usually expected, which most experience, and which require adjustment or adaptation
Health/Illness-Related Normative (HI-RN)	Events, situations, conditions, or cues which are related to health or to illness, and/or treatment for these, and which are usually expected, which most experience, and which require adjustment or adaptation
Life-Related Catastrophic (L-RC)	Events, situations, conditions, or cues which are generally unpredictable, usually infrequent, and commonly result in dire consequences in addition to requiring adjustment or adaptation
Health/Illness-Related (HI-RC)	Events, situations, conditions, or cues which are related to health or to illness, and/or treatment for these, and which are generally unpredictable, usually infrequent, and commonly result in dire consequences in addition to requiring adjustment or adaptation

SOURCE: From Werner (1993, pp. 17-18). Copyright © 1993 by Sigma Theta Tau International.

person escaping injury is dependent on the speed and efficiency of their protective actions; and (c) the danger-of-victimization phase, which occurs immediately after the impact of the danger has terminated or subsided. In addition to these early models of stress that introduced the importance of assigned meaning and coping options to understanding the origin of discomforts, there were psychosomatic stress models that incorporated personal perception as a determinant of organic processes (Alexander, 1950; Dunbar, 1947; Grinker & Speigel, 1945; Wolf, 1950; Wolf, Friedman, Hofer, & Mason, 1964).

Due in part to the early works of all the aforementioned researchers, by the 1960s stress had become a popular construct in psychological and psychosomatic research. Including his own research findings, Lazarus's 1966 book, *Psychological Stress and the Coping Process,* represents an elegant theoretical integration of all the research findings on stress and its interrelationship with health through the early 1960s. The theoretical framework that Lazarus presented to explain the complex phenomenon of stress was a major impetus for the field of cognitive psychology because his framework consistently emphasized the important role that "appraisal" plays in how a person reacts, feels, and behaves.

Lazarus (1967) and Lazarus and Folkman (1984) asserted that the primary mediator of person-environment transactions was appraisal. Three types of appraisal were identified: primary, secondary, and reappraisal. *Primary appraisal* is a judgment about what the person perceives a situation holds in store for him or her. Specifically, a person assesses the possible effects of demands and resources on well-being. If the demands of a situation outweigh available resources, then the individual may determine that the situation represents (a) a potential for harm or loss (threat) or that (b) actual harm has already occurred (harm) or (c) the situation has potential for some type of gain or benefit (challenge). It is important to note, however, that the perception of challenge in the absence of perceived potential for harm was not considered a stress appraisal.

The perception of threat triggers *secondary appraisal,* which is the process of determining what coping options or behaviors are available to deal with a threat. Often, primary and secondary appraisals occur simultaneously and interact with one another, which makes measurement very difficult (Lazarus & Folkman, 1984).

Reappraisal is the process of continually evaluating, changing, or relabeling earlier primary or secondary appraisals as the situation evolves. What was initially perceived as threatening may now be viewed as a challenge or as benign or irrelevant. Often, reappraisal results in the cognitive elimination of perceived threat.

There are many situational factors that influence appraisals of threat, including their number and complexity; person's values, commitments, and goals; availability of resources; novelty of the situation; self-esteem; social support; coping skills; situational constraints; degree of uncertainty and ambiguity; proximity (time and space), intensity, and duration of the threat; and the controllability of the threat. What occurs during appraisal processes determines emotions and coping behaviors (Lazarus, 1966; Lazarus & Folkman, 1984).

Other important concepts in Lazarus's transactional framework for stress include coping and stress emotions. Unlike the response-based or stimulus-based orientation to stress discussed earlier, the transactional model explicitly includes coping efforts. Coping is defined as "constantly changing cognitive and behavioral efforts to manage specific external and/or internal demands that are appraised as taxing or exceeding the resources of the person" (Lazarus & Folkman, 1984, p. 141). This definition clearly deems coping as a process-oriented phenomenon, not a trait or an outcome, and makes it clear that such effort is different from automatic adaptive behavior that has been learned. Furthermore, coping involves "managing" the stressful situation; therefore, it does not necessarily mean "mastery." Managing may include efforts to minimize, avoid, tolerate,

change, or accept a stressful situation as a person attempts to master or handle his or her environment.

Lazarus and Folkman (1984) warned against "stage"-type models of coping because they tend to create situations in which a person's behavior is judged to be inside or outside the norm by the way the person deals with a stressful situation over time. A common example of a stage model is that proposed by Kubler-Ross (1969) for death and dying. It is not uncommon for health care providers to inappropriately judge a person's grief response because of the expectation that a person must experience all the predicted stages and only cycle through them one time. Although there may be commonalties or patterns in certain situations that are similar in terms of both the nature of the situation and the cultural ways of responding, there is probably not a dominant pattern of coping.

In 1966, Lazarus identified two forms of coping: direct action and palliative. In 1984, Lazarus and Folkman changed the names of these two forms to problem-focused and emotion-focused, respectively. *Problem-focused coping* strategies are similar to problem-solving tactics. These strategies encompass efforts to define the problem, generate alternative solutions, weigh the costs and benefits of various actions, take actions to change what is changeable, and, if necessary, learn new skills. Problem-focused efforts can be directed outward to alter some aspect of the environment or inward to alter some aspect of self. Many of the efforts directed at self fall into the category of reappraisals—for example, changing the meaning of the situation or event, reducing ego involvement, or recognizing the existence of personal resources or strengths.

Emotion-focused coping strategies are directed toward decreasing emotional distress. These tactics include such efforts as distancing, avoiding, selective attention, blaming, minimizing, wishful thinking, venting emotions, seeking social support, exercising, and meditating. Similar to the cognitive strategies identified in problem-focused coping efforts, changing how an encounter is construed without changing the objective situation is equivalent to reappraisal. The following are common examples: "I decided that something a lot worse could have happened" or "I just decided there are more important things in life." Unlike problem-focused strategies, emotion-focused strategies do not change the meaning of a situation directly. For example, doing vigorous exercise or meditating may help an individual reappraise the meaning of a situation, but the activity does not directly change meaning. Emotion-focused coping is the more common form of coping used when events are not changeable (Lazarus & Folkman, 1984).

Lazarus (1966) and Lazarus and Folkman (1984) summarize a large body of empirical evidence supporting the distinction between emotion (palliative) and problem-focused (direct-action) coping. In addition, the evidence indicates that everyone uses both types of strategies to deal with stressful encounters or troublesome external or internal demands.

Folkman (1997), based on her work in studying AIDS-related caregiving, proposed an extension of the model regarding the theoretical understanding of coping. Her study involved measurement of multiple variables of psychological state (depressive symptomatology, positive states, and positive and negative affect), coping, and religious or spiritual beliefs and activities. Each caregiver participant was interviewed twice. Although participants reported a high level of negative psychological states as expected, they also reported high levels of positive affect. Interestingly, the interview data, when examined along with quantitative analyses, revealed that the coping strategies associated with positive psychological states had a common theme: "searching for and finding positive meaning. Positive reappraisal, problem-focused coping, spiritual beliefs and practices, and infusing ordinary events with positive meaning all involve the activation of beliefs, values, or goals that help define the positive significance of events" (p. 1215). Folkman cites many studies that support her conclusion that finding positive meaning in a stressful situation is linked to the experience of well-being.

Another important construct in Lazarus's (1966, 1991) transactional model is emotion—specifically emotions that are considered to be stress emotions. These include, but are not limited to, anxiety, fear, anger, guilt, and sadness (Lazarus, 1991, 1966; Lazarus & Folkman, 1984). Lazarus (1991) does not treat depression as an emotion but rather as a composite of several stress emotions, including anxiety, anger, sadness, and guilt.

Lazarus and Folkman (1984) present cogent arguments for the explanatory power of the cognitive theory of emotion. Although thoughts proceed emotions—that is, emotions are shaped by thought processes—emotions can in turn affect thoughts. The primary appraisal of threat and the specific meaning of the situation to the person trigger a particular stress emotion consistent with the meaning.

Lazarus (1966) and Lazarus and Folkman (1984) link stress-related variables to health-related outcomes. All of their constructs in the transactional model, when taken together, affect adaptational outcomes. Lazarus and Folkman propose three types of adaptational outcomes: (a) functioning in work and social living, (b) morale or life satisfaction, and (c) somatic health. They view the concept of health broadly to encompass physical (somatic conditions, including illness and physical functioning), psychological (cognitive functional ability and morale—including positive and negative effects regarding how people feel about themselves and their life, including life satisfaction), and social (social functioning) (Table 1.2).

➤ THE CONCEPT OF HEALTH

Each of the three theoretical perspectives on stress incorporate proposed links between stress and health. It is clear that both the stimulus-based and the response-based models were developed based on a biomedical orientation to health in which illness is operationalized as disease and health is viewed as the

TABLE 1.2 Stress, Coping, and Health Outcomes as Defined in Stress Theory

Scientific View	Conceptualization of Stress	Conceptualization of Coping	Health Outcomes
Response based (Selye, 1956, 1983)	Stress is the nonspecific response to any noxious stimulus. The physiological response is always the same regardless of stimulus—the general adaptation syndrome (GAS).	There is no conceptualization of coping per se. Instead, Selye used the concept of "resistance stage," the purpose of which is to resist damage (this concept is part of the GAS)	On the basis of the assumption that each person is born with a finite amount of energy and that each stress encounter depletes energy stores that cannot be rejuvenated, it was proposed that stress causes "wear and tear on the body" that can result in various diseases based on the person's genetic propensity.
Stimulus based (Holmes & Rahe, 1967)	The term stress is synonymous with "life event." Life events are "stress" that require adaptation efforts.	Coping is not defined.	A summative accumulation of adaptation efforts over a threshold level makes a person vulnerable to developing a physical or mental illness (operationalized as disease) within 1 year.
Transaction based (Lazarus, 1966; Lazarus & Folkman, 1984)	The term stress is "rubric" for a complex series of subjective phenomena, including cognitive appraisals (threat, harm, and challenge), stress emotions, coping responses, and reappraisals. Stress is experienced when the demands of a situation tax or exceed a person's resources and some type of harm or loss is anticipated.	Coping is conceptualized as efforts to ameliorate the perceived threat or to manage stress emotions (emotion-focused coping and problem-focused coping)	Adaptational health outcomes are conceptualized as short term and long term. Short-term outcomes include social functioning in a specific encounter, morale in the positive and negative affect during and after an encounter, and somatic health in symptoms generated by the stressful encounter. Long-term outcomes include social functioning, morale, and somatic health. Both short-term and long-term health outcomes encompass effective, affective, and physiological components.

absence of disease. The transaction model, however, views health as a subjective phenomenon that encompasses somatic sense of self and functional ability.

"Health" is an elusive term. It is a term that many people think they understand until they are asked to define or describe it and then asked how they would measure it. Health has been described as a value judgment, as an objective state, as a subjective state, as a continuum from illness to wellness, and as a utopian state (rarely achievable). Contributing to the confusion about health are the related concepts wellness, well-being, and quality of life.

Despite the common origin of the word health from "hoelth," an Old English word meaning safe or sound and whole of body (Dolfman, 1973), there is no one contemporary meaning for the term. During the twentieth century, many attempts have been made by the lay community to define health in a manner that has broad applicability. These global definitions, however, are confusing and make it difficult, if not impossible, to clearly operationalize. This confusion has particularly important ramifications when one considers that health is a target goal shared by many professions and the federal government.

The health-related professions offer definitions of health that give rise to discipline-specific foci for diagnosis and treatment. Such definitions are not necessarily problematic. In fact, these differences have probably contributed to targeted and efficient efforts to generate knowledge about different aspects of the human condition. However, there are three important problems with discipline-specific definitions for which we must use caution.

The first is that discipline-specific perspectives partition the holistic phenomenon of health in such a manner that the whole picture of a person's condition and how the person is feeling and doing is lost. The second is that too often the discipline's perspective on health is adopted by other disciplines when there is not a good match in terms of the disciplines' philosophical presuppositions and social mandate. An excellent example is the nursing field adopting the medical model definition of health as the absence of disease. A third problem is that the acceptance of a discipline-specific view of health by policy-making groups necessarily leads to health policy decisions that may not be in the best interest of the population as a whole.

The Biomedical View of Health

The most popular and widely held view of health is the biomedical view. Medicine has traditionally viewed health from an objective stance and defines it as the absence of disease or discernible pathology and defines illness as the presence of same (Engel, 1992; Kleinman, 1981; Millstein & Irwin, 1987). On the basis of this perspective, medicine's social mandate has been the diagnosis and treatment of disease. Public health professionals and government agencies commonly adopt the biomedical model and use morbidity and mortality statistics as an index of the population's health.

The biomedical model, as noted by Antonovsky (1979), is a dichotomous model. Consistent with this perspective, a person who has a chronic disease cannot have health or be considered well. Furthermore, a logical extension of the dichotomous model is that a person cannot be healthy in the presence of disease.

Nursing's View of Health

Nursing has been critical of the narrow confines of the biomedical model as a model for nursing practice and its adoption by government agencies (Hall & Allan, 1987; Leininger, 1994; Lyon, 1990). Many nurses in practice and nurse educators, however, commonly adopt the biomedical view and equate illness and disease using the terms interchangeably. Likewise, concepts of health and wellness are used interchangeably, resulting in the conclusion that persons who have chronic diseases are not and cannot be well. Because health and wellness are targeted outcomes, it is imperative that nursing be clear on how it defines these concepts. This is particularly important in developing theoretical models linking stress, coping, and health that can serve as a framework for nursing practice. Nursing must define health in a manner that (a) is consistent with its philosophical presuppositions, (b) is measurable, (c) is empirically based, and (d) captures outcomes that are sensitive to nursing interventions or therapeutics.

Currently, there is little unity regarding a definition of health as a central concept for nursing. Considered an essential ingredient of nursing's theoretical metaparadigm (i.e., person, environment, health, and nursing), nurse theorists have elected to define health in the context of their proposed models. Florence Nightingale (1860/1969) wrote that health is "not only to be well, but to be able to use well every power we have to use" (p. 26). Although one cannot be sure what Nightingale actually meant by the word "well," Selanders (1995) argues she meant "being the best you can be at any given point in time" (p. 26). This allows for an individual to be healthy even if not medically well. Some additional light is shed on the meaning of wellness because it is clear that Nightingale viewed disease and illness as distinctly different phenomena. It is interesting to speculate that if Florence Nightingale were writing *Notes on Nursing* today, she most certainly would have included stress as one of the many nondiseased-based causes of symptoms experienced by patients.

Tripp-Reimer (1984) proposes a two-dimensional health state with an *etic* perspective (disease-nondisease) that reflects an objective interpretation of health data and an *emic* perspective (wellness-illness) that represent the subjective experience. Four health states are possible within her model. Tripp-Reimer proposes that this approach is particularly useful cross-culturally when perceptions of heath state differ between scientifically educated providers and the client. Newman (1986) views health as the totality of life processes that are evolving toward expanded consciousness. Man represents only one stage of this evolution. Orem (1995) distinguishes health and wellness. She defines health as a state characterized by soundness or wholeness of human structure and bodily and mental

functions. Wellness, she notes, is a state characterized by experiences of contentment, pleasure, and movement toward maturation and achievement of the human potential (personalization). Engagement in self-care facilitates this process of personalization. Other nurses offering conceptualizations of health include Henderson (1966), King (1981), Lyon (1990), Newman (1986), Parse (1992), Paterson and Zderad (1976), Peplau (1952, 1988), and Rogers (1970). Health is defined in many ways within the discipline of nursing (Table 1.3). Commonly shared attributes of health inherent in these definitions, however, include that it is a subjective experience that encompasses how a person is feeling and doing. These commonly shared attributes are apparent in Keller's (1981) analysis of definitions of health. A subjective orientation to defining health is quite different from the medical definition of health as an objective phenomenon manifested by the absence of disease or pathology.

Regarding the possibility of a single definition of health for nursing, Meleis (1990) points out that, "although diversity should be accepted and reinforced, there is a need for unity in perspective that represents the territory of investigation, the territory for theoretical development" (p. 109). This unity in perspective would also help to shape the target goals of nursing's unique contributions to society and could serve as a practical guideline for assessment, diagnosis, and intervention. The importance of using a definition of health that can be operationalized and used to guide nursing practice cannot be overemphasized.

A nursing-oriented definition of health consistent with the theme that health is a subjective phenomenon that is operationalizable has been proposed by Lyon (1990). Lyon defined health as a subjective representation of a person's composite evaluation of somatic sense of self (how one is feeling) and functional ability (how one is doing). As such, health is manifested in the subjective judgment that one is experiencing wellness or illness. These subjective experiences are dynamic and are an outgrowth of person and

TABLE 1.3 Nursing-Focused Definitions of Health

Author	Definition of Health
Henderson (1966)	Health is viewed in terms of a person's ability to perform 14 self-care tasks and a quality of life basic to human functioning.
Peplau (1952, 1988)	Health is defined as forward movement of the personality that is promoted through interpersonal processes in the direction of creative, productive, and constructive living.
Rogers (1970, 1989)	Health is defined as a value term for which meaning is determined by culture or the individual. Positive health symbolizes wellness.
Orem (1971, 1980, 1995)	Health is defined as a "state" that is characterized by soundness or wholeness of bodily and mental functioning. It includes physical, psychological, interpersonal, and social aspects. Well-being is the individual's perceived condition of existence.
King (1971, 1981)	Health is defined as a dynamic state of the life cycle; illness is an interference in the life cycle. Health implies continuous adaptation to stress.
Neuman (1989)	Health is defined as reflected in the level of wellness.
Parse (1981, 1989)	Health is defined as a lived experience—a rhythmic process of being and becoming.
Tripp-Reimer (1984)	Health is defined as a person's subjective expression of the composite evaluation of somatic sense of self (how one is feeling) and functional ability (how one is doing). The resulting judgment is manifested in the subjective experience of some degree of illness or wellness.
Lyon (1990)	Health is defined as encompassing two dimensions, the etic (objective) and the emic (subjective), which include both disease/nondisease and illness/wellness.

environment interactions. As long as a person is capable of evaluating how he or she is feeling and doing at some level, the person has health. For example, an infant, although unable to utter words, is capable of evaluating somatic sensations and functional ability. Likewise, a fundamental assumption underlying nursing practice is that all persons who have brain waves have the capability of sensing their environment and the capability of experiencing discomfort or comfort. Therefore, even persons who are unconscious but have brain waves should be treated in a manner that assumes that they can sense discomfort and comfort. Defined in this manner, both illness and wellness are health outcomes. The target goals for nursing care are to promote and maintain wellness (comfortable somatic sensations and functional ability at capability level) and to prevent or alleviate illness (so-matic discomfort and a decline in functional ability below capability level). Illness and wellness are conceptualized as different phenomena, not as opposite or polar ends of the same phenomenon.

Illness is defined by Lyon (1990) as the subjective experience of somatic discomfort (emotional or physical or both) that is accompanied by some degree of functional decline below the person's perceived capability level. Illness occurs on a continuum from low ("I'm not feeling well.") to high ("I'm very ill or sick."). The experience of somatic discomfort and a decline in functional ability can be the consequence of both disease- and, importantly for nursing, nondisease-based factors that are amenable to nursing interventions (Figures 1.1 and 1.2).

Nursing's unique health-related contribution to society is the diagnosis and treatment

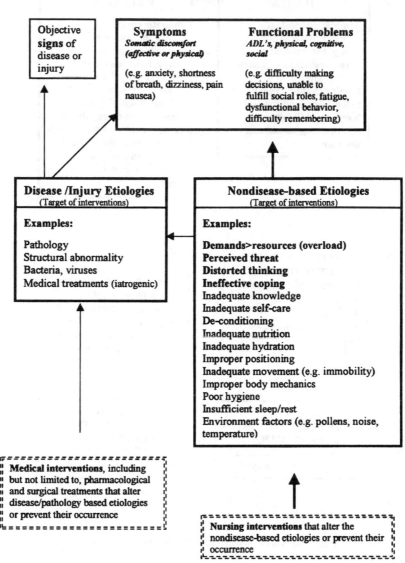

Figure 1.1. Disease-Based and Nondisease-Based Etiologies of Illness With Medical and Nursing Interventions (Reproduced with permission from B. L. Lyon © 1995)

of nondisease-based etiologies or factors contributing to or causing illness (Lyon, 1990). No other discipline focuses on the prevention or alleviation of nondisease-based etiologies of illness. In fact, it is interesting to note that the concept of "cure" is applicable to illness experiences. That is, in addition to preventing somatic discomforts and functional disability caused by nondisease-based factors, nursing therapeutics also can cure "illness" by eliminating or altering nondiseased-based factors that are causing symptoms. Symptoms such as pain, fatigue, nausea, and a decline in functional ability, such as skin breakdown, falling, and inability to swallow, need to be addressed.

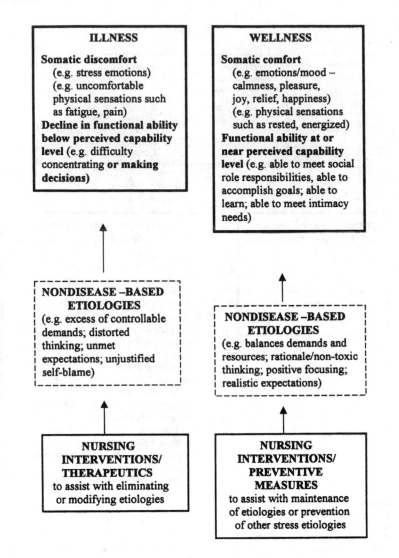

Figure 1.2. Linking Nursing Interventions to Health Outcomes

Wellness is characterized by Lyon (1990) as the experience of somatic comfort (emotional and physical) and a functional ability level at or near the person's perceived capability level. There is an abundance of research to demonstrate that people commonly judge themselves to feel well even in the presence of chronic, debilitating, or life-threatening diseases when they are somatically comfortable and can function at their perceived capability level (Dasback, Klein, Klein, & Moss, 1994; Long & Weinert, 1992; Okun, Zautra, & Rob-

inson, 1988; Stuifbergen, Becker, Ingalsbe, & Sands, 1990). Evaluation of somatic sense of self and functional ability is ongoing and can change from moment to moment. The important distinction in Lyon's (1990) definition of functional ability is that a person's subjective evaluation of functional ability is a comparison between what the person believes is his or her capability level and what he or she is actually able to do. This orientation allows for adjustments of perceived capability downward or upward. Therefore, during the early phases after diagnosis of rheumatoid arthritis, a person may not only be experiencing physical discomfort but also be viewing their self as not being able to measure up to previously held standards and expectations of functional ability. As a consequence, the person judges himself or herself to be experiencing some degree of illness. After a diminished level of functioning has become the person's norm (along with learning to live with some degree of discomfort), however, the individual with rheumatoid arthritis actually might judge himself or herself as quite well.

Some in nursing may, at first glance, be concerned about using a subjective definition of health as a framework to guide nursing practice. That is, what do you do with the person who has diagnosed hypertension or diabetes and yet perceives himself or herself as well? Nothing? Of course not. It is important to note, however, that the individual with hypertension or diabetes may not do anything unless he or she deems the actions (e.g., taking medications and controlling diet and weight) as both salient and important. Helping patients to elevate and to maximize their awareness of slight somatic discomforts (e.g., tiredness) or slight problems with functional ability (e.g., thinking clearly) can be beneficial in stimulating therapeutic self-care action (Figure 1.2).

The understanding that both illness and wellness can be experienced in the presence or absence of disease and that nursing's unique contribution is focusing on the diagnosis and treatment of nondisease-based factors contributing to illness is a fundamental cornerstone of nursing. Grasping this idea is what makes it possible for nurses to see possibilities for patients to experience wellness in the presence of a chronic or life-threatening disease or both. Knowledge about nondisease-based factors, such as stress, that contribute to somatic (physical or emotional) discomfort and declines in functional ability increases a nurse's repertoire of intervention possibilities to help patients. It is imperative that the nursing discipline adopt or develop measurements of health outcomes to demonstrate the efficacy of stress- and coping-related nursing in-terventions. In Chapter 23, Lyon and Rice present a conceptual model for nursing that links stress, coping, and health.

➤ REFERENCES

Alexander, F. (1950). *Psychosomatic medicine: Its practices and application*. New York: Norton.

Antonovsky, A. (1979). *Health, stress, and coping*. San Francisco: Jossey-Bass.

Antonovsky, A. A. (1987). *Unraveling the mystery of health: How people manage stress and stay well*. San Francisco: Jossey-Bass.

Arnold, M. B. (1967). Stress and emotion. In M. H. Appley & R. Trumbull (Eds.), *Psychological stress: Issues in research* (pp. 123-150). New York: Appleton-Century-Crofts.

Basowitz, H., Persky, H., Korchin, S. J., & Grinker, R. R. (1955). *Anxiety and stress*. New York: McGraw-Hill.

Bennett, E. J., Tennant, D. C., Piesse, C., Badcock, C. A., & Kellow, J. E. (1998). Level of chronic life stress predicts clinical outcome in irritable bowel syndrome. *Gut, 43*(2), 256-261.

Benschop, R. J., Greenen, R., Mills, P. J., Naliboff, B. D., Kiecolt-Glaser, J. K., Herbert, T. B., van der Pompe, G., Miller, G. E., Matthews, K. A., Godaert, G. L., Gilmore, S. L., Glaser, R., Heijnen, C. J., Dopp, J. M., Bijlsma, J. W., Solomon, G. F., & Cacioppo, J. T. (1998). Cardiovascular and immune responses to acute psychological stress in young and old women: A meta-analysis. *Psychosomatic Medicine, 60*(3), 290-296.

Brkovich, A. M., & Fisher, W. A. (1998). Psychological distress and infertility: Forty years of research. *Journal of Psychosomatic Obstetrics & Gynecology, 19*(4), 218-228.

Cannon, W. B. (1932). *The wisdom of the body* (2nd ed.). New York: Norton.

Cohen, S., Frank, E., Doyle, W. J., Skoner, D. P., Rabin, B. S., & Gwaltney, J. M. (1998). Types of stressors that increase susceptibility to the common cold in healthy adults. *Health Psychology, 17*(3), 214-223.

Cohen, S., & Rabin, B. S. (1998). Psychologic stress, immunity, and cancer. *Journal of the National Cancer Institute, 90*, 30-36.

Cohen, S., Tyrrell, D. A. J., & Smith, A. P. (1991). Psychological stress and susceptibility to the common cold. *New England Journal of Medicine, 325*, 606-612.

Cox, D. M., & Gonder-Frederick, L. (1992). Major developments in behavioral diabetes research. *Journal of Consulting and Clinical Psychology, 60*, 628-638.

Crofford, L. J., Jacobson, J., & Young, E. (1999). Modeling the involvement of the hypothalamic-pituitary-adrenal and hypothalamic-pituitary-gonadal axes in autoimmune and stress-related rheumatic syndromes in women. *Journal of Women's Health, 8*(2), 203-215.

Cummings, N. A., & Vandenbos, G. R. (1981). The twenty year Kaiser-Permanente experience with psychotherapy and medical utilization: Implications for national health policy and national health insurance. *Health Policy Quarterly, 1,* 159-175.

Dancey, J. C. P., Taghavi, M., & Fox, R. J. (1998). The relationship between daily stress and symptoms of irritable bowel: A time-series approach. *Journal of Psychosomatic Research, 44*(5), 537-545.

Dasback, E. J., Klein, R., Klein, E. K., & Moss, S. E. (1994). Self-rated health and mortality in people with diabetes. *American Journal of Public Health, 84,* 1775-1779.

Davis, P. A., Holm, J. E., Myers, T. C., & Suda, K. T. (1998). Stress, headache, and physiological disregulation: A time-series analysis of stress in the laboratory. *Headache, 38*(2), 116-121.

deCarteret, J. C. (1994). Occupational stress claims: Effects on workers' compensation. *American Association of Occupational Health Nursing Journal, 42*(10), 494-498.

Delongis, A. D., Coyne, J. C., Dakof, G., Folkman, S., & Lazarus, R. S. (1982). Relationship of daily hassles, uplifts, and major life events to health status. *Health Psychology, 1,* 119-136.

Dimsdale, J. E., Ruberman, W., & Carleton, R. A. (1987). Conference on behavioral medicine and cardiovascular disease: Task force 1: Sudden cardiac death, stress and cardiac arrhythmias. *Circulation, 76*(Suppl. 1), 198-201.

Dolfman, M. L. (1973). The concept of health: An historic and analytic examination. *Journal of School Health, 43*(8), 491-497.

Dunbar, H. F. (1947). *Mind and body.* New York: Random House.

Dyrehag, L. E., Widerstrom-Noga, E. G., Carlsson, S. G., Kaberger, K., Hedner, N., Mannheimer, C., & Andersson, S. A. (1998). Relations between self-rated musculoskeletal symptoms and signs and psychological distress in chronic neck and shoulder pain. *Scandinavian Journal of Rehabilitation Medicine, 30*(4), 235-242.

Engel, G. L. (1992). The need for a new medical model: A challenge for biomedicine. *Family Systems Medicine, 10*(3), 317-331.

Fanciullacci, C., Allessandri, M., & Fanciullacci, M. (1998). The relationship between stress and migraine. *Functional Neurology, 13*(3), 215-223.

Farr, L., Keene, A., Samson, D., & Michael, A. (1984). Alterations in circadian excretion of urinary variables and physiological indicators of stress following surgery. *Nursing Research, 33,* 140-146.

Folkman, S. (1997). Positive psychological states and coping with severe stress. *Social Science and Medicine, 45*(3), 207-221.

Fontana, A., & McLaughlin, M. (1998). Coping and appraisal of daily stressors predict heart rate and blood pressure levels in young women. *Behavioral Medicine, 24,* 5-16.

Fukunishi, I., Akimoto, M., Horikawa, N., Shirasaka, K., & Yamazaki, T. (1998). Stress, coping and social support in glucose tolerance abnormality. *Journal of Psychosomatic Research, 45*(4), 361-369.

Glaser, R., & Kiecolt-Glaser, J. K. (1998). Stress-associated immune modulation: Relevance to viral infections and chronic fatigue syndrome. *American Journal of Medicine, 105*(3A), 35S-42S.

Goleman, D., & Gurin, J. (1993). *Mind-body medicine: How to use your mind for better health.* New York: Consumer Report Books.

Gorman, J. M., & Kertzner, R. M. (1991). Psychoimmunology update. In *Progress in psychiatry* (No. 35). Washington, DC: American Psychiatric Press.

Grinker, R. R., & Speigel, J. P. (1945). *Men under stress.* Philadelphia: Blakiston.

Guzzetta, C. E., & Forsyth, G. L. (1979). Nursing diagnostic pilot study: Psychophysiologic stress. *Advances in Nursing Science, 2,* 27-44.

Hall, B. A., & Allan, J. D. (1987, June). Sharpening nursing's focus by focusing on health. *Nursing and Health Care,* 315-320.

Henderson, V. (1966). *The nature of nursing.* New York: Macmillan.

Holm, J. E., Lokken, C., & Myers, T. C. (1997). Migraine and stress: A daily examination of temporal relationships in women migraineurs. *Headache, 37*(9), 553-558.

Holmes, T., & Rahe, R. (1967). The social readjustment rating scale. *Journal of Psychosomatic Research, 12,* 213-233.

Holroyd, K. A., Nash, J. M., Pingel, J. D., Cordingley, G. E., & Jerome, A. (1991). A comparison of pharmacological (amitriptyline HCL) and nonpharmacologcial (cognitive-behavioral) therapies for chronic tension headaches. *Journal of Consulting and Clinical Psychology, 59,* 387-393.

Inui, J. A., Kitaoka, H., Majima, M., Takamiya, S., Uemoto, M., Yonenaga, C., Honda, M., Shirakawa, K., Ueno, N., Amano, K., Morita, S., Kawara, A., Yokono, K., Kasuga, M., & Taniguchi, H. (1998). Effect of the Kobe earthquake on stress and glycemic control in patients with diabetes mellitus. *Archives of Internal Medicine, 158*(3), 274-278.

Janis, I. (1954). Problems of theory in the analysis of stress behavior. *Journal of Social Issues, 10,* 12-25.

Johnson, J. H., & Sarason, I. G. (1979a). Moderator variables in life stress research. In I. G. Sarason & C. D. Spielberger (Eds.), *Stress and anxiety, Volume 6* (pp. 151-168). New York: John Wiley.

Johnson, J. H., & Sarason, I. G. (1979b). Recent developments in research on life stress. In V. Hamilton & D. Warburton (Eds.), *Human stress & cognition: An information processing approach* (pp. 205-233). New York: John Wiley.

Kanner, A. D., Coyne, J. C., Schaefer, J. C., & Lazarus, R. S. (1981). Comparison of two modes of stress measurement: Daily hassles and uplifts versus major life events. *Journal of Behavioral Medicine, 4*, 1-39.

Keller, M. J. (1981, October). Toward a definition of health. *Advances in Nursing Science*, 43-52.

King, I. (1971). *Toward a theory for nursing: General concepts of human behavior.* New York: John Wiley.

King, I. (1981). *A theory for nursing: Systems, concepts, process.* New York: John Wiley.

Kleinman, A. (1981). The failure of Western medicine. In P. R. Lee, N. Brown, & I. Red (Eds.), *The nation's health* (pp. 18-20). San Francisco: Boyd & Fraser.

Kobasa, S. C. (1979). Stressful life events, personality, and health: An inquiry into hardiness. *Journal of Personality and Social Psychology, 37*, 1-11.

Krantz, D. S., DeQuattro, V., Blackburn, H. W., Eaker, E., Hayes, S., James, S. A., Manuck, S. B., Meyers, H., Shekelle, R. B., & Syme, S. L. (1987). Psychosocial factors in hypertension. *Circulation, 76*(1, pt. 2), 184-188.

Kubler-Ross, E. (1969). *On death and dying.* New York: Macmillan.

Lacey, J. I. (1967). Somatic response patterning and stress: Some revisions of activation theory. In M. H. Appley & R. Trumbull (Eds.), *Psychological stress: Issues in research* (pp. 14-42). New York: Appleton-Century-Crofts.

Lazarus, R. S. (1966). *Psychological stress and the coping process.* New York: McGraw-Hill.

Lazarus, R. S. (1991). *Emotion and adaptation.* New York: Oxford University Press.

Lazarus, R. S., & Folkman, S. (1984). *Psychological stress and the coping process.* New York: Springer.

Lebwohl, M., & Tan, M. H. (1998). Psoriasis and stress. *Lancet, 351*(9096), 82.

Leininger, M. (1994). Nursing's agenda of health care reform: Regressive or advanced-discipline status? *Nursing Science Quarterly, 7*(2), 93-94.

Lindsey, A. M. (1993). Stress response. In V. Carrieri, A. M. Lindsey, & C. M. West (Eds.), *Pathophysiological phenomena in nursing: Human responses to illness* (pp. 397-419). Philadelphia: W. B. Saunders.

Long, K. A., & Weinert, C. (1992). Descriptions and perceptions of health among rural and urban adults with multiple sclerosis. *Research in Nursing and Health, 15*, 335-342.

Lorig, K., Seleznick, M., Lubeck, D., Ung, E., Chastain, R. L., & Holman, H. R. (1989). The beneficial outcomes of the arthritis self-management course are not adequately explained by behavior change. *Arthritis and Rheumatism, 32*, 91-95.

Lyon, B. (1990). Getting back on track: Nursing's autonomous scope of practice. In N. Chaska (Ed.), *The nursing profession: Turning points* (pp. 267-274). St. Louis, MO: C. V. Mosby.

Lyon, B., & Werner, J. S. (1987). Stress. In J. Fitzpatrick & R. L. Taunton (Eds.), *Annual review of nursing research* (Vol. 5, pp. 3-22). New York: Springer.

Manning, M. R., Williams, R. F., & Wolfe, D. M. (1988). Hardiness and the relationship between stressors and outcomes. *Work & Stress, 2*(3), 205-216.

Mason, J. W. (1971). A re-evaluation of the concept of "non-specificity" in stress theory. *Journal of Psychiatric Research, 8*, 323-333.

Mason, J. W. (1975a). A historical view of the stress field (Part I). *Journal of Human Stress, 1*, 6-12.

Mason, J. W. (1975b). A historical view of the stress field (Part II). *Journal of Human Stress, 1*, 22-36.

Masuda, M., & Holmes, T. H. (1967). Magnitude estimations of social readjustments. *Journal of Psychosomatic Research, 11*, 219-225.

Matteson, M. T., & Ivancevich, J. M. (1987). *Controlling work stress: Effective human resource and management strategies.* San Francisco: Jossey-Bass.

Mechanic, D. (1962). *Students under stress.* New York: Free Press.

Meleis, A. I. (1990). Being and becoming healthy: The core of nursing knowledge. *Nursing Science Quarterly, 3*(3), 107-114.

Millstein, S. G., & Irwin, C. E. (1987). Concepts of health and illness: Different constructs or variations on a theme? *Health Psychology, 6*, 515-524.

Neuman, B. (1989). *The Neuman systems model* (2nd ed.). Norwalk, CT: Appleton & Lange.

Newman, M. A. (1986). *Health as expanding consciousness.* St Louis, MO: C. V. Mosby.

Nightingale, F. (1969). *Notes on nursing: What it is and what it is not.* New York: Dover. (Original work published 1860)

Oken, D. (1967). The psychophysiology and psychoendocrinology of stress and emotion. In M. H. Appley & R. Trumbull (Eds.), *Psychological stress.* New York: Appleton-Century-Crofts.

Okun, M. A., Zautra, A. J., & Robinson, S. E. (1988). Hardiness and health among women with rheumatoid arthritis. *Personality and Individual Differences, 9*, 101-107.

Orem, D. E. (1971). *Nursing: Concepts of practice.* New York: McGraw-Hill.

Orem, D. E. (1980). *Nursing: Concepts of practice* (2nd ed.). New York: McGraw-Hill.

Orem, D. E. (1995). *Nursing: Concepts of practice* (5th ed.). New York: McGraw-Hill.

Ornish, D. M., Scherwitz, L. W., & Doody, S., Jr. (1983). Effects of stress management training and dietary changes in treating ischemic heart disease. *Journal of the American Medical Association, 249*, 54-59.

Ornstein, R., & Sobel, D. (1988). *The healing brain.* New York: Simon & Schuster.

Parse, R. R. (1981). *Man-living-health: A theory of nursing.* New York: John Wiley.

Parse, R. R. (1989). Man-living-health: A theory of nursing. In J. Riehl-Sisca (Ed.), *Conceptual models for nursing practice* (3rd ed.). Norwalk, CT: Appleton & Lange.

Parse, R. R. (1992). Human becoming: Parse's theory of nursing. *Nursing Science Quarterly, 5,* 35-42.

Pashkow, F. J. (1999). Is stress linked to heart disease? *Cleveland Clinic Journal of Medicine, 66*(2), 75-77.

Paterson, J. G., & Zderad, L. T. (1976). *Humanistic nursing.* New York: John Wiley.

Pelletier, K. R. (1992). Mind-body health: Research, clinical and policy implications. *American Journal of Health Promotion, 6,* 345-358.

Pelletier, K. R. (1995). Between mind and body: Stress, emotions, and health. In E. Goleman & J. Gurin (Eds.), *Mind body medicine: How to use your mind for better health* (pp. 18-38). New York: Consumer Reports Books.

Peplau, H. (1952). *Interpersonal relations in nursing.* New York: G. P. Putnam.

Peplau, H. (1988). The art and science of nursing: Similarities, differences and relations. *Nursing Science Quarterly, 1,* 8-15.

Rahe, R. H. (1978). Life change and illness studies: Past history and future directions. *Journal of Human Stress, 4,* 3-14.

Rahe, R. H., & Arthur, R. H. (1978). Life change and illness studies. *Journal of Human Stress, 4,* 3-15.

Ringsberg, K. C., & Akerlind, I. (1999). Presence of hyperventilation in patients with asthma-like symptoms but negative asthma test responses: Provocation with voluntary hyperventilation and mental stress. *Journal of Allergy and Clinical Immunology, 103*(4), 601-608.

Rogers, M. (1970). *The theoretical basis of nursing.* Philadelphia: F. A. Davis.

Rogers, M. (1989). Nursing: A science of unitary, irreducible, human beings: Update 1990. In E. A. M. Barrett (Ed.), *Vision of Rogers' science-based nursing* (Publication No. 15-2285, pp. 5-11). New York: National League for Nursing.

Sarason, I. G., Johnson, J. H., & Siegel, J. M. (1979). Development of the life experiences survey. In I. G. Sarason & C. D. Spielberger (Eds.), *Stress and anxiety, Volume 6* (pp. 131-149). New York: John Wiley.

Schachter, J. (1957). Pain, fear, and anger in hypertensives and normotensives: A psychophysiologic study. *Psychosomatic Medicine, 19,* 17-29.

Schalling, D. (1976). Anxiety, pain, and coping. In I. G. Sarason & C. D. Spielberger (Eds.), *Stress and anxiety, Volume 3* (pp. 49-71). New York: Hemisphere.

Schnall, P. L., Schwartz, J. E., Landsbergis, P. A., Warren, K., & Pickering, T. G. (1998). A longitudinal study of job strain and ambulatory blood pressure: Results from a three-year follow-up. *Psychosomatic Medicine, 60*(6), 697-706.

Schwartz, L. P., & Brenner, Z. R. (1979). Critical care unit transfer: Reducing patient stress through nursing interventions. *Heart & Lung, 8,* 540-546.

Selanders, L. C. (1995). Florence Nightingale: An environmental adaptation theory. In C. M. McQuiston & A. A. Webb (Eds.), *Foundations of nursing theory: Contributions of 12 key theorists.* Thousand Oaks, CA: Sage.

Selye, H. (1956). *The stress of life.* New York: McGraw-Hill.

Selye, H. (1983). The stress concept: Past, present, and future. In C. L. Cooper (Ed.), *Stress research: Issues for the eighties.* New York: John Wiley.

Siegel, B. (1986). *Love, medicine, and miracles.* New York: Harper & Row.

Sobel, D. S. (1995). Rethinking medicine: Improving health outcomes with cost-effective psychosocial interventions. *Psychosomatic Medicine, 52,* 234-244.

Stacy, C. B., Kaplan, A. S., & Williams, G. (1992). *The fight against pain.* Yonkers, NY: Consumer Reports Books.

Stuifbergen, A. K., Becker, H. A., Ingalsbe, K., & Sands, S. (1990). Perceptions of health among adults with disabilities. *Health Values, 14*(2), 18-26.

Suarez, E. C., & Williams, R. B. (1989). Situational determinants of cardiovascular and emotional reactivity in high and low hostile men. *Psychosomatic Medicine, 51,* 404-418.

Surwit, R. S., Schneider, M. S., & Feinglos, M. N. (1992). Stress and diabetes. *Diabetes Care, 15,* 1413-1422.

Syme, S. L. (1987). Conference on behavioral medicine and cardiovascular disease: Coronary artery disease, a sociocultural perspective. *Circulation, 76*(Suppl. 1), 112-116.

Tamez, E., Moore, M., & Brown, P. (1978). Relaxation training as a nursing intervention versus pro re nata medication. *Nursing Research, 27,* 160-165.

Toth, J. C. (1980). Effect of structure preparation for transfer on patient anxiety on leaving coronary care unit. *Nursing Research, 29,* 28-34.

Tripp-Reimer, T. (1984). Reconceptualizing the construct of health: Integrating emic and etic perspectives. *Research in Nursing and Health, 7,* 101-109.

Ursin, H., Baade, E., & Levine, J. S. (Eds.). (1978). *Psychobiology of stress: A study of coping man.* New York: Academic Press.

Vgontzas, A. M., Tsigos, C., Bixler, E. O., Stratakis, C. A., Sachman, K., Kales, A., Vela-Bueno, A., & Chrousos, G. P. (1998). Chronic insomnia and activity of the stress system: A preliminary study. *Journal of Psychosomatic Research, 45,* 21-31.

Volicer, B. J., & Bohannon, M. W. (1975). A hospital stress rating scale. *Nursing Research, 24,* 352-359.

Werner, J. S. (1993). Stressors and health outcomes: Synthesis of nursing research, 1980-1990. In J. Barfather & B. Lyon (Eds.), *Stress and coping: State of the science and implications for nursing theory, research, and practice* (pp. 11-38). Indianapolis, IN: Sigma Theta Tau International.

Whitehead, W. E., & Schuster, M. M. (1985). *Gastrointestinal disorders: Behavioral and physiological basis for treatment*. San Diego: Harcourt Brace Jovanovich.

Wolf, C. T., Friedman, S. B., Hofer, M. A., & Mason, J. W. (1964). Relationship between psychological defenses and mean urinary 17-hydroxycorticosteroid excretion rates: A predictive study of parents of fatally ill children. *Psychosomatic Medicine, 26*, 576-591.

Wolf, H. G. (1950). Life situations, emotions and bodily disease. In M. L. Reymert (Ed.), *Feelings and emotions* (pp. 284-335). New York: McGraw-Hill.

Wright, R. J., Rodriquez, M., & Cohen, S. (1998). Review of psychosocial stress and asthma: An integrated biopsychosocial approach. *Thorax, 53*(12), 1066-1074.

PART II

Response-Oriented Stress

CHAPTER 2

Theories of Stress and Relationship to Health

Virginia Hill Rice

onceptualizations of stress and the stress response have varied in form and context throughout the centuries. Florence Nightingale (1860/1969) wrote in *Notes on Nursing,*

> In watching disease, both in private houses and in public hospitals, the thing which strikes the experienced observer most forcibly is this, that the symptoms or the sufferings generally considered to be inevitable and incidental to the disease are very often not symptoms of disease at all, but of something quite different—of the want of fresh air, or of light, or of warmth, or of quiet, or of cleanliness, or of punctuality and care in the administration of diet, of each or of all of these. (p. 8)

Nightingale (1860/1969) believed that all patients were experiencing some "stress" (as it was later to be called) regardless of their illness. Nightingale wrote to nursing, "If you knew how unreasonably sick people suffer from reasonable causes of distress, you would take more pains about these things" (p. 104).

Nursing's challenge is to facilitate the "reparative process" (p. 9).

More than 70 years later, Hans Selye (1956), a young medical student at the University of Prague, noted,

> Whether a man suffers from a loss of blood, an infectious disease, or advanced cancer, he loses his appetite, his muscle strength, and his ambition to accomplish anything; usually the patient also loses weight and even his facial expression betrays that he is ill. (p. 19)

He labeled this phenomenon the "syndrome of just being sick" and pursued the catalysts and processes of the syndrome in the laboratory and in his medical practice for more than 50 years. He described it as "stress-response theory" and systematically examined its relationship with health. Other researchers of the stress-response phenomenon include Mason (1971) and McEwen and Mendelson (1983). This chapter examines, in depth, the development of stress response theory and the wealth of research, theory development, and clinical implications that have been derived from the work.

> ## STRESS RESPONSE THEORY

Selye initially proposed a triadic model as the basis for the stress response pattern. The elements included adrenal cortex hypertrophy, thymicolymphatic (e.g., the thymus, the lymph nodes, and the spleen) atrophy, and gastrointestinal ulcers. These three, he noted, were closely interdependent; they seemed to accompany most illnesses, and they were provoked no matter what the stimulus or illness. Selye could evoke the response in laboratory rats with agents such as formalin, enzymes, hormones, heat, and cold, and he observed it in patients with such diverse health problems as infections, cancer, and heart disease. He noted that the syndrome probably represented an expression of a generalized "call to arms" of the body's defensive forces in reaction to excessive demands or provocative stimuli. Selye (1936) called this "nonspecific" response to damage of any kind "stress." Later, he used the term *stressor* to designate the stimulus that provoked the stress response (Selye, 1976b).

To derive a conceptualization of stress, Selye (1976b) chose to delineate what it was not. He wrote that stress is not

1. Simply nervous tension: It can occur in organisms without nervous systems or in anesthetized or unconscious patients.
2. An emergency discharge of hormones from the adrenal medulla: Although catecholamines are a part of the stress reaction, they are not the only hormones activated, and they play no role in generalized inflammatory diseases or local stress reactions.
3. Everything that causes a secretion of the adrenal cortex (i.e., corticoids): Adrenocorticotropic hormone (ACTH) can stimulate the release of corticoids without producing a stress response.
4. Always the nonspecific result of damage: Normal activities, such as tennis or a pas-

sionate kiss, can produce a stress response without conspicuous damage.

5. The same as a deviation from homeostasis (Cannon, 1932), the body's steady state: Reactions to loud noises, blinking of the eye, or contracting a muscle may cause deviations from the resting state without evidence of a generalized stress reaction.
6. Anything that causes an alarm reaction: It is the stressor that is the stimulus and not the stress itself.
7. Identical with the alarm reaction: These reactions are characterized by certain end-organ changes caused by stress and, hence, cannot be stress.
8. Nonspecific reaction: The pattern of the stress response is specific, although its cause and effects may vary.
9. Necessarily bad: The stress of success, challenge, and creativity is positive, whereas that of failure, anxiety, and infection can be negative.
10. To be avoided: Stress cannot be avoided. It is ubiquitous; it is an essential ingredient of life (Selye, 1976b). Selye viewed stress as the common denominator of all adaptive reactions in the body and complete freedom from stress as death (Selye, 1974).

In his first publication on stress in *Nature* in 1936, Selye defined stress as "the nonspecific response of the body to any demand made on it" (p. 32). Following criticisms for being too vague, confusing, and ambiguous, he offered the following operational definition: Stress is "a state manifested by a specific syndrome which consists of all the nonspecifically induced changes within a biological system" (Selye, 1976b, p. 64). He proposed that such changes were measurable and occurred at both the system and the local level. The entire stress process at the system level, including the threat and the individual's reaction to it, he called the general adaptation syndrome (GAS). The regional response (e.g., localized inflammation where microbes have entered the body) he termed the local adaptation syndrome (LAS). The GAS and LAS are seen as closely coordinated, with the GAS acting as backup (Selye, 1976a). GAS is described in detail in the following sections.

General Adaptation Syndrome

Selye (1956) noted that throughout history aspects of stress and the stress phenomenon floated aimlessly like loose logs on the sea, periodically rising and falling in waves of popularity and disgrace. He attempted to bind together these loose logs of observable facts with solid cables (workable theories) and secure them with a resulting raft (GAS) by mooring it to generally accepted classical medicine in space and time. In space, the three fixed points were the triad of adrenal, thymicolymphatic, and intestinal changes. In time, three distinct phases were identified as the alarm reaction, stage of resistance, and stage of exhaustion. Bringing together these points of space and time, he reasoned, permitted stress to be less ethereal and more amenable to scientific inquiry.

Selye (1976b) labeled this process general "because it was produced only by agents which have a general effect upon large portions of the body," adaptive "because it stimulated defense and, thereby, helped in the acquisition and maintenance of a state of inurement," and syndrome "because its individual manifestations are coordinated and, even partly, dependent upon one another" (p. 38). This response to stimuli, he noted, included (a) the direct effect of the stress on the organism, (b) internal responses that stimulated tissue defense to destroy the damaging threat, and (c) internal responses that caused tissue surrender by inhibiting unnecessary or excessive defense. He noted, "Resistance and adaptation depend on a proper balance of these three factors that occur during the general adaptation syndrome" (p. 56).

In addition to the three theoretical stages of the GAS (alarm, resistance, and exhaustion), Selye (1976b) identified level of function and normal level of resistance as other constructs in his model. In routine day-to-day situations, he wrote, the organism functions within a level of normal resistance or homeostasis. Self-regulating and balancing devices, as well as problem solving, facilitate maintenance and adaptation to routine stressors and stress. Responses are automatic or habitual adaptations. When a stressor is encountered that exceeds current adaptive resources, an alarm is initiated. The alarm reaction involves activation of the hypothalamus-hypophysis-adrenal axis.

Alarm Stage

Selye (1976b) wrote that, even as a demand is being appraised and possible specific responses are being tested, certain cells in the hypothalamus are being alerted to a state of emergency. There is a generalized stimulation of the autonomic nervous system during this initial shock phase of the alarm reaction. A nonspecific breakdown of resistance occurs; sympathetic nervous system activity is suppressed, accompanied by a decrease in muscle tone, hypotension, and hypothermia. Other manifestations include hemoconcentration, hypocholoremia, hypoglycemia, and acidemia. Generalized protein catabolism occurs with altered capillary and cell membrane permeability. The initial shock stage can last from a few moments to as long as 24 hours depending on the intensity of the stressor and the vulnerability of the individual.

A countershock phase follows if the stressor persists or the individual is weak or both. This phase is characteristic of the "fight-or-flight" reaction described by Cannon (1932). It involves stimulation of the sympathoadrenal medullary system with the release of catecholamines (epinephrine and norepinepine). Epinephrine causes dilation of bronchi and pupils; increases in respirations, blood pressure, heart rate, blood volume, blood clotting, perspiration, alertness, blood supply to vital organs, and energy; and causes a decrease in peristalsis. Norepinephrine leads to peripheral vasoconstriction, renin secretion, and stimulation of aldosterone, which in turn causes sodium retention and potassium secretion. Simultaneously, the signal induces secretion of the corticotrophin-releasing factor (CRF) by median eminence cells in the hypothalamus. CRF is conveyed down the portal-venous system into the adenohypothysis, in which it triggers the release of the ACTH. ACTH, carried through the vascular system, acts directly on the adrenal cortex and regulates the secretions of a variety of hormones known collectively as the corticoids. Corticoids are carried to all parts of the body, inducing numerous effects, including gluconeogenesis, thymicolymphatic involution, eosinopenia, peptic ulcers, and decreased immune-inflammatory reactions.

Usually secreted in lesser amounts are proinflammatory cortocoids. These stimulate proliferative ability and reactivity of connective tissue to build strong barricades to resist invasion, increase the platelet count, and cause protein catabolism. The corticoid hormones are known as "syntoxic" because they facilitate coexistence with the stressor pathogen either by reducing sensitivity to it or by encapsulating it within a barricade of inflammatory tissue. These are distinguishable from the "catatoxic" hormones that enhance the destruction of potential pathogens, mostly through the induction of poison-metabolizing enzymes in the liver. The effects of all these substances can be modulated or conditioned by other hormones (e.g., thyroxin), nervous reactions, diet, heredity, health state, and tissue memories of previous experiences with stress.

Symptomatically, the individual may complain of chest pain, palpitations, a racing heart, headache, dysphagia, or all these. Other manifestations include intestinal cramping, dysmobility, dysnea, feelings of lightheadedness, muscle tremors, joint pain, and bruxism. If survival of the organism is at all possible, a stage of resistance follows the alarm reaction. It is called the "stage of resistance" because opposition to a particular stressor has been established, but resistance to most other stressors tends to be less than normal (Selye, 1976b). Manifestations of the second stage

are the antithesis of the alarm reaction stage. In the former, for example, the adrenal cortex discharges its hormone-containing secretions into the bloodstream; consequently, the stores of the gland are depleted. In the stage of resistance, the cortex accumulates an abundant reserve of secretory granules.

Resistance Stage

The resistance stage is evidenced by a dramatic reduction in the alarm reaction as full resistance to the stressor is being established. Developmental (homotrophic) adaptation occurs in the tissues that must intensify their characteristic functional activity for the body to transcend the stressor. There is an attempt to maintain a higher level of functioning in the presence of the stressor as enlargement and multiplication of preexisting cell elements occur without qualitative change. Heterotrophic adaptation, involving tissue readjustment and transformation to perform diverse functions, also occurs at this time. The stage of resistance may be viewed as an attempt at survival through a carefully balanced use of the body's syntoxic and catatoxic defense mechanisms to facilitate coexistence of the organism and the stressor (Selye, 1976a).

Exhaustion Stage

If the organism is not able to return to a normal level of resistance (i.e., prealarm reaction homeostasis) or the initial insult is too overwhelming, a third stage, the stage of exhaustion, ensues. At this time, endocrine activity is heightened; high circulating levels of cortisol begin to have pronounced negative effects on the circulatory, digestive, immune, and other systems. The symptoms are strikingly similar to those of the initial alarm reaction, but such a high level of resistance cannot be maintained indefinitely. Human resources become depleted, and permanent damage to the system through "wear and tear" or death or both is likely to occur. In the usual course of events, the organism would experience all the GAS stages. Surprisingly little has been written about this final stage of adaptation, and few studies have been performed.

GAS Assumptions

The following assumptions are foundational to the general adaptation syndrome theory: (a) Any demand, positive or negative, can provoke the stress response; (b) the stress response is characterized by the same chain of events and pattern of physiological correlates regardless of the stressor or stimulus that provoked it; (c) what occurs systematically in the GAS is evident to a much lesser degree in the LAS; (d) the occurrence of the LAS or GAS or both defines the occurrence of stress; (e) the theory deemphasizes differences among stimuli and organisms; and (f) the theory presumes adaptive resources are genetically determined and finite. According to Selye (1976a), every individual is endowed with a genetically predetermined quantity and quality of adaptive energy that may be spent with conservative discretion (producing a longer life) or with a reckless abandon (a shorter but more colorful existence).

Many criticisms of Selye's conceptualization of stress and the GAS have been raised by Mason (1971) and others. Mason identified the following: (a) Stress has too many ambiguous meanings (he thought that Selye should have coined a new word rather than selected one already in use); (b) stress is an abstraction—it has no real independent existence; (c) stress has been applied to both the agent and the consequence; (d) the stress response cannot be both specific and nonspecific; (e) there have been few attempts to arrive at a consensus definition and operationalization for the term stress; and (f) the stress definition and the GAS do not take into consideration cognition, perception, and interpretation of the stimulus.

Some of these concerns were addressed by Selye (1976c) in his article, "Forty Years of Stress Research: Principal Remaining Problems and Misconceptions." He argued that stress is the nonspecific response of the body to any demand, that the stressor is the agent that produces it, and that the GAS is the chronological development of the response to stressors when their action is prolonged. Selye wrote that the terms nonspecificity and specificity could be applied to both the eliciting agent and the response. By nonspecific is meant the generalized effects or responses that are characteristic of many stimuli or agents—that is, the manifestations of the alarm reaction with secretion of ACTH, the catecholamines, thymicolymphatic involution, and so on. These, he argued, are elicited by innumerable agents that make intense and systemic demands on the organism. Perception of a green light, however, is a highly specific response. It can occur only when given light wavelengths reach the retina. Selye noted that the stress response was affected by conditioning factors, such as age, genetic predisposition, sex, and exogenous treatments, and that these factors can cause the same stimulus to act differently in different individuals and to act differently in the same individual at different times.

Although "perception" and "cognition" were not identified in Selye's early work, he attempted to distinguish between agreeable (healthy) and disagreeable (pathogenic) stress as qualitatively different phenomenon. The first he called eustress and the latter, distress. He wrote that the body undergoes virtually the same nonspecific response during eustress and distress; in the former, however, there is much less damage. This notion of "appraisal" was addressed further by Selye's addition of perception, interpretation, and assessment to his 1985 model (Tache & Selye, 1985). According to Selye, perception and interpretation had not been developed because they were outside the realm of expertise of physiologists (such as himself) who had proposed the original theory (Tache & Selye, 1985).

Coping With Stress

Although not specified in his earlier works, Selye introduces the notion of coping in this later model (Tache & Selye, 1985). Coping he defined as "adapting" to stress situations. This is accomplished in our society, he wrote, "by removing stressors from our lives, by not allowing certain neutral events to become stressors, by developing a proficiency in dealing with conditions we do not want to avoid, and by seeking relaxation or diversion from the demand" (p. 20).

Tache and Selye (1985) summarized the essential points of Selye's model of stress as follows:

1. All life events cause some stress.
2. Stress is not bad per se, but excessive or unnecessary stress should be avoided whenever possible.
3. The stressor is the stimulus eliciting a need for adaptation; stress is the response.
4. The nonspecific aspects of the body's reaction to an agent may not be as obvious as the specific effects. Sometimes, only disease or dysfunction will make an individual realize that he or she is under stress.
5. Stress should be monitored through a battery of parameters.
6. Stress should not be equated with only ACTH, corticoid, or catecholamine secretions. These seem to manifest the main pathways of nonspecific adaptation; they are but a few of the elements of a very complex scheme, however.
7. Removal of the stressor eliminates stress.

Selye noted that stress is the price that organisms pay to survive as animals, and humans pay that same price to accomplish what they consider to be great things.

Stress, Disease, and Illness

According to Selye (Tache & Selye, 1985), the nervous and hormonal responses to stressors, as discussed previously, aid survival. He believed the demand-induced neurohormonal changes are carefully balanced to enhance the organism's capacity to meet challenges and, thus, are adaptive. If, however, there is an excess of defensive or submissive

bodily reactions, then diseases of adaptation can occur. Conditions in which such maladaption is a factor include high blood pressure, diseases of the heart and blood vessels, diseases of the kidney, eclampsia, rheumatic and rheumatoid arthritis, inflammatory diseases of the skin and eyes, infections, allergies and hypersensitivity diseases, nervous and mental diseases, sexual dysfunctions, digestive diseases, metabolic diseases, cancer, and diseases of a compromised immune system. Simonton, Simonton, and Creighton (1978) and Goodkin, Antoni, and Blaney (1986) proposed a strong relationship between stress and cancer. Matthews and Glass (1981) suggested a similar relationship between stress and heart disease.

Bryla (1996), a nurse researcher, reviewed the literature that addressed the relationship between stress and the development of breast cancer and the mediator effects of the immune system. She used published articles, book chapters, books, and workbooks from nursing and the medical literature as sources. Stress was defined as a somatic reaction to an environmental event, an adverse situation, mental frustration, or anxiety (Allen, 1983) and as the state manifested by a specific syndrome that consisted of all the nonspecifically induced changes within a biological system; a response that, although nonspecifically produced, has a very specific form (Selye, 1956).

Bryla (1996) noted that researchers tended to characterize women who developed breast cancer or who experienced progression of the disease or both as having certain personality traits and being overresponsive to emotional stress. These traits include emotional suppression, depression, conflict avoidance, repressive coping style, uncertainty, extroversion, sexual inhibitions, inability to manage anger (so-called "anger in"), masochism, aggressiveness, and hostility (masked with a facade of pleasantness) (Bahnson, 1981; Cooper, Cooper, & Faragher, 1989; Fox, 1983; Grassi & Cappellari, 1988).

Other studies have noted the connection between stress and breast cancer as a "stress-related" weakening of the immune system that, in turn, allows cancer cells to proliferate (Greer & Watson, 1985; Levy et al., 1990; Watson, Pettingale, & Greer, 1984). Measurable physiological effects include lymphocytopenia, thymus involution, and decreases in eosinophils, monocytes, macrophages, and T cells. Other changes are decreases in antibody production, inhibition of natural killer cells, and loss of tissue mass in the spleen and peripheral lymph nodes (Vitaliano, Scanlan, Ochs, Siegler, & Snyder, 1998).

Bryla (1996) concluded that there was a possibility of a "breast cancer personality"; she noted, however, that additional prospective studies are needed to clearly establish this relationship. To date, most studies have been correlational and retrospective in nature, involving women who have already been diagnosed with cancer. Not considered was the potential potent influence of the cancer diagnosis. Other methodological concerns included diverse "operationalization" of the stress concept. For the most part, stress has been measured as an emotion, such as anxiety, hostility, depression, or anger, or as physiological data. Linkages between manifest emotions and, for example, changes in heart rate and experienced stress have, at best, been inferred. Means to establish more direct links and measurements are necessary. Bryla points out the problem of isolating an individual's perception of stress from the extraneous factors that often coexist with it (e.g., fear and depression).

Bleiker and van der Ploeg (1999) reviewed 27 studies of the psychosocial factors in the etiology of breast cancer. Seven of the studies were retrospective, 12 were quasi-prospective, and 8 were prospective. The reviewers failed to find conclusive results and noted that there was a lack of specific knowledge on the relationship between breast cancer development and psychosocial factors, such as stressful life events, coping styles, depression, and the ability to express emotions. They concluded that at least three hypotheses have been described to explain a possible relationship between psychosocial variables and cancer development. The first proposes a biological pathway in which stress through the central nervous system and the endocrine system compromises the immune system leading to cancer development. The second assumes that psychological variables are related to high-risk lifestyle behaviors—for example, personality characteristics lead to cigarette smoking, which in turn leads to increased risk for cancer. A third hypothesis suggests that an unknown factor (possibly hormonal or genetic) may be responsible for the increased risk for cancer and for the increased chance of having a given personality trait. The authors concluded that much prospective research is needed to explicitly determine the personality-cancer relationship.

Leidy (1989) presented the physiological processes of stress as a useful framework for nursing to understand the dynamics of chronic illness, its evolution, and trajectory. She suggested that the manifestations of chronic health problems such as chronic obstructive lung disease can be interpreted as expressions of chronic stress that evolve as a consequence of environmental stressors, such as cigarette smoke or prolonged exposure to air pollutants, and individual pulmonary system vulnerability. She also noted the association between stress and nutritional imbalances, obesity, and diabetes mellitus.

Carrieri-Kohlman, Lindsey, and West (1993), in *Pathophysiological Phenomena in Nursing,* depict pathological consequences associated with the stress response and identify many conditions antecedent to it. These physiological manifestations include lipolysis, proteolysis, gluconeogenesis, and ureagenesis. Antecedent conditions include multiple traumatic insult, ischemia, hypoxia, burns, surgery, sepsis, and loss of a loved one and other catastrophic sociopsychological losses. Fauci et al. (1998), in *Harrison's Principles of Internal Medicine,* describe clinical manifestations of many stress-related disorders, including depression, ulcers, and hypertension. The proposed relationship between stress and health and illness is explicated further in this book.

Other Stress Response Theorists

Although Selye was the pioneer of stress response theory, other early contributors in the field include Mason (1971) and McEwen and Mendelson (1983). Mason believed that coping processes were constantly shaping the endocrine response to stressors and that this response varied with the particular properties of the stimuli. He disagreed with Selye that there was a nonspecific response to stimuli. Mason coined the term "psychoendocrinology," thus attributing to mental processes some of the variance in the endocrine response to stressful stimuli.

Like Selye, McEwen and Mendelson (1983) believed that a stressor was an event that challenged homeostasis, with disease the consequence of failure of the normal adapatative system. These scientists proposed that psychological stress (such as fear and anxiety) involved perceived threats to homeostasis and that these were likely to evoke psychosomatic reactions, such as gastric ulcers and immunosuppression. The focus of their work was on the neuroendocrine response of the brain to stressors and the development of depressive symptoms. They found glucocorticoids to be one of the body's natural antidepressants. These researchers believed the important first mediator of the GAS was psychological. This is discussed in more detail in subsequent chapters.

Stress Response Empirical Adequacy

During the past 60 to 70 years, thousands of studies have sought to explicate Selye's theory and the stress response. Selye (1979) wrote "30 books and about 15,000 technical articles on the subject" (p. xi) and produced *Selye's Guide to Stress Research* (1980) to present the then current state of the knowledge of the stress concept. Included in Volume 1 are a preface and epilogue by Selye and the seminal works of Dohrenwend and Dohrenwend on life events theory, Lazarus's psycho-

logical stress and adaptation model, and Frankenhaeuser's psychoneuroendocrine approaches to the study of stressful person-environment transactions. Studies of stress as a response have been conducted in such diverse fields as business, law, pharmacy, psychology, anthropology, education, sociology, physiology, and philosophy.

A major portion of the stress research has been conducted in the sciences of medicine and nursing because of the hypothesized relationships between stress and disease and stress and illness. A MedLine search of the literature (since 1966), using the general key word "stress," generated more than 95,000 citations. With "Selye" as the key word, 212 references resulted; when the focus-phase "general adaptation syndrome" was added, 100 studies were cited. Sampled literature indicates that stress as a response has been examined in such diverse situations as adults experiencing surgery (Lanuza, 1995), heart disease (Brown, 1976), panic (Lopez-Ibor, 1987), fatigue (Eidelman, 1980), cancer (Vitaliano et al., 1998), biofeedback (Zolten, 1989), antibody production (Herbert & Cohen, 1993), and chronic hypertension (Calhoun, 1992).

In the Cumulative Index for Nursing and Allied Health Literature (CINAHL) (dating from 1982), there were more than 11,000 references for the key word stress; there are 143 references for Selye and 58 for the general adaptation syndrome. A hand search produced several other important works from earlier years. In general, stress response nursing knowledge has been generated in theory development, nursing practice, and empirical research. Each of these content areas will be reviewed in the following sections.

➤ STRESS RESPONSE NURSING KNOWLEDGE

Theory Development

Conceptualization of stress as a response has contributed to the development of many theories and models in nursing science. Among those detailed here is Roy's Adaptation Model (RAM).

Roy's Adaptation Model

One of the earliest nursing theories was developed by Sister Callista Roy while still a graduate student. RAM has some of the characteristics of systems theory and some of the characteristics of stress and interaction theories. Roy borrowed and expanded on theories from others, including Seyle (1936), Helson (1964), and Maslow (1970). She has continued to expand her model from its inception to the present. RAM focuses on the individual (person) as a biopsychosocial adaptive system and describes nursing as a humanistic discipline that "places emphasis on the person's own coping abilities to achieve health" (Roy, 1984, p. 32).

This model relies heavily on stress theory, the notion of adaptation, and the ability of nursing to facilitate client adaptation to stress. From stress theory, Roy selected the concepts of stressor, stress, and adaptation for her model. She defines stress as "a constantly changing point, made up of focal, contextual, and residual stimuli, which represent the person's own standard of the range of stimuli to which one can respond with ordinary adaptive responses" (Roy, 1984, pp. 27-28). Focal stimuli are the internal and external demands immediately confronting the organism (e.g., a need for cancer surgery). Contextual stimuli are all other internal and external factors in the given situation (e.g., fear of dying). Residual stimuli are factors that may be affecting current emotions and behaviors but whose effects are not clearly validated (e.g., having a mother who died from cancer).

Stress, for Roy (1984), represents the person's adaptive level. She wrote, "The human system has the capacity to adjust effectively to changes in the environment and, in turn, to affect the environment" (p. 22). She defined adaptation as "that which promotes the integrity of the person in terms of survival, growth, reproduction, and mastery" (p. 51).

A person's adaptation level is determined by the combined effect of the three classes of stimuli (input). Health results when adaptation reaches the optimal level of the individual's potential to meet his or her physical, psychosocial, and self-actualization needs. The individual uses both innate and acquired biological, psychological, or social adaptive mechanisms or all three.

Roy's model postulates that there is an interchange between the adaptive system (individual) and various stimuli (input) from the environment and from the adaptive system. Responses to stimuli are processed through subsystems that include two control mechanisms (coping processes) and four adaptive modes. One control mechanism is the regulator subsystem. It responds automatically via neural, chemical, and endocrine processes. Stimuli from the internal and external environment (through the senses) act as inputs to the nervous, circulatory, and endocrine systems of the body. Automatic, unconscious (coping) responses are produced.

The second subsystem, the cognator, receives input from external and internal stimuli that involve psychological responses concerned with the process of perception (the link between the regulator and cognator), learning, judgment, and emotion. The four modes of the second subsystem are (a) physiological function (biological integrity derived from basic needs), (b) self-concept (interaction with others and the psychic integrity regarding perception of self), (c) role function (social integrity and the performance of duties based on positions within society), and (d) interdependence (seeking of help, affection, and attention along with relationships with significant others and support systems).

Adaptation, Roy (1984) noted, may occur predominantly in one mode or simultaneously in several. The output of the adaptive system is either adaptation or maladaptive (ineffective) responses. Ineffective responses (coping) result in illness. Adaptive coping results in health. The goal of nursing is to "maintain and enhance adaptive behavior and to change ineffective behavior to adaptive" (p. 59). According to Roy, each individual has finite adaptive potential that is affected by the conditions of the person or the individual's state of coping. This introduces the idea of control into stress, which goes beyond earlier theories of stress in which the individual was considered a passive recipient of stimuli. It also reflects a more optimistic view of the human capability and potential.

Roy's Adaptation Model
Empirical Adequacy

Roy's Adaptation Model has served to guide the development of nursing curriculum, the sophistication of nursing practice, and nursing research. A search of CINAHL revealed 324 references to Roy's Adaptation Model. Since its inception, the model has been supported through research in practice and education (Bower & Baker, 1976; Jones, 1978; Mitchell & Pilkington, 1990; Rambo, 1983; Ryan, 1996). Fawcett and Tulman (1990) built a program of research around the RAM, and many midrange theories have been derived from the model (Calvert, 1989; Ryan, 1996). Even Roy has authored seven books (Andrew & Roy, 1986; Roy, 1984; Roy & Andrews, 1991), 21 articles, and numerous book chapters. Summary reviews of Roy's work can be found in Alligood and Marriner-Tomey (1997) and Marriner-Tomey (1994).

Critical Analysis of RAM Theory

Evaluation of RAM in terms of its level of theory development (using criteria proposed by Walker, 1994, and Walker & Avant, 1988) has shown it to be appropriately meaningful for nursing, logically adequate with well-defined concepts, and useful for guiding nursing practice, education, and research. It has been shown to be generalizable across age groups, health conditions, and cultures (Jackson, 1990; White, Richter, & Fry, 1992). RAM is fairly complex with numerous components and proposed relationships, thus reducing its parsimony. The model has generated many hypotheses that have been subjected to empirical testing through research (Aaronson & Seaman, 1989; Innes, 1992; Inouye, Albert, Mohs, Sun, & Berkman, 1993).

Other theories for nursing that have incorporated stress response include Levine's (1973) four conservation principles, Betty Neuman's (1982) systems model, and King's (1971, 1981) theory of goal attainment. These models are critically examined in the text *Nursing Theorists and Their Work* (Marriner-Tomey, 1994), and their utility and application are described in *Nursing Theory: Utilization & Application* (Alligood & Marriner, 1997).

➤ STRESS RESPONSE AND MIDRANGE THEORY DEVELOPMENT

Many midrange theories for nursing have been derived from stress response theory. Some of the earliest conceptualizations were proposed by Sutterley (1979) and Frain and Valiga (1979).

Stress Level Behavior Model

Sutterley (1979) defined stress as a "dynamic state within the individual that results from any demand to adapt or to change . . . a perceived threat . . . a challenge to one's ability to cope or perform [and] . . . unmet needs" (p. 177). She noted that manifestations of stress were indications of the psychophysiological stress response as described by Selye. Sutterley proposed a model of stress level "behaviors" that paralleled Travis's seven stages of disease (Pelletier, 1977). She wrote that the stress response was not an "all-or-nothing" reaction but one that was a matter of degree; stress levels ranged from ataraxy to panic.

Sources of stress that Sutterley (1979) identified were biophysical-chemical (e.g., excessive heat and fatigue), psychosocial-cultural (e.g., hostility, frustration, and powerlessness), or both. Four self-regulation approaches suggested by the author are altering the environmental circumstances, attempting to change one's own behavior or beliefs, lowering physiological arousal, and enhancing one's resistance and immunity.

Sutterley (1979) noted that each of the self-regulation modalities fit well within Nightingale's (1890/1969) concept of nursing's goal to put the body in the best condition for nature to act on it. She wrote, however, that modern nursing needs to reach beyond Nightingale's model to promote mind-body-spirit integration to tap self-healing potentials.

Multilevel Stress Model

Frain and Valiga (1979) proposed a multilevel model and indicated that it reflected Selye's GAS stages. They, like Sutterley (1979), addressed differences in the severity of the stress response. They noted that Level I includes the day-to-day reactions that most people manifest as they experience "routine" stress. Responses are automatic or habitual or both and require a minimum of energy expenditure for adaptation. Although the alarm-resistance process is active, it is practically imperceptible. An example is the daily experience of an early morning commute to work in heavy traffic.

At Level II, mild stress can occur as less routine events are experienced (such as a job interview or a formal social evening). A heightened alarm reaction with increased alertness, cold and clammy hands, diaphoresis, and increased cardiac output, heart rate, and blood pressure may be evident.

At Level III, moderate stress occurs when the person encounters a persistently stressful event that the use of previous adaptive behaviors fail to resolve. The individual senses danger, may express concern about lack of control, and may hang precariously between successful and unsuccessful resolution of the encounter. Examples are when an individual

is facing surgery, unemployment, and marital difficulties. Frain and Valiga (1979) noted that "in Selye's terms there is a struggle between the resistance and exhaustion stages of the GAS" (p. 62).

At this level, manifestation of the alarm-resistance phenomenon is more obvious, and measurable changes occur. There is an increase in the levels of catecholamines and corticosteroids. Signs and symptoms include tachycardia, palpitations, tremors, weakness, cool and pale skin, and elevated blood pressure. Frain and Valiga termed this reaction the "intraorganismic" response to a stressor. No follow-up research was found for either of these early models.

Adaptive Potential Assessment Model

This midrange model for nursing was proposed by Erickson and Swain (1982). These theorists divided stress response into three states: arousal, equilibrium, and impoverishment. Each of these states represents a different potential for the mobilization of self-care resources—resources that are biophysical and psychosocial. During arousal, individuals show signs and symptoms similar to those found in Selye's alarm and resistance stages. In the equilibrium state, signs and symptoms of adaptation are observable (i.e., normal blood pressure, heart rate, etc.). With impoverishment comes a depletion of available resources and manifestations similar to those found in Selye's exhaustion stage. The authors describe a dynamism among these three states.

Erickson and Swain note that the Adaptive Potential Assessment Model (APAM) differs from Selye's conceptualization because coping resources are considered, not just stressors. Second, an interactive relationship is shown among the states of APAM rather than a unidirectional process, as in the GAS. Last, the developers suggest that APAM represents a holistic perspective that is more consistent with nursing, whereas Selye's model addresses only a biophysical stress response (Erickson, Tomlin, & Swain, 1983).

Critical Analysis of APAM

Evaluation of APAM in terms of its level of theory development (using criteria proposed by Walker & Avant, 1988) has shown it to be appropriately meaningful for nursing and logically adequate with well-defined concepts. It has been shown to be useful to guide dissertation research (Barnfather, 1988) and to direct nursing practice (Campbell, Finch, Allport, Erickson, & Swain, 1985; Kinney & Erickson, 1990).

Generalizability across age groups, health conditions, and culture is limited. APAM is parsimonious, having few well-defined concepts. The model has generated hypotheses that have been subjected to empirical testing through research; that is, adherence in hypertensives (Steckel & Swain, 1977; Swain & Steckel, 1981), active patient orientation (Schulman & Swain, 1982), and experienced perinatal loss (Krazewski, 1994). Empirical testing of the proposed relationships in APAM, however, has been limited to that the developers of the model.

Psychophysiological Stress Model

Another midrange theory model was created by Toth (1984) as a result of her dissertation and used to direct her program of research. Her Psychophysiological Stress Model (PSM) was designed to explain the interplay of multiple stressors on affective and physiologic behavior that increase the likelihood of relapse in acute myocardial infarction (AMI) patients. This model was based on the work of Selye (1956, 1980) and the physiologic consequences of stress (Guyton, 1986). Stress is theoretically defined as "a generalized stimulation of the autonomic nervous system that alerts a person to the presence of stressors arising from an actual or perceived threat" (Toth, 1993, p. 36). The response of AMI patients to psychophysiologic stressors

translates into the specific consequences analogous to Selye's stage of alarm.

Toth proposes that her model explains both the disease process that can result in an AMI and the negative consequences of multiple stressors in the recovering AMI patient. Key concepts in the model include stressors (physiological, psychological, environmental, and sociocultural), psychophysiological stress, and conditioning effects. Toth noted that with stressors there are increases in heart rate, blood pressure, and myocardial oxygen consumption that, in turn, leads to an increase in myocardial ischemia and the possibility of fatal dysrhythmias or reinfarction. Therefore, assessing stress level at hospital discharge for AMI patients is important to determine who may be at risk for a subsequent AMI. It is also essential for practitioners planning discharge patient care.

PSM Instrument Development

PSM was used by Toth (1988) to guide the development of a Stress of Discharge Assessment Tool (SDAT). SDAT is a 60-item, norm-referenced, self-report measure that is completed by AMI patients at the time of their hospital discharge. The first 46 items assess stressors common to most AMI patients; 14 additional items measure the effects of stressors that may be specific to some AMI patients (e.g., those that relate to employment).

Scoring is on a 5-point, Likert-type scale that assesses the degree of consensus with the items from "strongly agree" to "strongly disagree." Summative scores range from 60 to 300 points; the higher the score, the higher the experienced stress. Scale items were determined through a literature search and reviewed by an eight-member panel of expert clinicians for content validity. Construct validity was examined with a sample of 104 AMI patients who completed the SDAT 48 hours prior to hospital discharge. Scores ranged from 86 to 168; 72% were within one standard deviation of the mean. Internal consistency, using a Cronbach's alpha coefficient, was .85. Toth proposed that such assessment information is needed before initiation of interventions to reduce the stress response.

Six hypotheses, based on the PSM, were generated by Toth (1988). Each examined the value of factors measured by the SDAT to predict magnitude of stress following AMI prior to discharge in 104 adults. Variables included persistent symptoms, SES, age, previous AMI history, marital status, and severity of AMI. Only severity of AMI was found to be significantly related to the stress response at hospital discharge. Toth (1987) found that older and younger AMI patients generally experienced similar stressors; younger patients, however, were less worried about having another AMI and had felt less sick during their hospitalization. Both age groups believed their partners worried about them too much and this was a source of stress.

In a subsequent study, Toth (1993) found that women did not differ from men at hospital discharge in the magnitude of stress experienced, their most stressful concerns, the severity of AMI, or their age. Women, however, had and reported more persistent cardiac symptoms than men.

Findings from these studies serve to guide the nurse clinician in ensuring that AMI clients receive appropriate referrals for stress management or cardiac rehabilitation or both on discharge. Toth suggested that the SDAT be tested with other AMI samples and that SDAT scores be used as a dependent variable in assessing the effectiveness of different types of stress reduction and cardiac rehabilitation programs.

Critical Analysis of PSM

PSM, in terms of it's level of theory development using criteria proposed by Walker and Avant (1988), has been shown to be appropriately meaningful in identifying persons in need of nursing care. It is useful to guide nursing practice in the planning of discharge care for AMI patients and their families. The model has logical adequacy in that all its key concepts are defined or specified by Toth. The theory has generated testable hypotheses and an instrument (SDAT) to operationalize con-

cepts in the model. The PSM has shown generalizability across age groups and race (Toth, 1987) and gender (Toth, 1993). The PSM is fairly complex, with numerous components and proposed relationships when the physiological elements are explicated, thus reducing its parsimony. Empirical adequacy is limited; to date, much of the research has been conducted by the designer of the model.

➤ STRESS RESPONSE AND CLINICAL PRACTICE MODELS

Many clinical practice models have evolved from the work of Selye and from response theory. Some of these are described briefly in the following sections.

An Adaptation Model for Nursing Practice

This model was designed by Jones (1978). She proposed that the interaction among unmet basic needs (as identified by Maslow, 1970), adaptability (as described by Selye, 1976b), and location on a illness-wellness scale (Dunn, 1959) constituted relative health. She conceptualized each of these factors on a continuum from below average to a high level. Envisioned as a linear model, a line can be plotted from any point on the basic needs continuum to its opposite apex and intersect with another line similarly plotted on the adaptability continuum. Thus, a person's position on the illness-wellness continuum is determined by finding where the basic needs and adaptability lines intersect and drawing a vertical line from that point down to the illness-wellness continuum. As a person's position on either their basic needs or adaptability lines changes, so does their position on the illness-wellness continuum. For example, an older adult with hypertension who is low on adaptability but whose basic needs for normotension are being largely met may be placed at the point of average health. If the need to manage the hypertension increases, while adaptability remains the same, health will move in a direction below average.

Kidder (1989) offered a conceptual framework that examines five factors (stress, coping, development, social support, and immunocompetence) from a biopsychosocial perspective to gain a clearer understanding of why some children in intensive care recover faster than others. Her definition of physiological stress was derived from the work of Selye (1950). She concluded that a child's recovery from a critical illness is not merely a matter of providing the correct medical treatment at the appropriate time. Knowledge and analysis of the stressors in the child's environment, the child's ability to cope, developmental age, availability of social supports, and competence of the child's immune system are needed by nursing for understanding, planning, and implementing effective care.

➤ STRESS RESPONSE MEASUREMENT

Many physiological measures have been used by nursing in stress response research. Typically, measures are vital signs (Guzzeta & Forsyth, 1979), heart rate (Brown, 1976), urinary Na+/K+ ratios and 17-ketosteroids (Farr, Keene, Sampson, & Michael, 1984), and plasma cortisol (Page & Ben-Eliyahu, 1997). Chapter 4 presents detailed descriptions of the various stress measures, including their source, research, reliability, validity, sensitivity, and specificity.

➤ STRESS RESPONSE AND NURSING INTERVENTION RESEARCH

In this section, a sampling of the nursing research studies guided by stress response theory during the past 30 years are presented, followed by a summary of three reviews of stress response studies (Doswell, 1988; Lindsey, 1983; Werner, 1993). Some of the studies appear in more than one of the sources.

One of the earliest studies, conducted by Cleland (1965), examined the effects of stress on the performance of staff nurses. She found that those who scored highest on need for social approval reported a sharp decline in performance when situational stressors were increased. Nurses with low need for social approval increased their performance when situational stressors were increased.

In a descriptive study, Garbin (1979) asked 76 nurses to list significant stressors in their work environment. The ones identified as most stressful were "heavy workload, making total patient care impossible" and "making a mistake." The author created a "stress: individual/environment interaction model" as an outcome of her research. Topf (1994) and von Onciul (1996) also evaluated environmental stressors using a stress response perspective. Topf proposed several concepts to supplement stress theory with the goal of better understanding and management of environmental stressors. These constructs were "enhancement of the person-environmental compatibility," "societal and technological development," and "intrinsic sensitivity to ambient stressors."

In another area, many studies have examined therapeutic touch (TT) as an intervention to reduce the stress response. Krieger (1975) described TT as the laying on of hands to direct excess body energies from the person in the role of healer to another for the purpose of helping or healing that individual. Krieger, Peper, and Encoli (1979) used a pretest-posttest design to monitor the physiological relaxation effects of TT in adult patients for two consecutive days. The electroencephalogram, electromyographic, galvanic skin response, temperature, and heart rate indicators showed significantly lower reactivity levels with a greater abundance of large-amplitude alpha activity in both eyes-open and eyes-closed states. Participants also reported higher positive feelings during and after TT.

Wishing to determine if TT had an effect on emotions, Heldt (1981) examined the effects of TT on the anxiety of 90 adult cardio-vascular patients randomly assigned to three matched intervention groups. One group received therapeutic touch, one was given casual touch, and a third group received no touch at all. Anxiety, defined as a transitory negative emotional state, was measured on Spielberger's State-Trait Anxiety Inventory. Cannon's (1932) conceptualization of anxiety as a sympathetic nervous system reaction guided the study. Findings revealed that the 5-minute therapeutic touch resulted in a significant decrease in posttest anxiety 10 minutes after intervention. Unknown, however, are the long-term effects or the effects of repeated exposure to therapeutic touch on negative emotions. The researcher believed the use of therapeutic touch helped strengthen the interpersonal relationship between the patient and the nurse. Keller and Bzdek (1986) evaluated TT in 60 adults with tension headaches who were randomly assigned to TT treatment and placebo groups. They found a significant reduction in reported pain and distress for the TT group.

Lafreniere et al. (1999) experimentally evaluated the effects of TT on biochemical indicators and moods of 41 healthy women. Pretest and posttest urine samples were collected for nitric oxide levels, and mood inventories were assessed during three consecutive monthly sessions. Findings revealed that mood disturbance in the experimental group significantly decreased during the course of the three sessions compared to the mood disturbance of women in the control group. In addition, there was a significantly lower nitric oxide leveling in the TT group. The authors concluded that TT significantly reduced psychological and physiological distress in these women, and that it may have an impact on reducing symptom distress in breast cancer patients undergoing chemotherapy.

Two other authors proposed the use of stress response theory in relation to managing patients' experiencing endoscopy (Murphy, 1993) and to understanding patient stress in the intensive care unit setting (Sharp, 1996). In addition, Murphy suggested nursing inter-ventions, such as patient teaching, relaxation techniques, and communication skills, that could promote positive health outcomes for the patients experiencing endoscopy; none of these was tested.

Many nursing research studies have examined biochemical measures of the stress response following threatening health care procedures. Farr et al. (1984) found altered circadian excretion of urinary catecholamines in postoperative surgical patients. Lanuza and Marotta (1987) reported cortisol elevations in cardiac pacemaker implant patients, and Lanuza (1995) found elevated cortisol levels in both coronary artery bypass graft patients and patients undergoing implantation of an automatic cardioverter or defibrillator device.

➤ STRESS RESPONSE AND NURSING RESEARCH REVIEWS

Three reviews of stress response as a perspective for nursing research were examined. Lindsey (1983) reviewed nursing research studies of physiological phenomena between 1970 and 1980. She reported 141 studies divided into three categories: (a) phenomena investigated were primarily individual-related ($n = 66$), (b) phenomena studied were primarily related to the environment ($n = 25$), and (c) studies focused on some aspect of nursing therapeutics ($n = 50$).

Following a detailed examination of all the studies, Lindsey concluded that a wide variety of physiological phenomena have been studied with relatively small sample sizes. Most of the studies were either preliminary in nature or pilot studies, most were single investigations without follow-up, few were replications or extensions, and most were imprecise or lacking in theoretical underpinnings.

Doswell (1988) focused her review on nursing research studies conducted between 1977 and 1987 that had examined physiological responses to stress. She found 19 studies, which she divided into four subject categories: life events, vocal stress, hospitalization and environmental stressors, and miscellaneous (covering single studies). The majority of the physiological response variables were studied in cardiovascular patients. All subjects were adults. The reviewer concluded that nursing studies of physiological responses to stress were only nominally linked to a conceptual framework. In addition, the number of published nursing studies was too small and too disjointed to provide any consistent support for stress response relationships. She concluded that the research during the previous decade included a majority of single diverse studies measuring single cardiovascular variables using Selye's theory of stress. There was little attempt to build a systematic body of nursing knowledge in this area.

A third review was conducted by Werner (1993). She examined the nursing research literature for studies on stressors and health outcomes between 1980 and 1990; she found seven studies that had a stress response theoretical orientation. Werner noted that a diminishing number of nursing researchers were using Selye's perspective of physiological stress as a response. She reasoned that this may be the consequence of nursing taking a much broader view of the human condition in response to stress. It also may be related to the increasing interest in Lazarus's transactional model, with its heavy emphasis on cognition and appraisal. Lyon and Werner (1987) noted that response models of stress are incompatible with nursing's view of the wholistic human experience. Focusing on physiological phenomena without consideration of the person's perspective, psyche, and emotions was seen as only treating one half of the person.

➤ CONCLUSION

There is a very long history of stress response theory and its evolution in psychology, medicine, and nursing. It has led to numerous models, thousands of research studies and publications, and the development of health care provider curriculum. Selye (1936) was the "founding father" of stress response theory. Stress response theory was one of the most significant contributions to the field of stress and coping. Selye designed it to describe, predict, and explain living organisms' physiological reactions to ubiquitous life stressors. He gave it prominence and detail with his general adaptation syndrome. The GAS is able to describe and explain, in part, physiological responses to stressors. Noticeably absent, however, is the "connection" between the body and the mind. It is this missing "piece" that has given the theory limited usefulness for nursing.

Some of the early research in nursing also examined the stress response physiologically; in addition, nursing has sought to assess, predict, and explain both the physiological and the psychosocial components of stress. With the need to "see" the patient as a whole, nursing moved quickly toward using models and theories that took into consideration both components. This is reflected in the broad adoption of biopsychosocial models, measurements, and intervention arenas of research. These developments in stress, coping, and health are further explicated in this book.

➤ REFERENCES

Aaronson, L., & Seaman, L. (1989). Managing hypernatremia in fluid deficient elderly. *Journal of Gerontological Nursing, 15,* 29-36.

Allen, R. (1983). *Human stress: Its nature and control.* Minneapolis, MN: Burgess.

Alligood, M., & Marriner-Tomey, M. (1997). *Nursing theory: Utilization & application.* Norwalk, CT: Appleton-Century-Crofts.

Andrew, H., & Roy, C. (1986). *Essentials of the Roy Adaptation Model.* Norwalk, CT: Appleton-Century-Crofts.

Bahnson, C. (1981). Stress and cancer: The state of the art. *Psychosomatics, 22,* 207-220.

Barnfather, J. (1988). Testing a theoretical proposition from modeling and role modeling: Basic need and adaptive potential status. *Issues in Mental Health, 14,* 1-18.

Bleiker, E., & van der Ploeg, H. M. (1999). Psychosocial factors in the etiology of breast cancer: Review of a popular link. *Patient Education and Counseling, 37,* 201-214.

Bower, H., & Baker, B. (1976). The Roy Adaptation Model: Using the adaptation model in a practitioner curriculum. *Nursing Outlook, 24,* 686-689.

Brown, A. (1976). Effect of family visits on the blood pressure and heart rate of patients in CCU. *Heart & Lung, 5,* 291-296.

Bryla, C. (1996). The relationship between stress and the development of breast cancer: A literature review. *Oncology Nursing Forum, 23,* 441-448.

Calhoun, D. (1992). Hypertension in blacks: Socioeconomic stressors and sympathetic nervous system activity. *American Journal of Medical Sociology, 304,* 306-311.

Calvert, M. (1989). Human-pet interaction and loneliness: A test of concepts from Roy's Adaptation Model. *Nursing Science Quarterly, 2*(4), 194-202.

Campbell, J., Finch, D., Allport, C., Erickson, H. C., & Swain, M. A. (1985). A theoretical approach to nursing assessment. *Journal of Advanced Nursing, 10*(2), 111-115.

Cannon, W. B. (1932). *The wisdom of the body.* New York: Norton.

Carrieri-Kohlman, V., Lindsey, A., & West, C. (1993). *Pathophysiological phenomena in nursing: Human responses to illness* (2nd ed.). Philadelphia: W. B. Saunders.

Cleland, V. (1965). The effect of stress on performance: A study of the effect of situational stressors on the performances of nurses—Modified by need for social approval. *Nursing Research, 14,* 4-10.

Cooper, C., Cooper, R., & Faragher, E. (1989). Incidence and perception of psychosocial stress: The relationship with breast cancer. *Psychological Medicine, 19,* 415-422.

Doswell, W. (1988). Physiological responses to stress. *Annual Review of Nursing Research, 7,* 51-69.

Dunn, H. (1959). *High level wellness.* Arlington, VA: R. W. Beatty.

Eidelman, D. (1980). Fatigue toward an analysis and unified definition. *Medical Hypotheses, 6,* 517-526.

Erickson, H., & Swain, M. (1982). A model for assessing potential adaptation to stress. *Research in Nursing & Health, 5,* 93-101.

Erickson, H., Tomlin, E., & Swain, M. (1983). *Modeling and role modeling: A theory and paradigm for nursing.* Englewood Cliffs, NJ: Prentice Hall.

Farr, L., Keene, A., Sampson, D., & Michael, A. (1984). Alterations in circadian excretion of urinary variables and physiological indicators of stress following surgery. *Nursing Research, 33,* 140-146.

Fauci, A., Braunwald, E., Isselbacher, K. J., Wilson, J., Martin, J., Kasper, D., Hauser, S., & Longo, D. (Eds.). (1998). *Harrison's principles of internal medicine, 14th edition.* New York: McGraw-Hill.

Fawcett, J., & Tulman, L. (1990). Building a programme of research from the Roy Adaptation Model of nursing. *Journal of Advanced Nursing, 15,* 720-725.

Fox, B. (1983). Current theory of psychogenic effects on cancer incidence and prognosis. *Journal of Psychosocial Oncology, 1,* 17-31.

Frain, M., & Valiga, T. (1979). The multiple dimensions of stress. *Topics in Clinical Nursing, 1,* 43-52.

Garbin, M. (1979). Stress research in clinical settings. *Topics in Clinical Nursing, 1,* 87-95.

Goodkin, K., Antoni, M., & Blaney, P. (1986). Stress and hopelessness in the promotion of cervical intraepithelial neoplasia to invasive squamous cell carcinoma of the cervix. *Journal of Psychosomatic Research, 30,* 67-76.

Grassi, L., & Cappellari, L. (1988). State and trait psychological characteristics of breast cancer patients. *New Trends in Experimental and Clinical Psychiatry, 4,* 99-109.

Greer, S., & Watson, M. (1985). Towards a psychobiological model of cancer. Psychological considerations. *Social Science and Medicine, 20,* 773-777.

Guyton, A. (1986). *Textbook of medical physiology* (7th ed.). Philadelphia: W. B. Saunders.

Guzzeta, C., & Forsyth, G. (1979). Nursing diagnostic pilot study: Psychophysiological stress. *Advances in Nursing Science, 2,* 27-44.

Heldt, P. (1981). Effect of therapeutic touch on anxiety level in hospitalized patients. *Nursing Research, 30,* 32-37.

Helson, H. (1964). *Adaptation level theory.* New York: Harper & Row.

Herbert, T., & Cohen, S. (1993). Stress and immunity in humans: A meta-analytic review. *Psychosomatic Medicine, 55,* 364-379.

Innes, M. (1992). Managing upper airway obstruction. *British Journal of Nursing, 9*(14), 732-735.

Inouye, S., Albert, M., Mohs, R., Sun, K., & Berkman, L. (1993). Cognitive performance in a high-functioning community-dwelling elderly population. *Journal of Gerontology, 48,* 146-151.

Jackson, B. (1990). Social support and life satisfaction of black climacteric women. *Western Journal of Nursing Research, 12,* 25-27.

Jones, P. (1978). An adaptation model for nursing practice. *American Journal of Nursing, 78,* 1900-1906.

Keller, E., & Bzdek, V. (1986). Effects of therapeutic touch on tension headache pain. *Nursing Research, 35,* 101-106.

Kidder, C. (1989). Reestablishing health: Factors influencing the child's recovery in pediatric intensive care. *Journal of Pediatric Nursing, 4,* 96-103.

King, I. (1971). *Toward a theory for nursing: General concepts of human behavior.* New York: John Wiley.

King, I. (1981). *A theory for nursing: Systems, concepts, process.* New York: John Wiley.

Kinney, C. K., & Erickson, H. C. (1990). Modeling the client's world: A way to holistic care. *Issues in Mental Health Nursing, 11*(2), 93-108.

Krazewski, A. (1994). *Coping with miscarriage: Use of adaptive potential.* Unpublished master's thesis, Wayne State University, College of Nursing, Detroit, MI.

Krieger, D. (1975). Therapeutic touch: The imprimatur of nursing. *American Journal of Nursing, 75,* 784-787.

Krieger, D., Peper, E., & Encoli, S. (1979). Therapeutic touch: Searching for evidence of physiological change. *American Journal of Nursing, 79*(4), 660-662.

Lafreniere, K., Mutus, B., Camerson, S., Tannous, M., Giannotti, M., Abu-Zahra, H., & Laukkanen, E. (1999). Effects of therapeutic touch on biochemical and mood indicators in women. *Journal of Alternative and Complementary Medicine, 5,* 367-370.

Lanuza, D. (1995). Postoperative circadian rhythms and cortisol stress response to two types of cardiac surgery. *American Journal of Critical Care, 4,* 212-220.

Lanuza, D., & Marotta, S. (1987). Endocrine and psychologic responses of patients to cardiac pacemaker implantation. *Heart & Lung, 16,* 496-505.

Leidy, N. (1989). A physiological analysis of stress and chronic illness. *Journal of Advanced Nursing, 14,* 868-876.

Levine, M. (1973). *Introduction to clinical nursing* (2nd ed.). Philadelphia: F. A. Davis.

Levy, S., Herberman, R., Lee, J., Whiteside, T., Kirkwood, J., & McFeeley, S. (1990). Estrogen receptor concentration and social factors as predictors of natural killer cell activity in early-stage breast cancer patients. *Natural Immune Cell Growth Regulation, 9,* 313-324.

Lindsey, A. (1983). Stress response. In V. Carrieri-Kohlman, A. Lindsey, & C. West (Eds.), *Pathophysiological phenomena in nursing: Human responses to illness* (2nd ed.). Philadelphia: W. B. Saunders.

Lopez-Ibor, J. (1987). The meaning of stress, anxiety, and collective panic in clinical settings. *Psychotherapy and Psychosomatic, 47,* 168-174.

Lyon, B., & Werner, J. (1987). Stress. In J. Fitzpatrick & R. Taunton (Eds.), *Annual review of nursing research.* New York: Springer.

Marriner-Tomey, M. (1994). *Nursing theorists and their work.* Norwalk, CT: Appleton-Century-Crofts.

Maslow, A. H. (1970). *Motivation and personality* (2nd ed.). New York: Harper & Row.

Mason, J. W. (1971). A re-evaluation of the concept of "non-specificity" in stress theory. *Journal of Psychiatric Research, 8,* 323-333.

Matthews, K., & Glass, D. (1981). Type A behavior, stressful life events, and coronary heart disease. In B. Dohrenwend & B. Dohrenwend (Eds.), *Stressful life events and their context.* New York: Prodist.

McEwen, B., & Mendelson, S. (1983). Effects of stress on the neurochemistry and morphology of the brain: Counterregulation versus damage. In L. Goldberger & S. Breznitz (Eds.), *Handbook of stress: Theoretical and clinical aspects* (3rd ed.). New York: Free Press.

Mitchell, G., & Pilkington, B. (1990). Theoretical approaches to nursing practice: A comparison of Roy and Parse. *Nursing Science Quarterly, 3,* 81-87.

Murphy, D. (1993). Managing patient stress in endoscopy. *Gastroenterology Nursing, 16,* 72-74.

Neuman, B. (1982). *The Neuman Systems Model.* Norwalk, CT: Appleton-Century-Crofts.

Nightingale, F. (1969). *Notes on nursing: What it is and what it is not.* New York: Dover. (Original work published 1860)

Oster, C. (1979). Sensory deprivation and homeostasis. *Journal of the American Geriatric Society, 8,* 364-367.

Page, G. G., & Ben-Eliyahu, S. (1997). The immune-suppressive nature of pain. *Seminars in Oncology Nursing, 13,* 10-15.

Pelletier, K. (1977). *Mind as healer, mind as slayer.* New York: Dell.

Rambo, B. (1983). *Adaptation nursing: Assessment and intervention.* Philadelphia: W. B. Saunders.

Roy, C. (1984). *Introduction to nursing: An adaptation model* (2nd ed.). Englewood Cliffs, NJ: Prentice Hall.

Roy, C., & Andrews, H. (1991). *The Roy Adaptation Model: The definitive statement.* Norwalk, CT: Appleton & Lange.

Ryan, M. (1996). Loneliness, social support, and depression as interactive variables with cognitive status: Testing Roy's model. *Nursing Science Quarterly, 9,* 107-114.

Schulman, B., & Swain, M. (1980). Active patient orientation. *Patient Counseling and Health Education, 2,* 32-37.

Selye, H. (1936). A syndrome produced by diverse nocuous agents. *Nature, 138,* 32.

Selye, H. (1950). Forty years of stress research: Principal remaining problems and misconceptions. *CMA Journal, 115,* 53-55.

Selye, H. (1956). *The stress of life.* New York: McGraw-Hill.

Selye, H. (1974). *Stress without distress.* Philadelphia: J. B. Lippincott.

Selye, H. (1976a). *Stress in health and disease.* Reading, MA: Butterworth's.

Selye H. (1976b). *The stress of life* (Rev. ed.). New York: McGraw-Hill.

Selye, H. (1976c). Forty years of stress research: Principal remaining problems and misconceptions. *CMA Journal, 115,* 53-55.

Selye, H. (1979). *The stress of my life: A scientist's memoirs.* New York: Van Nostrand Reinhold.

Selye, H. (1980). *Selye's guide to stress research.* New York: Van Nostrand Reinhold.

Sharp, S. (1996). Understanding stress in the ICU setting. *British Journal of Nursing, 5,* 369-373.

Simonton, C., Simonton, S., & Creighton, J. (1978). *Getting well again.* Los Angeles: Tarcher.

Sutterley, D. (1979). Stress & health: A survey of self-regulation modality. *Topics in Clinical Nursing, 1,* 1-26.

Swain, M. A., & Steckel, S. B. (1981). Influencing adherence among hypertensives. *Research in Nursing & Health, 4,* 213-222.

Tache, J., & Selye, H. (1985). On stress and coping mechanisms. *Issues in Mental Health Nursing, 7,* 3-24.

Topf, M. (1994). Theoretical considerations for research on environmental stress and health. *Image, 26,* 289-293.

Toth, J. (1984). Variables associated with the stressful experience of hospital discharge during acute myocardial infarction [Doctoral dissertation, The Catholic University of America, 1984). *Dissertation Abstracts International,* A82857.

Toth, J. (1987). Stressors affecting older versus younger AMI patients. *Dimensions of Critical Care Nursing, 6,* 147-157.

Toth, J. (1988). Measuring the stressful experience of hospital discharge following acute myocardial infarction. In C. Waltz & O. Strickland (Eds.), *Measurement of nursing outcomes* (pp. 3-23). New York: Springer.

Toth, J. (1993). Is stress at hospital discharge after acute myocardial infarction greater in women than in men? *American Journal of Critical Care, 2,* 35-40.

Vitaliano, P., Scanlan, J., Ochs, H., Siegler, I., & Snyder, E. (1998). Psychosocial stress moderates the relationship of cancer history with natural killer cell activity. *Annals of Behavioral Medicine, 20,* 199-208.

von Onciul, J. (1996). Stress at work. *British Medical Journal, 313,* 745-749.

Walker, L. O., (1994). *Strategies for theory construction in nursing* (3rd ed.). Norwalk, CT: Appleton & Lange.

Walker, L. O., & Avant, K. C. (1988). *Strategies for theory construction in nursing.* Norwalk, CT: Appleton & Lange.

Watson, M., Pettingale, K., & Greer, S. (1984). Emotional control and autonomic arousal in breast cancer patients. *Journal of Psychosomatic Research, 28,* 467-474.

Werner, J. S. (1993). Stressors and health outcomes: Synthesis of nursing research, 1980-1990. In J. Barnfather & B. Lyon (Eds.), *Stress and coping: State of the science and implications for nursing theory, research, and practice* (pp. 11-38). Indianapolis, IN: Sigma Theta Tau International.

White, N. E., Richter, J. M., & Fry, C. (1992). Coping, social support, and adaptation to chronic illness. *Western Journal of Nursing Research, 14*(2), 211-224.

Zolten, A. (1989). Constructive integration of learning theory and phenomenological approaches to biofeedback training. *Biofeedback Self Regulation, 14,* 89-99.

CHAPTER 3

Stress, Immunity, and Health Outcomes

Linda Witek-Janusek and Herbert L. Mathews

 he assumption that psychological stress, physical stress, mood, and behavior modulate the immune system, and predispose an individual to illness, is centuries old. In the sixteenth century, the Greek physician Galen observed that melancholy women were more predisposed to the development of tumors. Today, the assumption is widely held that stress, emotions, and behavior affect health, well-being, and predisposition to disease. For example, a character proclaims in Woody Allen's film *Manhattan,* "I can't express anger, I grow a tumor instead." Only recently, however, has this mind-immune relationship been subjected to rigorous scientific inquiry.

The organized establishment of the science of psychoneuroimmunology is often credited to Robert Ader, who first introduced this term in his presidential address to the American Psychosomatic Society (Ader, 1980). Ader defined *psychoneuroimmunology* as the study of the interactions among behavioral, neural, endocrine (neuroendocrine), and immunological processes of adaptation. The central premise is that an individual's response and adaptation to the environment is an integrated process involving interactions among the nervous, endocrine, and immune systems. This is in contrast to the traditional view of the immune system in which it is autonomous and functions independently of the other organ systems of the body. Today, psychoneuroimmunology is a multidisciplinary science that includes nurses, psychologists, immunologists, microbiologists, neuro-

AUTHORS' NOTE: This chapter is dedicated to the memory of my (LWJ) mentor and my friend, Dr. Sabath F. Marotta (1929-1996), who introduced me and numerous other nurses to scientific inquiry and stress physiology. May his memory live on in our collective contributions to the field of stress. This work was supported in part by the Department of the Army (DAMD-98-8120), the National Cancer Institute (CA-77120-01), the National Institute of Nursing Research (NR-00085), the National Institute of Allergy and Infectious Disease (AI-31127), Catholic Health Partners, and the Cancer Federation. The expertise of Josh Takagishi and Maribel Barrigan is gratefully acknowledged. The content of this chapter does not reflect the position or the policy of the Department of the Army or the U.S. government.

scientists, endocrinologists, and others. The collective aims of these scientists are to explore and explain the common belief that one's behavior and emotions can influence stress, immunity, and health outcome.

Despite the recent development of psychoneuroimmunology as a discipline, initial evidence that linked stress to the immune system was reported by Hans Selye in the 1930s. In his general adaptation syndrome, Selye described a triad of responses to acute physical stress that consisted of adrenal gland enlargement, gastric erosion, and thymic involution (Selye, 1936, 1976). Since then, scientific evidence confirming biological links among the nervous, endocrine, and immune systems has accumulated. These links include direct innervation of lymphatic tissue by the central nervous system and a shared communication network in which cells of the nervous, endocrine, and immune systems use common molecules and receptors to reciprocally modulate biologic activity. Thoughts, emotions, and behavior are known to activate anatomical and biochemical pathways, and these pathways in turn modulate immune function (La Via & Workman, 1998). Such observations and demonstrations have permitted advocates of psychoneuroimmunology to suggest that biobehavioral interventions aimed at strengthening immunocompetence may be an important component of holistic health care (Kiecolt-Glaser & Glaser, 1992).

➤ NEURAL-IMMUNE INTERACTIONS

The connection between the brain and the immune system is through direct innervation of lymphoid tissue and through the release of products from the brain that bind to membrane receptors on immunologically competent cells. It is clear that primary and secondary lymphoid tissues are innervated with noradrenergic and peptidergic nerve fibers (Felten et al., 1987). The Feltens's immunohistochemical studies provide direct evidence of the close association between presynaptic sympathetic nerve endings and lymphocytes and macrophages (Felten, Felten, Carlson, Olschowka, & Livnat, 1985). Experimentally produced brain lesions of the hypothalamus, hippocampus, and cerebral cortex alter immune function, suggesting a neural-immune interactive network of connections. Those areas of the brain that exert immunomodulatory effects are areas concerned with emotions and with visceral, autonomic, and neuroendocrine regulation, thus establishing the "hardwiring" between neural centers that process emotions and immune cells. Further verification of a neural-immune network or axis was provided when lymphocytes and macrophages were shown to bear receptors for adrenergic substances (both α- and β-adrenergic receptors) and various neuropeptide hormones, including vasoactive intestinal polypeptide, somatostatin, calcitonin gene-related peptide, substance P, and opioids (Stevens-Felten & Bellinger, 1997). The presence of such receptors on immune cells provides a mechanism whereby the immune system can respond to biochemical signals from the brain. Activation of these receptors leads to functional changes in immune response (i.e., lymphocyte proliferation, cytotoxicity, antibody production, and cytokine secretion).

A pivotal step in firmly establishing that the brain and immune system interact was accomplished by psychologists who, using animal models, demonstrated that classical psychological (Pavlovian) conditioning could produce immunologic changes (Ader & Cohen, 1993). Such conditioning and its effect on the immune system have been demonstrated clinically. For example, research has documented the occurrence of anticipatory immunosuppression prior to the administration of chemotherapy (Bovbjerg et al., 1990; Fredrikson, Furst, Lekander, Rothstein, & Blomgren, 1993).

Investigators continue to unravel the intricate interplay among the nervous, endocrine, and immune systems. The associated immunologic changes that occur in response to neuroendocrine mediators, however, are highly complex, and often the characterization of putative interactions has been measured only *in vitro,* in which one variable is manipulated. *In vivo,* however, immunologically competent cells respond to multiple stimuli, including numerous so-called molecules of emotion, within a microenvironment. Ultimately, the net immune response is an integration of these stimuli. The multiple levels and complexity of such immune modulation are remarkable, considering that numerous peptide and hormonal mediators can augment and diminish immune function (Wang, Fiscus, Yang, & Mathews, 1995; Witek-Janusek & Mathews, 1999a). It remains to be determined how these peptides and mediators fit within a homeostatic framework or are altered by environmental perturbation.

Adding additional complexity, it is well established that not only do nerves and secretory products from the brain influence immune function but also the converse is true. Immune activation can modulate central nervous system activity. Hugo Besedovsky and collaborators conducted seminal studies, which demonstrated that antigenic challenge of the immune system can produce an increase in neural firing within the medial hypothalamus (Besedovsky, Felix, & Haas, 1977). A peak immune response was associated with a decrease in norepinephrine turnover. Cytokines produced by antigen-activated lymphoid cells altered the turnover of norepinephrine (Besedovsky, del Rey, Prada, Burri, & Honegger, 1983).

It is now understood that alterations in cytokine secretion subsequent to immune activation mediate behavioral effects often associated with illness. For example, interleukin-1 (IL-1), IL-6, and tumor necrosis factor-α (TNF-α) mediate sickness behavior (the fatigue, lethargy, and decreased appetite associated with infectious illness) (Dantzer et al., 1998). Because they are large protein molecules, cytokines do not readily cross the blood-brain barrier. They are believed to signal the brain by entering neural structures that do not possess tight capillary endothelial barriers, such as the organum vasculosum

laminae terminalis and area postrema. In addition, recent evidence indicates that cytokines released in the periphery can activate sensory afferents, such as vagal afferents, and signal central nervous system (CNS) areas involved in immune-related behavioral responses (Watkins, Meier, & Goehler, 1995).

Collectively, this evidence supports the concept of a dynamic neuroendocrine-immune network whereby soluble products of immunologically competent cells affect the CNS following antigenic challenge. It is this conceptualization that led Blalock to liken the immune system to a sensory organ capable of informing the CNS of an antigenic challenge (Blalock & Smith, 1985).

Both psychological and physical stressors are known to activate neuroendocrine pathways that interact with the immune system (Chrousos, 1998). Stressor activation leads to increased secretion of neurosecretory hormones from the hypothalamus, such as corticotropin-releasing hormone (CRH). In turn, these hypothalamic hormones regulate secretion of pituitary hormones, such as adrenocorticotropin hormone (ACTH) and endorphins. Because there are shared hormonal receptors on cells of the immune and neuroendocrine systems, reciprocal interactions between these systems are possible (Reichlin, 1993; Weigent & Blalock, 1999). Neuroendocrine secretory products have immunomodulatory effects and alter leukocyte function (e.g., the immunologic effects of glucocorticoids, endorphins, ACTH, growth hormone, and prolactin). These effects include the regulation of cytokine secretion, antibody synthesis, natural killer cell (NK) activity, and lymphocyte proliferation (Weigent & Blalock, 1999). The complex interactions between the neuroendocrine and immune systems are believed to, in part, downregulate inflammatory responses and limit continuous proliferation of lymphoid cells or excessive production of immune cell products or both (Munck & Guyre, 1986).

Interestingly, neuroendocrine hormones can be produced by leukocytes, the most well studied of which is proopiomelanocorticotropin (POMC). POMC is a precursor molecule for the hormones ACTH and endorphin. Although the role of hormones produced by immune cells is under investigation, it is likely that they function by autocrine/paracrine mechanisms within the local lymphoid microenvironment (Weigent & Blalock, 1999). The finding that immune cells can produce hormones normally secreted from the anterior pituitary emphasizes the close relationship of the immune and endocrine systems. Finally, immune cell secretory products (e.g., cytokines) alter neuroendocrine cell secretion. For instance, cytokines have actions at both the hypothalamic and pituitary levels. Cytokines, such as IL-1, IL-2, IL-6, and TNF, activate the adrenal axis, whereas IL-1 and TNF inhibit the gonadal axis and TNF and interferon-gamma (IFN-γ) suppress the thyroid axis (Weigent & Blalock, 1999).

The bidirectional nature of the neuroendocrine and immune systems likely accounts for the effect of stress on the immune system (Figure 3.1). Regulatory hormones and neuropeptides once believed to be confined to the brain or endocrine system or both are now known to be mutually expressed by all three systems (nervous, endocrine, and immune), and as a result each system may be capable of modulating the function of the other.

In summary, during the past 15 years empirical evidence has emerged that supports the existence of a communication network linking the nervous, endocrine, and immune systems. Psychological stimuli modulate the immune response either through direct activation of neural pathways that terminate in lymphoid tissue or by activation of neuroendocrine circuits leading to the release of molecules that bind to immunologically competent cells. Conversely, the immune system recognizes noncognitive stimuli, such as bacteria, fungi, and viruses, resulting in the secretion of an array of cytokines that act on receptors of the neuroendocrine system. Collectively, cognitive and noncognitive stimuli form a network, which is the basis for behaviorally induced alterations in immune function (Weigent & Blalock, 1999). It is likely that this neuroendocrine-immune network mediates the effect of stress on the development or progression or both of immune-based disease.

➤ STRESS AND IMMUNITY

Stressful life events, and the subsequent emotional and behavioral responses to these events, are commonly believed to alter immunity. When external demands (i.e., stressors) exceed an individual's adaptive capabilities, a stress response ensues (Lazarus & Folkman, 1984). It is the subsequent neurological and endocrinological changes that are believed to produce stress-elicited immune alterations. Studies during the past decade provide convincing evidence that psychological stress can affect the immune system (e.g., lymphocyte proliferation, NK activity, antibody synthesis, and cytokine production). These studies have been accomplished with animal models and in human stress situations, including both experimentally produced stress and naturalistic paradigms for stress evaluation. This chapter focuses on the major human stress paradigms.

Early studies supporting the effects of stress on immunity were conducted by the research team of Glaser and Kiecolt-Glaser. These investigators conducted a series of stress studies in medical students that demonstrated the immunosuppressive effects of in-class examinations (Kiecolt-Glaser, Garner, Speicher, Penn, & Glaser, 1984). The results of these studies indicate that the stress that accompanies examinations leads to a wide range of immunosuppressive effects, including decreased NK cell activity (Glaser, Rice, & Speicher, 1986), lymphocyte proliferation (Glaser et al., 1987), IFN-γ production (Glaser et al., 1986), IL-2 production (Glaser et al., 1990), and latent viral activation as evidenced by increased antibody titer to the virus (Glaser et al., 1992).

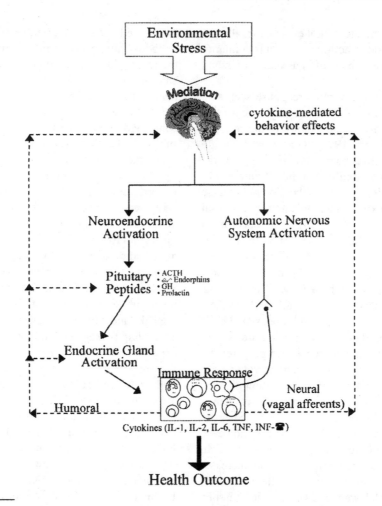

Figure 3.1. Summary and possible interconnections by which environmental stimuli, or stress, can affect the immune response and health outcomes. Perceived environmental stress is mediated by the central nervous system and can lead to neuroendocrine and autonomic nervous system activation. As a result, the immune response can be altered by autonomic nerve fibers that directly synapse with immune cells and by circulating catecholamines released from the adrenal medulla. In addition, further alteration can be produced by secretory products (hormones and neuropeptides) released from the pituitary and endocrine target glands (adrenal cortex, thyroid, ovaries, and testes). In turn, feedback (dashed lines) from immune cell products (cytokines) can modulate endocrine and central nervous system activity by either humoral or neural communication networks.

Furthermore, medical students with lower anxiety levels had faster and stronger immune responses to hepatitis B vaccination than did students with higher levels of anxiety (Glaser et al., 1992; Glaser, Kiecolt-Glaser, Malarkey, & Sheridan, 1998). Recently, examination stress was shown to alter cytokine production that shifts the cytokine pattern away from a Th1 to a Th2 type of response (Maes et al., 1998). This shift is characterized by a decrease in secretion of IFN and an increased secretion of IL-10. The authors suggest that the shift in cytokine production may partially explain the increased incidence of viral infection, latent viral expression, allergic and asthmatic reactions, and autoimmunity reported during times of high stress (Marshall et al., 1998).

The type of immune response seen as a result of stress is dependent on the acute versus chronic or repeated nature of the stressful event (McEwen, 1998). For example, acute stressors, such as parachute jumping, are correlated with a mobilization in the numbers of NK cells; this is likely attributable to a change in cell trafficking related to adrenergic arousal (Schedlowski et al., 1993) or glucocorticoid secretion (McEwen, 1998) or both. Studies such as these suggest that acute stress produces a redistribution of lymphocytes and macrophages in the body. These cells marginate on blood vessel walls and compartmentalize in the skin, lymph nodes, and bone marrow. It is theorized that acute stress activates the immune response and prepares the organism for potential encounters with an immunologic challenge. This activation may exacerbate autoimmune or allergic responses (Dhabhar, Miller, McEwen, & Spencer, 1996). Repeated or chronic stress, however, suppresses immune responsiveness, particularly cell-mediated immunity, and increases susceptibility to infectious challenge and tumor cells (McEwen, 1998). Chronic stressors, such as bereavement, caregiving, marital conflict, and divorce, impair the ability of NK cells to be lytic and to respond to cytokines (IFN-γ or IL-2) *in vitro* (Esterling, Kiecolt-Glaser, & Glaser, 1996; Herbert & Cohen, 1993; Kiecolt-Glaser, Dura, Speicher, Trask, & Glaser, 1991; Kiecolt-Glaser, Glaser, Cacioppo, & Malarkey, 1998). Other aspects of cellular immunity are also affected by chronic stress (Herbert & Cohen, 1993), including decreased lymphoproliferation, NK cell activity, numbers of circulating lymphocytes, as well as salivary and serum immunoglobulin levels.

The impact of chronic stress has been poignantly illustrated by assessing the immune response of individuals caring for relatives with Alzheimer's disease. Kiecolt-Glaser et al. (1987) found that such caregiving was accompanied by greater distress and heightened levels of herpes virus-specific antibody (suggesting viral reactivation). Furthermore, elderly individuals experiencing the chronic stress of caring for a spouse with Alzheimer's disease had attenuated responses to the influenza vaccine and more physician-confirmed respiratory infections than control subjects. Health behaviors did not differ between the two groups.

Conversely, Irwin et al. (1991) reported no differences in NK cell activity between caregivers and control subjects. Esterling et al. (1996), however, found that both caregivers and former caregivers (those whose relative had died at least 2 years previously) had blunted NK cell activity compared to nonstressed control subjects. Interestingly, the results of this study suggested that the psychological and immunological aftermath of caregiving persists beyond the actual stressful experience. In an attempt to reverse the immunosuppressive effects of stress in the elderly, these investigators enrolled subjects in a 1-month stress-reduction program that used progressive muscle relaxation. This form of stress reduction produced a 30% increase in NK cell activity (Kiecolt-Glaser et al., 1985).

The type and magnitude of stress-elicited effects on the immune system are influenced by many factors. Such factors may relate to the stressor, such as the type, intensity, and duration of the stressful stimulus. The sampling time frame between the stressor and the immune response can also influence whether an effect can be measured. Furthermore, not all components of the immune system may respond to a stressor. Therefore, it is important that the immune parameter to be measured be carefully chosen within the context of the population or illness studied or both. A variety of host or subject factors will also influence the immune response to stress, such as age, preexisting illness, nutritional status, substance abuse, exercise habits, adequacy of sleep, coping, and social support (Kiecolt-Glaser & Glaser, 1988; Zeller, McCain, McCann, Swanson, & Colletti, 1996).

The primary criticism of many stress-immune studies is that although the immune change observed is often statistically significant, the magnitude of the change is small and often within normal limits. Whether or not such a change in immune function is significant to health outcomes remains to be determined. There are studies, however, that have found that stress-induced immune changes can increase susceptibility to infectious disease and may also influence the course of disease (Cohen, Tyrel, & Smith, 1991; Spiegel, Bloom, Kraemer, & Gottheil, 1989). Such studies support the contention that even small changes in immune function may have health-related significance.

> ## STRESS-IMMUNITY AND HEALTH OUTCOMES

One fundamental question that remains unanswered in the field of psychoneuroimmunology is whether or not stress-induced alteration in immune function plays a role in disease development or disease progression or both. Numerous studies, although inconclusive, have shown stress to influence the course or progression of illness or disease (e.g., cancer, infectious disease, and HIV). Few studies, however, provide definitive evidence that links stress, immunity, and health outcomes. This area remains a challenge for researchers in psychoneuroimmunology.

One of a handful of well-controlled studies that examined the effect of psychological stress on susceptibility to illness was conducted by Cohen et al. (1991). They investigated the relationship between stress and the common cold using a viral challenge paradigm. Following extensive health and psychological assessment (for the previous 12 months), 394 volunteers were randomized to receive either a low infectious dose of a respiratory virus or saline. For 2 days prior to viral challenge and 7 days postchallenge, volunteers were quarantined. Rhinovirus infection was based on the development of clinical symptoms of a cold, the development of virus-specific antibodies, and the culture and isolation of the inoculated virus. The results revealed that psychological stress predicted susceptibility to colds among the initially healthy people exposed to the respiratory virus. Psychological stress was operationalized as an index of the number of negative life events, the perceived impact of these negative life events, perceived stress, and negative affect. In a related study, Cohen et al. analyzed the relationship of an individual's social contacts to the development of the common cold. In 276 volunteers exposed to rhinovirus, a greater resistance to upper respiratory infection was exhibited in subjects who had the greatest diversity of social contacts (friends, family, and community). Interestingly, greater resistance to infection was related to increased numbers of social contacts and not to the absolute number of individuals involved in the social contacts (Cohen, Doyle, Skoner, Rabin, & Gwaltney, 1997). Recently, these investigators reported that acute stressful life events (less than 1 month in duration) were not associated with the onset of colds. Severe chronic stressors (1 month or longer in duration), however, were associated with the risk of cold development. The most prevalent chronic stressors for this study group were under- or unemployment or enduring interpersonal difficulties with family or friends (Cohen et al., 1998).

> ## STRESS AND WOUND HEALING

Studies of the effects of stress on wound healing and tissue repair have suggested that stress-induced neuroendocrine activation impairs healing and delays recovery. Both animal and human models of wound healing have been used to examine the effects of stress. In one study (Padgett, Marucha, & Sheridan, 1998), the effects of restraint stress on the healing of a sterile punch wound in rats were studied. Rats were subjected to restraint stress for 3 days prior to and for 5 days after wounding. Wound healing was measured using photography and image analysis. Compared to control rats, which were wounded but not restrained, healing was delayed an average of 3 days in the restraint stressed group. Treatment of the restraint stressed group with a glucocorticoid receptor antagonist produced healing rates that were similar to those of control animals. These results demonstrate that restraint stress delayed wound healing. Because the glucocorticoid antagonist reversed this effect, the delay was likely due to a stress-induced increase in glucocorticoids. Padgett et al. (1998) hypothesized that the stress-induced elevation in glucocorticoids prevented the early part of wound healing in which macrophages move into the area to remove cellular debris and secrete growth factors, cytokines, and chemotactic factors needed for tissue repair. Glucocorticoids are well-known to suppress the inflammatory response, including the production of IL-1, IL-6, and TNF-α (Bendrups, Hilton, Meager, & Hamilton, 1993). The results of this study provide compelling evidence, albeit in an animal model, that disruption of neuroendocrine homeostasis by a stressor modulates wound healing.

The ability of stress to delay wound healing has also been shown in human stress paradigms. Kiecolt-Glaser, Marucha, Malarkey, Mercado, and Glaser (1995) studied the effects of chronic stress on caregivers (spouses) for patients suffering from Alzheimer's disease. Punch biopsy wounds were applied to caregivers and age-matched control subjects. The results indicated that wound healing was markedly delayed in the caregivers compared to control subjects. These differences were not related to other covariates, such as nutrition, sleep, or the presence of other illnesses. In another study, wound healing was delayed by the more acute and benign stress of academic examinations. Two punch biopsy wounds were placed on the hard palate of dental students during summer vacation and then on the contralateral side 3 days prior to the first major exam of the term. Mucosal wound healing took 3 days longer to complete during the exam period. The production of mRNA for IL-1β was also reduced during the stress of examination (Marucha, Kiecolt-Glaser, & Favagehi, 1998).

In summary, the previously discussed studies provide compelling evidence suggesting that stress can impair tissue repair and wound healing. This can have significant implications for recovery from injury and surgery, especially in vulnerable populations, such as individuals with diabetes, impaired tissue perfusion, and advanced age. Delayed healing of wounds increases the risk for wound complication by infectious pathogens, which can further prolong recovery and length of hospital stay. Nurses are in a pivotal position to recognize and reduce stress and to teach stress management skills. This has the potential to promote both healing and recovery and enhance health outcomes.

➤ STRESS-IMMUNITY AND CANCER

The immune system is believed to play a role in surveillance against malignantly transformed cells. It has been hypothesized that stress-induced suppression of immune cell activity (e.g., NK cell activity) may alter the clinical course of cancer. The relationship between NK cell activity and cancer is complex (Rosenberg & Lotze, 1986). NK cells, however, are also important in the control of viral infections (Trinchieri, 1989; Whiteside & Herberman, 1989). As such, NK cells may prevent the development of infectious complications in cancer patients who are often immunosuppressed.

There are a few highly intriguing studies that have examined the relationship between stress and immunity in cancer patients. Levy et al. (1990) found that estrogen receptor status predicted NK cell activity in 66 women with Stage I or II breast cancer 3 months after surgery with or without adjuvant therapy. These researchers also showed that social support contributed significantly to a regression model predicting higher NK cell activity. That is, the greater an individual's social support, the higher the individual's NK cell activity.

Andersen et al. (1998) studied stress-immune parameters in 116 women who were diagnosed with invasive breast cancer (Stages II and III). Women were enrolled within 4 months of their breast surgery but prior to adjuvant therapy initiation. Stress was measured using the Impact of Event Scale, which is a self-report measure of intrusive and avoidance thoughts and behaviors (Horowitz, Wilner, & William, 1979). Using hierarchical multiple regression analysis, their results revealed that higher stress levels significantly predicted lower NK cell activity, diminished NK cell response to IFN-γ, and decreased lymphocyte proliferation (Andersen et al., 1998). It is noteworthy that this study controlled for extraneous variables that might also affect immunity, including age, stage of disease, nutritional status, and days since surgery. The results are intriguing and suggest that stress may play a pivotal role in women with cancer, possibly resulting in more susceptibility to cancer progression or infectious complications or both.

Researchers have begun to address the definitive question as to whether psychosocial interventions can produce health effects that slow cancer progression and promote survival (Fawzy, Fawzy, Arndt, & Pasnau, 1995; Greer & Brady, 1988; Speigel, 1996). Randomized prospective trials have shown protective effects of psychosocial interventions on cancer progression (Spiegel, Sephton, Terr, & Stites, 1998). Fawzy et al. (1993) studied the effects of a behavioral intervention in patients with malignant melanoma. Subjects were randomized to an intervention consisting of six 90-minute sessions including health education, stress management, coping skills, and group discussion. Six months later, the intervention group showed reduced psychological distress and enhanced immune function (increased IFN-α and augmented NK cell activity) compared to the nonintervention group. Although no association between survival and NK cell activity was found, individuals with higher baseline NK cell activity had a decreased incidence of disease recurrence.

In another study, the effects of a home visit and educational intervention program for lymphoma and leukemia patients were investigated (Richardson, Shelton, Krailo, & Levine, 1990). The results showed that patients in the intervention group were more compliant with their medical treatment. More important, when controlling for this difference, members of the intervention group lived significantly longer than members of the control group.

A landmark study that assessed the effect of behavioral intervention on cancer survival was conducted by David Spiegel and colleagues (1989). They reported compelling results suggesting that an intervention, characterized as supportive-expressive group therapy, increased the survival of women with advanced breast cancer. Fifty of 86 women with advanced breast cancer were randomly assigned to support groups. The groups were designed to build strong supportive bonds, encourage "emotional expressiveness" about cancer, confront fears of dying and death, reorder life's priorities, improve relationships with family and friends, enhance communication with and development of shared problem solving with physicians, and teach self-hypnosis for pain control (Spiegel et al., 1998). The women were followed for 10 years, and a significant 18-month increase in survival for women in the intervention group was observed. Further analysis of the results of this study, in which medical records were reviewed, showed no difference in therapeutic treatment that could account for the differences in survival. Rather, a correlation was found between group support and survival. Spiegel's research team is currently replicating this study with a larger group in which endocrine markers of stress and cellular immune response, including NK cell activity, are being measured in addition to survival. It is hypothesized that psychosocial support will buffer the immunological consequences of cancer-associated stress and thereby improve disease outcomes (Spiegel et al., 1998).

In addition to the ongoing study of Spiegel, Andersen and colleagues (1998) are conducting a prospective, randomized study evaluating the effectiveness of stress-reduction interventions on psychological, immunological, and survival outcomes in women with advanced breast cancer. The structured intervention includes several stress-reduction strategies, such as progressive muscle relaxation, social and emotional interventions designed to increase the quality of life, and healthy living habits. The intervention is provided weekly for the first 4 months and monthly for an additional 8 months. Psychological and immunological variables are being measured, with survival being the ultimate end point of this ongoing longitudinal study (McNeil, 1998; Voelker, 1997).

The role of psychological stress in cancer progression or response to treatment or both remains controversial, as was expressed in an editorial by Cohen and Rabin (1998). They contend that it is not clear if the effects of behavioral interventions are due to an individual's greater adherence to a healthy lifestyle or to the behavioral intervention therapy or both. The results of behavioral-based intervention studies are highly provocative and difficult to ignore, however. Indeed, the results of the ongoing clinical trials will provide further data that will aid in the understanding of the importance of stress, its impact on the immune system, and cancer control.

➤ STRESS-IMMUNITY AND HIV

Individuals living with HIV face numerous stressors, such as family discord, change in occupation, economic hardship, social isolation, and bereavement (McCain & Zeller, 1996; Robinson, Mathews, & Witek-Janusek, 2000). Because the immune system plays a dominant role in the prevention of viral infections and in the suppression of latent viral infections, stress-induced changes in immune function may alter disease progression. Evidence suggests that stress-induced modulation of immunity may alter the course of HIV infection (McCain & Zeller, 1996; Robinson et al., 2000). Psychological variables are hypothesized to mediate host resistance to the HIV virus by modifying behavioral practices and by promoting an optimal neuroendocrine and immune milieu. Overall, most of these

studies are fraught with methodological difficulties, such as small and nonhomogeneous samples, lack of control for treatment and disease stage variables, inability to document or measure the presence of psychosocial stress in the sample, and lack of sensitive and relevant indices of immune measures. Nevertheless, the results are intriguing.

Goodkin, Fuchs, Feaster, Leeka, and Rishel (1992) studied stress-immune correlates in asymptomatic HIV-positive males. Although the sample size was small, the results suggested that men with a lower ability to cope with stress had lower total lymphocyte counts, whereas men with higher coping abilities had greater numbers of CD4+ T lymphocytes. A series of stress-immune studies have originated from the University of Miami's Center for the Biopsychosocial Study of AIDS; some of these studies have evaluated the psychoimmune effects of the stress of HIV antibody testing (i.e., test notification stress). This research team reported a significant relationship between increased anxiety (State Trait Anxiety Index [STAI]) at the time of notification of test results and decreased NK cell activity. No association with lymphocyte proliferation was found (Ironson et al., 1990).

In a similar study, during a 5-week period before and after HIV testing, seropositive subjects reported higher anxiety (STAI), higher depression, increased intrusive thoughts, and lower lymphocyte proliferation rates than seronegative subjects. Although plasma cortisol levels declined significantly in the seropositive group during the study period, they were within normal limits (Antoni et al., 1991). McCain and Cella (1995) found a significant relationship between high stress and lower CD4+ cell numbers in their study of a heterogeneous group (heterosexuals, minorities, injecting drug users, and those with various stages of disease progression) of 53 men with HIV disease. These same investigators examined the effect of a stress management intervention in HIV-positive individuals. Although a reduction in stress was demonstrated, they failed to show any significant accompanying change in immune function (McCain, Zeller, Cella, Urbanski, & Novak, 1996). In another intervention study, however, Esterling and colleagues (1992) measured antibody titers to Epstein-Barr virus (EBV) as the immune end point. Both HIV-positive and HIV-negative men in the 10-week program had significant decreases in anti-EBV viral encapsulated antigen when compared to their matched controls (Esterling et al., 1992). Because of the intriguing nature of these intervention studies, similar lines of research will likely be pursued in the future.

Although there is no clear mechanism for how stress influences HIV disease progression, Clerici and colleagues (1994) proposed an "immunoendocrinological" hypothesis implicating the potential role of elevated cortisol in the progression of HIV disease through modulatory effects on viral replication, cytokine modulation, and increased induction of apoptosis. Supportive evidence for this theory has been provided by reports that cortisol enhances HIV viral infections when added to cell culture medium containing human lymphocytes (Markham, Salahuddin, Veren, Orndorff, & Gallo, 1986) and HIV viral replication when added to monocyte cultures (Swanson, Zeller, & Spear, 1998). Norepinephrine, a major catecholamine released during stress, also accelerates HIV replication (Cole, Korin, Fahe, & Zack, 1998).

It is likely that studies examining psychoneuroimmune parameters in HIV disease are limited by the immune outcome variables measured. It is possible that psychological effects may not have a measurable impact on indices of HIV disease development or progression or both. More important, stress may play an important role in the HIV-infected person's susceptibility to opportunistic infection. Consequently, there is a need to design and implement studies aimed at determining the role of psychological stress on immune system indices designed to measure defense mechanisms important in host defense against opportunistic infection (Robinson et al., 2000). The nature of the stress-immune relationship in HIV disease needs to be carefully evaluated within the context of currently used antiretroviral therapy and within the context of future therapeutic approaches. Such therapies may not only alter immune responsiveness in those with HIV but also influence the type of stress they encounter as they live with HIV.

➤ STRESS-IMMUNITY AND INFECTION

Vulnerable populations, such as cancer patients and persons with HIV, face a multitude of stressors. These stressors can influence the immune system and increase susceptibility to infectious diseases. Psychological stress seems to alter the susceptibility of individuals to infectious agents and influences the onset, course, and outcome of the pathology associated with infection (Biondi & Zannino, 1997). Moreover, infectious disease can be a stressor. The human body's response to infection and to immunological challenge resembles both physical and psychological stress (Dunn, Powell, Meitin, & Small, 1989).

Infection can activate the hypothalamic-pituitary-adrenal axis (HPA) axis and increase the synaptic release of norepinephrine and serotonin in the brain (Dunn, 1993). Thus, by physiological criteria, infection can be regarded as stressful. The activation of the HPA axis associated with immune responses has been interpreted as a signal to the brain indicating the presence of an infectious threat from the external environment, triggering a stress response (Blalock & Smith, 1985). Once an effective immune response has been initiated, the HPA axis is thought to negatively regulate the immune system by the release of glucocorticoids that limit the inflammatory response and prevent overreactivity and autoimmune phenomena (Besedovsky, del Rey, Sorkin, & Dinarello, 1986; Munck & Guyre, 1986). Thus, the effects of stress on the immune system and the effects of the immune system on the neurologic response to infection are a complex and interrelated series of physiologic events with many reciprocal interactions. Many specific infectious states appear to have a clear association with stress.

Tuberculosis

Stress has long been associated with the pathogenesis of tuberculosis. With the recent resurgence of tuberculosis, understanding the potential role of stress in susceptibility to and progression of this infectious disease has become even more important. In previous studies, high rates of tuberculosis have been reported among socially isolated individuals and in schoolchildren and their teachers during periods of emotional stress, such as during war (Guyre, Girard, Morganelli, & Manganiello, 1988; Ishigami, 1919). These studies showed a reduced capacity of the infected individuals to phagocytize the infectious agent and suggested that stressful situations might serve as cofactors in the development of tuberculosis. Until recently, very little evidence existed to support this suggestion. Work using experimental animals has shown that HPA axis activation, induced by restraint stress, increased the growth of the tubercle bacillus (Zwilling et al., 1990). Adrenalectomy and treatment with the glucocorticoid receptor antagonist RU486 abrogated this effect. Furthermore, HPA axis activation suppressed phagocyte function and decreased the capacity of the animals to produce immune augmenting cytokines in response to the mycobacteria (Brown, Sheridan, Pearl, & Zwilling, 1993).

The effects of stress in experimental animals may have important implications in human disease. In an extensive study, tubercular patients were shown to have a dramatic increase in the number of stressful life events approximately 2 years prior to their hospitalization (Homes, Hawkins, Bowerman, Clarke, & Joffe, 1957). Likewise, mortality due to tuberculosis has been shown to be higher in subjects who have experienced divorce (Somers, 1979). It is possible that the reactivation of tuberculosis may be a consequence of suscepti-

ble populations being affected by stressors. Stress, mediated by neuroendocrine-immune interactions, may significantly contribute to this infectious disease, which continues to be a serious health hazard worldwide.

Viral Infections

Colds and influenza have been useful models to evaluate the role of psychoneuroimmunology in human disease. As discussed previously, Cohen et al. (1991) evaluated the significance of psychosocial factors on the common cold. Subjects were inoculated with respiratory viruses, and the risk of developing the infectious disease was directly associated with chronic stress. This study and many others showed similar effects of stress on the development of colds and influenza but no direct effect of stress on the immune system of the more susceptible individuals (Clover, Abell, Becker, Crawford, & Ramsey, 1989).

Many other studies have evaluated the effects of stress on latent viral infections caused by herpes simplex virus, EBV, and HIV. These viruses are typically latent in humans, and the hypothesis that stress favors viral reactivation has been evaluated. These studies have shown that exposure to acute psychological stressors (e.g., examinations and spousal discord) and chronic psychological stressors (e.g., nuclear disaster and caregiving) is associated with high antibody titers to these viruses. These viruses are thought to be controlled by normal host cell-mediated immune response. When stress reduces the cell-mediated immune response, the virus replicates and stimulates an antibody response that is typically nonprotective (Kiecolt-Glaser et al., 1991). In the case of genital herpes, Kemeny, Cohen, Zegans, and Conant (1989) showed that a negative mood state was correlated with a decrease in CD8+ lymphocytes (the principal effector against herpesvirus) and herpetic lesion recurrence. Likewise, psychological stress has been shown to predispose an individual to the onset of infectious mononucleosis (Glaser et al., 1991). This work remains controversial, however, and the role of psychoneuroimmunology in latent viral infections, viral reactivation, and immune stimulation requires further investigation.

Fungal Infections

Although the association between emotional stress and infectious mycological disease has been long suspected, only recently has considerable attention been paid to this association. Fungal infections are well-known to be associated with the stressful conditions of pregnancy, surgical trauma, cancer, organ transplants, long-term antibiotic use, corticosteroid therapy, diabetes mellitus, critical illness, and prematurity (Reszel, Mishra, Mishra, & Pierson, 1993; Shareef, Myers, Nagabhushan, Mathews, & Witek-Janusek, 1998; Witek-Janusek, Cusack, & Mathews, 1998).

Stress hormones such as cortisol and adrenaline are known to enhance pathogenesis of experimental fungal disease (Odds, 1988). For example, *Candida albicans* and related fungi are endogenous opportunists, and infections with these fungi are typically associated with debilitating or predisposing conditions or both. *Candida* infections are the first symptom of active AIDS to appear in HIV-positive individuals. One factor shared by AIDS patients and the other susceptible individuals described previously is hormonal imbalance resulting from HPA axis activation. Furthermore, emotionally affected women who perceive their situation to be stressful have a higher incidence of vaginal *Candida* infections (Reszel et al., 1993). Candidiasis also appears frequently in people undergoing surgery, a unique form of stress that involves emotional stressors (anxiety), chemical stressors (anesthesia), and physical stressors (surgery) (Mishra et al., 1994). Similarly, the emotional stress of divorce has been positively correlated with increased incidence of the carriage of *Candida* (Reszel et al., 1993). Such associations of stress and fungal infection in vulnerable populations are only beginning to be understood.

➤ STRESS-IMMUNITY AND NURSING SCIENCE

The holistic view of human nature ascribed to by the discipline of nursing is harmonious with the philosophical underpinnings of psychoneuroimmunology (McCain & Smith, 1994; Zeller, McCain, & Swanson, 1996). As a result, nurse researchers have used a psychoneuroimmunological framework in their research and have made significant contributions to the scientific growth of this field. Nurse investigators have examined stress-immune interactions in a variety of immune-based illnesses, including asthma, HIV, and cancer. In addition, nurse scientists have documented the immunosuppressive nature of postoperative pain and the effects of stress on wound healing. A psychoneurouimmunologic framework has also been used to understand the immunologic implications of child birth and postpartal stress on maternal-infant well-being. Some of these studies are addressed in the following discussion.

Asthmatic symptoms can often be initiated and potentiated by stressful life events. Kang et al. studied the effect of examination stress in asthmatic and nonasthmatic adolescents. Their results revealed that examination stress produces significant alterations in circulating immune cell subsets and in both proliferative and cytolytic activities. No differences were found between the asthmatic and nonasthmatic adolescents, however. Both healthy and asthmatic adolescents reported similar levels of stress and similar changes in immune cell numbers and function (Kang, Coe, Karaszewski, & McCarthy, 1998; Kang, Coe, & McCarthy, 1996). The lack of a relationship between asthma status and social support was believed to be due to the stability and well-managed nature of this asthmatic population (Kang, Coe, McCarthy, & Ershler, 1997). In a similar study, examination stress in adolescent asthmatics produced a bias toward a Th2-like pattern of cytokine production compared to that of nonasthmatic adolescents (Kang, Coe, McCarthy, et al., 1997). These studies are suggestive and need to be replicated in asthmatics with less stable disease and in naturalistic situations of more intense or chronic stress or both.

The laboratory of Gayle Page conducted a series of compelling experiments in rodents that showed that untreated postoperative pain led to impaired NK cell activity and enhanced tumor metastases (Ben-Eliyahu, Page, Yirmiya, & Shakhar, 1999; Page & Ben-Eliyahu, 1997; Page, Ben-Eliyahu, & Liebeskind, 1994; Page, Ben-Eliyahu, Yirmiya, & Liebeskind, 1993). In her model, rats were subjected to laparotomy and injected with NK cell-sensitive radiolabeled tumor cells that metastasized to the lung. Rats that were treated with morphine, and that exhibited signs of pain relief, had significantly less radiolabeled tumor in the lung, fewer metastatic lesions on the lung, and higher postoperative NK cell activity (Page et al., 1993, 1994). These results suggest that untreated postoperative pain leads to impaired immune function (e.g., reduced NK cell activity) and potentially increased organ localization of tumor emboli. In addition, this research group has demonstrated that the degree of postoperative pain immunosuppression is related to the estrus stage of the rat, suggesting that reproductive hormones may affect the stress-immune response to surgical stress (Ben-Eliyahu, Page, Shakhar, & Taylor, 1996). As a whole, the studies of Page and colleagues indicate that the treatment of pain is necessary not only to alleviate suffering but also to prevent pain-induced immunosuppression and possible tumor metastatic spread. Although these observations have been made in animal models, others have shown in humans that surgery for tumor resection leads to a postoperative reduction in NK cell activity compared to preoperative levels (Pollack, Lotzova, & Stanford, 1992). Evidence that healing and recovery from surgery are potentially altered by stress has also been provided by Wysocki (1996), who found that noise stress delayed wound healing in an animal model. Also, McCarthy, Ouimet, and Daun (1991) have provided evidence that noise stress alters lymphoid cell function needed for tissue repair. The previously discussed results support the supposition that an individual's psychological state can influence surgical recovery by altering various aspects of immunity (Kiecolt-Glaser, Page, Marucha, MacCullum, & Glaser, 1998).

Immunity and HIV Progression

Living with HIV is replete with multiple stressors, and nurse scientists have contributed to the supposition that the stress-endocrine-immune axis is implicated in HIV disease progression (McCain & Cella, 1995; McCain & Gramling, 1992; Robinson, Matthews, & Witek-Janusek, 1999a; Robinson et al., 1999b). Stress-induced neuroendocrine activation leads to elevations in plasma cortisol. *In vitro,* physiological concentrations of cortisol increase HIV replication in monocyte-derived macrophages, suggesting a potential role for stress hormones in HIV disease activation and progression (Swanson et al., 1998). The effectiveness of stress-reducing interventions in HIV disease has been evaluated by McCain et al. In a pretest-posttest design, the effect of a 6-week stress management program in HIV disease was evaluated (McCain et al., 1996). Outcome measures at 6 weeks and 6 months included perceived stress, quality of life, psychological distress, illness-related uncertainty, and CD4+ T lymphocyte levels. Although the program improved measures of emotional well-being, no significant changes in CD4+ lymphocyte levels were detected. It is likely that CD4+ lymphocyte number may not be a sensitive indicator of improvement in immune function, and other types of immunological assessment may yield more positive results.

In an ongoing intervention study, Robinson and colleagues are examining the efficacy of an 8-week, mindfulness meditation-based stress-reduction program on psychoimmune variables in HIV-positive individuals. These investigators are measuring NK cell activity, which is an important host defense mechanism against viral infections, and opportunistic microbial infections, which cause significant morbidity and mortality in HIV-positive patients. Preliminary data from the study suggest a positive effect of this program on psychological well-being and immune status (Robinson et al., 1999a). Undoubtedly, nurse investigators will continue to explore the role of stress in HIV disease management and progression.

Stress-induced immunosuppression may have special relevance to the nursing care of cancer patients who undergo immunosuppressive therapies. The emotional stress of undergoing breast biopsy for cancer diagnosis has been clearly demonstrated and presents a useful human paradigm to study psychologic stress (Hooper, Mathews, & Witek-Janusek, 1997; Witek-Janusek & Mathews, 1999b). Anticipation of breast cancer diagnosis has been shown to alter immune cell subsets (Fillion, Lemyre, Mandeville, & Piche, 1996) and TH1 and TH2 cytokine production (Witek-Janusek & Mathews, 1999b). The effect of stress on gene transcription factors has been investigated in women undergoing diagnostic breast biopsy. Gene transcription factors play a significant role in the immune response and can regulate the production of cytokines (Wulczyn, Krappmann, & Scheidereit, 1996). In the diagnostic breast biopsy paradigm, nuclear localization in lymphocytes of two transcription factors, NF-kapB and AP-1, was decreased in women experiencing significant emotional stress, whereas when stress was relieved (post-biopsy) the nuclear localization of these gene transcription factors was similar to those of age-matched control women (Nagabhushan, Mathews, & Witek-Janusek, 2000). If and how these factors relate to the modification of immune function and to cancer outcome remain to be determined, but such studies will move this field to a molecular understanding of the effects of stress.

Nurse researchers have used a psycho-neuroimmunologic approach toward understanding the impact of childbirth and postpartal stress on maternal child health. Maureen Groer and her research team at the University of Tennessee College of Nursing have demonstrated that childbirth stress leads to a reduction in maternal secretory immuno-globulin A (sIgA). This reduction was most pronounced in women who reported an increased state of anxiety. Women with very low or undetectable levels of sIgA had a greater incidence of postpartal complications, and their infants had more illnesses. These results indicate that the stress of childbirth can have profound effects on maternal immune function, which can alter the clinical course of mothers and that of their infants (Annie & Groer, 1991). Interestingly, Groer, Mozingo, et al. (1994) demonstrated that touch, provided by a 10-minute slow-stroke effleurage back rub, was shown to increase sIgA levels in elderly adults. It remains to be determined if such an intervention may blunt the decrease in sIgA observed during parturition. Other nurse investigators have demonstrated that gluco-corticoid hormones can profoundly influence the pattern of cytokine production (i.e., colony-stimulating factors) from neonatal mononuclear cells obtained from umbilical cord blood. Such immunomodulation may alter the newborn's ability to resist infectious pathogens (Witek-Janusek & Mathews, 1999b).

The unique psychologic and immuno-logic relationship between a breast-feeding mother and her infant is an intriguing paradigm in which to evaluate the stress-immune relationship. Stress-induced alterations in maternal immunity in breast-feeding mothers could potentially alter their capability to provide optimal levels of immunoglobulins for their infants. Postpartal mothers of preterm infants report high levels of mood disturbance compared to the general population. Mothers who score higher on negative mood subscales of the Profile of Mood States produce less milk sIgA than those who report lower negative mood states. Conversely, mothers who report higher vigor and anger produce greater amounts of milk sIgA (Groer, Droppleman, & Mozingo, 1999). Interestingly, an inverse relationship between cortisol levels and sIgA in breast milk has been reported, such that the higher milk cortisol was associated with lower milk sIgA. It is plausible that increased maternal stress leads to elevated plasma and milk cortisol. Higher levels of milk cortisol may impair milk immune cell production of immunoglobulins or other immune cell functions or both (Groer, Humenick, & Hill, 1994; Groer et al., 1999). Such stress-induced alterations in milk endocrine and immune composition may potentially impact the immunologic benefits that infants receive from breast milk and certainly require additional investigation. This is especially relevant to premature and low-birth-weight infants, who are at high risk for infectious illness.

➤ FUTURE DIRECTIONS AND NURSING IMPLICATIONS

The guiding premise of psychoneuroimmunology is that stress-induced impairment of immune function influences disease progression or response to therapy or both. These types of investigations are directed toward an understanding of the effect of the psychoendocrine stress response on the immune system, particularly within the context of cancer, autoimmune disease, infectious disease, and maternal child health. Nurses must recognize the potential effectiveness of biobehavioral approaches to the care of patients with immune-based disease. Such approaches to stress management may not only improve the quality of life and emotional well-being of targeted populations but also halt disease progression or complications from opportunistic infection or both.

Complementary and alternative therapies integrate preventive and curative therapies that consider the whole person and are used to "complement" traditional approaches to illness. The use of complementary and alternative therapies by American health care consumers has markedly increased; rigorous scientific testing of such practices has lagged behind, however (Eisenberg et al., 1998; Fontanarosa & Lundberg, 1998). Increased use of massage, touch, meditation, acupuncture, yoga, botanical herbs, guided imagery, and behavioral-based stress reduction programs has spurred a renewed interest in understanding the scientific basis for such approaches toward healing and health maintenance. This integrative biobehavioral, mind-body, therapeutic approach is harmonious with the view of psychoneuroimmunology and that of nursing science.

As discussed previously, the links among one's emotional state, neuroendocrine activity, and immune response are well described. Future emphasis needs to be placed on understanding the mechanism(s) of stress-induced immune dysregulation and the relationship between stress-induced immune dysregulation and health outcome. That is, do stress-induced changes in immunity alter health, and can stress-reducing interventions that strengthen immunity halt disease progression and improve health? These are critical questions that require intensive empirical investigations using human paradigms of stress. Such approaches will lead to a better understanding of disease and to better diagnosis, treatment, or both of stress-induced immune dysfunction. The results will provide the scientific foundation that will lead to the identification of individuals "at risk" for psychological distress and altered immune reactivity. Such identification will permit the development of psychologically based interventions designed to reduce stress, promote immunocompetence, and hence improve health. Such interventions may prove to be cost-effective additions to traditional forms of treatment or therapy or both and hold promise for disease control. Ultimately, this will serve to enhance the quality and the quantity of life.

➤ REFERENCES

Ader, R. (1980). Presidential address: Psychosomatic and psychoimmunologic research. *Psychosomatic Medicine, 42,* 307-321.

Ader, R., & Cohen, N. (1993). Psychoneuroimmunology: Conditioning and stress. *Annual Review of Psychology, 44,* 53-85.

Andersen, B. L., Farrar, W. B., Golden-Kreutz, D., Kutz, L. A., MacCallum, R., Courtney, M. E., & Glaser, R. (1998). Stress and immune responses after surgical treatment for regional breast cancer. *Journal of the National Cancer Institute, 90,* 30-36.

Annie, C. L., & Groer, M. W. (1991). Childbirth stress: An immunologic study. *Journal of Obstetrics and Gynecological Neonatal Nursing, 20,* 391-397.

Antoni, M. H., Schneiderman, N., Klimas, N., LaPerriere, A., Ironson, G., & Fletcher, M. A. (1991). Disparities in psychological, neuro-endocrine, and immunological patterns in asymptomatic HIV-1 seropositive and seronegative gay men. *Biological Psychiatry, 29,* 1023-1041.

Bendrups, A., Hilton, A., Meager, A., & Hamilton, J. A. (1993). Reduction of tumor necrosis factor alpha and interleukin-1-beta levels in human synovial tissue by interleukin-4 and glucocorticoids. *Rheumatology International, 12,* 217-220.

Ben-Eliyahu, S., Page, G. G., Shakhar, G., & Taylor, A. N. (1996). Increased susceptibility to metastasis during pro-oestrus in rats: Possible role of estradiol and natural killer cells. *British Journal of Cancer, 74,* 1900-1907.

Ben-Eliyahu, S., Page, G. G., Yirmiya, R., & Shakhar, G. (1999). Evidence that stress and surgical interventions promote tumor development by suppressing natural killer cell activity. *International Journal of Cancer, 80,* 880-888.

Besedovsky, H., del Rey, A., Prada, M. D., Burri, R., & Honegger, C. (1983). The immune response evokes changes in brain noradrenergic neurons. *Science, 221,* 564-565.

Besedovsky, H., Felix, D., & Haas, H. (1977). Hpothalamic changes during the immune response. *European Journal of Immunology, 7,* 323-325.

Besedovsky, H. O., del Rey, A., Sorkin, E., & Dinarello, C. A. (1986). Immunoregulatory feedback between interleukin-1 and glucocorticoid hormones. *Science, 233,* 652-654.

Biondi, M., & Zannino, L. G. (1997). Psychological stress, neuroimmunomodulation, and susceptibility to infectious diseases in animals and man: A review. *Psychotherapy Psychosomatics, 66,* 3-26.

Blalock, J. E., & Smith, E. M. (1985). A complete regulatory loop between the immune and neuroendocrine systems. *Federation Proceedings, 44,* 108-111.

Bovbjerg, D. H., Redd, W. H., Maier, L. A., Holland, J. C., Lesko, L. M., Niedzwiecki, D., Rubin, S. C., & Hakes, T. B. (1990). Anticipatory immune suppression and nausea in women receiving cyclic chemotherapy for ovarian cancer. *Journal of Consulting Clinical Psychology, 58,* 153-157.

Brown, D. H., Sheridan, J. F., Pearl, D., & Zwilling, B. S. (1993). Regulation of mycobacterial growth by the hypothalamus-pituitary-adrenal axis: Differential responses of mycobacterium bovis BCG-resistant and -susceptible mice. *Infection and Immunity, 61,* 4793-4800.

Chrousos, G. P. (1998). Stressors, stress, and neuro-endocrine integration of the adaptive response. *Annals of the New York Academy of Science, 851,* 311-335.

Clerici, M., Bevilacqua, M., Vago, T., Villa, M. L., Shearer, G., & Norbinato, G. (1994). An immunoendocrinological hypothesis of HIV infection. *Lancet, 343,* 1552-1553.

Clover, R. D., Abell, T., Becker, L. A., Crawford, S., & Ramsey, J. C. N. (1989). Family functioning and stress as predictors of influenza B infection. *Journal of Family Practice, 28,* 535-539.

Cohen, S., Doyle, W. J., Skoner, D. P., Rabin, B., & Gwaltney, J. M. (1997). Social ties and susceptibility to the common cold. *Journal of the American Medical Association, 277,* 1940-1944.

Cohen, S., Frank, E., Doyle, W. J., Skoner, D. P., & Rabin, B. (1998). Types of stressors that increase susceptibility to the common cold in healthy adults. *Health Psychology, 17,* 214-223.

Cohen, S., & Rabin, B. (1998). Psychologic stress, immunity, and cancer. *Journal of the National Cancer Institute, 90,* 3-4.

Cohen, S., Tyrel, D. A. J., & Smith, A. P. (1991). Psychological stress and susceptibility to the common cold. *New England Journal of Medicine, 325,* 606-612.

Cole, S., Korin, Y., Fahe, J., & Zack, J. (1998). Norepinephrine accelerates HIV replication via protein kinase-A-dependent effects of cytokine production. *Journal of Immunology, 161,* 610-616.

Dantzer, R., Bluthe, R. M., Laye, S., Bret-Dibat, J., Parnet, P., & Kelley, K. (1998). Cytokines and sickness behavior. *Annals of the New York Academy of Science, 840,* 586-683.

Dhabhar, F. S., Miller, A. H., McEwen, B. S., & Spencer, R. L. (1996). Stress-induced changes in blood leukocyte distribution: Role of adrenal steroid hormones. *Journal of Immunology, 157,* 1638-1644.

Dunn, A. J. (1993). Role of cytokines in infection-induced stress. *Annals of the New York Academy of Science, 697,* 189-197.

Dunn, A. J., Powell, M. L., Meitin, C., & Small, P. A. (1989). Virus infection as a stressor: Influenza virus elevates plasma concentrations of corticosterone, and brain concentrations of MHPG and tryptophan. *Physiology of Behavior, 45,* 591-594.

Eisenberg, D. M., Davis, R. B., Ettner, L., Appel, S., Wilkey, S., Van Rompay, M., & Kessler, R. C. (1998). Trends in alternative medicine use in the United States, 1990-1997: Results of a follow-up national survey. *Journal of the American Medical Association, 280,* 1569-1575.

Esterling, B. A., Antoni, M. H., Schneiderman, N., LaPerriere, A., Ironson, G., Klimas, N. G., & Fletcher, M. A. (1992). Psychological modulation of antibody to Epstein-Barr viral capsid antigen and human herpes virus type 6 in HIV-1 infected and at-risk gay men. *Psychosomatic Medicine, 54,* 354-371.

Esterling, B. A., Kiecolt-Glaser, J. K., & Glaser, R. (1996). Psychosocial modulation of cytokine-induced natural killer cell activity in older adults. *Psychosomatic Medicine, 58,* 264-272.

Fawzy, F. I., Fawzy, N. W., Arndt, L., & Pasnau, R. O. (1995). Critical review of psychosocial interventions in cancer care. *Archives of General Psychiatry, 52,* 100-113.

Fawzy, F. I., Fawzy, N. W., Hyun, C. S., Elashoff, R., Guthrie, R., Fahey, J. L., & Morton, D. L. (1993). Malignant melanoma: Effects of an early structured psychiatric intervention, coping, and affective state on recurrence and survival six years later. *Archives of General Psychiatry, 50,* 681-689.

Felten, D., Felten, S., Carlson, S., Olschowka, J., & Livnat, S. (1985). Noradrenergic and peptidergic innervation of lymphoid tissue. *Journal of Immunology, 135*(Suppl. 2), 755S-765S.

Felten, D. L., Felten, S. Y., Bellinger, D. L., Carlson, S. L., Ackerman, K. D., Madden, K. S., Olschowka, J. A., & Livnat, S. (1987). Noradrenergic sympathetic neural interactions with the immune system: Structure and function. *Immunological Reviews, 100,* 225-260.

Fillion, L., Lemyre, L., Mandeville, R., & Piche, R. (1996). Cognitive appraisal, stress state, and cellular immunity responses before and after diagnosis of breast tumor. *International Journal of Rehabilitation Health, 2,* 169-187.

Fontanarosa, P. B., & Lundberg, G. D. (1998). Alternative medicine meets science. *Journal of the American Medical Association, 280,* 1618-1619.

Fredrikson, M., Furst, C. J., Lekander, M., Rothstein, S., & Blomgren, H. (1993). Trait anxiety and anticipatory immune reactions in women receiving adjuvant chemotherapy for breast cancer. *Brain, Behavior, & Immunity, 7,* 79-90.

Glaser, R., Kennedy, S., Lafuse, W. P., Bonneau, R. H., Speicher, C., Hillhouse, J., & Kiecolt-Glaser, J. (1990). Psychological stress-induced modulation of interleukin 2 receptor gene expression and interleukin 2 production in peripheral blood leukocytes. *Archives of General Psychiatry, 47,* 707-712.

Glaser, R., Kiecolt-Glaser, J. K., Bonneau, R. H., Malarkey, W., Kennedy, S., & Hughes, J. (1992). Stress-induced modulation of the immune response to recombinant hepatitis B vaccine. *Psychosomatic Medicine, 54,* 22-29.

Glaser, R., Kiecolt-Glaser, J. K., Malarkey, W. B., & Sheridan, J. F. (1998). The influence of psychological stress on the immune response to vaccines. *Annals of the New York Academy of Sciences, 840,* 649-655.

Glaser, R., Pearson, G. R., Jones, J. F., Hillhouse, J., Kennedy, S., Mao, H., & Kiecolt-Glaser, J. K. (1991). Stress related activation of Epstein Barr virus. *Brain, Behavior, & Immunity, 5,* 219-232.

Glaser, R., Rice, J., Sheridan, J., Fertel, R., Stout, J., Speicher, C. E., Pinksy, D., Kotur, M., Post, A., Beck, M., & Kiecolt-Glaser, J. K. (1987). Stress-related immune suppression: Health implications. *Brain, Behavior, & Immunity, 1,* 7-20.

Glaser, R., Rice, J., & Speicher, C. E. (1986). Stress depresses interferon production by leukocytes concomitant with a decrease in natural killer cell activity. *Behavioral Neuroscience, 100,* 675-678.

Goodkin, K., Fuchs, I., Feaster, D., Leeka, J., & Rishel, D. D. (1992). Life stressors and coping style are associated with immune measures in HIV-1 infection—A preliminary report. *International Journal of Psychiatry and Medicine, 22,* 155-172.

Greer, S., & Brady, M. (1988). Natural killer cells: One possible link between cancer and the mind. *Stress Medicine, 4,* 105-111.

Groer, M. W., Droppleman, P. G., & Mozingo, J. (1999). Behavioral states and milk immunology in preterm mothers. *Journal of Applied Biobehavioral Research, 4,* 13-26.

Groer, M. W., Humenick, S., & Hill, P. D. (1994). Characterizations and psychoneuroimmunologic implications of secretory immunoglobulin A and cortisol in preterm and term breast milk. *Journal of Perinatal Nursing, 7,* 42-51.

Groer, M. W., Mozingo, J., Droppleman, P., Davis, M., Jolly, M. L., Boynton, M., Davis, K., & Kay, S. (1994). Measures of salivary secretory immunoglobulin A and state anxiety after a nursing back rub. *Applied Nursing Research, 7,* 2-6.

Guyre, P. M., Girard, M. T., Morganelli, P. M., & Manganiello, P. D. (1988). Glucocorticoid effects on the production and actions of immune cytokines. *Journal of Steroid Biochemistry, 30,* 89-93.

Herbert, T., & Cohen, S. (1993). Stress and immunity in humans: A meta-analytic review. *Psychosomatic Medicine, 55,* 364-379.

Homes, T. H., Hawkins, N. G., Bowerman, C. E., Clarke, E. R., & Joffe, J. R. (1957). Psychosocial and physiological studies of tuberculosis. *Psychosomatic Medicine, 19,* 134-143.

Hooper, P. J., Mathews, H. L., & Witek-Janusek, L. (1997, April). *Stress-immune interactions pre and post breast biopsy.* Paper presented at the Proceedings of the Midwest Nursing Research Society, Detroit, MI.

Horowitz, M., Wilner, N., & William, A. (1979). Impact of event scale: A measure of subjective stress. *Psychosomatic Medicine, 41,* 209-218.

Ironson, G., LaPerriere, A., Antoni, M. H., O'Hearn, P., Schneiderman, N., Klimas, N., & Fletcher, M. A. (1990). Changes in immune and psychological measures as a function of anticipation of and reaction to news of HIV-1 antibody status. *Psychosomatic Medicine, 52,* 247-270.

Irwin, M., Brown, M., Patterson, T., Hauger, R., Mascovich, A., & Grant, I. (1991). Neuropeptide Y and natural killer cell activity: Findings in depression and Alzheimer caregiver stress. *FASEB Journal, 5,* 3100-3107.

Ishigami, T. (1919). The influence of psychic acts on the progress of pulmonary tuberculosis. *American Review of Tuberculosis, 2,* 470-475.

Kang, D. H., Coe, C. L., Karaszewski, J., & McCarthy, D. O. (1998). Relationship of social support to stress responses and immune function in healthy and asthmatic adolescents. *Research in Nursing Health, 21,* 117-128.

Kang, D. H., Coe, C. L., & McCarthy, D. O. (1996). Academic examinations significantly impact immune responses, but not lung function, in healthy and well-managed asthmatic adolescents. *Brain, Behavior, & Immunity, 10,* 164-181.

Kang, D. H., Coe, C. L., McCarthy, D. O., & Ershler, W. B. (1997). Immune responses to final exams in healthy and asthmatic adolescents. *Nursing Research, 46,* 12-19.

Kang, D. H., Coe, C. L., McCarthy, D. O., Jarjour, N. N., Kelly, E. A., Rodriguez, R. R., & Busse, W. W. (1997). Cytokine profiles of stimulated blood lymphocytes in asthmatic and healthy adolescents across the school year. *Journal of Interferon and Cytokine Research, 17,* 481-487.

Kemeny, M. E., Cohen, F., Zegans, L. A., & Conant, M. A. (1989). Psychological and immunological predictors of genital herpes recurrence. *Psychosomatic Medicine, 51,* 195-208.

Kiecolt-Glaser, J. K., Dura, J. R., Speicher, C. E., Trask, O. J., & Glaser, R. (1991). Spousal caregivers of demintia victims: Longitudinal changes in immunity and health. *Psychosomatic Medicine, 53,* 345-362.

Kiecolt-Glaser, J. K., Garner, W., Speicher, E., Penn, G., & Glaser, R. (1984). Psychosocial modifiers of immunocompetence in medical students. *Psychosomatic Medicine, 46,* 7-14.

Kiecolt-Glaser, J. K., & Glaser, R. (1988). Methodological issues in behavioral immunology research with humans. *Brain, Behavior, & Immunity, 2,* 67-78.

Kiecolt-Glaser, J. K., & Glaser, R. (1992). Psychoneuroimmunology: Can psychological interventions modulate immunity? *Journal of Consulting Clinical Psychology, 40,* 569-575.

Kiecolt-Glaser, J. K., Glaser, R., Cacioppo, J. T., & Malarkey, W. B. (1998). Martial stress: Immunologic, neuroendocrine, and autonomic correlates. *Annals of the New York Academy of Sciences, 840,* 656-663.

Kiecolt-Glaser, J. K., Glaser, R., Dyer, C., Shuttleworth, E., Ogrocki, P., & Speicher, C. E. (1987). Chronic stress and immunity in family caregivers for Alzheimer's disease victims. *Psychosomatic Medicine, 49,* 523-535.

Kiecolt-Glaser, J. K., Glaser, R., Wiliger, D., Stout, J., Messick, G., Sheppard, S., Richer, D., Romisher, D., Briner, W., & Bonnel, W. (1985). Psychosocial enhancement of immunocompetence in a geriatric population. *Health Psychology, 4,* 25-41.

Kiecolt-Glaser, J. K., Marucha, P. T., Malarkey, W. B., Mercado, A. M., & Glaser, R. (1995). Slowing of wound healing by psychological stress. *Lancet, 346,* 1194-1196.

Kiecolt-Glaser, J. K., Page, G. G., Marucha, P. T., MacCallum, R. C., & Glaser, R. (1998). Psychological influences on surgical recovery. Perspectives from psychoneuroimmunology. *Annals of Psychology, 53,* 1209-1218.

La Via, M. F., & Workman, E. A. (1998). Stress-induced immunodepression in humans. In J. Hubbard & E. Workman (Eds.), *Handbook of stress medicine: An organ system approach* (pp. 153-164). Boca Raton, FL: CRC Press.

Lazarus, R. S., & Folkman, S. (1984). *Stress, appraisal and coping.* New York: Springer.

Levy, S. M., Herberman, R. B., Lee, J., Whiteside, T., Kirkwood, J., & McFeeley, S. (1990). Estrogen receptor concentration and social factors as predictors of natural killer cell activity in early-stage breast cancer patients. *Natural Immune Cell Growth Regulation, 9,* 313-324.

Maes, M., Song, C., Lin, A., De Jongh, R., Van Gastel, A., Kenis, G., Bosmans, E., De Meester, I., Benoy, I., Neels, H., Demedts, P., Janca, A., Scharpe, S., & Smith, R. S. (1998). The effects of psychological stress on humans: Increased production of pro-inflammatory cytokines and a Th1-like response in stress-induced anxiety. *Cytokine, 10,* 313-318.

Markham, P. D., Salahuddin, S. Z., & Veren, K., Orndorff, S., & Gallo, R. C. (1986). Hydrocortisone and some other hormones enhance the expression of HTLV-III. *International Journal of Cancer, 37,* 67-72.

Marshall, G. D., Agarwal, S. K., Lloyd, C., Cohen, L., Henninger, M., & Morris, G. J. (1998). Cytokine dysregulation associated with exam stress in healthy medical students. *Brain, Behavior, & Immunity, 12,* 297-307.

Marucha, P. T., Kiecolt-Glaser, J. K., & Favagehi, M. (1998). Mucosal wound healing is impaired by examination stress. *Psychosomatic Medicine, 60,* 362-365.

McCain, N. L., & Cella, D. F. (1995). Correlates of stress in HIV disease. *Western Journal of Nursing Research, 17,* 141-155.

McCain, N. L., & Gramling, L. F. (1992). Living with dying: Coping with HIV disease. *Issues in Mental Health Nursing, 13,* 271-284.

McCain, N. L., & Smith, J. C. (1994). Stress and coping in the context of psychoneuroimmunology: A holistic framework for nursing practice and research. *Archives of Psychiatric Nursing, 8,* 221-227.

McCain, N. L., & Zeller, J. M. (1996). Psychoneuroimmunological studies in HIV disease. *Annual Review of Nursing Research, 14,* 23-55.

McCain, N. L., Zeller, J. M., Cella, D. F., Urbanski, P. A., & Novak, R. M. (1996). The influence of stress management training in HIV disease. *Nursing Research, 45,* 246-253.

McCarthy, D. O., Ouimet, M. E., & Daun, J. M. (1991). Shades of Florence Nightingale: Potential impact of noise stress on wound healing. *Holistic Nursing Practice, 5,* 39-48.

McEwen, B. S. (1998). Protective and damaging effects of stress mediators. *New England Journal of Medicine, 338,* 171-179.

McNeil, C. (1998). Stress reduction: Three trials test its impact on breast cancer progression. *Journal of the National Cancer Institute, 90,* 12-14.

Mishra, S. K., Segal, E., Gunter, E., Kurup, V. P., Mishra, J., Murali, P. S., Pierson, D. L., Sandovsky-Losica, H., & Stevens, D. A. (1994). Stress, immunity and mycotic diseases. *Journal of Medical and Veterinary Mycology, 32,* 379-406.

Munck, A., & Guyre, P. (1986). Glucocorticoid physiology, pharmacology and stress. *Advances in Experimental Medicine and Biology, 196,* 81-96.

Nagabhushan, M., Mathews, H. L., & Witek-Janusek, L. (2000). Aberrant nuclear expression of AP-1 and NfκB in lymphocytes of women stressed by the experience of breast biopsy. *Brain Behavior & Immunity.*

Odds, F. C. (1988). *Candida and candidosis* (2nd ed.). London: Bailliere Tindall.

Padgett, D. A., Marucha, P. T., & Sheridan, J. F. (1998). Restraint stress slows cutaneous wound healing in mice. *Brain, Behavior, & Immunity, 12,* 64-73.

Page, G. G., & Ben-Eliyahu, S. (1997). The immunesuppressive nature of pain. *Seminars in Oncology Nursing, 13,* 10-15.

Page, G. G., Ben-Eliyahu, S., & Liebeskind, J. (1994). The role of LGL/NK cells in surgery-induced promotion of metastasis and its attenuation by morphine. *Brain, Behavior, & Immunity, 8,* 241-250.

Page, G. G., Ben-Eliyahu, S., Yirmiya, R., & Liebeskind, J. (1993). Morphine attenuates surgeryinduced enhancement of metastatic colonization in rats. *Pain, 54,* 21-28.

Pollack, R. E., Lotzova, E., & Stanford, S. D. (1992). Surgical stress impairs natural killer cell programming of tumor for lysis in patients with sarcomas and other solid tumors. *Cancer, 70,* 2192-2202.

Reichlin, S. (1993). Neuroendocrine-immune interactions. *New England Journal of Medicine, 329,* 1246-1253.

Reszel, E. M., Mishra, S. K., Mishra, A., & Pierson, D. L. (1993). Stress, immunity and mucocutaneous candidiasis. *Journal of Osteopathic Medicine, 7,* 26-28.

Richardson, J. L., Shelton, D. R., Krailo, M., & Levine, A. M. (1990). The effect of compliance with treatment on survival among patients with hematologic malignancies. *Journal of Clinical Oncology, 8,* 356-364.

Robinson, F. P., Matthews, H. L., & Witek-Janusek, L. (1999a, November). *Psycho-endocrine-immune responses to a mindfulness-based stress reduction program in HIV infected individuals.* Paper presented at the 11th Annual Conference of the Association of Nurses AIDS Care, San Diego.

Robinson, F. P., Matthews, H. L., & Witek-Janusek, L. (1999b). Stress and HIV disease progression: Psychoneuroimmunological framework. *Journal of the Association of Nurses in AIDS Care, 10,* 21-31.

Robinson, F. P., Matthews, H. L., & Witek-Janusek, L. (2000). Stress reduction and HIV disease: A review of intervention studies utilizing a psychoneuroimmunology framework. *Journal of the Association of Nurses in AIDS Care, 11,* 56-65.

Rosenberg, S. A., & Lotze, M. T. (1986). Cancer immunotherapy using interleukin-2 and interleukin-2-activated lymphocytes. *Annual Review of Immunology, 4,* 681-709.

Schedlowski, M., Jacobs, R., Stratmann, G., Richter, S., Hadicke, A., Tewes, U., Wagner, T. O., & Schmidt, R. E. (1993). Changes of natural killer cells during acute psychological stress. *Journal of Clinical Immunology, 13,* 119-126.

Selye, H. (1936). A syndrome produced by diverse nocuous agents. *Nature, 138,* 132-135.

Selye, H. (1976). *Stress in health and disease.* Reading, MA: Butterworth's.

Shareef, M. J., Myers, T. F., Nagabhushan, M., Mathews, H. L., & Witek-Janusek, L. (1999). Reduced capacity of neonatal lymphocytes to inhibit the growth of *Candida albicans. Biology of the Neonate, 75,* 31-39.

Somers, A. R. (1979). Marital status, health, and use of health services: An old relationship revisited. *Journal of the American Medical Association, 241,* 1818-1822.

Spiegel, D. (1996). Psychological distress and disease course for women with breast cancer: One answer, many questions. *Journal of the National Cancer Institute, 88,* 629-631.

Speigel, D., Bloom, J. R., Kraemer, H. C., & Gottheil, E. (1989). Effects of psychosocial treatment on survival of patients with metastatic breast cancer. *Lancet, 2,* 888-891.

Spiegel, D., Sephton, S. E., Terr, A. I., & Stites, D. P. (1998). Effects of psychosocial treatment in prolonging cancer survival may be mediated by neuroimmune pathways. *Annals of the New York Academy of Science, 840,* 674-683.

Stevens-Felten, S. Y., & Bellinger, D. L. (1997). Noradrenergic and peptidergic innervation of lymphoid organs. *Chemical Immunology, 69,* 99-131.

Swanson, B., Zeller, J. M., & Spear, G. T. (1998). Cortisol upregulates HIV p24 antigen production in cultured human monocyte-derived macrophages. *Journal of the Association of Nurses AIDS Care, 9,* 78-83.

Trinchieri, G. (1989). Biology of natural killer cells. *Advances in Immunology, 47,* 187-376.

Voelker, R. (1997). Study examines stress-immune system links in women with breast cancer. *Journal of the American Medical Association, 278,* 534.

Wang, X., Fiscus, R. R., Yang, L., & Mathews, H. L. (1995). Suppression of the functional activity of IL-2 activated lymphocytes by CGRP. *Cellular Immunology, 162,* 105-113.

Watkins, L. R., Maier, S. F., & Goehler, L. E. (1995). Cytokine-to-brain communication: A review and analysis of alternative mechanisms. *Life Sciences, 57,* 1011-1026.

Weigent, D. A., & Blalock, J. E. (1999). Bidirectional communication between the immune and neuroendocrine systems. In N. Plotnikoff, R. Faith, A. Murgo, & R. Good (Eds.), *Cytokines—Stress and immunity* (pp. 173-186). New York: CRC Press.

Whiteside, T. L., & Herberman, R. B. (1989). The role of natural killer cells in human disease. *Clinical Immunology and Immunopathology, 53,* 1-23.

Witek-Janusek, L., Cusack, C., & Mathews, H. L. (1998). *Candida albicans:* An opportunistic threat to critically ill low birth weight infants. *Dimensions in Critical Care, 17,* 243-255.

Witek-Janusek, L., & Mathews, H. L. (1999). Differential effects of glucocorticoids on colony stimulating factors (CSFs) produced by neonatal mononuclear cells. *Pediatric Research, 46,* 1-6.

Witek-Janusek, L., & Mathews, H. L. (1999b, December). *THI/TH2 cytokine production during the stress of breast cancer diagnosis.* Paper presented at the 7th Annual Conference of the International Cytokine Society Meeting, Hilton Head, SC.

Wulczyn, F. G., Krappmann, D., & Scheidereit, C. (1996). The NF-kappa B/Rel and I kappa B gene families: Mediators of immune response and inflammation. *Journal of Molecular Medicine, 74,* 749-769.

Wysocki, A. B. (1996). The effect of intermittent noise exposure on wound healing. *Advances in Wound Care, 9,* 35-39.

Zeller, J. M., McCain, N. L., McCann, J. J., Swanson, B., & Colletti, M. A. (1996). Methodological issues in psychoneuroimmunology research. *Nursing Research, 45,* 314-318.

Zeller, J. M., McCain, N. L., & Swanson, B. (1996). Psychoneuroimmunology: An emerging framework for nursing research. *Journal of Advanced Nursing, 23,* 657-664.

Zwilling, B. S., Dinkins, M., Christner, R., Faris, M., Griffin, A., Hilburger, M., McPeek, M., & Pearl, D. (1990). Restraint stress induced suppression of major histocompatibility complex class II expression by murine peritoneal macrophages. *Journal of Neuroimmunology, 29,* 125-131.

CHAPTER 4

Physiological Measurement of the Stress Response

Jill M. White and Carol Mattson Porth

Many renowned scholars have attempted to describe and delineate stress. Although Cannon (1939) did not directly define it, he discussed stress as a stimulus that results in increased activity of the sympathetic nervous system as a compensatory process in response to the perception of aversive or threatening situations. This increased sympathetic nervous system activity reflects an effort to regain a sense of homeostasis. Years later, Hans Selye, a world-renowned endocrinologist, popularized stress as a scientific and medical phenomenon. He described stress as the nonspecific response of the body to any demands placed on it (Selye, 1974). This response enables the body to resist stressors by enhancing the function of specific systems in an effort to defend against threats against it. During a stress response, changes from the normal resting state may be manifested in cognitive functioning, emotions, behavior, physiological functioning, or all these. This chapter addresses a variety of methods that can be employed to measure the physiological consequences of the stress response.

A normally functioning stress response system interprets and integrates numerous incoming signals and responds accordingly. These signals may originate from the external environment or the internal milieu. When these signals are interpreted as threatening to the organism, a stress response ensues with resultant activation of the autonomic nervous system, the sympatho-adreno-medullary system, the hypothalamic-pituitary-adrenal-cortical system, the immune system, or all these (Guyton & Hall, 1996; Porth, 1998) (Figure 4.1). The effects are further modulated by various neuropeptides, vagal (parasympathetic) outflow, circadian influences, adaptive strategies, genetic factors, and the presence of disease or defects (Elliot & Morales-Ballejo, 1994).

Three categories of human reaction have been described: (a) effort without distress, (b) effort with distress, and (c) distress without effort (Frankenhaeuser, 1983; Peters et al., 1998). Effort without distress occurs during complex coping attempts with a stressor (Frankenhaeuser, 1983). The sympatho-

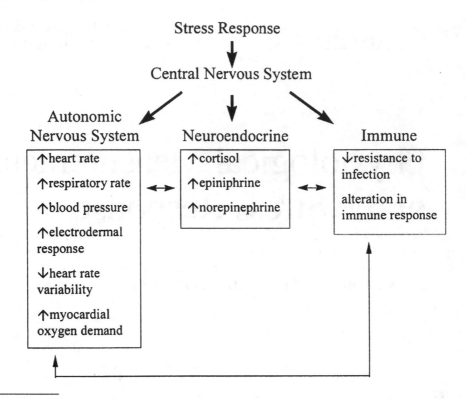

Figure 4.1. Stress Response

adreno-medullary system is activated with increases in heart rate and blood pressure as well as release of epinephrine and norepinephrine (Frankenhaeuser, 1983; Henry, 1992; Peters et al., 1998). In contrast, activation of the hypothalamic-pituitary-adrenal-cortical system is associated with distress without effort. In this situation, the individual's inability to cope, feelings of helplessness, and perceptions of powerlessness (Peters et al., 1998; Weiner, 1992) result in the release of adrenocorticotrophic hormone (ACTH) and cortisol (Weiner, 1992), with associated increases in blood pressure and total peripheral resistance and reductions in heart rate and cardiac output. Situations involving effort with distress would activate both systems simultaneously (Frankenhaeuser, 1983).

Physiologic manifestations of the stress response can be measured by a variety of methods, many of which include the use of bioinstrumentation techniques or biochemical analyses. Bioinstrumentation methods such as electrocardiograph recording equipment or blood pressure monitoring machines are commonly used to measure cardiovascular responses to stress. Many of the biochemical analyses incorporate the use of chromatography, radioimmunoassay, or enzyme-linked immunoabsorbent assay to study neuroendocrine or immune system manifestations of stress. Many of these methods require expensive supplies and equipment. Some methods involve invasive procedures and can introduce additional stress to the experimental situation. The insertion of a needle to draw blood, for example, can introduce an element of both physiological and psychological stress. All techniques require thorough understanding of the procedure and underlying theoretical base of the measure employed.

Although many authors have extolled the high degree of objectivity, reliability, and validity associated with physiological measures

(Polit & Hungler, 1995; Waltz, Strickland, & Lenz, 1991; Woods & Cantanzaro, 1988), measurement error remains a prominent concern. Investigators choosing to use physiological measures of the stress response must attend closely to issues of validity, reliability, selectivity, sensitivity, specificity, cost, and availability.

When physiological measures are employed, reliability is directly related to the precision of the method, consistency of the measurements with repeated sampling, and the reproducibility of the measurements made by the method. Measures of reliability reflect the amount of random error introduced into the measurements (Waltz et al., 1991). Validity reflects the difference between a given value and the true value and whether the measure is carrying out its intended purpose. Closely related to validity are the concepts of selectivity, sensitivity, and specificity. The ability of an instrument to identify signals under study correctly and to distinguish them from all other signals is known as selectivity (Rubin, 1987). Sensitivity can be interpreted two different ways, depending on the type of physiological measurement being used. For example, when bioinstrumentation is used, sensitivity refers to the smallest amount of change in a parameter or variable that can be detected or measured precisely (Cromwell, Weibell, & Pfeiffer, 1980). In a clinical laboratory situation, sensitivity generally is defined as the likelihood that an individual with a given condition will have a positive test result (Waltz et al., 1991). In contrast, specificity refers to the probability that an individual without a specified condition will have a negative test result. The levels of validity, selectivity, sensitivity, and specificity provide information about systematic error introduced by a particular method of measurement. For additional reading with respect to these factors, several authors have provided excellent discussions (Burns & Grove, 1997; Cook & Campbell, 1979; Cromwell et al., 1980; Polit & Hungler, 1995; Rubin, 1987; Waltz et al., 1991; Woods & Cantanzaro, 1988).

➤ AUTONOMIC NERVOUS SYSTEM MEASURES OF THE STRESS RESPONSE

The first physiological axis to become activated during the stress response is the autonomic nervous system. During a stress response, the balance between sympathetic and parasympathetic activity is disrupted, with sympathetic nervous system activity being dominant. Activation of the sympathetic nervous system is oriented toward performance, with little regard to the physiological "costs" of this demand. The primary neurotransmitter that is released is norepinephrine, resulting in increased heart rate, blood pressure, blood glucose levels, pupil dilation, bronchial dilation and respiratory rate, and myocardial oxygen (MVO_2) consumption. At the same time, reductions in heart rate variability, gastric motility, pancreatic activity, and blood flow to the skin, stomach, and kidneys occur.

The primary autonomic nervous system indicators of the stress response used in research are heart rate, respiratory rate, blood pressure, heart rate variability, cardiac output, and electrodermal activity. In addition, rate pressure product has been used as a reliable noninvasive indicator of myocardial oxygen demand. Recently, impedance cardiography has been employed to determine noninvasive estimates of cardiac output and peripheral vascular resistance.

Measurement of Heart Rate

Heart rate refers to the number of ventricular contractions per minute. Measurement of heart rate can be accomplished by use of electrocardiographic equipment that records the electrical events associated with cardiac contraction or through methods that trace the pulse wave that is generated as blood is ejected from the heart with each contraction. Heart rate also can be determined by auscultation with a stethoscope over the chest wall. Accuracy of this method depends on correct detection of heart sounds and time keeping. Another approach to measuring heart rate is palpation of peripheral pulses. Reliability of this method is dependent on perfusion of ventricular contractions to the periphery and on precise identification and counting of pulse waves. In human stress research, heart rate should be regarded as a highly labile state-dependent measure. When using heart rate as an indicator of autonomic nervous system activity in stress research, consideration must be given to the impact of circadian variation, body position, environmental conditions, and medications.

Electrocardiographic Methods

Passive electrocardiogram (ECG) provides a graphic display or recording or both of the time-variant voltages produced by the myocardium during the cardiac cycle. To record ECG data, electrodes are affixed to the body. The electrodes are connected to an ECG machine, telemetry box, or Holter recorder by means of lead wires. When examining the ECG recording, the QRS complex corresponds with ventricular depolarization. In a normally functioning heart, ventricular depolarization results in contraction of the ventricles. Under pathological conditions, QRS complexes may not have a corresponding peripheral pulse wave. Many types of ECG monitoring equipment provide a digital display of heart rate. The computer-generated digitally displayed heart rate, however, is dependent on accurate detection of QRS complexes, and the displayed numbers represent an average heart rate from a given sampling period. A more reliable method involves generating a hard copy of 1 minute of ECG data and having the investigator identify and tabulate the number of ventricular depolarizations recorded during a given time frame. A decision must be made regarding inclusion of ectopic complexes. Placement of electrodes, condition of lead wires, and movement of the individual under study can produce artifact, making interpretation of the ECG complexes more difficult (Schlant & Sonnenblick, 1994).

Pulse Wave Methods

Examination of the pulse wave can be accomplished in a variety of ways: (a) photoplysmography, (b) audiometry, and (c) oscillometry.

Photoelectric plethysmography involves the application of a light source in an opaque chamber that transmits light through a fingertip or other body region to which the transducer is applied. Light is scattered and transmitted through the capillaries of the region and sensed by the photocell, which is shielded from all other light. With each pulse wave, the capillaries are filled with blood and the blood density increases, thereby reducing the amount of light reaching the photocell. Resistance changes are sensed by the photocell and can be measured and recorded. This type of measurement is limited primarily to detecting pulsations in the finger. In addition, the slightest movement of the finger with respect to the photocell or light source results in a severe amount of movement artifact. Moreover, if the light source produces heat, changes in local circulation beneath the light source and photocell may occur (Cromwell et al., 1980).

When audiometric methods are employed, a microphone is positioned over an artery to detect each pulse wave. In contrast, the oscillometric approach to measuring heart rate employs a pressure sensor that detects the distention of the arterial wall as a pulse wave moves through it. The brachial artery is the most frequently used artery for these purposes. These approaches generally are used in conjunction with blood pressure measurements, whereby the artery being sampled is compressed by an inflatable cuff. Compression of the artery produces more accurate sensing of the Korotkoff sounds and arterial distentions (Everly & Sobelman, 1987). These methods introduce the potential for movement artifact. In addition, if the microphone or pressure sensor are not placed directly over the artery, pulse waves may not be detected accurately.

The optimal method for determining heart rate is by means of an ECG recording. This approach provides a hard copy of heart rate and allows for intrarater or interrater reliability checks or both. Because heart rate is a reflection of state-dependent changes, test-retest reliability is not appropriate.

Heart Rate Variability Measurement

In the absence of any neurohumoral influences, normal intrinsic heart rate is approximately 100 to 120 beats per minute (Hainsworth, 1995). With an intact, unblocked autonomic nervous system, heart rate provides a representation of the net effect of parasympathetic nervous system and sympathetic nervous system influences on the sinoatrial (SA) node. During normal resting periods, heart rate is primarily controlled by vagal (parasympathetic) influences (Schlant & Sonnenblick, 1994). As vagal outflow increases, greater cardiac interbeat variability is evident. Conversely, with increased sympathetic nervous system arousal, a reduction in cardiac variability occurs (Fuller, 1992).

Traditionally, it has been suggested that normal sinus rhythm (NSR), with all intervals between successive QRS complexes (R-R intervals) nearly identical in duration, is the optimal cardiac rhythm. Respiratory sinus arrhythmia is an alteration in NSR that reflects the cholinergic influences on waxing and waning of SA node activity that is entrained to the respiratory rate as a result of afferent input from bronchopulmonary receptors (Grossman, vanBeek, & Wientjes, 1990). Today, it is accepted that respiratory sinus arrhythmia is the optimal heart rhythm, and beat-to-beat heart rate should not be completely regular.

Respiratory sinus arrhythmia is a major component of heart rate variability, and it reflects alterations in vagal function (Berntson, Cacioppo, & Quigley, 1993; Grossman et al., 1990; Saul & Cohen, 1994). Heart rate varies in a phase relationship with inspiration and expiration. Vagal cardiometer neurons are inhibited during inspiration and appear to be mildly activated during the expiratory phase of respiration. In contrast, excitation of sympathetic motor neurons occurs during the inspiratory phase, whereas mild inhibition occurs during expiration (Richter & Spyer, 1990; Saul & Cohen, 1994). Therefore, heart rate is increased during inspiration and reduced during expiration. Both voluntary and involuntary alterations in respiratory patterns influence heart rate variability (Hirsch & Bishop, 1981).

Analysis of heart rate variability produces indirect measures of cardiovascular responsiveness to alterations in autonomic nervous system reactivity. Heart rate variability measures provide quantification of modulations in heart periods, or R-R intervals, resulting from cyclical fluctuations in autonomic nervous system control of the SA node. That is, heart rate variability analysis yields information about the variation from one cardiac cycle to the next. Distinct changes in heart rate are expected in response to physiological and mental stressors (Pagani et al., 1995).

To perform heart rate variability analyses, a continuous ECG recording and sophisticated computer software are required. The ECG recording must be examined, and the morphology of each QRS complex must be identified and categorized. Identification is accomplished by computer program, and data are edited by trained personnel. Then, either instantaneous heart rate or intervals between successive sinus QRS complexes are determined. When performing heart rate variability analysis, only sinus complexes are used. In the event that ECG complexes are generated from other areas of the cardiac conduction system, or short sequences of bad or missing data are identified, interpolation techniques generally are employed in heart rate variability determinations. Although other methods of heart rate variability analysis are sometimes used, time and frequency domain measures are employed most frequently.

Time Domain Measures of Heart Rate Variability

Time domain measures of heart rate variability are perhaps the simplest to perform and involve determination of either instantaneous heart rate or interval lengths between successive ECG complexes originating from depolarization of the SA node. Simple time domain measures generally are examined in many ways, including measurements of variance, standard deviations, log units, counts, and percentages.

Most time domain variables can be categorized into two classes—one based on interbeat intervals and the other on comparisons of adjacent cycle lengths (Hatch, Borcherding, & Norris, 1990). Interbeat interval-based measures are broad based and are influenced by both short-term (e.g., respiratory) and long-term (e.g., circadian) factors. Comparisons of adjacent cycle lengths are virtually independent of long-term trends and predominantly reflective of vagal tone (Kleiger et al., 1991). Measures based on interbeat intervals include standard deviation of all normal sinus R-R intervals (SDNN) and the standard deviation of 5-minute mean heart periods during a 24-hour period (SDANN). SDNN is sensitive to both short- and long-term variations, whereas SDANN is insensitive to short-term sources of variation.

The second category of time domain measures is based on the differences between lengths of adjacent cycles. This category includes the pNN50 and rMSSD. The pNN50 is a measure of the proportion of adjacent normal sinus R-R intervals of more than 50 ms. It is computed by examining triplets of normal complexes. Each triplet defines two adjacent coupling intervals. The difference between the two coupling intervals is compared to 50 ms, and a count is maintained. When the analysis has been completed, a proportion is computed and is expressed as a percentage. The rMSSD is the root mean square difference of successive normal sinus R-R intervals. It is determined by examining triplets of normal complexes as well. In this analysis, the difference between the two coupling intervals is squared and summed. Then, the sum is divided by the number of triplets, and the square root is determined. Both pNN50 and rMSSD are most sensitive to vagal influences.

Two other commonly employed time domain measures are the mean of all coupling intervals between normal complexes (mean NN) and the mean standard deviations of normal sinus R-R intervals of successive 5-minute blocks during a 24-hour period (*SD*). The mean NN interval is determined by using only coupling intervals that contain no ectopy or noise. *SD* is less sensitive to posture and activity changes than SDANN but is sensitive to all other vagal influences. Furthermore, SDANN is sensitive to long-term changes, whereas *SD* is insensitive to circadian variations.

Frequency Domain Measures of Heart Rate Variability

Data analysis in the frequency domain is mathematically more complex than in the time domain. Frequency domain measurement, also known as power spectral analysis, provides information about the amount of overall variance in heart rate resulting from periodic oscillations of heart rate at various frequencies (Stein, Bosner, Kleiger, & Conger, 1994). Power spectral analysis breaks down the natural oscillations of heart rate into their component frequencies, and the amplitude or power of each oscillation is plotted over a range of frequencies. From the resultant frequency components, inferences can be drawn regarding the influence of physical activity, baroreceptors, and circadian rhythms (Akselrod et al., 1981; Ebert, 1992; Task Force, 1996).

When power spectral analysis is performed, the power of each contributing component is generally displayed over the frequency range of 0 to 0.5 Hz (Figure 4.2). When displayed in this manner, there are three primary frequencies of heart rate oscillations that contain the majority of the heart rate power: very-low-frequency (VLF), low-frequency (LF), and high-frequency (HF) bands. Power spectral densities can be examined over specified time periods, such as 2-minute, 1-hour, or 24-hour epochs. The VLF oscillations occur at frequencies ranging from 0 to 0.04 Hz. This band is the least understood of the

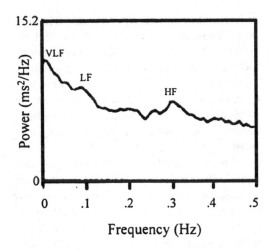

Figure 4.2. Power Spectrum of Instantaneous Heart Rate Fluctuations Featuring Three Main Peaks: Very Low Frequency (0-0.04 Hz), Low Frequency (0.04-0.15 Hz), and High Frequency (0.15-0.40 Hz)

three regions and is believed to reflect thermoregulatory feedback mechanisms (Hyndman, Kitney, & Sayers, 1971), renin-angiotensin activity (Akselrod et al., 1981), and circulating neurohormone levels (Saul, 1990).

The LF component extends over the range of 0.04 to 0.15 Hz. This band reflects both sympathetic and vagal input to the heart (Akselrod et al., 1981; Ebert, 1992; Task Force, 1996). Both chemoreceptors and baroreceptors are involved in generating these oscillations.

The HF band appears to originate from the parasympathetic nervous system exclusively (Akselrod et al., 1981; Appel, Berger, Saul, Smith, & Cohen, 1989; Pagani et al., 1986; Pomeranz et al., 1985). Respiratory sinus arrhythmia is contained within this band. Heart rate oscillations occurring with respiration are believed to be controlled by the medullary respiratory centers, baroreceptors in the large thoracic capacitance vessels, and the Bainbridge reflex (Ebert, 1992).

Power spectral analysis is generally performed by either fast Fourier transform (FFT)

(nonparametric) or autoregressive (AR) (parametric) spectral models. When both methods have been employed on the same data set, correlations of the integral of the power spectral density between AR and FFT techniques within LF and HF bands ranged from $r = .97$ to $r = .99$, when 4-minute, 1-hour, and 24-hour segments were analyzed (Cowan, Kogan, Burr, Hendershot, & Buchanan, 1990). Therefore, both methods appear to provide comparable results.

Spectral density of the HF component of heart rate variability provides a reliable estimate of parasympathetic nervous system influence on the SA node. As parasympathetic nervous system influences dominate, HF heart rate variability increases. Sympathetic nervous system activity is more difficult to display and quantify (Akselrod, 1995). Some have suggested that the ratio of power of LF:HF heart rate variability may provide a measure of sympathovagal balance (Malliani, Pagani, Lombardi, & Cerutti, 1991). It may be a valid estimate in a variety of physiological situations, particularly when the purpose of evaluation is to determine changes in sympathovagal balance under various conditions (Akselrod, 1995).

Although heart rate variability measures may provide valuable insights into autonomic outflow, many extraneous variables or conditions may impact the reliability of these measures. The magnitude of heart rate variability decreases with age (Hrushesky, Fader, Schmitt, & Gilbertsen, 1984; O'Brien, O'Hare, & Corrall, 1985; Schwartz, Gibb, & Tran, 1991). In addition, changes in body position can have a profound effect on short-term measures of heart rate variability (Malliani et al., 1991; Vybiral, Bryg, Maddens, & Boden, 1989). As with other cardiovascular measures, consideration must be given to the possible impact medications might have on measures of heart rate variability, particularly bet-adrenergic blocking agents. In addition, these measures are generally performed only on individuals whose underlying cardiac rhythm is sinus in origin. When more than 10% of the ECG data in any segment are not sinus complexes, or are un-readable, the segment should be discarded from the analysis. Heart rate variability mea-sures have been used as indicators of psycho-logical and physiological stress in many stud-ies (Cowan et al., 1990; DeBenedittis, Cigada, Bianchi, Signorini, & Cerutti, 1994; Hatch et al., 1990; Sakakibara, Takeuchik, & Hayano, 1994; White, 1999).

Blood Pressure Measurement

Blood pressure is a product of cardiac output and tone of the peripheral resistance vessels in the arterial system. Both heart rate, a determinant of cardiac output, and periph-eral vascular resistance are regulated by the autonomic nervous system; as a result, they are strongly influenced by both physiological and psychological stressors. During periods of acute stress, the systolic blood pressure changes more rapidly than diastolic blood pressure. For example, changes in systolic blood pressure can be observed within 1 or 2 minutes of the cold-pressor stress test in which the hand is immersed in cold water (Porth, 1976; Tassorelli, Micieli, Osipova, Rossi, & Nappi, 1995). Thus, methods that can detect rapid changes in blood pressure are often needed to demonstrate the effect of acute stress. The effects of chronic stress on blood pressure are less obvious, presumably because there is an adaptation of blood pres-sure control mechanisms.

Blood pressure can be measured directly using an arterial catheter and a pressure trans-ducer or indirectly using a blood pressure cuff and a method for detecting the arterial pres-sure wave as it travels through the arterial sys-tem (Andrew & Scott, 1985; Gorny, 1993; O'Brien, Fitzgerald, & O'Malley, 1985). Di-rect and indirect methods of blood pressure monitoring measure different phenomenon. Direct monitoring methods use the arterial pressure wave to determine the blood pres-sure. Because these methods require insertion of an arterial catheter, they are seldom used in stress studies. Indirect methods, which are noninvasive, determine blood pressure by vol-ume displacement or by flow detection. Noninvasive blood pressure measurement methods include the auscultatory method, oscillometric method, Doppler technique, and the finger blood pressure cuff. A modification of the auscultatory method uses a microphone to detect the auscultatory sounds during cuff inflation and deflation.

The accuracy of blood pressure measure-ments obtained by the different methods of measurement are subject to user-related and instrumentation-related errors that correspond to the technique and measurement assump-tions of each type of instrumentation. Non-invasive blood pressure equipment should meet the standards of the Advancement of Medical Instrumentation or the British Hyper-tension Society (Pickering, 1995). Most noninvasive blood pressure machines that are purchased by patients for home blood pres-sure monitoring are not adequate for use in re-search studies.

The Auscultatory Method
of Blood Pressure Measurement

The auscultatory method relies on arterial occlusion by an inflated cuff and, as the cuff is deflated, detection of the auscultatory sounds by means of a stethoscope. Accurate measure-ment of blood pressure requires that the cuff be deflated at a rate of 2 mm/second. Investi-gators are referred to the American Heart As-sociation or British Hypertension Society guidelines for blood pressure measurement (Working Party, 1997). This method generally limits the frequency with which blood pres-sure measurements can be obtained every 2 or 3 minutes and may be inadequate for studies that require beat-by-beat measurements of blood pressure. The use of proper cuff size as determined by the arm circumference of the subject is essential for accurate measurements (Banner & Gavenstein, 1991). Because this method requires listening to auscultatory sounds, data collectors need to be trained in the skills of blood pressure monitoring, and observer accuracy must be established if more than one investigator is involved in data collection (O'Brien, Mee, Tan, Atkins, & O'Malley, 1991). The mercury sphygmomanometer is usually considered more accurate than the anaeroid manometer. If an anaeroid manometer is used, frequent calibration checks are required.

The Oscillometric Method of Blood Pressure Measurement

The oscillometric method employs a cuff that compresses the limb and underlying vasculature and measures blood pressure by sensing arterial pulsations as a function of cuff pressure. This is the method used with many of the automatic noninvasive blood pressure machines. Cuff deflation usually is determined by heart rate. The oscillometric devices have the advantage of serial measurement capabilities through automatic cycling without investigator intervention. As with the auscultatory method, accuracy of measurement depends on use of proper cuff size and instrument calibration.

Doppler Techniques of Blood Pressure Measurement

Doppler techniques require placement of a sensor over an artery distal to an inflatable cuff or between the cuff and the limb. The sensor consists of a transmitter that projects ultrasound waves into the limb and a transducer that picks up the reflected ultrasound from the various soft tissue interfaces. The sound transmitted from the blood moving through the artery is converted to an audible sound from which the listener can determine maximum cuff pressure for blood flow distal to the cuff. As with other noninvasive blood pressure methods, the accuracy of blood pressure measurements is dependent on proper cuff size. Systolic measurements are more accurate than diastolic.

Finger Arterial Measurement of Blood Pressure

The finger arterial blood pressure monitoring method (Finapres, Datex Ohmeda) facilitates continuous finger arterial pressure waveform (Imholz, Wieling, van Montfrans, & Wessling, 1998). The equipment is easy to use and provides a method for continuous measurement of blood pressure changes. Although there are conflicting reports regarding their utility in the clinical setting in which treatment options are determined by blood pressure measurements (Jagomagi, Talts, Raamat, & Lansimes, 1996; Latman, 1992; Lyew & Jamieson, 1994; Nesselroad, Flacco, Phillips, & Kruse, 1996; Ristuccia, Grossman, Watkins, & Lown, 1997), they provide a noninvasive method for tracking momentary blood pressure changes in stress studies (Imholz et al., 1988).

Rate Pressure Product

When a stress response is elicited, there is a concomitant increased release of epinephrine and norepinephrine. Increased circulating levels of epinephrine and norepinephrine result in increases in heart rate, peripheral vascular resistance, and force of myocardial contraction. These protective mechanism are initiated to meet the increased demands of the body, but they are accompanied by an increase in the myocardial oxygen demand of the heart (MVO_2 demand).

Rate pressure product (RPP) is a reliable noninvasive indicator of myocardial oxygen demand (Amersterdam, Hughes, DeMaria, Zelis, & Mason, 1974; Gobel, Nordstrom, Nelson, Jorgenson, & Wang, 1978). It is calculated by multiplying heart rate by systolic blood pressure. Gobel et al. (1978) reported a correlation of $r = .83$ when calculated RPPs were compared to direct measures of myocardial oxygen demand. Measures of RPP are only as reliable as the measures of heart rate and systolic blood pressure obtained to calculate this value. RPP has been used as a noninvasive measure of myocardial oxygen demand in response to physiologic and psychological stressors in numerous studies (Bairey Merz et al., 1998; Belkic, Emdad, & Theorell, 1998; Hattori et al., 1998; Jain et al., 1998; Kavanagh, Matosevic, Thacker, Belliard, & Shephard, 1998; Villella, Villella, Barlera, Franzosi, & Maggioni, 1999; White, 1999).

Cardiac Output Measurements

Impedance cardiography provides a noninvasive method for obtaining data related to cardiac function (Jensen, Yakimets, & Teo, 1995; Woltjer, Bogaard, & deVries, 1997). This method uses the electrical impedance or resistance changes that occur as a low-voltage (2.5-4.0 mA), high-frequency (70-100 kHz), alternating electrical current is passed through the thorax using spot or band electrodes. The electrical impedance changes are detected by sensing electrodes. Pulsatile blood flow through the thoracic aorta causes shifts in the thoracic impedance as a function of changes in blood volume. There is a decrease in electrical impedance as the blood volume in the aorta increases; as blood volume decreases, electrical impedance increases.

The impedance cardiac output method was originally developed by Kubicek and colleagues (Kubicek, Karnegis, Patterson, Witssoe, & Mattson, 1966). Assumptions of the impedance cardiograph include that the thorax acts as a cylinder that is homogeneously perfused with blood of specific resistivity (p) in ohms, which can vary with hematocrit. The thorax is thought to have a steady-state base impedance (Z_0) between the electrodes (ohms) with pulsatile variations in aortic blood flow and electrical impedance (ΔZ), which is further expressed as its first derivative (dZ/dt). This derivative has been shown to be proportional to the stroke volume (SV) of the heart. When the heart rate is known, cardiac output can be derived. According to Kubicek et al. (1996), stroke vol-

ume can be determined using the following equation:

$$SV = \frac{p \bullet L^2 \bullet (dZ/dt)\max \bullet LVET}{Z_0^2},$$

where L^2 is the length between the sensing electrodes (cm), and $LVET$ (seconds) is the left ventricular ejection time. The LVET is determined from an ECG tracing. Heart sounds are often used to confirm the markings for LVET.

Computerized methods of impedance cardiograph monitoring have been developed that provide a means for continuous measurement of stoke volume and cardiac output during research of the stress response. Measurement of blood pressure permits determination of changes in peripheral vascular resistance. Impedance cardiography has been used to study the cardiovascular responses to both physical and emotional stress (Probst, Bulbulian, & Knapp, 1997).

Respiratory Rate Measurement

Respiratory rate is controlled by brain stem sensors that monitor blood oxygen and carbon dioxide levels. The pattern of breathing can also be altered by emotional responses to conditions such as fear and anxiety by other parts of the brain, including the limbic system and hypothalamus.

Respiratory rate can be measured by means of impedance pneumography, visual inspection, or auscultation with a stethoscope over the chest wall. An impedance pneumograph senses changes in resistance across the chest that are caused by the act of breathing. Reliability of this measure is dependent on accurate placement of the electrodes. Visual inspection of the act of breathing is more accurate when both the chest and abdomen can be viewed directly. Combining visual inspection with chest auscultation may provide a better alternative to either visual inspection or auscultation alone. Some impedance pneumographs are capable of providing a hard copy of respirations, but the expense of this equipment makes visual inspection and auscultation a viable option for consideration.

Electrodermal Activity Measurement

The notion that changes in electrical activity of the skin can be produced by a variety of physical and emotional stimuli was first reported by Charles Fere in 1888 (Woodworth & Schlosberg, 1954). He passed a small current between two electrodes on the surface of the skin and noted changes in electrodermal activity when individuals were presented with various stimuli.

From a psychophysiological perspective, electrodermal activity refers to the bioelectrical attributes of the skin or the neurons directly associated with the skin. The skin is supplied by two types of sweat glands: the eccrine and apocrine sweat glands. The eccrine sweat glands are particularly abundant on palms of the hands, the soles of the feet, and the forehead. Eccrine gland secretion, which is a hypotonic electrolyte solution, functions in regulation of body temperature. In contrast, the apocrine sweat glands secrete more fatty acids and proteins, empty into hair follicles, and are more abundant in the axillary and anogenital areas. The eccrine sweat glands located in the soles of the feet and the palms of the hands are believed to respond to psychological stimulation rather than to temperature changes (Everly & Sobelman, 1987). The sympathetic fibers innervating these glands are adrenergic in nature (Guyton & Hall, 1996), making skin conductance (SC) and skin potential (SP) indices of sympathetic nervous system activity. A delay time between the time stimulation occurs and the actual response of electrodermal activity has been estimated to range from 1.5 to 2.5 seconds (Edelberg, 1972). The activity of sympathetic neurons innervating the sweat glands and the moisture produced by eccrine gland sweating form the physiological basis for measurement of electrodermal activity.

There are two basic techniques for measuring electrodermal activity: exosomatic and endosomatic (Everly & Sobelman, 1987). The exosomatic approach involves introduction of a mild electrical current to the skin. This technique is sometimes referred to as *galvanic skin response.* The measurement obtained is that of SC. Because moist skin conducts current more readily than dry skin, skin conductance varies with eccrine gland sweating. In contrast, the endosomatic method consists of passive reception of the electrical activity of sympathetic neurons of the dermal substrate (skin). This approach is referred to as SP.

There are two basic types of circuits used to measure skin conductance: those that apply a constant voltage and those that employ a constant current (Andreassi, 1989). The SC method uses bipolar placement of electrodes placed on the medial phalanxes of two adjacent fingers (either the second and third or the fourth and fifth) (Venables & Christie, 1973). This approach maintains the voltage across the electrodes constant, and the current through the skin varies with changes in conductance. As sympathetic nervous system activity increases, sweat production increases and thus SC increases. The changes in conductance are recorded. When current through the skin is held constant, the voltage necessary to maintain this current varies with resistance. Increased sweat production reduces resistance. When this method is employed, changes in resistance are recorded. With increased sympathetic nervous system activity, resistance is lowered and SC increases. For additional information with respect to these techniques, the reader is referred to Edelberg (1967, 1972), Venables and Christie (1973), and Venables and Martin (1967).

When SP is measured, a unipolar method is employed (Andreassi, 1989). The active electrode is placed on the palm of the hand and is referred to an essentially inactive site (reference) on the forearm. To prepare the site for the inactive electrode, the skin is abraded prior to electrode application. The active electrode must be placed in an area that is free from cuts or other skin lesions because their presence can interfere with the measured response. The SP may be measured by means of a sensitive DC amplifier.

Measures of electrodermal activity may be useful indicators of arousal states (Andreassi, 1989; Everly & Sobelman, 1987). Their utility in reflecting relaxation is questionable, however (Andreassi, 1989). In addition, electrodermal activity possesses both tonic status and phasic propensities (Everly & Sobelman, 1987). Therefore, it is critical that the investigator establish a reliable baseline (situational tone) prior to attempting to determine any reactionary states (phasic activity). In addition, electrode size can affect skin potential and skin conductance measures. Electrodermal response has been used to evaluate responses to physiological and psychological stress in many studies (Guzzetta, 1989; Rief, Shaw, & Fichter, 1998; Seibt, Boucsein, & Schuech, 1998; Steptoe, Cropley, & Joekes, 1999; Steptoe, Evans, & Fieldman, 1997; Vogele, 1998).

➤ NEUROENDOCRINE MEASURES OF THE STRESS RESPONSE

It has long been recognized that the psychoneuroendocrine manifestations of stress reflect the activity of the hypothalamic-pituitary-adrenal-cortical and sympatho-adreno-medullary systems. Thus, methods for studying the stress response often focus on measurement of cortisol, which can be used as a marker of hypothalamic-pituitary-adrenal-cortical activity, and on the catecholamines as measures of sympatho-adreno-medullary activity. Stress is commonly considered a generalized response; as such, there is interaction among other hormones (e.g., prolactin and growth hormone) and with other neurotransmitters (e.g., dopamine and serotonin). In stress studies, cortisol levels are commonly obtained from saliva samples, whereas catecholamines are generally measured from plasma samples or urine specimens.

Because of their invasive nature, tests used in the diagnosis of clinical disease may be inappropriate for research studies. For example, introduction of a venipuncture procedure introduces a stress of its own, thereby imposing extraneous influences on measures obtained in this manner. Intraindividual variations such as changes in body position and baroreflex activity, as well as circadian influences, affect cortisol and catecholamine levels.

Salivary Cortisol

Cortisol, which is produced by the adrenal cortex, is commonly regarded as a marker of activity in the hypothalamic-pituitary-adrenal-cortical system. The measurement of cortisol in saliva has become an acceptable alternative to blood analysis (Kirschbaum & Hellhammer, 1994; Kirschbaum, Read, & Hellhammer, 1992). Because cortisol is thought to enter the saliva by passive diffusion or other means independent of active transport mechanisms, it approximates the level of free cortisol in the plasma and is not affected by the salivary flow rate. Also, the ease of sample collection allows for almost unlimited frequency of sample collection in a variety of research settings. The cortisol response to acute psychological stress is thought to peak after 20 to 30 minutes; thus, momentary changes in cortisol can be measured using this method (Kirschbaum & Hellhammer, 1989). The method has been used for studying stress in infants and children (Schmidt, 1998), adults (Kirschbaum et al., 1995), and the elderly (Samuels, Furlan, Boyce, & Katz, 1997).

There are several methods for collecting salivary samples. Whole saliva can be sampled in wide, disposable containers that provide adequate material for analysis. Another method of sampling is the "Salivette," a small cotton swab that fits into a standard centrifuge tube. The gentle chewing of the swab stimulates salivary flow at a rate that provides a sufficient sample within 30 to 60 seconds. The use of the Salivette facilitates pipetting of the sample because the debris is separated from the clear water saliva supernatant (Kirschbaum & Hellhammer, 1994).

A relatively new sampling device called the "oral diffusion sink" (ODS) allows for the collection of time-integrated measures of cortisol (Wade & Haegele, 1991). This device consists of a 2 mul 15-mm radio-opaque polycarbonate resin shell with 12 perforations (ports) that are covered by a membrane that allows salivary components to diffuse into the device according to their molecular weights. The ODS is secured to a tooth in the subject's mouth with dental floss. Cortisol molecules are bound inside the ODS by either specific antibodies (Wade & Haegele, 1991) or β-cyclodextrin (Wade, 1992). The binding capacity allows for sampling intervals of 1 to 8 hours, thus permitting measurement over prolonged periods. The validity of the ODS has been studied both *in vitro* (Shipley, Alessi, Wade, Haegele, & Helmbold, 1992) and *in vivo* (Gehris & Kathol, 1992).

In infants, saliva can be obtained by gently swabbing the baby's mouth with a cotton dental roll (Gunnar, Connors, & Isenee, 1989) or by aspirating saliva with a small pipette (Hanecke & Haeckel, 1992). Hanecke and Haeckel described a method in which modified feeding bottles containing absorption material within the nipple were used.

Plasma and Urinary Measures of Catecholamines

The catecholamines, epinephrine and norepinephrine, are sympathetic neurotransmitters of the stress response. Norepinephrine is the neurotransmitter released at the postganglionic synapses of the sympathetic nervous system. The adrenal medulla, which is part of the sympathetic nervous system, secretes both epinephrine and norepinephrine in a ratio of approximately 3:1 (Dimsdale & Ziegler, 1991). Two methods have been used to measure catecholamine response to stress: One measures the catechol-

amines in the plasma and the other measures urinary catecholamines.

The measurement and interpretation of the catecholamine response to stress are complicated by the fact that most of the norepinephrine that is released from nerve endings is taken back up into the presynaptic neuron through the reuptake process, with only a small percentage making its way into the bloodstream. Once in the bloodstream, approximately 10% is filtered into the urine, but most is rapidly cleared from the body (Dimsdale & Ziegler, 1991). Each organ rapidly clears and adds norepinephrine to the plasma. Furthermore, the various organs add and remove norepinephrine from the blood at different rates. Organs with the largest blood flow contribute the largest amount of norepinephrine. The sampling site for blood has a marked effect on catecholamine levels. Arterial blood has higher epinephrine and lower norepinephrine levels. Catecholamine levels from venous blood more accurately reflect catecholamines released from all body organs.

Plasma venous catecholamines are exquisitely sensitive to stress. Venipuncture, however, can increase catecholamine levels by more than 50% (Carruthers, Taggart, Conway, Bates, & Somerville, 1990). Thus, venous catheterization is usually done when multiple samples are required. Plasma catecholamines also are affected by diet, caffeine, nicotine, posture, and the stress of the experimental protocol. Because of the assay variability, the numerous confounding variables, and the modest effect of the stressors, relatively large sample sizes may be needed to perceive stress effects of 100 pg/ml in venous epinephrine (Dimesdale & Ziegler, 1991).

Catecholamine levels are commonly measured using high-performance liquid chromatography (HPLC). Although radioimmunoassays (RIAs) can be performed on small blood volumes and they are fairly sensitive, the methods are difficult to perform and require expensive agents. The HPLC methods use electrochemical detectors to quantify the catecholamines after HPLC separation. The

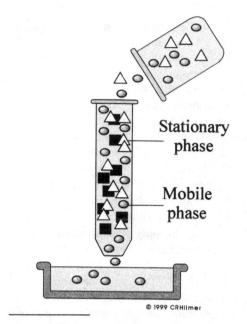

© 1999 CRHilmer

Figure 4.3. Column chromatography separates compounds according to their ability to move through a column containing an adsorbent material. Compounds that adhere to adsorbent material (stationary phase) are separated from those that are mobile and move through the column (reproduced with permission from C. R. Hilmer. Copyright © 1999).

detectors lack the sensitivity to measure low levels of epinephrine and suffer from instability and electrical interference at their most sensitive setting. Therefore, investigators using this method are advised to use an already established catecholamine laboratory.

Biochemical Measurement Methods

Among the biochemical methods used to measure the neuroendocrine responses to stress response are chromatography, RIA, and enzyme-linked immunoabsorbent assay (ELISA). These assays usually require sophisticated methods and less experienced investigators often find it advantageous to collaborate with laboratories that are experienced in performing these tests. In the process of de-

veloping a research protocol that uses the services of any laboratory, it is recommended that the investigator understand the assay method that will be used and receive an assurance that the same method and reagents will be used for all samples that will be submitted. Research protocols frequently require that samples be collected, stored, and transported to the laboratory that has been contracted with to carry out the studies.

Chromatography

Chromatography methods use differences in the solubility of compounds to achieve their separation. In all forms of chromatography, substances are introduced into a column containing an absorbent material that interacts with the compound passing through the column (Figure 4.3). When molecules of a compound are introduced in the top of the column, they are subjected to two opposing forces—that of the mobile forces that tend to move them through the column and that of the stationary phase that has a tendency to keep them within the column (DuFour, 1990). There are several types of chromatography separation methods, including thin layer and column chromatography, which separate polar and nonpolar substances; ion exchange, which separates cations and anions; molecular sieve column chromatography, which separates compounds based on differences in size; and gas-liquid chromatography, which separates an absorbed liquid into an inert support (stationary phase) and an inert gas (mobile phase).

Column chromatography is used for purification of urine vanillylmandelic acid and fractionalization of urine androgens; gas-liquid chromatography is used to separate estrogens and progestagins. In HPLC, the mobile phase is liquid (Allenmark, 1988). It is used to separate catecholamines and catecholamine metabolites (DuFour, 1990). HPLC can be automated and has the advantage of relatively rapid separation, but it is more expensive than other methods and requires experience in performing the assays.

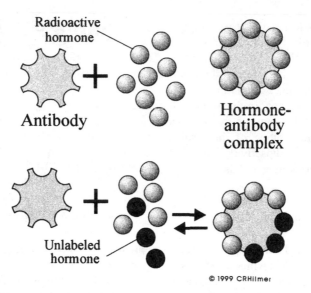

Figure 4.4. Radioimmunoassay (RIA) uses a specific antibody for the hormone being measured and a radiolabeled hormone. The test relies on competitive binding between the unlabeled hormone in the sample being tested and the radiolabeled hormone. The hormone-antibody complexes from samples containing a high concentration of unlabeled hormone will have a lower radiation count than samples containing a low concentration of hormone (reproduced with permission from C. R. Hilmer. Copyright © 1999).

Gas-liquid chromatograph requires high capitol outlay and expert technical assistance as well.

Once separated, the substance being measured can be detected by monitoring specific physical or chemical properties of substances that remain in the column or by analyzing material removed by the mobile phase of the process. The ultraviolet spectrophotometer commonly is used for this purpose.

Radioimmunoassay

Radioimmunoassay, which was developed in the late 1950s and early 1960s, is a major tool in endocrine research (Rhoades & Tanner, 1995). Since its inception, RIA has revolutionized the quantification of hormone levels. It is a competitive binding assay that uses a specific antibody for the hormone being measured and a radioactively labeled hormone (Figure 4.4). The hormone is measured *in vitro* in a series of test tubes. Fixed amounts

of hormone antibody and the radiolabeled antibody are added to all the test tubes. A given volume of the sample to be tested (plasma, saliva, or urine) is then added to one series of tubes. Varying concentrations of the hormone being tested, added to a second series of test tubes, provide the standard for the test. In each series of test tubes, the amount of radioactive hormone bound to the antibody is measured. The response produced by the radiolabeled hormone in the standard series is used to generate a standard curve, and the response produced by the hormone level in the sample is compared to the standard curve.

The assay is based on the principle that the unlabeled hormone in the sample and the radiolabeled hormone in the test tube will compete for the limited number of binding sites present in the antibody that has been added to the test tubes. The amount of each hormone that is bound to the antibody is an indicator of the proportion present in the test tube solution. In a sample with a high concentration of hormone, less radioactive hormone will be bound to antibody and vice versa.

One of the limitations of the RIA is that it measures immunoreactivity rather than biologic activity. The presence of an immunologically related but different hormone or heterogeneous forms of the same hormone can complicate the interpretation of the results. The RIA generates radioactive waste that poses a disposal problem and adds to the expense of the test.

Enzyme-Linked Immunoabsorbent Assay

The enzyme-linked immunoabsorbent assay is a solid-phase, enzyme-based assay whose use and application have increased greatly during the past few years. A typical ELISA is a colorimetric or fluorometric assay that does not use radioactive materials and thus does not produce radioactive waste. This procedure eliminates the increasing environmental concerns and cost of radioactive waste disposal. Because the ELISA is a solid-phase assay, it can be automated to a great extent, which also has served to reduce the cost of this procedure.

The typical ELISA is performed on a 3 × 5-in. plastic plate containing small wells that are precoated with an antibody that is specific for the hormone being measured. A sample of the specimen being tested is introduced into the wells, followed by the addition of a second hormone-specific antibody that binds to the hormone contained in the specimen (Figure 4.5). A third antibody, which recognizes the second antibody, is then added. The third antibody is coupled to an enzyme that will convert an appropriate substrate into a colored or fluorometric product. The amount of product that is formed can be determined using optical methods. After addition of each antibody or sample to the wells, the plates are incubated for an appropriate amount of time to allow the antibodies and hormones to bind. Any unbound hormone is washed out of the well before the addition of the next reagent. The amount of colored or fluorometric product produced is directly proportional to the

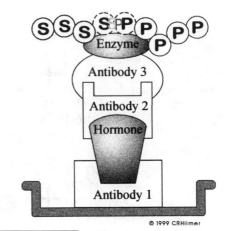

© 1999 CRHilmer

Figure 4.5. The ELISA relies on a change in color or fluorometric properties of a hormone (or antigen). The typical test uses a plastic plate containing small antibody (antibody 1)-coated wells that binds the hormone in the sample being tested. A second hormone (antibody 2) binds to the antibody-hormone complex and to a third antibody (antibody 3). Antibody 3, in turn, activates an enzyme that converts an appropriate substrate (S) to a colored or fluorometric product (P) that can be seen or measured (reproduced with permission from C. R. Hilmer. Copyright © 1999).

amount of hormone present in specimen. As with the RIA, this test is conducted using a standard sample. Concentrations are determined using a standard curve.

➤ IMMUNE MEASURES OF THE STRESS RESPONSE

The precise mechanism by which stress produces its effect on immune function is unknown. It has been suggested that the immune and neuroendocrine cells share common signal pathways, and that hormones and neuropeptides can alter the function of immune cells. Furthermore, the immune system and its products can impact neuroendocrine function (Falaschi, Martocchia, Proietti, Pastore, & D'urso, 1994). The nervous and immune systems are comparable in several ways. Both systems are characterized by a diversity of cell types and by cell-to-cell transmission of information by soluble factors, including lymphokines (immune system) and neurotransmitters (nervous system) (Terr, Dubey, Yunis, Slavin, & Waldman, 1991). Lymphocytes and macrophages have receptors that are capable of responding to the neurotransmitters norepinephrine, acetylcholine, endorphins, enkephalins, ACTH, corticosteroids, insulin, prolactin, growth hormone, estradiol, and testosterone. Likewise, lymphocytes are capable of producing and secreting ACTH and endorphin-like compounds.

The human immune response can be divided into two categories: nonspecific and specific responses (Cacioppo, 1994). Nonspecific response refers to the general bodily defenses that result from pathogen exposure and include activation of natural killer (NK) cells, which monitor the body and destroy virally infected and tumor cells. Also included in this category is the activation of macrophages that engulf and destroy foreign substances. Specific immune responses include antibody production by B lymphocytes and T lymphocyte-mediated responses involving helper/inducer and suppressor/cytotoxic T lymphocytes.

There are five classes of antibodies or immunoglobulins (Igs): IgA, IgD, IgE, IgG, and IgM. IgA, a secretory immunoglobulin, is found in tears, saliva, breast milk, and bronchial, gastrointestinal, prostatic, and vaginal secretion. IgG (gamma globulin), the most abundant of the immunoglobulins, is present in body fluids and is the only immunoglobulin to cross the placenta. It displays antiviral, antitoxin, and antibacterial properties. IgM, a large antibody, is predominant in early immune responses. IgD is found on the cell membrane of B lymphocytes and functions in their maturation. IgE is involved in combating parasitic infections, inflammation, allergy, and hypersensitivity responses.

The technique of producing virtually unlimited quantities of a single antibody specific for a particular antigenic determinant has revolutionized immunology. Known as monoclonal antibodies, these laboratory-generated antibodies interact with specific antigenic markers or immune cells. The modern classification of immune cells is based on the development of population-specific monoclonal antibodies and on the discovery that functionally distinct subpopulations, such as helper T lymphocytes, express different cell membrane proteins called clusters of differentiation (CD).

Generally, two methods are employed to examine cellular immune status (Cacioppo, 1994). First, the percentage of various kinds of blood cells can be quantified *in vitro* by using commercially available monoclonal antibodies. Flow cytometry using monoclonal antibodies is used routinely for determination of NK, CD4+, and CD8+ cell counts. For example, the CD4+ marker on the cell surface identifies helper/inducer lymphocytes, whereas CD8+ markers identify suppressor/cytotoxic lymphocytes (Stites, 1991). Because the balance between helper/inducer and suppressor/cytotoxic T lymphocytes is important in mounting an effective immune response (Herbert & Cohen, 1993), the ratio of CD4+:CD8+ cells is also frequently reported.

The second method provides insight into the functional status of cellular immunity. This procedure involves quantification of the blastogenic response to mitogens *in vitro*. Specific mitogens are introduced in an effort to stimulate B and T lymphocyte proliferation (Stites, 1991). In addition, NK cell function can be tested *in vitro* by means of radioactively labeled targets. Measurement of the radioactivity released from the lysed cells provides data about the NK cytotoxicity (Stites, 1991).

When examining measures of immune function, there are three issues that deserve consideration (Rabin, Kusnecov, Shurin, Zhou, & Rasnick, 1994). First, a laboratory value may indicate that a particular component is not functioning normally. It may only appear abnormal, however, as a result of actions being exerted by another component of the interactive system that is functioning abnormally. For example, with common variable immunodeficiency, immunoglubulin production becomes markedly reduced when it previously had been normal. This situation is not caused by an abnormality of B lymphocytes but rather by increased activity of the T-suppressor lymphocyte population that acts to inhibit B lymphocytes from producing antibody (Ammann, 1991).

A second consideration demanding attention is that it may be difficult to determine when a statistical abnormality is a biologically abnormal (Rabin et al., 1994). When the immune system is evaluated, a statistically significant reduction in immune measures may not be sufficient to have clinical relevance. For example, an IgG concentration of 300 mg/dl is markedly lower than the lower limits of normal range, but it remains adequate to protect an otherwise healthy individual from many infectious diseases.

The third concern that must be taken into account when evaluating measures of immune function is that a laboratory value that appears normal, and is an accumulation of multiple parts, actually may be abnormal (Rabin et al., 1994). An example of this situation is the analysis of IgG levels. There are four subclasses that comprise IgG: IgG_1, IgG_2, IgG_3, and IgG_4. Although the total IgG may appear to be normal, it may be composed of an abnormal subcomponent mixture. Therefore, a statistically normal value may be biologically abnormal.

Many studies have been reported in which the influence of chronic stress and mood on salivary IgA has been investigated. Salivary IgA (sIgA) concentrations or secretion rates or both have been reduced in conjunction with relatively high levels of stress or in the absence of positive mood states (Evans, Bristow, Hucklebridge, Clow, & Walters, 1993; Graham, Chiron, Bartholomeusz, Taboonpong, & LaBrooy, 1988; McClelland, Alexander, & Marks, 1982). In contrast, when the immunological response to acute stress has been investigated, almost invariably an increase in sIgA during or immediately after the stressor has been reported

(Bristow, Hucklebridge, Clow, & Evans, 1997; Carroll et al., 1996; Deinzer & Schuller, 1998; Evans, Bristow, Hucklebridge, Clow, & Pang, 1994; Willemsen et al., 1998; Zeier, Brauchli, & Joller-Jemelka, 1996). Results from these studies suggest that different mechanisms may control acute and chronic regulation of sIgA. Cacioppo (1994) suggested that reductions in sIgA in the long term may reflect involvement of the hypothalamic-pituitary-adrenal-cortical system, whereas short-term increases in sIgA may be a result of sympatho-adreno-medullary activation. In contrast, McClelland, Ross, and Patel (1985) proposed that reductions in sIgA associated with chronic stress may represent receptor downregulation resulting from repeated exposure to short-term challenges. Further investigation into the role of autonomic nervous system influences on sIgA is necessary to provide a better understanding of the meaningfulness of sIgA measures.

For sIgA measurement, saliva generally is collected by means of a Salivette. Before collection of the sample, subjects are asked to swallow until their mouths are dry. Then, a cotton wool swab is placed under the tongue for 2 to 5 minutes. Next, the swab is placed into a Salivette tube. The saliva can be analyzed within 48 hours of collection, or the Salivette can be sealed and frozen at −20° C for later analysis. Both sIgA secretion rate and concentration can be determined.

Until recently, the most commonly employed method for quantifying IgA was the radial immunodiffusion (RID) technique. Secretory IgA (11S) has different diffusion properties than those found in serum (7S), which is used as the standard for the RID assay. Therefore, results obtained from the RID assay for sIgA must be multiplied by a factor of three to correct for this difference in diffusion properties (Samson, McClelland, & Shearman, 1973). When there is a mixture of 7S, 9S, and 11S IgA, as well as IgA fragments, the correction factor method is less accurate (Sack, Neogi, & Alam, 1980).

The purpose of RID is to detect the reaction of antigen and antibody by the precipitation reaction (Stites & Rodgers, 1991). RID is based on the principle that a quantitative relationship exists between the amount of antigen placed in a well cut in an agar-antibody plate and the resulting ring of precipitation. The area circumscribed by the precipitation ring is proportionate to the concentration of antigen. This method requires that the precipitation ring be allowed to reach its maximal size. This method may require 48 to 72 hours of diffusion. A standard curve is experimentally determined with known antigen standards. The equation that describes the standard curve then can be used for determining the antigen concentration corresponding to any diameter size. The sensitivity of these methods ranges from 1 to 3 μg/ml of antigen.

Another method used to determine these measures is the nephelometric technique (Deinzer & Schuller, 1998). Using this technique, samples are spun for 2 minutes at 3000 rpm. Specific human anti-IgA and a buffer are added to the sample. The suspension is stirred and after 6 seconds a blank value for determining diffuse light scattering is obtained. After a 30-minute incubation period, the solution is stirred again to obtain response values. To determine sIgA concentration, the difference between blank and response light scattering is compared with a previously calculated standard curve between 0.5 and 150 mg/dl. Concentration rate can then be determined by multiplying the concentration by one fifth of the sampled saliva volume.

ELISA methods, described previously, are also frequently used in the determination of sIgA concentrations. These methods produce rapid (same day), sensitive, and reproducible results, and they do not require a correction factor when measuring sIgA (Sack et al., 1980). When sIgA measures determined by ELISA methods have been compared with quantifications obtained by RID techniques, very high correlations have been reported ($r =$ .875 to $r =$ .992) (Miletic, Schiffman, Miletic, & Sattely-Miller, 1996; Sack et al., 1980). Likewise, when sIgA measures obtained by means of nephelometric techniques have been compared with quantifications determined by

RID methods, correlations of $r =$ .93 have been reported (Deinzer & Schuller, 1998).

Studies of stressor-induced alterations in human immune function have focused on activation of the sympathetic nervous system as the mediator of immune changes. In a recent meta-analysis of cardiovascular and immune responses to acute psychological stress in young and old women, a medium to large significant correlation between NK cell numbers and heart rate responses and small to medium correlations between NK cell number changes and blood pressure response were obtained (Benschop et al., 1998). The positive correlation between changes in heart rate and NK cell numbers was consistently observed across studies, independent of age or type of stressor. This finding was consistent with reports using male subjects (Benschop et al., 1995, 1994; Naliboff et al., 1995).

➤ RELIABILITY AND VALIDITY CONSIDERATIONS

Manifestations of the stress response can be measured in a variety of ways. Some methods require invasive procedures; many approaches demand expensive equipment; all techniques require thorough understanding of the procedure and underlying theoretical base of the measure employed. Many measurement methods can introduce additional stress to the experimental situation. The insertion of a needle to draw blood, for example, can introduce an element of both physiological and psychological stress.

Time

The time at which measurements are completed also demands consideration. Variables such as catecholamine release and heart rate undergo rapid changes during an acute stress challenge. In studies of acute stress, a beat-by-beat recording of heart rate may be required to ensure that the entire response is included in the analysis. Other variables such as changes in immune cells occur over a longer period of time. Thus, an understanding of the physiologic events being studied and the time sequence during which measurements should be made can be critical in designing a research protocol.

Many physiologic variables follow a circadian rhythm (Mathias & Alam, 1995; Moore, 1997). For example, cortisol peaks during early morning hours (Turton & Deegan, 1974). Other physiologic variables, such as norepinephrine and epinephrine, are influenced by the hypothalamic-pituitary-adrenal-cortical system. The body may be more susceptible to stresses imposed at certain phases of the circadian cycle than others. Thus, stress studies is which physiologic measurements are employed are best conducted at the same time each day to avoid variability among subject responses to circadian influences.

Although heart rate and blood pressure often are used in evaluating the effects of physical and emotional stressors, there are methodological problems associated with using these variables in the laboratory setting (Parati et al., 1991). Blood pressure and heart rate responses to laboratory-induced stressors are limited by within-subject variability, poor correlation between blood pressure and heart rate responses to different stressors, and the fact that these responses bear only a limited relation to 24-hour patterns of variability in these measures.

Gender and Age

Both gender and age can influence physiologic responses to stress. Because of their different body size and composition and different hormonal profiles, women may recruit and use physiologic mechanisms differently than men (Frey & Porth, 1990). With aging, there is a general decline in adaptive capacity, in addition to changes in the ability to respond to stress.

The physiologic responses of women and men to physical and psychological stressors reflect the autonomic nervous system, the central nervous system, the responsiveness to hormones, and the function of the cardiovascular system. For example, men reportedly secrete more catecholamines during mental and other exercise stresses, whereas women secrete more catecholamines during exercise (Frankenhaeuser, 1983). Until recently, published data about women were integrated into a study with the data of men, and samples consisted predominantly of male subjects. As a result, many of the differences and similarities in the physiologic responses to stress between the sexes remain unclear.

Differences in hormones, particularly the reproductive hormones, provide one possible explanation for differences in responses of men and women to stress. When measuring the effects of the stress response in women, consideration must be given to the women's station in the menstrual cycle (Heitkemper et al., 1996). Responses to experimental and naturally occurring stress in daily life can be influenced by these hormonal fluctuations. For example, heart rate and systolic blood pressure were reported to be significantly greater during the luteal phase of the menstrual cycle when compared to the follicular phase (Manhem & Jern, 1994). Ovulation can be determined by use of a 9-day test kit (OvuQuick) to track the urinary luteinizing hormone surge (Rudy & Estok, 1992).

There is a reported decline in autonomic nervous system and cardiovascular responsiveness to stress associated with advancing age (Smith & Porth, 1990). The effects of aging on cardiovascular responsiveness, reaction time, and the ability to respond to stress are all factors that need to be addressed when designing a research study.

➤ SUMMARY

Physiologic measures can prove to be a reliable method for studying the consequences of physiological and psychological stress. Technologic advances that have led to the development of noninvasive measurement methods favor their use in stress research. These measurements can be used singly, in combination, or as an adjunct to other more subjective methods of measuring the stress response.

Many of these noninvasive measures require expensive equipment and a thorough understanding of their underlying scientific principles and of the physiologic phenomenon that they measure. Furthermore, many of the physiologic parameters that these methods measure are subject to the impact of circadian, gender, and age influences, changes in posture or body position, and investigator or operator error or both. In addition, proper use of the equipment requires special training. Interrater and intrarater variability can impose threats to the reliability of these measures. Controlling for time of day, body position, and phase of menstrual cycle can increase validity of these measures.

As with any laboratory tests, accuracy or validity of test results relies on the use of proper procedures and reagents in the laboratory. It is advisable to determine the reliability of the laboratory, its personnel, and equipment in use. When multiple laboratories are used, the possibility of additional measurement error is introduced. Laboratory procedures are expensive. Frequently, venipuncture is involved, making these approaches less attractive to potential subjects. If repeated measures are employed, repeated venipuncture may be necessary. In addition, it is very important that careful consideration be given to the specificity and sensitivity of these measures in relation to the questions being posed. The cost:benefit ratio of using any physiological measures must also be examined.

The value of physiologic measures of the stress response will be enhanced by using multiple physiological measures in conjunction with psychometric instruments. Inclusion of interrater or intrarater reliability checks or both is imperative. All equipment used to determine physiological responses must meet professionally set specifications that ensure reliability and validity of determined measures.

➤ REFERENCES

Akselrod, S. (1995). Components of heart rate variability: Basic studies. In M. Malik & A. J. Camm (Eds.), *Heart rate variability* (pp. 147-163). Armonk, NY: Futura.

Akselrod, S., Gordon, D., Ubel, F. A., Shannon, D. C., Barger, A. C., & Cohen, R. J. (1981). Power spectrum analysis of heart rate fluctuation: A quantitative probe of beat-to-beat cardiovascular control. *Science, 213,* 220-222.

Allenmark, S. (1988). High-performance liquid chromatography of catecholamines and their metabolites in biological material. *Monographs in Endocrinology, 30,* 32-65.

Amersterdam, E. A., Hughes, J. L., DeMaria, A. N., Zelis, R., & Mason, D. T. (1974). Indirect assessment of myocardial oxygen consumption in the evaluation of mechanisms and therapy of angina pectoris. *American Journal of Cardiology, 33,* 737-743.

Ammann, A. J. (1991). Antibody (B cell) immunodeficiency disorders. In D. P. Stites & A. I. Terr (Eds.), *Basic and clinical immunology* (7th ed., pp. 322-334). Norwalk, CT: Appleton & Lange.

Andreassi, J. L. (1989). *Psychophysiology: Human behavior and physiological response* (2nd ed.). Hillsdale, NJ: Lawrence Erlbaum.

Andrew, W., & Scott, C. (1985). Haemodynamic monitoring: Measurement of system blood pressure. *Canadian Anaesthesia Society Journal, 32,* 294-298.

Appel, M. L., Berger, R. D., Saul, J. P., Smith, S. M., & Cohen, R. J. (1989). Beat to beat variability in cardiovascular variables: Noise or music? *Journal of the American College of Cardiology, 14,* 1139-1148.

Bairey Merz, C. N., Kop, W., Krantz, D. S., Helmers, K. F., Berman, D. S., & Rozanski, A. (1998). Cardiovascular stress response and coronary artery disease: Evidence of an adverse postmenopausal effect in women. *American Heart Journal, 135* (5, Pt. 1), 881-887.

Banner, T. E., & Gavenstein, J. S. (1991). Comparative effects of cuff size and tightness of fit on accuracy of blood pressure measurements. *Journal of Clinical Monitoring, 7,* 281-284.

Belkic, K., Emdad, R., & Theorell, T. (1998). Occupational profile and cardiac risk: Possible mechanisms and implications for professional drivers. *International Journal of Occupational Medicine and Environmental Health, 11,* 37-57.

Benschop, R. J., Geenen, R., Mills, R. J., Naliboff, B. D., Giecolt-Glaser, J. K., Herbert, T. B., van der Pompe, G., Miller, G. E., Matthews, K. A., Godaert, G. L. R., Gilmore, S. L., Glaser, R., Heijnen, C. J., Dopp, J. M., Bulsma, W. J., Solomon, G. F., & Cacioppo, J. T. (1998). Cardiovascular and immune responses to acute psychological stress in young and old women: A meta-analysis. *Psychosomatic Medicine, 60,* 290-296.

Benschop, R. J., Godaert, G. L. R., Geenen, R., Brosschot, J. R., deSmet, J. B. M., Olff, M., Hiijnen, C. J., & Ballieux, R. E. (1995). Relationships between cardiovascular and immunologic changes in an experimental stress model. *Psychological Medicine, 25,* 323-327.

Benschop, R. J., Nieuwenhuis, E. E. S., Tromp, E. A. M., Godaert, G. L. R., Ballieux, R. E., & van Doornen, L. J. P. (1994). Effects of beta-adrenergic blockade on immunologic and cardiovascular changes induced by mental stress. *Circulation, 89,* 762-769.

Berntson, G. G., Cacioppo, J. T., & Quigley, K. S. (1993). Respiratory sinus arrhythmia: Autonomic origins, physiological mechanisms, and psychophysiological implications. *Psychophysiology, 30,* 183-196.

Bristow, M., Hucklebridge, F., Clow, A., & Evans, P. (1997). Modulation of secretory immunoglobulin A in saliva in relation to an acute episode of stress and arousal. *Journal of Psychophysiology, 11,* 248-255.

Burns, N., & Grove, S. K. (1997). *The practice of nursing research: Conduct, critique, & utilization.* Philadelphia: W. B. Saunders.

Cacioppo, J. T. (1994). Social neuroscience: Autonomic, neuroendocrine, and immune responses to stress. *Psychophysiology, 31,* 113-128.

Cannon, W. B. (1939). *The wisdom of the body.* New York: Norton.

Carroll, D., Ring, C. L., Shrimpton, J., Evans, P., Willemsen, G., & Hucklebridge, F. (1996). Secretory immunoglobulin A and cardiovascular responses to acute psychological challenge. *International Journal of Internal Medicine, 3,* 266-279.

Carruthers, M., Taggart, P., Conway, N., Bates, D., & Somerville, W. (1990). Validity of plasma catecholamine estimation. *Lancet, 2,* 62-67.

Cook, T. D., & Campbell, D. T. (1979). *Quasi-experimental design: Design & analysis issues for field setting.* Boston: Houghton Mifflin.

Cowan, M. J., Kogan, H., Burr, R., Hendershot, S., & Buchanan, L. (1990). Power spectral analysis of heart rate variability after biofeedback training. *Journal of Electrocardiology, 23*(Suppl.), 85-94.

Cromwell, L., Weibell, F. J., & Pfeiffer, E. A. (1980). *Biomedical instrumentation and measurements* (2nd ed.). Englewood Cliffs: NJ: Prentice Hall.

DeBenedittis, G., Cigada, M., Bianchi, A., Signorini, M. G., & Cerutti, S. (1994). Autonomic changes during hypnosis: A heart rate variability power spectrum analysis as a marker of sympatho-vagal balance. *International Journal of Clinical and Experimental Hypnosis, 17,* 140-152.

Deinzer, R., & Schuller, N. (1998). Dynamics of stress-related decrease in salivary immunoglobulin A (sIgA): Relationship to symptoms of the common cold and studying behavior. *Behavioral Medicine, 23,* 161-169.

Dimsdale, J. E., & Ziegler, M. G. (1991). What do plasma and urinary measures of catecholamines tell us about human response to stressors. *Circulation, 83*(Suppl. II), II-36-II-42.

DuFour, D. R. (1990). Reference values in endocrinology. In K. L. Becker, J. P. Bilezikian, W. J. Bremmer, W. Hung, C. R. Kahn, D. L. Loriaux, R. W. Rebar, G. L. Robertson, & L. Wartofsky (Eds.), *Principles and practice of endocrinology and metabolism* (pp. 1723-1765). Philadelphia: J. B. Lippincott.

Ebert, T. J. (1992). Autonomic balance and cardiac function. *Current Opinions in Anaesthesiology, 5,* 3-10.

Edelberg, R. (1967). Electrical properties of the skin. In C. C. Brown (Ed.), *Methods in psychophysiology* (pp. 1-53). Baltimore, MD: Williams & Wilkins.

Edelberg, R. (1972). Electrodermal activity of the skin. In N. S. Greenfield & R. A. Sternbach (Eds.), *Handbook of psychophysiology* (pp. 367-418). New York: Holt, Rinehart & Winston.

Elliot, R. S., & Morales-Ballejo, H. M. (1994). The heart, emotional stress, and psychiatric disorders. In R. C. Schlant & R. W. Alexander (Eds.), *Hurst's the heart* (8th ed., pp. 2087-2097). New York: McGraw-Hill.

Evans, P., Bristow, M., Hucklebridge, F., Clow, A., & Pang, F. Y. (1994). Stress arousal, cortisol, and secretory immunoglobulin A in students undergoing assessment. *British Journal of Clinical Psychology, 33,* 575-576.

Evans, P., Bristow, M., Hucklebridge, F., Clow, A., & Walters, N. (1993). The relationship between secretory immunity, mood and life events. *British Journal of Clinical Psychology, 32,* 227-236.

Everly, G. S., Jr., & Sobelman, S. A. (1987). *Assessment of the human stress response: Neurological, biochemical, and psychological foundations.* New York: AMS Press.

Falaschi, P., Martocchia, A., Proietti, A., Pastore, R., & D'urso, R. (1994). Immune system and the hypothalamus-pituitary-adrenal axis. *Annals of the New York Academy of Sciences, 741,* 223-231.

Frankenhaeuser, M. (1983). The sympathetic-adrenal and pituitary-adrenal response to challenge: Comparison between the sexes. In T. M. Dembroski, T. H. Schmidt, & G. Blumchen (Eds.), *Biobehavioral bases of coronary heart disease* (pp. 91-105). Basel: Karger.

Frey, M. A. B., & Porth, C. M. (1990). Sex differences in response to orthostatic and other stresses. In J. J. Smith (Ed.), *Circulatory response to the upright position* (pp. 141-167). Boca Raton, FL: CRC Press.

Fuller, B. F. (1992). The effects of stress—Anxiety and coping styles on heart rate variability. *International Journal of Psychophysiology, 12,* 81-86.

Gehris, T. L., & Kathol, R. G. (1992). Comparison of time-integrated measurement of salivary corticosteroids by oral diffusion sink technology to plasma cortisol. *Endocrine Research, 18,* 77-89.

Gobel, F. L., Nordstrom, L. A., Nelson, R. R., Jorgenson, C. R., & Wang, Y. (1978). The rate-pressure product as an index of myocardial oxygen consumption during exercise in patients with angina pectoris. *Circulation, 57,* 549-556.

Gorny, D. A. (1993). Arterial pressure measurement techniques. *AACN Clinical Issues in Critical Care Nursing, 4,* 66-78.

Graham, N. M. H., Chiron, R., Bartholomeusz, A., Taboonpong, N., & LaBrooy, J. T. (1988). Does anxiety reduce the secretion rate of secretory IgA in saliva? *Medical Journal of Australia, 148,* 131-133.

Grossman, P., vanBeek, J., & Wientjes, C. (1990). A comparison of three quantification methods for estimation of respiratory sinus arrhythmia. *Psychophysiology, 27,* 702-714.

Gunnar, M. R., Connors, J., & Isenee, J. (1989). Lack of stability in neonatal adrenocortical reactivity because of rapid habituation of the adrenocortical response. *Developmental Psychobiology, 22,* 221-233.

Guyton, A. C., & Hall, J. E. (1996). *Textbook of medical physiology* (9th ed.). Philadelphia: W. B. Saunders.

Guzzetta, C. E. (1989). Effects of relaxation and music therapy on patients in a coronary care unit with presumptive acute myocardial infarction. *Heart & Lung, 18,* 609-616.

Hainsworth, R. (1995). The control and physiological importance of heart rate. In M. Malik & A. J. Camm (Eds.), *Heart rate variability* (pp. 3-19). Armonk, NY: Futura.

Hanecke, P., & Haeckel, R. (1992). A method to collect saliva from infants. In C. Kirschbaum, G. F. Read, & D. H. Hellhammer (Eds.), *Assessment of hormones and drugs in saliva in biobehavioral research* (pp. 33-35). Seattle: Hogrefe & Huber.

Hatch, J. P., Borcherding, S., & Norris, L. K. (1990). Cardiopulmonary adjustments during operant heart rate control. *Psychophysiology, 27,* 641-648.

Hattori, N., Tamaki, N., Kudoh, T., Masuda, I., Magata, Y., Kitano, H., Inubushi, M., Tadamura, E., Nakao, K., & Konishi, J. (1998). Abnormality of myocardial oxidative metabolism in noninsulin-dependent diabetes mellitus. *Journal of Nuclear Medicine, 39,* 1835-1840.

Heitkemper, M., Jarrett, M., Cain, K., Shaver, J., Bond, E., Woods, N. F., & Walker, E. (1996). Increased urine catecholamines and cortisol in women with irritable bowel syndrome. *American Journal of Gastroenterology, 91,* 906-913.

Henry, J. P. (1992). Biological basis of the stress response. *Integrative Physiology and Behavioural Science, 27,* 66-83.

Herbert, T. B., & Cohen, S. (1993). Stress and immunity in humans: A meta-analytic review. *Psychosomatic Medicine, 55,* 364-379.

Hirsch, J. A., & Bishop, B. (1981). Respiratory sinus arrhythmia in humans: How breathing pattern modulates heart rate. *American Journal of Physiology, 241,* H620-H629.

Hrushesky, W. J. M., Fader, D., Schmitt, O., & Gilbertsen, V. (1984). The respiratory sinus arrhythmia: A measure of cardiac age. *Science, 224,* 1001-1004.

Hyndman, B. W., Kitney, R. I., & Sayers, B. M. (1971). Spontaneous rhythms in physiological control systems. *Nature, 233,* 339-342.

Imholz, B. P., Wieling, W., van Montfrans, G. A., & Wessling, K. H. (1998). Fifteen years experience with finger arterial pressure monitoring: Assessment of the technology. *Cardiovascular Research, 38,* 605-616.

Imholz, B. P. M., van Montfrans, G. A., Settels, J. J., Gerard, M. A., VanDerHoeven, G. M. A., Karemaker, J. M., & Wieling, W. (1988). Continuous non-invasive blood pressure monitoring: Reliability of Finapres device during the Valsalva maneuver. *Cardiovascular Research, 22,* 390-397.

Jagomagi, K., Talts, J., Raamat, R., & Lansimes, E. (1996). Continuous non-invasive measurement of mean blood pressure in finger by volume-clamp and differential oscillometric method. *Clinical Physiology, 16,* 551-560.

Jain, D., Shaker, S. M., Burg, M., Wackers, F. J., Soufer, R., & Zaret, B. L. (1998). Effects of mental stress on left ventricular and peripheral vascular performance in patients with coronary artery disease. *Journal of the American College of Cardiology, 31,* 1314-1322.

Jensen, L., Yakimets, J., & Teo, K. K. (1995). A review of impedance cardiography. *Heart & Lung, 24,* 183-193.

Kavanaugh, T., Matosevic, V., Thacker, L., Belliard, R., & Shephard, R. J. (1998). On-site evaluation of bus drivers with coronary heart disease. *Journal of Cardiopulmonary Rehabilitation, 18,* 209-215.

Kirschbaum, C., & Hellhammer, D. H. (1989). Salivary control in psychobiological research. An overview. *Neuropsychology, 22,* 150-169.

Kirschbaum, C., & Hellhammer, D. H. (1994). Salivary cortisol in psychoneuroendocrine research: Recent developments and applications. *Psychoneuroendocrinology, 19,* 313-333.

Kirschbaum, C., Prussner, J. C., Stone, A. A., Federenko, I., Gaab, J., Lintz, D., Schommer, N., & Hellhammer, D. H. (1995). Persistent high cortisol responses to repeated psychological stress in a subpopulation of healthy men. *Psychosomatic Medicine, 57,* 468-474.

Kirschbaum, C., Read, G. F., & Hellhammer, D. H. (1992). *Assessment of hormones and drugs in saliva in biobehavioral research.* Seattle: Hogrefe & Huber.

Kleiger, R. E., Bigger, J. T., Bosner, M. S., Chung, M. K., Cook, J. R., Rolnitzky, L. M., Steinman, R., &

Fleiss, J. L. (1991). Stability over time of variables measuring heart rate variability in normal subjects. *American Journal of Cardiology, 68,* 626-630.

Kubicek, W. G., Karnegis, J. N., Patterson, R. P., Witssoe, D. A., & Mattson, R. H. (1966). Development and evaluation of an impedance cardiac output system. *Aerospace Medicine, 37,* 1208-1212.

Latman, N. S. (1992). Evaluation of finger blood pressure monitoring instruments. *Biomedical Instrumentation and Technology, 26,* 52-57.

Lyew, M. A., & Jamieson, J. W. (1994). Blood pressure measurement using oscillometric finger cuffs in children and young adults. *Anesthesia, 49,* 895-899.

Malliani, A., Pagani, M., Lombardi, F., & Cerutti, S. (1991). Cardiovascular neural regulation explored in the frequency domain. *Circulation, 84,* 482-492.

Manhem, K., & Jern, S. (1994). Influence of daily-life activation on pulse rate and blood pressure changes during the menstrual cycle. *Journal of Human Hypertension, 8,* 851-856.

Mathias, C. J., & Alam, M. (1995). Circadian changes of the cardiovascular system and the autonomic nervous system: Observations in autonomic disorders. In M. Malik & A. J. Camm (Eds.), *Heart rate variability* (pp. 21-30). Armonk, NY: Futura.

McClelland, D. C., Alexander, C., & Marks, E. (1982). The need for power, stress, immune function and illness among male prisoners. *Journal of Abnormal Psychology, 91,* 61-70.

McClelland, D. C., Ross, G., & Patel, V. (1985). The effect of an academic examination on salivary norepinephrine and immunoglobulin levels. *Journal of Human Stress, 11,* 52-59.

Miletic, I. D., Schiffman, S. S., Miletic, V. D., & Sattely-Miller, E. A. (1996). Salivary IgA secretion rate in young and elderly persons. *Physiology & Behavior, 60,* 243-248.

Moore, R. Y. (1997). Circadian rhythms: Basic neurobiology and clinical applications. *Annual Review of Medicine, 48,* 253-260.

Naliboff, B. D., Solomon, G. F., Gilmore, S. L., Fahey, J. L., Benton, D., & Pine, J. (1995). Rapid changes in cellular immunity following a confrontational role-play stressor. *Brain, Behavior, & Immunity, 9,* 207-219.

Nesselroad, J. M., Flacco, V. A., Phillips, D. M., & Kruse, J. (1996). Accuracy of automated finger blood pressure devices. *Family Medicine, 28,* 189-192.

O'Brien, E., Fitzgerald, D., & O'Malley, K. (1985). Blood pressure measurement: Current practice and future trends. *British Medical Journal, 290,* 729-734.

O'Brien, E., Mee, F., Tan, S., Atkins, N., & O'Malley, K. (1991). Training and assessment of observers for blood pressure measurement in hypertension research. *Journal of Human Hypertension, 5,* 7-10.

O'Brien, I. A. D., O'Hare, P., & Corrall, R. J. M. (1985). Heart rate variability in healthy subjects: Effects of age and the derivation of normal ranges for tests of autonomic function. *British Heart Journal, 55,* 348-354.

Pagani, M., Lombardi, F., Guzzetti, S., Rimoldi, U., Furlan, R., Pizzinelli, P., Sandrone, G., Malfatto, G., Dell'Orto, S., Piccaluga, E., Turiel, M., Baselli, G., Cerutti, S., & Malliani, A. (1986). Power spectral analysis of heart rate and arterial pressure variabilities as a marker of sympatho-vagal interaction in man and conscious dog. *Circulation Research, 59,* 178-193.

Pagani, M., Lucini, D., Rimoldi, O., Furlan, R., Piazza, S., & Biancardi, L. (1995). Effects of physical and mental exercise on heart rate variability. In M. Malik & A. J. Camm (Eds.), *Heart rate variability* (pp. 245-266). Armonk, NY: Futura.

Parati, G., Trazzi, S., Ravogli, A., Casadei, R., Omboni, S., & Manacia, G. (1991). Methodological problems in evaluation of cardiovascular effects of stress in humans. *Hypertension, 17*(Suppl. III), III-50-III-55.

Peters, M. L., Godaert, G. L. R., Ballieux, R. E., van Vliet, M., Willemsen, J. J., Sweep, F. C. G. J., & Heijnen, C. J. (1998). Cardiovascular and endocrine responses to experimental stress. *Psychophysiology, 23,* 1-17.

Pickering, T. (1995). Recommendations for use of home (self) and ambulatory blood-pressure monitoring. American Society for Blood Pressure Ad Hoc Panel. *American Journal of Hypertension, 9,* 1-11.

Polit, D. F., & Hungler, B. P. (1995). *Nursing research: Principles and methods* (5th ed.). Philadelphia: J. B. Lippincott.

Pomeranz, B., Macaulay, J. B., Caudill, M. A., Kutz, I., Adam, D., Gordon, D., Kilborn, K. M., Barger, A. C., Shannon, D. C., Cohen, R. J., & Benson, H. (1985). Assessment of autonomic function in humans by heart rate spectral analysis. *American Journal of Physiology, 17,* H151-H153.

Porth, C. M. (1976). *A comparison of cardiovascular responses to cold pressor and isometric handgrip exercises in normal young males.* Unpublished master's thesis, Medical College of Wisconsin, Milwaukee.

Porth, C. M. (1998). *Pathophysiology: Concepts of altered health states* (5th ed.). Philadelphia: J. B. Lippincott.

Probst, M., Bulbulian, R., & Knapp, C. (1997). Hemodynamic responses to stroop and cold pressor test after submaximal cycling exercise in normotensive males. *Physiology & Behavior, 62,* 1283-1290.

Rabin, B. S., Kusnecov, A., Shurin, M., Zhou, D., & Rasnick, S. (1994). Mechanistic aspects of stressor-induced immune alteration. In R. Glaser & J. Kiecolt-Glaser (Eds.), *Handbook of human stress and immunity* (pp. 23-51). San Diego: Academic Press.

Rhoades, R. A., & Tanner, G. A. (1995). *Medical physiology*. Boston: Little, Brown.

Richter, D. W., & Spyer, K. M. (1990). Cardiorespiratory control. In A. D. Loewy & K. M. Spyer (Eds.), *Central regulation of autonomic function* (pp. 189-207). New York: Oxford University Press.

Rief, W., Shaw, R., & Fichter, M. M. (1998). Elevated levels of psychophysiological arousal and cortisol in patients with somatization syndrome. *Psychosomatic Medicine, 60*, 198-203.

Ristuccia, H. L., Grossman, P., Watkins, L. L., & Lown, B. (1997). Incremental bias in Finapres estimation of baseline blood pressure levels over time. *Hypertension, 19*, 1039-1043.

Rubin, S. A. (1987). Measurement theory and instrument errors. In S. A. Rubin (Ed.), *The principles of biomedical instrumentation* (pp. 50-74). Chicago: Year Book Medical.

Rudy, E. B., & Estok, P. (1992). Professional and lay interrater reliability of urinary luteinizing hormone surges measured by OvuQuick test. *Journal of Obstetrics and Gynecological and Neonatal Nursing, 21*, 407-411.

Sack, D. A., Neogi, P. K. B., & Alam, M. D. K. (1980). Immunobead enzyme-linked immunosorbent assay for quantifying immunoglobulin A in human secretions and serum. *Infection and Immunity, 29*, 281-283.

Sakakibara, M., Takeuchik, S., & Hayano, J. (1994). Effect of relaxation training on cardiac parasympathetic tone. *Psychophysiology, 31*, 223-238.

Samson, R. R., McClelland, D. B. L., & Shearman, D. J. C. (1973). Studies on the quantification of immunoglobulin in human intestinal secretions. *Gut, 14*, 616-626.

Samuels, S. C., Furlan, P. M., Boyce, A., & Katz, I. R. (1997). Salivary cortisol and daily events in nursing home residents. *American Journal of Geriatric Psychiatry, 5*, 172-176.

Saul, J. P. (1990). Beat-to-beat variations of heart rate reflect modulation of cardiac autonomic outflow. *NIPS, 5*, 32-37.

Saul, J. P., & Cohen, R. J. (1994). Respiratory sinus arrhythmia. In M. N. Levy & P. J. Schwartz (Eds.), *Vagal control of the heart: Experimental basis and clinical implications* (pp. 511-536). Armonk, NY: Futura.

Schlant, R. C., & Sonnenblick, E. H. (1994). Normal physiology of the cardiovascular system. In R. C. Schlant & R. W. Alexander (Eds.), *Hurst's the heart* (8th ed., pp. 113-151). New York: McGraw-Hill.

Schmidt, N. A. (1998). Salivary cortisol testing in children. *Issues in Comprehensive Pediatric Nursing, 20*, 183-190.

Schwartz, J. B., Gibb, W. J., & Tran, T. (1991). Aging effects on heart rate variability. *Journal of Gerontology, 46*, M99-M106.

Seibt, R., Boucsein, W., & Schuech, K. (1998). Effects of different stress settings on cardiovascular parameters and their relationship to daily life blood pressure in normotensives, borderline hypertensives and hypertensives. *Ergonomics, 41*, 634-648.

Selye, H. (1974). *Stress without distress*. New York: New American Library.

Shipley, J. E., Alessi, N. E., Wade, S. E., Haegele, A. D., & Helmbold, B. (1992). Utility of an oral diffusion sink (ODS) device for quantification of saliva corticosteroids in human subject. *Journal of Clinical Endocrinology and Metabolism, 71*, 639-644.

Smith, J. J., & Porth, C. J. M. (1990). Age and the response to orthostatic stress. In J. J. Smith (Ed.), *Circulatory response to the upright posture* (pp. 121-139). Boca Raton, FL: CRC Press.

Stein, P. K., Bosner, M. S., Kleiger, R. E., & Conger, B. M. (1994). Heart rate variability: A measure of cardiac autonomic tone. *American Heart Journal, 127*, 1376-1381.

Steptoe, A., Cropley, M., & Joekes, K. (1999). Job strain, blood pressure and response to uncontrollable stress. *Journal of Hypertension, 17*, 193-200.

Steptoe, A., Evans, O., & Fieldman, G. (1997). Perceptions of control over work: Psychophysiological responses to self-paced and externally paced tasks in an adult population sample. *International Journal of Psychophysiology, 25*, 211-220.

Stites, D. P. (1991). Laboratory evaluation of immune competence. In D. P. Stites & A. I. Terr (Eds.), *Basic and clinical immunology* (7th ed., pp. 312-318). Norwalk, CT: Appleton & Lange.

Stites, D. P., & Rodgers, R. P. C. (1991). Clinical laboratory methods for detection of antigens and antibodies. In D. P. Stites & A. I. Terr (Eds.), *Basic and clinical immunology* (7th ed., pp. 217-262). Norwalk, CT: Appleton & Lange.

Task Force of the European Society of Cardiology and the North American Society of Pacing and Electrophysiology. (1996). Heart rate variability: Standards of measurement, physiological interpretation, and clinical use. *European Heart Journal, 60*, 1239-1245.

Tassorelli, C., Micieli, G., Osipova, V., Rossi, F., & Nappi, G. (1995). Pupillary and cardiovascular responses to cold-pressor test. *Journal of the Autonomic Nervous System, 55*(1/2), 45-49.

Terr, A. I., Dubey, D. P., Yunis, E. J., Slavin, R. G., & Waldman, R. H. (1991). Physiologic and environmental influences on the immune system. In D. P. Stites & A. I. Terr (Eds.), *Basic and clinical immunology* (7th ed., pp. 187-199). Norwalk, CT: Appleton & Lange.

Turton, M. B., & Deegan, T. (1974). Circadian variations of plasma catecholamines, cortisol, and immunoreactive insulin concentrations in supine subjects. *Clinica Chimica Acta, 55*, 389-397.

Venables, P. H., & Christie, M. J. (1973). Mechanism, instrumentation, recording techniques and quantification of responses. In W. F. Prokasy & D. C. Raskin (Eds.), *Electrodermal activity in psychological research* (pp. 1-124). New York: Academic Press.

Venables, P. H., & Martin, I. (1967). Skin resistance and skin potential. In P. H. Venables & I. Martin (Eds.), *Manual of psycho-physiological methods* (pp. 53-102). Amsterdam: North-Holland.

Villella, M., Villella, A., Barlera, S., Franzosi, M. G., & Maggioni, A. P. (1999). Prognostic significance of double product and inadequate double product response to maximal symptom-limited exercise stress testing after myocardial infarction in 6,296 patients treated with thrombolytic agents. *American Heart Journal, 137,* 443-452.

Vogele, C. (1998). Serum lipid concentrations, hostility and cardiovascular reactions to mental stress. *International Journal of Psychophysiology, 28,* 167-179.

Vybiral, T., Bryg, R. J., Maddens, M. E., & Boden, W. E. (1989). Effect of passive tilt on sympathetic and parasympathetic components of heart rate variability in normal subjects. *American Journal of Cardiology, 53,* 1117-1120.

Wade, S. E. (1992). An oral-diffusion-sink device for extended sampling of multiple steroid hormones from saliva. *Clinical Chemistry, 38,* 1878-1882.

Wade, S. E., & Haegele, A. D. (1991). Time-integrated measurement of corticosteroids in saliva by oral diffusion sink technology. *Clinical Chemistry, 37,* 1166-1172.

Waltz, C. F., Strickland, O. L., & Lenz, E. R. (1991). *Measurement in nursing research.* Philadelphia: F. A. Davis.

Weiner, H. (1992). *Perturbing the organism: The biology of the stressful experience.* Chicago: University of Chicago Press.

White, J. M. (1999). Effects of relaxing music on cardiac autonomic balance and anxiety after acute myocardial infarction. *American Journal of Critical Care, 8,* 220-230.

Willemsen, G., Ring, C., Carroll, D., Evans, P., Clow, A., & Hucklebridge, F. (1998). Secretory immunoglubulin A and cardiovascular reactions to mental arithmetic and cold pressor. *Psychobiology, 35,* 252-259.

Woltjer, H. H., Bogaard, H. J., & deVries, P. M. J. M. (1997). The technique of impedance cardiography. *European Heart Journal, 18,* 1396-1403.

Woods, N. F., & Cantanzaro, M. (1988). *Nursing research: Theory and practice.* St. Louis, MO: C. V. Mosby.

Woodworth, R. S., & Schlosberg, H. (1954). *Experimental psychology.* New York: Holt.

Working Party on Blood Pressure Measurement of the British Hypertension Society. (1997). *Blood pressure measurement: Recommendations of the British Hypertension Society* (3rd ed.). Plymouth, UK: British Medical Journal Publishing Group.

Zeier, H., Brauchli, P., & Joller-Jemelka, H. I. (1996). Effects of work demands on immunoglobulin A and cortisol in air traffic controllers. *Biological Psychology, 42,* 413-423.

PART III

Stimulus-Oriented Stress

CHAPTER 5

Major Life Stressors and Health Outcomes

Joan Stehle Werner and Marlene Hanson Frost

S tress is a broad area of study and knowledge development involving many disciplines, presumably in search of describing, understanding, and predicting stressors and their consequences for health and well-being. Ultimately, for some disciplines such as nursing, the goal is to be able to mitigate the ill effects of stress with individuals, families, communities, and even societies. Stress has relatively recently been portrayed as a process, including a stimulus, individual characteristics and perception, a response, and long-term consequences (Elliott & Eisdorfer, 1982). For example, Cohen, Kessler, and Gordon (1995) describe a model they call a "unifying model of the stress process" (p. 10) that includes the following factors: (a) environmental demands, (b) cognitive evaluation of the threat potential of the demand and coping abilities available, (c) perception of stress, (d) negative emotional reactions, followed by (e) "behavioral or physiological responses that put a person under risk for psychiatric and physical illness" (p. 10). Many factors have been studied to understand this process better, including genetic predisposition, personality, appraisal, resources, social support, control, vulnerability, and context.

Within the broad rubric of stress, three major traditions or spheres of scholarly work have historically flourished, each engendering voluminous amounts of research. Knowledge within these spheres has often been cultivated separately, with little attention paid to other parts of the overall process. Cohen and colleagues (1995), in discussing stress and disease risk, refer to these three traditions as the environmental stress perspective, biological stress perspective, and psychological stress perspective (pp. 4-8). The environmental perspective emphasizes elements of the environment or stressful events that happen to people that have an impact that brings about need for adjustment. The biological perspective encompasses processes within the body following exposure to a stressor. The psychological perspective focuses on perception, subjective meaning, and interpretation as crucial parts of the stress process.

Others have coined different labels for these perspectives. In theoretical terms, these spheres have been labeled stimulus, response, and relational (Lazarus & Folkman, 1984) or stimulus based, response based, and transactional (Cox, 1978; Derogatis & Coons, 1993; Lazarus & Folkman, 1984; Lyon & Werner, 1987). The stimulus-based orientation views stress as the initiator or spark of the stress process. Often, stress is viewed as originating outside of the individual. The response-based orientation posits that stress occurs within the individual and consists of complicated physiological changes that essentially serve to bring about adaptation but that, when overused, produce ill effects. This maladaptive functioning is often conceptualized as a precursor to disease or disorder. The transactional orientation focuses on individual differences, mainly through emphasis on cognitive and emotional aspects of the individual. The appraisal process is central to this perspective (Lazarus, 1966; Lazarus & Folkman, 1984).

In this chapter, we discuss one of these traditions of stress research and theorizing— the environmental or stimulus-based orientation. The chapter recounts the development and testing of this perspective on stress beginning with its historical origins. Following information on current conceptualizations, various dimensions underlying stressors are addressed. The chapter also discusses the relevance of stimulus-based stress knowledge, or the environmental perspective, for nursing. Next, measurement issues are discussed, along with various instruments designed to capture stress as stimulus. Finally, interventions are addressed as they relate to the stimulus-based perspective of stress.

➤ DEFINITION

No matter what the discipline or theoretical perspective of stress, all traditions have a concept of initiator of the stress process. In the environmental or stimulus-based perspective, this initiator is presumed to be the stress it-self. In addition to stress, this initiator is often alternately called the stressor (Breznitz & Goldberger, 1993; Elliott & Eisdorfer, 1982; Selye, 1956), the stimulus (Cox, 1978; Derogatis & Coons, 1993), or the activator or potential activator (Elliott & Eisdorfer, 1982). Stressors in the environmental or stress-as-stimulus perspective include both specific events and environmental conditions (Cohen et al., 1982).

As a result of the 1982 Institute of Medicine/National Academy of Sciences study on stress and health, Elliott and Eisdorfer (1982) defined *activator* as "internal or external environmental events or conditions that change an individual's present state" (p. 20). They included in their explanation that the absence of a certain condition or event can also be an activator. They differentiated activators from potential activators, which they stated had been shown by research to be activators in certain conditions. Furthermore, they stated that activators are not necessarily stressors, but that stressors are activators that are "sufficiently intense or frequent . . . to produce significant physical or psychosocial reactions" (p. 20). On the basis of an extensive review of the nursing research regarding stressors in patient-client populations, and Elliott and Eisdorfer's concept of reaction (1982, p. 20), Werner (1993) defined *stressor* as "an external or internal event, condition, situation, and/or cue, that has the potential to bring about, or actually activates significant physical or psychosocial reactions" (p. 15). The four variants or subconcepts are further elaborated in Table 5.1.

For the purposes of this chapter, the initiator of the stress process is termed stressor or stress-as-stimulus. Several other terms have also been used to denote stress-as-stimulus and are often based on the underlying dimension of stress portrayed. Examples include stressful life event, life-change event, life change, life event, and life stressor. Most embrace the idea that these stressors come from outside the individual, and that there is stress inherent in certain environmental events, regardless of individual differences.

TABLE 5.1 Four Stressor Subconcepts With Definitions and References

Subconcept	Definition With Corroboration From Literature	Reference
Event	A noteworthy happening, occasion, or occurrence	Kort and Weijma (1991)
	"Objective occurrences of sufficient magnitude"	Dohrenwend, Krasnoff, Askenasy, and Dohrenwend (1982, p. 336)
Situation	The sum total of internal and external stimuli that act on an organism within a given time interval; combination of circumstances at a certain moment	
	"Environmental circumstances that have stress-eliciting properties"	Suter (1986, p. 68)
	"Constellations of related events and conditions"	Lepore (1995, p. 103)
Condition	A state of being with attendant circumstances	
	"Demands made on the person by his environment"	Cox (1978, p. 15)
	"Forces of a deleterious nature"	Kort and Weijma (1991, p. 523)
	"Demands impinging on a person"	Mechanic (1968, p. 301)
Cue	A feature indicating the nature of something perceived	
	"Characteristics of environments which are recognized as disturbing or disruptive"	Cox (1978, p. 12)
	Intrusive thoughts or cues as stressors	Costa, Somerfield, and McCrae (1996); Hobfoll, Green, and Solomon (1996)

SOURCE: From Werner (1993, p. 15). Copyright © 1993 by Sigma Theta Tau International. Adapted with permission.

➤ HISTORICAL BACKGROUND

Inception of Stress-as-Stimulus

The origins of the stress-as-stimulus conceptualization appear to have begun in ancient history. Lazarus and Folkman (1984) related that as early as the 1300s, the term stress was used to describe adversity or hardship. In the 1600s, Hooke employed the term stress to refer to an external force in the physical science sense of load that produced strain in an object. These ideas are still employed in engineering today (Cox, 1978). Hinkle (1973) stated that in the 1800s in medicine, physicians such as Osler noted that intensity of life was thought to contribute to angina pectoris or heart pain.

In the 20th century, Cannon was known for studying physical and emotional stimuli and the resulting disruption in the internal environment of the body in the form of the fight-or-flight response. From early in the century to the 1930s, Adolf Meyer, a psychiatrist interested in the precursors of disease, developed a life chart that served as part of the medical examination and interview (as cited in Cohen et al., 1995). His biographies suggested that patients became ill shortly after clusters of major changes in their lives more often than patients without these clusters. Additional work stemming from this type of stressor or event interview in medical practice led to research in the 1940s that began to illuminate relationships between stressful life events and illness.

Also in the 1930s, Hans Selye began his work that has led to a large body of physiological stress research. As a medical student, Selye noticed the "syndrome of just being sick" in response to varying disease states (Selye, 1993, p. 9). Selye is known for his response-based definition of stress. Mason (1975), however, observed that Selye, in his early writings, appeared to use the term stress in the stimulus sense of the word and later changed his idea of stress to the nonspecific bodily response that has been his signature definition. Wolff was also known for his pioneering studies in the area of "life stress and disease in the 1940s and 1950s" (Lazarus & Folkman, 1984, p. 3). For example, in 1950, Wolff, Wolff, and Hare investigated stressful aspects of the telephone operator occupation and documented periods of stress that were associated with various illnesses (as cited in Cohen et al., 1995). Wolff and colleagues emphasized the dynamic state of the organism as a centerpiece of their conceptualization of stress. In the 1950s and 1960s, there were also several key pieces of research done focusing on war and combat, stemming from both the Korean and the Vietnamese conflicts. Effects of many major stressors were investigated, including bombing (Janis, 1951) and concentration camp experience (Bettelheim, 1960).

Social sources of stress began to gain in importance in the 1970s. Levine and Scotch's (1970) book *Social Stress* laid out many social stressors, such as work organization, the family life cycle, race, social class, social isolation, and role conflict. Incorporated in Levine and Scotch's volume are life stressors, including marriage and divorce. These topics as social stressors were the forerunners of the current area of life transitions as stressors.

In most of these historical conceptualizations and examinations of stress-as-stimulus, the other important factor contributing to stress is the adaptive capability of the person. Mechanic (1968) advocated that stress occurs in the presence of a stressor but also when the individual's adaptive capacities or resources either fail or are not able to completely handle the threatening episode. He defined stress as "a discrepancy between the demands impinging on a person—whether these demands be external or internal, whether challenges or goals—and the individual's potential responses to these demands" (p. 301). This view is one in which negative consequences such as illness occur when the adaptive response, or the ability to readjust, is of an inappropriate kind or insufficient in the face of a stressor.

Recent Conceptualizations of Stress-as-Stimulus

The theme of adaptation or readjustment leads quite clearly to perhaps the most often investigated and cited work in the area of stressors—that of Holmes and colleagues. Drawing on Meyers's use of the life chart to indicate major life disruptions that affect medical status, Holmes and colleagues (Holmes & Masuda, 1974; Holmes & Rahe, 1967) conceptualized stress as amount of life change, based on life experiences, that brings about the need for readjustment. Accordingly, their checklist measurement device was called the Social Readjustment Rating Scale (SRRS) (Holmes & Rahe, 1967). This tool is based on several assumptions concerning stress-as-stimulus. First, change, whether positive or negative, denotes stress. Second, various life events result in different degrees of necessary readjustment; across individuals, however, these levels are relatively similar. To reflect this assumption in their scale, the researchers used a panel of raters to establish average or normative levels of adjustment called life change units (LCUs) associated with each of 42 predetermined events, which were then added to obtain a score representing stress as life change. This summation indicates the third assumption—that stress in the form of life changes is cumulative.

The stress-as-stimulus perspective previously described became the dominant paradigm of stress research from the early 1970s to the present. This, in part, resulted from the ease of using the checklist measurement device as a quick and easy way to measure stress. It also resulted from the viewpoint that the change associated with certain events was stressful to everyone experiencing them. This viewpoint is reflected in Dohrenwend's often quoted definition of stressful life events as "objective occurrences of sufficient magnitude to bring about changes in the usual activities of most individuals who experience them" (Dohrenwend, Krasnoff, Askenasy, & Dohrenwend, 1982, p. 336).

For the past three decades, the stressful life event or stress-as-stimulus theoretical underpinnings have changed very little. Measurement (discussed in detail later), however, has taken on many variations. Theoretical assumptions still include that it is the degree of change or readjustment necessary that is stressful. Recent developments, however, denote that positive and negative events are not equivalent. Rather, negative life events call for more readjustment. Other recent conceptual modifications reflected in a variety of measurement instruments include elaboration of specific events for particular life roles or developmental stages, impact, context, importance, and vulnerability factors (Cohen et al., 1995).

Probably the most important theoretical premise of this stress-as-stimulus tradition is that an accumulation of life changes or of stressors is associated with subsequent probability of disease or negative health consequences. Cohen et al. (1995), in discussing the research immediately following the development of the SRRS, report that there was "documentation of dramatic associations" (p. 5) with regard to stressful life events and illness. Most research in this area, however, yields modest associations, usually in the correlational range from .10 to .30. Of course, these results yield up to 10% of the variance explained that otherwise might not be attributable. Although these correlations are too low to be considered extraordinary, they are consistently and sometimes substantially present in most studies of stressful life events with many health outcome measures.

The body of knowledge regarding stressful life events and their effects on health and illness has been developed in and is important to many disciplines, including psychology, sociology, nursing, medicine, psychiatry, occupational therapy, and physiology. The reason for this widespread interest stems from the large body of evidence supporting the fact that stressful life events and environmental conditions do have an impact on physical and psychological reactions and, in some cases, on health and illness (Turner & Wheaton, 1995). They have been shown to influence the risk for, the initiation of, and the course of a wide range of physical and emotional disorders from colds and infections (Cohen, Tyrrell, & Smith, 1991) to major health crises such as myocardial infarction, sudden cardiac death (Rahe & Lind, 1971), and posttraumatic stress disorder (American Psychiatric Association, 1994). Because of the substantial body of knowledge supporting this stress-illness relationship, it is no wonder many dimensions and aspects of stress-as-stimulus have been examined.

➤ CLASSIFICATIONS OF STRESS-AS-STIMULUS

Dimensions

There are many categorization and classification schemes that detail organizing systems for stressors. Each of these classifications could be characterized by the dimension that underlies the classification schema. Consideration of underlying dimensions is important as researchers attempt "to identify characteristics of the environment that promote illness" (Cohen et al., 1995, p. 6). For example, in a review of the nursing research on stressors, Werner (1993) discussed the dimensions of locus, duration, temporality, forecasting, tone, and impact as representative of the underpinnings of many of the available classifications of stressors. Major current classification systems and their underlying dimensions are described in the following sections (Table 5.2).

TABLE 5.2 Examples of Underlying Stressor Dimensions and Concomitant Stressor Classifications

Underlying Dimension	Stressor Classification	Reference
Locus	Internal: within the individual	Vogel and Bower (1991)
	External: outside of the individual	
Forecasting	Predictable: able to be foretold, anticipated	Paterson and Neufeld (1989)
	Unpredictable: not able to be foretold, unanticipated	
Tone	Positive: pleasant or desirable events or occurrences	Rose (1980)
	Negative: unpleasant or undesirable events or occurrences	Thoits (1983)
Temporality	Acute: severe but of short duration	Cohen, Kessler, and Gordon (1995)
	Chronic: lasting a long time, recurring	
Duration and frequency	Acute: time limited, usually of short duration	Cohen et al. (1982, p. 150)
	Stressor sequence: "series of events that occur over an extended period of time" usually as a result of an initiating stressor	Cohen et al. (1982, p. 150)
	Chronic intermittent: occurring regularly at intervals over a period of time	Cohen et al. (1982, p. 151)
	Chronic: "persist continuously for a long time"; "may or may not be initiated by a discrete event"	Cohen et al. (1982, p. 151)
Impact (global—family)	Normative (life transitions): expected and predictable changes	Figley and McCubbin (1983)
	Catastrophe: sudden, unexpected, often life threatening	McCubbin and Figley (1983)
Impact (social roles)	Scheduled events: life stage junctures with fair degree of certainty	Pearlin (1993)
	Unscheduled events: not expected, occur without warning, more severe	

SOURCE: From Werner (1993, p. 16). Copyright © 1993 by Sigma Theta Tau International. Adapted with permission.

Locus

One of the most prevalent underlying dimensions is locus—that is, whether the stressor is external or internal. Most stress theorists focusing on stress-as-stimulus or on stressful life events state that all stressors are external, objective, outside of the individual, or environmental in nature (Dohrenwend et al., 1982). For example, Turner and Wheaton (1995) defined "eventful stress" as having three distinct characteristics: "(1) discreteness, (2) observability in principle, and (3) a self-limiting time course" (pp. 32-33). Others, however, include internal "event" in their definition of stressor. For example, McEwen and Mendelson (1993) defined stressor as "an event that challenges homeostasis" (p. 101).

They relate that internal cues such as fear may have this same effect and therefore should be included in the rubric of stressor. In addition, Costa, Somerfeld, and McCrae (1996), citing the work of Palmer, Tucker, Warren, and Adams in 1993, related that traumatic or unexpected events of great magnitude such as the death of a loved one "often produce intrusive thoughts" (p. 46) that then become stressors (cues) in and of themselves. Although these internal conceptualizations of stressor are rare, they are present in the scholarly discourse on stress-as-stimulus (Table 5.2).

Forecasting

The underlying dimension of forecasting refers to the predictability of the stressor. Predictability is the ability to "foretell a future event or events" (Neufeldt & Guralnik, 1996, p. 1062). Obviously, this dimension could be categorized as predictable or unpredictable (Table 5.2). In reviewing several previous human studies, Paterson and Neufeld (1989) reported that there is "less behavioral or physiological evidence of stress with predictable stressor onset" (p. 34). They cite conflicting results, however. Therefore, the preparatory response hypothesis of Perkins (as cited in Paterson & Neufeld, 1989) that being able to predict stressors prepares the individual for impact is not wholly supported by previous research. An alternate hypothesis by Seligman and colleagues (as cited in Paterson & Neufeld, 1989) suggests that perhaps it is not the predictability of impact that reduces stress but rather that the ability to predict also communicates to the affected person that he or she is safe, therefore reducing stress in the period anticipatory to stressor impact. Whatever the mechanism of action, predictability has been shown to be an important characteristic in several stressor studies when it has been included as a variable.

Tone

Another underlying dimension for stressors or life events is tone or "the prevailing or predominant style, character, spirit, trend, or morale" (Neufeldt & Guralnik, 1996, p. 1408). For stress-as-stimulus research, tone refers to whether the stressor is positive or negative. Positive tone alludes to the event being pleasant or desired. Negative tone concerns unwanted, unpleasant, or undesirable occurrences (Table 5.2). In the early work by Holmes and colleagues (Holmes & Masuda, 1974; Holmes & Rahe, 1967), both positive and negative events were considered important in determining the level of life change or stress because both were thought to require readjustment. Evidence has accumulated, however, showing that it is more often the negatively toned events and conditions that bring about deleterious health outcomes (Cohen et al., 1982; Rose, 1980; Thoits, 1983; Zautra & Reich, 1983).

Temporality

Another underlying dimension that has been used to differentiate types of stressors is temporality. Temporality refers to the quality or state of being transitory or limited in time, together with a connotation of intensity. In addition to life event stressors being discrete and of short but influential impact, there has recently been an emphasis on studying ongoing, constant stressors. The terms most often associated with this dimension are acute and chronic. *Acute* is defined as "severe and sharp . . . but of short duration" (Neufeldt & Guralinik, 1996, p. 14), whereas *chronic* is defined as "lasting a long time or recurring often" (p. 250).

Cohen and colleagues (1995) report that although the terms acute and chronic are used frequently in the scholarly literature and research on stressors, there is little explanation of what these terms actually mean. They note that, depending on the outcome, these terms might be defined differently. For example, even 6 months of experiencing a certain stressful life event such as unemployment might be considered acute in comparison to a health or illness outcome that develops over a period of years such as coronary artery disease. This same stressor, however, most likely would be considered chronic when considering the development of reactive depression.

Duration and Frequency

Two other dimensions, related to temporality, that have been used to differentiate types of stressors are duration and frequency. *Duration* refers to the time something continues, whereas *frequency* refers to "the number of times any action or occurrence is repeated in a given period" (Neufeldt & Guralnik, 1996, p. 539). For example, in the report of the Institute of Medicine's study of stress and human health, Cohen et al. (1982) used duration and frequency as their dimensions of interest in developing four "broad types of stressors" (p. 150) affecting humans. These groupings consist of (a) acute stressors, or time-limited events or conditions or both such as waiting for surgery; (b) stressor sequence, or succession of events often following a more major stressor such as job loss (e.g., subsequent stressors might consist of financial problems, bankruptcy, and searching for a new job); (c) chronic intermittent stressors, which refer to events or conditions that occur intermittently during a period of time (e.g., conflict with supervisor and periodic need for allergy shots); and (d) chronic stressors, which might be exemplified by ongoing conflict with spouse. These stressors "may or may not be initiated by a discrete event and . . . persist continuously for a long time" (Cohen et al., 1982, p. 151). Therefore, this classification takes into account the characteristics of continuousness and repetitiveness (Cohen et al., 1995). This schema of stressors can also be found in Table 5.2.

Repetitiveness

The characteristic of repetitiveness has been reviewed by Lepore and Evans (1996), who described arrangements of multiple exposures to environmental stressors. They address the occurrence of more than one stressor in the patterns that follow: (a) One major stressful life event precedes one or more other secondary events or stressors. This pattern for individuals is similar to the stressor pileup that families experience that is conceptualized in the Double ABCX Model of Family Adaptation to Stress developed by McCubbin and colleagues (McCubbin & Patterson, 1983); (b) two or more unrelated events occur at or nearly at the same time, both affecting the individual; (c) two or more unrelated events occur either at the same time or temporally close in time, with either one or all having secondary event sequences stemming from the original discrete stressors; and (d) there may be several combinations of stressor event sequences, with many stressors interacting with other events and secondary events. For example, an individual may be experiencing secondary stressors from an event in the past when another discrete event occurs. It is unclear how the stressor patterns described previously affect individuals because research on these patterns is rare (Lepore & Evans, 1996) (Figure 5.1).

Lepore and Evans offered possible ways that effects of these stressor patterns might vary (Figure 5.1). In one, called simple main effects, the effect of two stressors is equal only to the effect that either one of them would have independently. A second model, termed additive, refers to the possibility that the effect of two stressors experienced at one time results in the combined effects of each of the stressors were they experienced independently. Their third model is called attenuated and posits that perhaps "the joint effect of stressors A and B is less than would be expected from the additive model" (p. 356). Finally, Lepore and Evans described a potentiation effect in which the concomitant effect of the two stressors is more than expected from the addition of the separate effects. One can see how these possibilities become very complicated if two or more stressors are experienced simultaneously.

An additional development of the role of duration in the stress process was described by Baum, Cohen, and Hall (1993). They discussed combinations of (a) duration of stressor

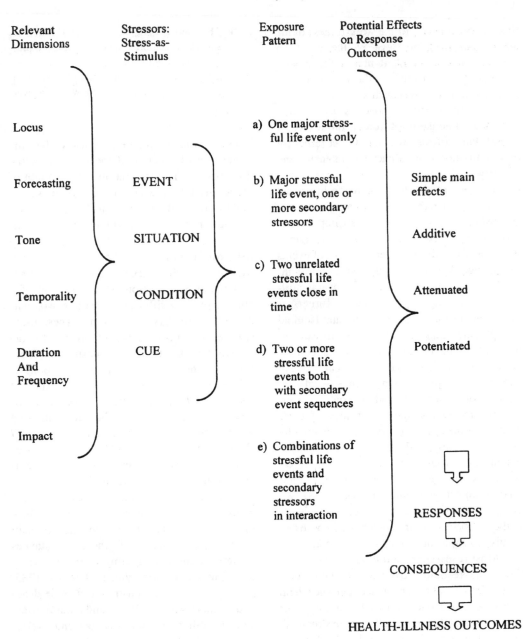

Figure 5.1. Model Depicting Potential Stressor Dimensions, Stress-as-Stimulus Subconcepts, Potential Patterns of Exposure, and Potential Response Outcome Effects

or event exposure, (b) duration of the resulting appraisal or perception of the threat, and (c) duration of the stress response. They represented these interrelationships in a 2 × 2 × 2 matrix.

Impact

Impact is a very important and often cited and studied dimension of stressful life events and other stressors. It can have two connotations. First, it refers to the stressfulness or the power, strength, or force of the event on the person(s). Second, it means the precise timing of the occurrence of the stressor (Lazarus & Folkman, 1984) such as in "time of impact." In this section, impact is used to discuss the dimension of force, influence, or stressfulness of the stimulus. Other terms for this connotation of impact are intensity and severity.

It is essentially the dimension of impact or intensity that researchers attempt to measure when they obtain ratings of importance, seriousness, or stressfulness by judges, raters, or those affected. Observers' ratings of events in this regard estimate stressfulness across individuals and therefore yield an "average difference in impact potential" (Turner & Wheaton, 1995, p. 43). Paterson and Neufeld (1989) stated that the severity of stressor impact is "one of the most fundamental considerations in the appraisal of a threat" (p. 26) and appears to be influenced by several subjective components, including goals or ideas of expected states, the importance of these goals, and the degree of threat engendered by goals not being attained. They conclude by explaining that greater stressfulness or severity can be affected by an increase in "magnitude of impact" or longer duration (p. 28). Degrees of stressfulness or impact are included in the classification of stressors by Lepore and Evans (1996) as described in Table 5.2.

Most researchers and theorists agree that there is a threshold above which certain events affect virtually everyone who experience them (Costa et al., 1996). Terms for this type of stress-as-stimulus include "extreme stressors" (Hobfoll, Freedy, Green, & Solomon, 1996, p. 322), disasters (Weisaeth, 1993), and cataclysms (Lepore & Evans, 1996). Hobfoll et al. (1996) noted the following properties of extreme stressors that differentiate them from less severe stressful events:

1. They attack people's most basic values (e.g., life and shelter).
2. They make excessive demands.
3. They often occur without warning.

4. They are outside the realm for which resource utilization strategies have been practiced and developed.
5. They leave a powerful mental image that is evoked by cues associated with the event (p. 328).

These characteristics help conceptualize the dimension of severity of the stressor, or the dimension of impact, that may be thought of as occurring on a continuum of lesser to greater stressfulness or intensity.

Another, more global connotation of impact has been offered by family stress theorists McCubbin and colleagues (Figley & McCubbin, 1983; McCubbin & Figley, 1983; McCubbin & Patterson, 1983). Instead of a continuum, this differentiation cites two qualitatively distinct types of events. These theorists separate major family stressors into normative life transitions and catastrophe (Table 5.2). They define *normative life transitions* as "changes or transitions which are expected and predictable, which most or even all families will experience over the life cycle, and which require adjustment and adaptation" (McCubbin & Figley, 1983, p. xxi). Examples include a family member leaving to go to college or to work and the addition of a new member. They define *catastrophe* as "an event which is sudden, unexpected, often life-threatening (to us or to someone we care deeply about), and due to the circumstances renders the survivors feeling an extreme sense of helplessness" (Figley & McCubbin, 1983, p. 6). Examples of catastrophe include death of a member, severe illness, and natural disasters and other extreme changes and events. These theorists explain that both of these types of stressors can have great impact on families and family life.

Similarly, Pearlin (1993), in discussing types of developmental and social stressors, categorizes life changes, what he terms "eventful experiences" (p. 312), into scheduled events and unscheduled events (Table 5.2). He defined *scheduled events* as those that are usually "junctures between life stages" that have a fair degree of certainty of occurring (p. 312). Examples include death of spouse and retirement. He described *unscheduled events* as those that are not expected and therefore "descend without prior warning" (p. 312). Examples include divorce and premature death of a loved one. Pearlin reported that the unscheduled events are associated with considerably more stress than the scheduled events, even though both types often engender large amounts of change. The unscheduled events therefore have greater impact.

The dimension of impact as discussed by McCubbin and colleagues was adapted by Werner (1993; Werner, Frost, & Orth, in press) to describe groupings of stressors targeted in the nursing research for the decade of 1980 to 1990 and the years 1991 to 1995, respectively. Stressors studied were found to focus in two broad areas. The first included the more predictable and often developmental life stress experiences and transitions, called life-related normative. The second overall grouping included catastrophic life stressors, or unexpected and often life-threatening situations, termed life-related catastrophic. Two other categories were subsets of the previous two. In this regard, Werner states,

> Because nursing is centrally concerned with health and departure from health, specific stressors related to health, illness, disease, and/or treatment were targeted, forming a subset within each major category. These subcategories were termed: *Health/ Illness-Related Normative . . .* and *Health/ Illness-Related Catastrophic.* (p. 17)

Table 5.3 contains these stressor categories, working definitions, examples, and percentages of studies in each category for each of the aforementioned reviews.

Context

Finally, another dimension that can be used to classify stressful life events is context. Context refers to "the whole situation, background, or environment relevant" (Neufeldt & Guralnik, 1996, p. 301). A classification of

environmental stressors based on context has been developed by Lepore and Evans (1996), who developed the following "general categories" (p. 352):

1. Cataclysms: These events are defined as "sudden, tumultuous, irrevocable events that impose great adaptive demands on many people" (p. 353). These events are generally severe in impact. Examples include floods, earthquakes, hurricanes, and war.

2. Major life events: These events are defined as being severe in impact to most people. They are described as being "episodic" and "irrevocable," calling for substantial adaptation (p. 353). Examples include death of partner, divorce, and unemployment.

3. Daily stressors: These stressors are the daily, ongoing, often minor stressors that occur repeatedly. They may, however, also be severe in nature. Often, they occur in tandem with other ongoing stressors. These stressors are similar to "daily hassles," a concept developed by Kanner, Coyne, Schaefer, and Lazarus (1981). Examples include lost car keys, "words" with the boss or partner, and lateness for an appointment.

4. Ambient stressors: Ambient stressors are defined as characteristics of the environment that are difficult to change and that have an ongoing effect on those in the environment ranging from minor to severe. Examples include overcrowding, noise, and pollution.

5. Role stressors: These stressors are generally ongoing and are related to the social obligations of the person experiencing them. When these stressors occur in important social roles, such as marriage or work, they can be severe (Lepore & Evans, 1996).

Lepore and Evans note that any of the stressors described previously can interact with any of the other types, generating some of the stressor patterns previously mentioned. Often, according to these researchers, cataclysmic or major life events give way to a host of daily and role stressors, complicating the research conducted on, and the understanding of, the effects of the various stressor types.

TABLE 5.3 Classification of Stressor Research in Nursing, Working Definitions, Examples, and Percentages of Studies From Two Extensive Reviews

Stressor Category	Working Definition	Example	Percentages of Studies	
			1980-1990	1991-1995
Life-Related Normative	Events, situations, conditions, or cues that are usually expected, that most experience, and that require adjustment or adaptation	Adolescence Role adjustment	16.3	10.5
Health/Illness-Related Normative	Events, situations, conditions, or cues that are related to health or to illness, and/or treatment for these, and that are usually expected, that most experience, and that require adjustment or adaptation	Menstruation Normal pregnancy	17.5	7.5
Life-Related Catastrophic	Events, situations, conditions, or cues that are generally unpredictable, usually infrequent, and commonly result in dire consequences in addition to requiring adjustment or adaptation	Involuntary relocation of elderly Loss of spouse	11.2	10.0
Health/Illness-Related Catastrophic	Events, situations, conditions, or cues that are related to health or to illness, and/or to treatment for these, and that are generally unpredictable, usually infrequent, and commonly result in dire consequences in addition to requiring adjustment or adaptation	Acute myocardial infarction Breast biopsy Hospitalization Surgery	55.0	72.0

SOURCE: From Werner (1993, pp. 17-18). Copyright © 1993 by Sigma Theta Tau International. Adapted with permission.

➤ STRESS-AS-STIMULUS IN NURSING KNOWLEDGE

Nursing has a long tradition of studying stress and stressors as they relate to life, health, and illness. Nursing stress studies date back to 1956 when the first indexed reference to stress appeared in the Cumulative Index for Nursing and Allied Health Literature (CINAHL). In a review and critical examination of nursing research regarding stress for the years 1974 to 1984, 28% ($n = 23$) of the 82 studies meeting inclusion criteria focused on stress-as-stimulus (Lyon & Werner, 1987). In a later comprehensive review and synthesis of findings in nursing for the years spanning 1980 through 1990, there were 133 studies focused on stressors, 81 of which met criteria for inclusion in the evaluation (Frost, 1993; Werner, 1993). Yet another review for the years 1991 through 1995 yielded an overall total of 362 studies fitting within the rubric of nursing research on stressors (Frost, Orth, & Werner, in press; Werner et al., in press). The tremendous growth in the number of stress-as-stimulus studies in nursing mirrors the large number of these studies in related disciplines and indicates nursing's increasing interest in stressors and life change.

Theoretical and Conceptual Development

Nursing has also included stress-as-stimulus in the theoretical work of the discipline. Theories developed by Neuman, Erickson, Tomlin, and Swain, Roy, and Johnson have all focused to different degrees on stressors and stress. For example, Neuman (1989) adapted a systems framework and incorporated primary, secondary, and tertiary prevention. The goal of her model is to guide nurses to protect and fortify the individual, family, or community from noxious stressors. Erickson, Tomlin, and Swain (1983) adapted Selye's view of stress as a reaction with basic needs as described by Maslow, psychosocial and cognitive development, loss and attachment, and object relations to assist nurses in understanding clients and their health. Their process of modeling is useful in understanding the world of the client including stressors.

Roy's theory (1984) focuses on adaptation as a person-environment interaction, which if successful contributes to health. People are depicted as adapting to internal and external stimuli called focal stimuli or stressors. Stressors as explained by Roy lead to a stress response that is explained by Selye's theory. The nurse's role is to promote effective adaptation. Johnson (1980) focused on nursing care for people who are experiencing stress related to health or illness. Similar to the work of Roy, Johnson proposed that stressors, or internal or external stimuli, disrupt the equilibrium of the person's system. The goal of nursing is to promote equilibrium and thereby facilitate system integrity.

All these theoretical frameworks emphasize the importance of stress and stressors in the nursing care of patients. Their importance lies in the fact that they underscore the need for nurses to attend to the human experience of stress to promote health and to mitigate illness. None of them, however, are able to assist in understanding stressors or stress-as-stimulus at an empirical level. Blegen and Tripp-Reimer (1997) noted that these early nursing models, although "essential in nursing's articulation of its identity . . . evolved parallel to, rather than interwoven with, research" (p. 38). Blegen and Tripp-Reimer underscore the need for middle-range theories to account for what is observed in a generalizable way. No such theories regarding stress-as-stimulus have been developed in nursing. Adaptations of stress theories focusing on other aspects of the stress process, however, have been developed (Scott, Oberst, & Dropkin, 1980). Regarding stress-as-stimulus, nursing has largely to this point conducted research that stems from and contributes to the theoretical knowledge base from other disciplines, mainly psychology, sociology, and family studies. In addition, much of the nursing research conducted to describe and explain stress-as-stimulus has been atheoretical (Frost, 1993; Lyon & Werner, 1987; Werner, 1993).

Research

Despite the great interest in examining stressors of human beings in nursing, few substantial ongoing programs of research have been sustained. One clear-cut exception to this is the program of research on hospital stressors carried out by Volicer in the 1970s. This program could be classified as focusing on health or illness-related catastrophic stressors (Table 5.3). Volicer and colleagues (Volicer, 1974, 1977; Volicer & Bohannon, 1975; Volicer & Burns, 1977; Volicer & Volicer, 1977) based their studies on the assumption that hospitalization is a stressful experience that occurs in the lives of most people. They also assumed that there were many concerns associated with hospitalization that could be considered stressful. To mitigate any untoward effects of these stressors on recovery during hospitalization, these stress factors needed to be measured and assessed. Volicer and colleagues further reasoned that unfamiliar procedures, equipment, unfamiliar personnel, routines, and jargon might be stressful for patients.

Therefore, Volicer and Bohannon (1975) designed an instrument to assess stressors in the hospital environment. Their procedure was modeled after the tool development strategies of Holmes and Rahe (1967). First, these researchers interviewed 23 people about their hospitalization experiences. From these interviews, they developed 45 potential stressors. Then, a sample of 216 nonhospitalized individuals were assigned scores for all items using a scaling procedure similar to that of Holmes and colleagues. Volicer (1977) stated, however, that instead of the change required, events were scored on their "level of stress produced or readjustment required" (p. 56). Once rankings and scores were assigned, items were revised and added, increasing the total number of items to 77. The tool was then used with 216 actual hospital patients using a card-sort procedure. Interestingly, findings from this study indicated that three of the five highest ranking items involved loss or potential loss (loss of sight, kidney, and hearing). One of the most clear factors in a subsequent factor analysis was labeled "Threat of Severe Illness" (Volicer, 1977, p. 64) and included all the loss items.

Although the procedure for measuring stressors associated with hospitalization is not free of limitations, Volicer and colleagues clearly identified many stressful hospital-associated characteristics and events that may affect a patient. Stressors identified by these researchers included unfamiliar surroundings, loss of independence, separation from loved ones and supportive others, and isolation, in addition to the loss issues already mentioned. Because hospitalization in the current health care system has changed dramatically (in-creased acuity and shorter hospital stays), however, it is unclear if the stressors identified by Volicer and colleagues are still relevant. New studies are warranted to identify the current hospital-associated stressors.

Another Health/Illness-Related Catastrophic program of research concerning hospitalization was conducted by Carter and Miles and colleagues (Carter & Miles, 1982; Carter, Miles, Buford, & Hassanein, 1985; Eberly, Miles, Carter, Hennessey, & Riddle, 1985; Graves & Ware, 1990; Miles & Carter, 1982; Miles, Carter, Spicker, & Hassanein, 1984). Their series of studies focused on illuminating stressors associated with being the parent of a child hospitalized in a pediatric intensive care unit (ICU). Findings of several of these studies supported the hypothesis that hospital-related factors were not as severe in stressor intensity as other factors, including role and relationship with the child in addition to the child's feelings, behavior, and appearance. Werner (1993, p. 27) provided the following generalizations gleaned from the studies cited previously:

1. Stressors associated with parental role and parent-child relationships are more powerful than other types of stressors facing these parents.
2. Stressors associated with the child's behavior, emotions, and appearance have more impact than environmental stressors.
3. Parents perceiving themselves inadequately prepared for ICU experience report more stress from stressors than those who believe themselves to be adequately prepared.
4. Parents of children admitted under emergency conditions are more stressed than parents of children admitted for planned surgery or for relapse of disease.
5. Although Perehudoff (1990) found that mothers reported greater overall stress than fathers, the more consistent finding is that mothers and fathers are equally stressed, but most salient types of stressors differ.

Another program of research deserving of mention is the research of Murphy, who studied the Life-Related Catastrophic stressors associated with disaster in the 1980s (Murphy, 1984, 1986a, 1986b, 1987, 1988, 1989). Murphy's focus was the survivors of the Mount St. Helens disaster, and her longitudinal research program spanned nearly a decade. In 1983, for example, Murphy collected data on disaster-bereaved subjects from her previous study and nondisaster-loss control participants. She found that among other variables, including age, sex, education, social support, and self-efficacy, negative life stress was a predictor for the outcome variable of mental distress. This finding, however, pertained only to the control group, accounting for 19% of the variance. For the disaster bereaved, only mental distress reported 2 years earlier and self-efficacy explained mental distress (Murphy, 1988). Murphy's results contribute to the conceptualizations of cataclysmic stressors and their relationships with related factors and outcomes.

There are several other areas of important stress-as-stimulus research in nursing, including the focus on stressors regarding pregnancy, birth, and the postpartum period being conducted by Mercer, Ferketich, and colleagues (Ferketich & Mercer, 1990, 1995; Mercer & Ferketich, 1990). Another Health/Illness-Related Catastrophic body of findings that is increasing concerns the severe stressor of cardiac surgery, such as coronary artery bypass surgery, valve replacement, pericardectomy, and cardiac transplant. For example, in 1986, Carr and Powers studied stressors pertinent to patients having coronary artery bypass graft surgery (CABG). They found that the four most intense stressors (the prospect of having surgery on the heart, worry about resuming lifestyle, pain, and fear of dying) were related to the illness, whereas one of the most severe stressors concerned the hospitalization (being absent from home and business). This study was replicated by Yarcheski and Knapp-Spooner (1994), who found, as did Carr and Powers, that (a) nurses generally rated most stressors, particularly hospital related and illness related, as more stressful for CABG patients than did patients and (b) both patients and nurses rated illness-related items as more

stressful than hospital-related items. This replication also indicated that stressfulness of stressors for CABG patients was considerably higher than that for patients in the original study. This result was believed to be due to timing because Yarcheski and Knapp-Spooner measured stressor impact on the third postoperative day versus the sixth to eighth day as in the original study. This difference suggests stressor severity diminishes as time from surgery increases.

The findings of two extensive reviews regarding stressors are pertinent in summarizing some of the nursing research conducted on stress-as-stimulus and stressful life events. The previously mentioned 10-year (1980-1990) review (Frost, 1993; Werner, 1993) yielded the following generalizations: First, the five areas of most intense Health/Illness-Related Catastrophic stressors among those areas studied included pediatric ICU hospitalization of one's own child, acute myocardial infarction, renal transplant, coronary bypass surgery, and hemodialysis and continuous ambulatory peritoneal dialysis. Second, in people experiencing catastrophic stressors related to health and illness, the health or illness losses and potential losses as well as treatment issues were found to be more severely stressful than were concomitant stressful life events. Third, nurses consistently rated most illness- and hospital-related stressors as more stressful than did patients or family members. This generalization persisted with many different patient and family groups, including CABG surgery patients (Carr & Powers, 1986), hospitalized elderly individuals (Davies & Peters, 1983), and parents of patients in pediatric units (Miles & Carter, 1982). The reason for this finding is unclear. It is plausible, however, that patients and family members experienced greater stress from events and situations not captured by the measurement devices used.

The fourth major generalization regarding stressors was that illness and disease-related stressors were generally rated as more stressful than any other types of stressors such as environmental conditions. Regarding this conclusion, "there is strong evidence that environmental aspects of hospitalization and/or the ICU are relatively minor when compared with the impact of the illness or disease conditions being dealt with" (Werner, 1993, p. 26). This finding held true for patients, clients, and family members. Finally, the loss-related stressors, such as threat of role functioning loss, loss of life, and loss of function, were the most powerful stressors in Health/Illness-Related Catastrophic studies (Werner, 1993).

➤ MEASUREMENT

Background

In 1984, Norbeck asserted that the popularity of measuring stress by life events had not waned despite unresolved methodological and theoretical questions. This assertion continues to be true today. A recent search of the literature revealed that the research on stressful life events has increased dramatically in the past few years. Although there were 7,207 articles identified using a Medline search of life events between the years 1963 and 1998, less than 10% ($n = 515$) were published before 1980. In addition, there was an increase in the number of articles identified in the 9-year period 1990 to 1998 ($n = 3,611$) compared to the previous 10-year period of time ($n = 3,073$). This same trend was identified with a CINAHL search in which fewer than 1% of the stressful life event articles were published before 1980. A larger number of articles were published from 1990 to 1998 ($n = 335$) compared to 1980 to 1989 ($n = 182$).

Self-Report Methods

The initiation of stressful life event measurements, and theoretical orientation of stress-as-stimulus as already addressed, is often credited to Holmes and Rahe with the development of the SRRS in 1967. Work in the area of life events, however, began long before the development of the SRRS. As far back as 1949, Homes and Rahe used a life chart modeled after the work of Adolph Meyer. In the 1930s, Meyer, building on the science of psychobiology, used a life chart device to organize medical data that he envisioned as dynamic, involving a relationship between biological, psychological, and sociological phenomena (Holmes & Rahe, 1967). By the late 1940s, Meyer's data provided support for associations between stressful life events and physical health or illness outcomes (Wolff et al., 1950).

In 1957, Hawkins, Davies, and Holmes developed the Schedule of Recent Experiences (SRE) to systematize Meyer's life chart. In 1967, Holmes and Rahe modified the SRE by assigning weights to represent the amount of difficulty or change created by each event (Holmes & Masuda, 1974). Holmes and Rahe made this change because they believed the addition of estimating the magnitude of various life events would advance the precision of their research. They developed this aspect of their research by providing individuals a list of life changes and asking them to score each event using as a pivot point an arbitrary score of 500 for marriage. This methodology resulted in a weighted score, an average, referred to as a LCU, for each event. The resulting SRRS measured changes in sleep, eating, social life, recreation, personal activities, and interpersonal habits (Rahe, 1968, 1972). Adding LCUs for each event experienced yielded a total SRRS score, which was used as a predictor of illness in the next 2 years. Interestingly, the process of developing the SRRS led Holmes and Rahe (1967) to note that "as expected, the psychological significance and emotions varied widely with the patient" (p. 216). They chose, however, to focus on what they termed the high degree of consensus in assigned scores to indicate the amount of stress created by each life change event, in turn sacrificing the individual perspective.

Several basic assumptions were used in the development of the SRRS: (a) Life-change events are normative, requiring a similar amount of adjustment across individuals and time; (b) the positive or negative tone of the event is irrelevant; (c) there is a common threshold beyond which disruption occurs; and (d) stress is an additive phenomenon (Rahe, 1977). These assumptions imply that individuals are passive recipients of stress.

The basic assumptions used in the development of the SRRS served as a basis for many life event instruments developed in the 1970s and even in the present. Various researchers have revised Holmes and Rahe's tool and measurement methodology by making changes in weighting of items, the specific events included, and the significance of negative and positive events. Researchers have also placed emphasis on events that are unique to specific populations for whom stressors or life events may be different from those of the general population. For instance, Coddington (1972a, 1972b) modified the SRRS to measure stressful life events in childhood. Volicer and Bohannon (1975) based the development of the Hospital Stress Rating Scale for use with medical, surgical, and psychiatric patients on Holmes and Rahe's work. Lengthier life event scales were developed, such as the Psychiatric Epidemiological Research Interview-Life Events Scale developed by Dohrenwend, Krasnoff, Askenasy, and Dohrenwend (1978, 1982) for a psychiatric population, allowing individuals to assign their own weight or score, and the Universal and Group Specific Events Scale by Hough (as cited in Miller, 1981) to incorporate differences based on ethnic group. Other numerous life event and stressor instruments identified as a result of the recent search of the literature previously mentioned can be found in Table 5.4.

Interview Methods

The use of interview methods to obtain information on life events was also introduced in the 1970s. The interview approach has generally been semistructured, with the interviewer requesting information about experiences with various events. For any event experienced by the participant, the interviewer probes the response to obtain contextual data and the level of significance. The most frequently used interview technique is the Life Events and Difficulties developed by Brown and Harris (1978). Other instruments using an interview approach are identified in Table 5.4.

Other

Recently, life event measurements have focused on individuals' subjective appraisals of particular events. Specifically, instead of predetermined weights given to events, individuals are asked to rate the amount of stress that they have experienced as a result of a particular event or stressor. For example, Budd, Workman, Lemsky, and Quick (1994) focused on headaches in children, whereas Gupta and Gupta (1995) emphasized stressors related to psoriasis.

Methodological Concerns

Terminology

Several terms are used in the life events literature, including life events, life change events, and life change. The Medline and CINAHL search term is "life change events." It is not clear how life change differs from life events. These terms are used interchangeably at times. It is also not clear how use of the term event differs from use of the term stressor because many items on life change event inventories are of smaller magnitude than one would associate with an event. For example, on the Hospital Stress Rating Scale (Volicer & Bohannon, 1975), "your call light answered" was considered an event. Cohen et al. (1995) assert the importance of distinguishing between events and other possible sources of stress. This is not possible if terminology is not consistent among researchers.

An examination of definitions reveals that an event is defined as something that happens, and change is defined as making something different (Kidney, 1993). Although

TABLE 5.4 Stressful Life Events, Life Change Events, and Stressor Instruments

Instrument	Measurement Focus
Adolescent-Family Inventory of Life Events and Changes (McCubbin, Patterson, Bauman, & Harris, 1981)	Recent family, adolescent, and youth life events and changes; chronic stressors and strains; the family's and youth's vulnerability and cumulative life events
Adolescent Life Change Event Scale (Yeaworth, York, Hussey, Ingle, & Goodwin, 1980)	Adolescent life change events
Adolescent Life Experiences (Towbes, Cohen, & Glyshaw, 1989)	Life stress inventory for adolescents
Adolescent Perceived Events Scale (Compas, Davis, Forsythe, & Wagner, 1987)	Adolescents rate life events according to desirability, impact, and frequency
Childhood Life Events and Family Characteristics Questionnaire (Byrne, Velamoor, Cernovsky, Cortese, & Losztyn, 1990)	Childhood life events and parent-child relationship
Children's Life Event Questionnaire (Deutsch & Erickson, 1989)	Early childhood life events
Childhood Unwanted Sexual Events (Lange, Kooiman, Huberts, & van Oostendorp, 1995)	Incidence of childhood experiences with sexual threat or abuse or both
Children's Headache Assessment Scale (Budd, Workman, Lemsky, & Quick, 1994)	Environmental events and variables associated with pediatric headache
Chronicity Impact and Coping Instrument: Parent Questionnaire (Hymovich, 1983)	Parent concerns in caring for a child with a chronic health problem
Detroit Couples Study Life Events Method (Kessler & Wethington, 1991)	Checklist of life events with semistructured interview probes
Family Inventory of Life Events and Changes (McCubbin, Patterson, & Wilson, 1980)	Life events and changes experienced by the family in the preceding year
General Life Events Schedule for Children (Sandler, Nolichuk, Brauer, & Fogas, 1986)	Events of children of divorce
Geriatric Social Readjustment Rating Scale (Amster & Krauss, 1974)	Life events of geriatric population
Hemodialysis Stressor Scale (Murphy, Powers, & Jalowiec, 1985)	Stressors associated with hemodialysis
Henderson, Byrne, & Duncan-Jones List of Recent Experiences (Henderson, Byrne, & Duncan-Jones, 1981)	Interview to obtain life events
High School Social Readjustment Scale (Tolor, Murphy, Wilson, & Clayton, 1983)	Stressful events in high school students
Hospital Stress Rating Scale (Volicer & Bohannon, 1975)	Events related to the experience of hospitalization
Impact of Event Scale (Horowitz, 1979)	Degree of subjective impact experienced during the preceding week as a result of a specific life event
Interview for Recent Life Events (Paykel, 1997)	Semistructured interview to establish life events and month in which they occurred
Interview Schedule for Events and Difficulties (Brown & Harris, 1978)	Life events and stressors
Junior High Life Events Survey (Swearingen & Cohen, 1985)	Life events of junior high school students

TABLE 5.4 Continued

Instrument	Measurement Focus
Life Change Inventory (Costantini, Braun, Davis, & Ivervolino, 1974)	Quantification of life events experienced by college students
Life Crisis History (Antonovsky & Kats, 1967)	Life crisis
Life Events and Difficulties Schedule (Brown & Harris, 1982)	Interview to obtain life events
Life Events Checklist (Johnson & McCutcheon, 1980)	Life stress in older children and adolescents
Life Events Inventory (Cochrane & Robertson, 1973)	Psychosocial stressors and the distress created
Life Event Questionnaire (Norbeck, 1984)	Life event questionnaire modified for adult female population of child-bearing age
Life Events Questionnaire (Horowitz, Schaefer, Hiroto, Wilner, & Levin, 1977)	Life events
Life Event Scale for Adolescents (Coddington & Troxell, 1980)	Life events of adolescents
Life Experiences Survey (Sarason, Johnson, & Siegel, 1978)	Life events experienced in the past 12 months
Life Stress Inventory (Cohen-Sandler, Berman, & King, 1982)	Life stress of children
Louisville Older Person Event Scale (Murrell, Norris, & Hutchins, 1984)	Life events in older adults
Modified SRRQ (Coddington, 1972a)	Life events in children
Munich Events List (Wittchen, Essau, Hecht, Teder, & Pfister, 1989)	Life events interview in which context is explored
Paykel Brief Life Event List (Paykel, 1983)	Interview of life events and difficulties with contextual probes
Psoriasis Life Stress Index (Gupta & Gupta, 1995)	Checklist of psoriasis-related events and rating of effect of each event
Psychiatric Epidemiological Research Interview-Life Events Scale (PERI-LES) (Dohrenwend, Krasnoff, Askenasy, & Dohrenwend, 1978)	Life events scale for psychiatric population
Psychosocial Assessment of Childhood Experiences (Glen, Simpson, Drinnan, McGuinness, & Sandberg, 1993)	Life events and experiences in childhood
Questionnaire on Resources and Stress (Glidden, 1993)	Demands, stresses, strains, and resources of families raising children with developmental disabilities
Questionnaire on Stress in Patients With Diabetes—Revised (Herschbach et al., 1997)	Sources of stress and the amount of distress experienced with each source
Recent Life Change Questionnaire (Rahe, 1975)	Life changes
Review of Life Events (Hurst, Jenkins, & Rose, 1978)	Life change stress
Schedule of Recent Life Events (SRE) (Holmes & Rahe, 1967)	Life changes listed by year of occurrence
Social Readjustment Rating Scale (Holmes & Rahe, 1967)	Quantification of experienced life events

(continued)

TABLE 5.4 Continued

Instrument	Measurement Focus
Social Readjustment Scale for Children (Coddington, 1972b)	Quantification of experienced life events of children
Spouse Transplant Stressor Scale (Collins, White-Williams, & Jalowiec, 1996)	Stressors associated with heart transplant
Stokes-Gordon Stress Scale (Stokes & Gordon, 1988)	Stressors of adults 65 years old or older
Student Life Stress Inventory (Gadzella, 1994)	Undergraduate college student stressors
Subjective Stress Scale (Bramston & Fogarty, 1995)	Stressors of people with intellectual disabilities
Symptom Severity Index (Black, Griffiths, & Pope, 1996)	Severity of stress incontinence and bothersome symptoms
The Children of Alcoholics Life-Events Schedule (Roosa, Sandler, Gehring, Beals, & Cappo, 1988)	Life events and stressors of children of alcohol-abusing parents
The Standardized Event Rating System (Dohrenwend, Raphael, Schwartz, Stueve, & Skodol, 1993)	Interview derived from the PERI and to be used with a variety of populations
The Universal and Group-Specific Event Scale (Hough as cited in Miller, 1981)	Incorporated life event differences based on ethnic group
Undergraduate Stress Questionnaire (Crandall, Preisler, & Aussprung, 1992)	Life event stress in college students
War Events Scale (Unger, Gould, & Babich, 1998)	Experiences with war-time atrocities and the distress associated with them

obviously two different concepts, the interchangeable use of these terms is consistent with the stress-as-stimulus model, in which events are assumed to create change in individuals regardless of their appraisal of those situations.

Life events were originally defined by Holmes and Rahe (1967) as changes that are indicative of or require significant readjustment. They accentuated change from a steady state and not the psychological meaning, emotion, or social desirability associated with the change. A favorable event was assumed to require as much of an adjustment as an unfavorable event, and similarity in individuals' responses was emphasized while ignoring the diversity that exists. Similar to Holmes and Rahe's definition, Dohrenwend and colleagues (1978, 1982) defined stressful life events as objective occurrences that are of a magnitude that require changes in the usual activities of most individuals.

Despite the continued use of terminology similar to that of Holmes and Rahe (1967), there is movement toward exploring life events as a concept influenced by individuals' appraisals of events and factors that influence life events. The theoretical underpinnings of stress-as-stimulus, however, still influence the methodology chosen by many researchers. This was apparent in the aforementioned 5-year review of identified stressors in nursing research in which very few researchers identified individuals' appraisals of how disruptive or significant, identified stressors were to their lives (Frost et al., in press).

Other

Several other methodological concerns have also been posed. One is the unidimensional nature of most of the life event scales, in which many of the factors that may affect the significance of a life event are ignored. For instance, potential factors often not measured include individuals' coping abilities, understanding of the event, social networks, cultural bias, personality, clustering with other events, biological variables, socioeconomic status, and interpersonal support systems (Werner, 1996; Werner & O'Neill, 1992). The lack of examining life events from a multidimensional perspective may explain why the relationships between life events and illness onset are often weak (Lyon & Werner, 1987; Norbeck, 1984) and results among studies are conflicting.

The significance of including positive events is not fully understood. Although correlations between negative events and health distress have been fairly consistent, the associations between positive events and health or distress have not (Zautra & Reich, 1983). It is possible that the effects of positive events are not captured with current theoretical models that do not account for the multiple factors that influence outcomes.

Comparison of results across life event studies is difficult due to variations in the life events included in the instrument, the time reference, weights given to each event, and decisions regarding what is a positive compared to a negative event. Specifically, some of the life events instruments are very specific to a given population and thus not transferable to other populations. Even among the general life event instruments, there is a lack of consistency in the events measured and the inclusion of positive events. Items rated differently result in score differences. Likewise, omission of any potential events may result in the underestimation of an individual's risk for detrimental health outcomes. Some researchers have accounted for the potential omission of an event significant to the study participant

through the addition of an opportunity for the participant to list additional events at the end of the scale.

Available instruments reference a variety of time intervals, such as last week, last month, and last year. The names of the instruments provide little if any guidance with regard to the time period that they reference. For instance, the SRE (Hawkins et al., 1957), the forerunner of the SRRS (Holmes & Rahe, 1967), actually measures events during the past 12 months and not the past week or past few days as the name suggests. The most appropriate time period for referencing of items is not clear. The 1-year time reference initially used in life event instruments was chosen because it was thought that it was the period of time needed to allow health outcomes to manifest (Holmes, 1979; Holmes & Masuda, 1974). The 12-month time interval, however, has been debated. Some researchers have reported that the time interval before health outcomes are manifested is approximately 6 months rather than 1 year (Rutter, 1989), whereas others note that a time interval of at least 6 months is important (Brown & Harris, 1978). A related issue has been raised by Cohen and colleagues (1995), who pointed out that it is unclear how long events have an effect on health outcomes. It is likely that events such as parental conflict, divorce, and physical or sexual abuse leave lifelong scars. Other events have an effect for a much shorter period of time, and these effects may not be evident 1 year after the event. Time of measurement is also important in terms of recall. A fallout rate of 1% to 5% per month has been identified with the recall of major events. When dealing with less important events, the fallout is higher (Brown & Harris, 1982; Funch & Marshall, 1984).

Artificial differences between study findings can also be found as a result of researchers providing different weights for various events. Although some researchers weight undesirable events stronger than desirable events, others weigh them identically. Some researchers assign negative and positive valences to an event. It is generally the researcher who makes judgments regarding the positive or negative effect of various events (Levenstein et al., 1993). Another area of concern is that illness may influence the report of a real or artificially high number of events (Cohen et al., 1995). There is also evidence suggesting that individuals may report a stressor as a result of a relatively minor event as if it was a significant event (Dohrenwend, Link, Kern, Shrout, & Markowitz, 1990).

Comparison of results is often confounded by the inclusion of various concepts in a life event measurement. Glidden (1993) reported theoretical difficulties in the development of life event tools due to the mixing of demands, stresses, and strains. Glidden identified each of these concepts as distinct, with a demand defined as a separate concept. He defined *demand* as a potential stressor created by the external environment, *stress* as the relationship between an external force and that to which the force is applied, and *strain* as the negative effect of stress on an individual. Other researchers include a mixture of stressors, stress reactions such as emotions, psychological function, and physical effects in their life event scales (Levenstein et al., 1993). The mixture of concepts results in the inability to make clear and specific conclusions about any of the included concepts.

Measurement: Future Directions

Little is known about the influence of timing of an event on health outcomes. For instance, if an event occurs during one developmental stage compared to another, are the effects more detrimental? Likewise, the result of the interaction of events is relatively unknown. If several events occur within a short time period, the effects on health outcomes may be different than if they occur months apart.

The majority of the life event research that exists is focused on acute health outcomes, with little emphasis on long-term chronic effects. In addition, there may be vul-

nerability factors (Cohen et al., 1995) by which some individuals are more susceptible to the physical and mental effects of stress than others. Exploration of factors that predict vulnerability would be useful in the development of life event models to guide research. Although individuals' appraisal of the situation has been added to several of the life event scales, many researchers continue to ignore the significance of this concept.

➤ IMPLICATIONS FOR NURSING PRACTICE

Interventions

Potential interventions associated with life change events and stressors are still in need of testing through research; therefore, they cannot be identified with certainty. Interventions vary for every stressor and with knowledge of the factors influencing individuals' appraisal of stressors. Therefore, it is not feasible to list all potential associated interventions. Obviously, there are some life change events and other stressors that are not predictable, avoidable, or changeable. Examples include death and weather-related catastrophic events. In these situations, focus needs to be placed on cognitive interventions that influence appraisal or on supporting the individual(s) in obtaining resources to meet related challenges.

In some situations, reframing can be used, in which the appraisal of the situation is refocused so that the situation is viewed from a more positive perspective. For situations that are obviously not positive, and cannot be reframed as such, stress management techniques can be taught to mitigate the distress resulting from the stressor and stress process. Interventions shown to be effective include relaxation techniques, massage therapy, journaling, music therapy, art therapy, and guided imagery. Support groups may be useful for individuals who have experienced similar types of events, and assisting individuals in seeking social support may be of assistance.

Purposeful priority setting and purposeful problem solving may be useful techniques for individuals who are overwhelmed by the number of life change events or stressors to which they have been exposed. Another intervention with potential to assist persons facing one or more meaningful stressors or changes is values clarification. Assisting individuals to identify life changes that are best delayed until the level of stress they are experiencing diminishes may also be a useful intervention. Assisting individuals to proactively examine the number of planned significant events (such as the purchase of a house and marriage) or to anticipate foreseeable events (such as an expected death) may be useful in giving individuals control over the number of events or stressors to which they are simultaneously exposed. At times when an individual is unable to prioritize for himself or herself, such as when comatose, the health care provider may need to play a more active role in limiting the number of stressors that are impinging on the person.

The level of stress experienced by individuals is dependent on the stressors they face and on their appraisal of any given situation. Assessment skills are needed to thoroughly evaluate not only the life change events or stressors experienced by individuals but also their perception of the stressors and the level of distress they are experiencing as a result of these stressors. Of great importance is the caveat that what may appear to be a benign or insignificant event or stressor to health care professionals may have great significance for others, and what health professionals view as potentially most stressful may have little significance for patients or clients.

➤ CONCLUSION

Several issues concerning stimulus-oriented stress in general and in nursing research have been addressed. This chapter provided definitions of stressor, including several types and dimensions. Also, selected findings from nursing research in this area have been summarized. To some extent, this chapter reflects a fleeting glance of work in progress because there have been many studies on stressors and presumably many more to come. Many promising areas of stress research in nursing are just beginning to be reported. Despite the many questions that remain, it is clear that stressors do have the ability to influence the health and well-being of people, and therefore they are worthy of our dedicated efforts.

➤ REFERENCES

American Psychiatric Association. (1994). *Diagnostic and statistical manual of mental disorders* (4th ed.). Washington, DC: Author.

Amster, L., & Kraus, H. (1974). The relationship between life crises and mental deterioration in old age. *International Journal of Aging and Human Development, 5,* 51-55.

Antonovsky, A., & Kats, R. (1967). The life crisis history as a tool in epidemiological research. *Journal of Health and Social Behavior, 8,* 15-21.

Baum, A., Cohen, L., & Hall, M. (1993). Control and intrusive memories as possible determinants of chronic stress. *Psychosomatic Medicine, 55,* 274-286.

Bettelheim, B. (1960). *The informed heart.* New York: Free Press.

Black, N., Griffiths, J., & Pope, C. (1996). Development of a symptom severity index and a symptom impact index for stress incontinence in women. *Neurology & Urodynamics, 15*(6), 630-640.

Blegen, M. A., & Tripp-Reimer, T. (1997). Implications of nursing taxonomies for middle-range theory development. *Advances in Nursing Science, 19*(3), 37-49.

Bramston, P., & Fogarty, G. J. (1995). Measuring stress in the mildly intellectually handicapped: The factorial structure of the Subjective Stress Scale. *Research in Developmental Disabilities, 16*(2), 117-131.

Breznitz, S., & Goldberger, L. (1993). Stress research at a crossroads. In L. Goldberger & S. Breznitz (Eds.), *Handbook of stress: Theoretical and clinical aspects.* New York: Free Press.

Brown, G. W., & Harris, T. O. (1978). *Social origins of depression.* New York: Free Press.

Brown, G. W., & Harris, T. (1982). Fall off in the reporting of life events. *Social Psychiatry, 17,* 23-28.

Budd, K. S., Workman, D. E., Lemsky, C. M., & Quick, D. M. (1994). The Children's Headache Assessment

Scale (CHAS): Factor structure and psychometric properties. *Journal of Behavioral Medicine, 17*(2), 159-179.

Byrne, C. P., Velamoor, V. R., Cernovsky, Z. Z., Cortese, L., & Losztyn, S. (1990). A comparison of borderline and schizophrenic patients for childhood life events and parent-child relationships. *Canadian Journal of Psychiatry, 35*(7), 590-595.

Carr, J. A., & Powers, M. J. (1986). Stressors associated with coronary bypass surgery. *Nursing Research, 35,* 243-246.

Carter, M. C., & Miles, M. S. (1982). Parental stressor scale: Pediatric intensive care units. *Nursing Research, 31,* 121.

Carter, M. C., Miles, M. S., Buford, T., & Hassanein, R. (1985). Parental environmental stress in pediatric intensive care units. *Dimensions of Critical Care Nursing, 4,* 180-188.

Cochrane, R., & Robertson, A. (1973). The life events inventory: A measure of the relative severity of psychosocial stressors. *Journal of Psychosomatic Research, 17,* 135-139.

Coddington, R. D. (1972a). The significance of life events as etiologic factors in the diseases of children. I. A survey of professional workers. *Journal of Psychosomatic Research, 16,* 7-18.

Coddington, R. D. (1972b). The significance of life events as etiologic factors in the diseases of children. II. A survey of a normal population. *Journal of Psychosomatic Research, 16,* 205-213.

Coddington, R. D., & Troxell, J. R. (1980). The effect of emotional factors on football injury rates: A pilot study. *Journal of Human Stress, 6,* 3-5.

Cohen, F., Horowitz, M. J., Lazarus, R., Moos, R., Robins, L., Rose, R., & Rutter, M. (1982). Panel report on psychosocial assets and modifiers of stress. In G. R. Elliott & C. Eisdorfer (Eds.), *Stress and human health: Analysis and implications of research* (pp. 147-188). New York: Springer.

Cohen, S., Kessler, R. C., & Gordon, L. U. (1995). *Measuring stress: A guide for health and social scientists.* New York: Oxford University Press.

Cohen, S., Tyrrell, D. A., & Smith, A. P. (1991). Psychological stress in humans and susceptibility to the common cold. *New England Journal of Medicine, 325,* 606-612.

Cohen, S., Tyrrell, D. A., & Smith, A. P. (1993). Negative life events, perceived stress, negative affect, and susceptibility to the common cold. *Journal of Personality and Social Psychology, 64,* 131-140.

Cohen-Sandler, R., Berman, A. L., & King, R. A. (1982). Life stress and symptomatology: Determinants of suicidal behavior in children. *Journal of the American Academy of Child Psychiatry, 21,* 178-186.

Collins, E. G., White-Williams, C., & Jalowiec, A. (1996). Spouse stressors while awaiting transplanta-

tion. *Heart & Lung: Journal of Acute & Critical Care, 25,* 1-13.

Compas, B. E., Davis, G. E., Forsythe, C. J., & Wagner, B. M. (1987). Assessment of major and daily stressful events during adolescence: The Adolescent Perceived Event Scale. *Journal of Consulting and Clinical Psychology, 55*(4), 534-543.

Costa, P. T., Somerfield, M., & McCrae, R. R. (1996). Personality and coping: A reconceptualization. In M. Zeidner & N. S. Endler (Eds.), *Handbook of coping.* New York: John Wiley.

Costantini, A. F., Braun, J. R., Davis, J., & Ivervolino, A. (1974). The life change inventory: A device for quantifying psychological magnitude of changes experienced by college students. *Psychological Reports, 34,* 991-1000.

Cox, T. (1978). *Stress.* Baltimore, MD: University Park Press.

Crandall, C. S., Preisler, J. J., & Aussprung, J. (1992). Measuring life event stress in the lives of college students: The Undergraduate Stress Questionnaire (USQ). *Journal of Behavioral Medicine, 15*(6), 627-662.

Davies, A. D., & Peters, M. (1983). Stresses of hospitalization in the elderly: Nurses' and patients' perceptions. *Journal of Advanced Nursing, 8,* 99-105.

Derogatis, L. R., & Coons, H. L. (1993). Self-report measures of stress. In L. Goldberger & S. Breznitz (Eds.), *Handbook of stress: Theoretical and clinical aspects.* New York: Free Press.

Deutsch, L. J., & Erickson, M. T. (1989). Early life events as discriminators of socialized and undersocialized delinquents. *Journal of Abnormal Child Psychology, 17*(5), 541-551.

Dohrenwend, B. S., Krasnoff, L., Askenasy, A. R., & Dohrenwend, B. P. (1982). The psychiatric epidemiology research interview life events scale. In L. Goldberger & S. Breznitz (Eds.), *Handbook of stress: Theoretical and clinical aspects.* New York: Free Press.

Dohrenwend, B. P., Link, B. G., Kern, R., Shrout, P. E., & Markowitz, J. (1990). Measuring life events: The problem of variability within event categories. *Stress Medicine, 6,* 179-187.

Dohrenwend, B. P., Raphael, K. G., Schwartz, S., Stueve, A., & Skodol, A. (1993). The structured event probe and narrative rating method for measuring stressful life events. In L. Goldberger & S. Breznitz (Eds.), *Handbook of stress: Theoretical and clinical aspects* (pp. 174-199). New York: Free Press.

Dohrenwend, B. S., Krasnoff, L., Askenasy, A. R., & Dohrenwend, B. P. (1978). Exemplification of a method for scaling life events: The PERI Life Events Scale. *Journal of Health Social Behavior, 19,* 205-229.

Eberly, T. W., Miles, M. S., Carter, M. C., Hennessey, J., & Riddle, I. (1985). Parental stress after the unexpected admission of a child to the intensive care unit. *Critical Care Quarterly, 8,* 57-65.

Elliott, G. R., & Eisdorfer, C. (1982). *Stress and human health.* New York: Springer.

Erickson, H., Tomlin, E., & Swain, M. (1983). *Modeling and role-modeling: A theory and paradigm for nursing.* Englewood Cliffs, NJ: Prentice Hall.

Ferketich, S. L., & Mercer, R. T. (1990). Effects of stress on health status during early motherhood. *Scholarly Inquiry for Nursing Practice, 4,* 127-149.

Ferketich, S. L., & Mercer, R. T. (1995). Predictors of role competence for experienced and inexperienced fathers. *Nursing Research, 44*(2), 89-95.

Figley, C. R., & McCubbin, H. I. (1983). *Stress and the family, Volume II: Coping with catastrophe.* New York: Brunner/Mazel.

Frost, M. H. (1993). Commentary on stressors and health outcomes: Implications for nursing research, theory, practice and policy agendas. In J. S. Barnfather & B. L. Lyon (Eds.), *Stress and coping: State of the science and implications for nursing theory, research, and practice* (pp. 43-64). Indianapolis, IN: Sigma Theta Tau Center Nursing Press.

Frost, M. H., Orth, K., & Werner, J. (in press). Stressors and chronic conditions. In J. S. Werner & M. H. Frost (Eds.), *Stress and coping: State of the science and implications for nursing theory, research and practice, Volume II.* Glenview, IL: Midwest Nursing Research Society Press.

Funch, D. P., & Marshall, J. R. (1984). Measuring life stress: Factors affecting fall-off in the reporting of life events. *Journal of Health and Social Behavior, 15,* 453-464.

Gadzella, B. M. (1994). Student-life stress inventory: Identification of and reactions to stressors. *Psychological Reports, 74,* 395-402.

Glen, S., Simpson, A., Drinnan, D., McGuinness, D., & Sandberg, S. (1993). Testing the reliability of a new measure of life events and experiences in childhood: The Psychosocial Assessment of Childhood Experiences (PACE). *European Child and Adolescent Psychiatry, 2*(2), 98-110.

Glidden, L. M. (1993). What we do not know about families with children who have developmental disabilities: Questionnaire on resources and stress as a case study. *American Journal of Mental Retardation, 97*(5), 481-495.

Graves, J. K., & Ware, M. E. (1990). Parents and health professionals' perceptions concerning parental stress during a child's hospitalization. *Child Health Care, 19,* 37-42.

Gupta, M. A., & Gupta, A. K. (1995). The Psoriasis Life Stress Inventory: A preliminary index of psoriasis-related stress. *Acta Dermato-Venereologica, 75*(3), 240-243.

Hawkins, N. G., Davies, R., & Holmes, T. H. (1957). Evidence of psychosocial factors in the development of pulmonary tuberculosis. *American Review of Tuberculosis and Pulmonary Diseases, 75,* 768-780.

Henderson, S., Byrne, D. G., & Duncan-Jones, P. (1981). *Neurosis and the social environment.* New York: Academic Press.

Herschbach, P., Duran, G., Waadt, S., Zettler, A., Amm, C., & Marten-Mittag, B. (1997). Psychometric properties of the Questionnaire on Stress in Patients with Diabetes—Revised (QSD-R). *Health Psychology, 16*(2), 171-174.

Hinkle, L. E. (1973). The concept of "stress" in the biological and social sciences. *Science, Medicine, and Man, 1,* 31-48.

Hobfoll, S. E., Freedy, J. R., Green, B., & Solomon, S. (1996). Coping in reaction to extreme stress: The roles of resource loss and resource availability. In M. Zeidner & N. S. Endler (Eds.), *Handbook of coping.* New York: John Wiley.

Holmes, T. H. (1979). Development and application of a quantitative measure of life change magnitude. In J. E. Barrett, R. M. Rose, & G. I. Klerman (Eds.), *Stress and mental disorder.* New York: Raven Press.

Holmes, T. H., & Masuda, M. (1974). Life change and illness susceptibility. In B. S. Dohrenwend & B. P. Dohrenwend (Eds.), *Stressful life events: Their nature and effects* (pp. 45-72). New York: John Wiley.

Holmes, T. H., & Rahe, R. (1967). The Social Readjustment Rating Scale. *Journal of Psychosomatic Research, 12,* 213-218.

Horowitz, M. (1979). *Impact of Event Scale (IES).* San Francisco: University of California Press.

Horowitz, M. J., Schaefer, C., Hiroto, D., Wilner, N., & Levin, B. (1977). Life event questionnaires for measuring presumptive stress. *Psychosomatic Medicine, 39,* 413-431.

Hurst, M. W., Jenkins, C. D., & Rose, R. M. (1978). The assessment of life change stress: A comparative and methodological inquiry. *Psychosomatic Medicine, 40,* 126-141.

Hymovich, D. (1983). The Chronicity Impact and Coping Instrument: Parent Questionnaire. *Nursing Research, 32*(5), 275-281.

Janis, I. L. (1951). *Air war and emotional stress.* New York: McGraw-Hill.

Johnson, D. E. (1980). The behavioral system model for nursing. In J. P. Riehl & C. Roy (Eds.), *Conceptual models for nursing practice* (2nd ed.). New York: Appleton-Century-Crofts.

Johnson, J. H., & McCutcheon, S. M. (1980). Assessing life stress in older children and adolescents: Preliminary findings with the life events checklist. In I. B. Sarason & C. C. Spielberger (Eds.), *Stress and anxiety* (Vol. 7, pp. 111-125). Washington, DC: Hemisphere.

Kanner, A. D., Coyne, J., Schaefer, C., & Lazarus, R. (1981). Comparison of two modes of stress measurements: Daily hassles and uplifts versus major life events. *Journal of Behavioral Medicine, 4,* 1-39.

Kessler, R. C., & Wethington, E. (1991). The reliability of life event reports in a community survey. *Psychological Medicine, 21,* 723-738.

Kidney, W. C. (1993) *Webster's 21st century dictionary.* Nashville, TN: T. Nelson.

Kort, W. J., & Weijma, I. M. (1991). Chronic stress and the immune response. In N. Plotnikoff, A. Mungo, R. Faith, & J. Wyban (Eds.), *Stress and immunity.* Boca Raton, FL: CRC Press.

Lange, A., Kooiman, K., Huberts, L., & van Oostendorp, E. (1995). Childhood unwanted sexual events and degree of psychopathology of psychiatric patients: Research with a new anamnestic questionnaire (CHUSE). *Acta Psychiatrica Scandinavia, 92*(6), 441-446.

Lazarus, R. S. (1966). *Psychological stress and the coping process.* New York: McGraw-Hill.

Lazarus, R. S., & Folkman, S. (1984). *Stress, appraisal, and coping.* New York: Springer.

Lepore, S. J. (1995). Measurement of chronic stressors. In S. Cohen, R. Kessler, & L. U. Gordon (Eds.), *Measuring stress.* New York: Oxford University Press.

Lepore, S. J., & Evans, G. W. (1996). Coping with multiple stressors in the environment. In M. Zeidner & N. S. Endler (Eds.), *Handbook of coping.* New York: John Wiley.

Levenstein, S., Prantera, C., Varvo, V., Scribano, M. L., Berto, E., Luzi, C., & Andreoli, A. (1993). Development of the Perceived Stress Questionnaire: A new tool for psychosomatic research. *Journal of Psychosomatic Research, 37,* 19-32.

Levine, S., & Scotch, N. A. (1970). *Social stress.* Chicago: Aldine.

Lyon, B. L., & Werner, J. S. (1987). Stress. *Annual Review of Nursing Research, 5,* 3-22.

Mason, J. W. (1975). A historical view of the stress field: Part I. *Journal of Human Stress, 1,* 6-12.

McCubbin, H. I., & Figley, C. R. (1983). *Stress and the family, Volume I: Coping with normative transitions.* New York: Brunner/Mazel.

McCubbin, H. I., & Patterson, J. M. (1983). The family stress process: The Double ABCX Model of Adjustment and Adaptation. *Marriage and Family Review, 6,* 7-35.

McCubbin, H. I., Patterson, J., Bauman, E., & Harris, L. (1981). *Adolescent-Family Inventory of Life Events and Changes (A-FILE).* Madison, WI: Family Stress, Coping and Health Project.

McCubbin, H. I., Patterson, J., & Wilson, L. (1980). *Family Inventory of Life Events and Changes (FILE).* Madison, WI: Family Stress, Coping and Health Project.

McEwen, B. S., & Mendelson, S. (1993). Effects of stress on the neurochemistry and morphology of the brain: Counterregulation versus damage. In L. Goldberger & S. Breznitz (Eds.), *Handbook of stress: Theoretical and clinical aspects.* New York: Free Press.

Mechanic, D. (1968). *Medical sociology.* New York: Free Press.

Mercer, R. T., & Ferketich, S. L. (1990). Predictors of family functioning eight months following birth. *Nursing Research, 39,* 76-82.

Miles, M. S., & Carter, M. C. (1982). Sources of parental stress in pediatric care units. *Child Health Care, 11,* 65-69.

Miles, M. S., Carter, M. C., Spicker, C., & Hassanein, R. (1984). Maternal and paternal stress reactions when a child is hospitalized in a pediatric intensive care unit. *Issues in Comprehensive Pediatric Nursing, 7,* 333-342.

Miller, T. W. (1981). Life events scaling: Clinical methodological issues. *Nursing Research, 30*(5), 316-320.

Murphy, S. A. (1984). Stress levels and health status of victims of a natural disaster. *Research in Nursing and Health, 7,* 205-215.

Murphy, S. A. (1986a). Perceptions of stress, coping and recovery one and three years after a natural disaster. *Issues in Mental Health Nursing, 8,* 63-77.

Murphy, S. A. (1986b). Status of natural disaster victims' health and recovery three years later. *Research in Nursing and Health, 9,* 331-340.

Murphy, S. A. (1987). Self-efficacy and social support: Mediators of stress on mental health following a natural disaster. *Western Journal of Nursing Research, 9,* 58-86.

Murphy, S. A. (1988). Mental distress and recovery in a high-risk bereavement sample three years after untimely death. *Nursing Research, 37,* 30-35.

Murphy, S. A. (1989). An explanatory model of recovery from disaster loss. *Research in Nursing and Health, 12,* 67-76.

Murphy, S. P., Powers, M. J., & Jalowiec, A. (1985). Psychometric evaluation of the Hemodialysis Stressor Scale. *Nursing Research, 34*(6), 368-371.

Murrell, S. A., Norris, F. H., & Hutchins, G. M. (1984). Distribution and desirability of life events in older adults: Population and policy implications. *Journal of Community Psychology, 12,* 301-311.

Neufeldt, V., & Guralnik, D. B. (1996). *Webster's new world college dictionary.* New York: Macmillan.

Neuman, B. (1989). *The Neuman systems model: Applications in nursing education and practice* (2nd ed.). Norwalk, CT: Appleton-Lange.

Norbeck, J. S. (1984). Modification of life event questionnaires for use with female respondents. *Research in Nursing and Health, 7,* 61-71.

Palmer, A. G., Tucker, S., Warren, R., & Adams, M. (1993). Understanding women's responses to treatment for cervical interepithelial neoplasia. *British Journal of Clinical Psychology, 32,* 101-112.

Paterson, R. J., & Neufeld, R. W. (1989). The stress response and parameters of stressful situations. In R. W. Neufeld (Ed.), *Advances in the investigation of psychological stress.* New York: John Wiley.

Paykel, E. S. (1983). Methodological aspects of life event research. *Journal of Psychosomatic Research, 27,* 341-352.

Paykel, E. S. (1997). Interview for recent life events. *Psychological Medicine, 27,* 301-310.

Pearlin, L. I. (1993). The social contexts of stress. In L. Goldberger & S. Breznitz (Eds.), *Handbook of stress: Theoretical and clinical aspects.* New York: Free Press.

Perehudoff, B. (1990). Parents' perceptions of environmental stressors in the special care nursery. *Journal of Neonatal Nursing, 9,* 39-44.

Rahe, R. H. (1968). Life-change measurement as a predictor of illness. *Proceedings of Research in Social Medicine, 61,* 1124-1126.

Rahe, R. H. (1972). Subjects' recent life changes and their near-future illness reports. *Annals of Clinical Research, 4,* 250-265.

Rahe, R. H. (1975). Epidemiological studies of life change and illness. *International Journal of Psychiatry in Medicine, 6,* 133-146.

Rahe, R. H. (1977). Life change measurement clarification. *Psychosomatic Medicine, 40,* 95-98.

Rahe, R. H., & Lind, E. (1971). Psychosocial factors and sudden cardiac death: A pilot study. *Journal of Psychosomatic Research, 15,* 19-24.

Roosa, M. W., Sandler, I. N., Gehring, M., Beals, J., & Cappo, L. (1988). The children of alcoholics life-events schedule: A stress scale for children of alcohol abusing parents. *Journal of Studies on Alcohol, 49*(5), 422-429.

Rose, R. M. (1980). Endocrine responses to stressful psychological events. *Psychiatric Clinics of North America, 3,* 251-276.

Roy, C. (1984). *Introduction to nursing: An adaptation model* (2nd ed.). Englewood Cliffs, NJ: Prentice Hall.

Rutter, M. (1989). Pathways from childhood to adult life. *Journal of Child Psychology and Psychiatry, 30,* 23-51.

Sandler, I. N., Nolichuk, S., Brauer, S. L., & Fogas, B. (1986). Significant events of children of divorce: Toward the assessment of a risky situation. In S. M. Averback & A. Stolberg (Eds.), *Crisis intervention with children and families* (pp. 65-87). New York: Hemisphere.

Sarason, I. G., Johnson, J. H., & Siegel, J. M. (1978). Assessing the impact of life changes: Development of Life Experiences Survey. *Journal of Consulting and Clinical Psychology, 46,* 932-946.

Scott, D. W., Oberst, M., & Dropkin, M. (1980). A stress coping model. *Advances in Nursing Science, 3,* 9-23.

Selye, H. (1956). *The stress of life.* New York: McGraw-Hill.

Selye, H. (1993). History of the stress concept. In L. Goldberger & S. Breznitz (Eds.), *Handbook of stress: Theoretical and clinical aspects.* New York: Free Press.

Stokes, S. A., & Gordon, S. E. (1988). Development of an instrument to measure stress in the older adult. *Nursing Research, 37,* 16-19.

Suter, S. (1986). *Health psychophysiology: Mind-body interactions in wellness and illness.* Hillsdale, NJ: Lawrence Erlbaum.

Swearingen, E. M., & Cohen, L. H. (1985). Life events and psychological distress: A prospective study of young adolescents. *Developmental Psychology, 21,* 1045-1054.

Thoits, P. A. (1983). Multiple identities and psychological well-being: A reformulation and test of the social interaction hypothesis. *American Sociological Review, 48,* 174-187.

Tolor, A., Murphy, V., Wilson, L. T., & Clayton, J. (1983). The High School Readjustment Scale: An attempt to quantify stressful events in young people. *Research Communication in Psychology, Psychiatry and Behavior, 8,* 85-111.

Towbes, L. C., Cohen, L. H., & Glyshaw, K. (1989). Instrumentality as a life-stress moderator for early versus middle adolescents. *Journal of Personality and Social Psychology, 57,* 109-119.

Turner, R. J., & Wheaton, B. (1995). Checklist measurement of stressful life events. In S. Cohen, R. C. Kessler, & L. U. Gordon (Eds.), *Measuring stress: A guide for health and social scientists.* New York: Oxford University Press.

Unger, W. S., Gould, R. A., & Babich, M. (1998) The development of a scale to assess war-time atrocities: The War Events Scale. *Journal of Traumatic Stress, 11*(2), 375-383.

Vogel, W. H., & Bower, D. B. (1991). Stress, immunity, and cancer. In N. Plotnikoff, A. Murgo, R. Faith, & J. Wybran (Eds.), *Stress and immunity.* Boca Raton, FL: CRC Press.

Volicer, B. J. (1974). Patients' perceptions of stressful events associated with hospitalization. *Nursing Research, 23,* 235-238.

Volicer, B. J. (1977). Stress factors in the experience of hospitalization. In M. V. Batey (Ed.), *Communicating nursing research, Volume 8* (pp. 53-67). Boulder, CO: Western Interstate Commission for Higher Education.

Volicer, B. J., & Bohannon, M. W. (1975). A hospital stress rating scale. *Nursing Research, 24*(5), 352-359.

Volicer, B. J., & Burns, M. W. (1977). Preexisting correlates of hospital stress. *Nursing Research, 26,* 408-415.

Volicer, B. J., & Volicer, L. (1977). Cardiovascular changes associated with stress during hospitalization. *Journal of Psychosomatic Research, 22,* 159-168.

Weisaeth, L. (1993). Disasters: Psychological and psychiatric aspects. In L. Goldberger & S. Breznitz (Eds.), *Handbook of stress: Theoretical and clinical aspects.* New York: Free Press.

Werner, J. S. (1993). Stressors and health outcomes: Synthesis of nursing research, 1980-1990. In J. S. Barnfather & B. L. Lyon (Eds.), *Stress and coping: State of the science and implications for nursing theory, research, and practice* (pp. 11-41). Indianapolis, IN: Sigma Theta Tau Center Nursing Press.

Werner, J. S. (1996). Stress: Nursing assessment and role in management. In S. M. Lewis, I. Collier, & M. Heitkemper (Eds.), *Medical surgical nursing: Assessment and management of clinical problems.* St. Louis, MO: C. V. Mosby.

Werner, J. S., Frost, M. H., & Orth, K. (in press). Stressors and health outcomes: Synthesis of nursing research, 1991-1995. In J. S. Werner & M. H. Frost (Eds.), *Stress and coping: State of the science and implications for nursing theory, research and practice, Volume II.* Glenview, IL: Midwest Nursing Research Society Press.

Werner, J. S., & O'Neill, S. E. (1992). Stress: Nursing assessment and role in management. In S. M. Lewis & I. Collier (Eds.), *Medical-surgical nursing: Assessment and management of clinical problems.* St. Louis, MO: C. V. Mosby.

Wittchen, H., Essau, C. A., Hecht, H., Teder, W., & Pfister, H. (1989). Reliability of life event assessments: Test-retest reliability and fall-off effects of the Munich Interview for the Assessment of Life Events and Conditions. *Journal of Affective Disorders, 16,* 77-91.

Wolff, H. G., Wolff, S. G., & Hare, C. (Eds.). (1950). *Life stress and bodily disease.* Baltimore, MD: Williams & Wilkins.

Yarcheski, A., & Knapp-Spooner, C. (1994). Stressors associated with coronary bypass surgery. *Clinical Nursing Research, 3,* 57-68.

Yeaworth, R., York, J., Hussey, M., Ingle, M., & Goodwin, T. (1980). The development of an adolescent life changes event scale. *Adolescence, 15,* 91-97.

Zautra, A. J., & Reich, J. W. (1983). Life events and perceptions of life quality: Developments in a two-factor approach. *Journal of Community Psychology, 1,* 121-132.

CHAPTER 6

Microstressors and Health

Carol L. Macnee and Susan McCabe

➤ **THE ORIGIN AND EVOLUTION OF THE HASSLES AND UPLIFTS MODEL**

Some researchers (Lazarus, 1984) would argue that it is not the major life events and changes that weigh on people's minds and bodies and cause them stress and illness but rather the day-to-day chronic buildup of minor life demands or hassles. Hassles and uplifts reflect relatively "minor" daily experiences and conditions that have been appraised as salient to an individual. They can be perceived as potentially harmful or threatening (hassles), or they can be perceived as positive or favorable (uplifts) (Lazarus, 1984). As such, hassles and uplifts are day-to-day irritants and momentary joys that reflect the stress of daily living in relation to how the individual psychologically and subjectively experiences a situation. Within the hassles and uplifts theory inputs are the day-to-day events, and the outputs or health outcomes depend on the subjective saliency and threat of the inputs. Because hassles and uplifts depend on cognitive appraisal or assessment, the same event can be a hassle for one

person and an uplift for another or even become an uplift for the same individual at a different point in time. Theoretically, hassles and uplifts should equally affect health outcomes, such as somatic, psychological, and affective symptoms, because they are thought to potentially balance one another (Lazarus, 1984).

The Theoretical Context for the Model

The Hassles and Uplifts Model reflects a cognitive perceptual approach to understanding the effects of stress on health. The model derives from the broader transactional theory of stress and coping (TTSC), which was developed in the late 1960s and 1970s by Lazarus and colleagues (Lazarus, 1993). Lazarus's TTSC takes a psychological view of the effects of stress on health by considering individual differences in motivation and cognitive appraisal as intervening variables between a potential external stressor and the stress reaction. The theory takes a relational approach to understanding the effects of stress on health rather than the more linear perspective of inputs (or stress as a stimulus) and outputs (or stress as a response), which is best reflected in the early work of Selye (1950).

According to Lazarus (1993), the TTSC has its origins in Lewin's (1951) writing about positively and negatively valenced situations, in which the environment is viewed as a product of perceptions and reactions rather than objective reality. The TTSC proposes that stress is the product of transactions between individuals and their environments, with two major concepts mediating the dynamics: (a) primary and secondary cognitive appraisal and (b) coping. The TTSC is described in greater detail in Chapter 9.

Concurrent with the development of the TTSC, the theory of life events as stressors that affect health outcomes was proposed and broadly accepted (Holmes & Rahe, 1967). As described in Chapter 5, life events theory is linear and stimulus oriented, and it assumes that major changes in life, whether positive or negative, are stressful and that the accumulation of life changes leads to changes in health (Holmes & Rahe, 1967). The Hassles and Uplifts Model reflects the view that microstressors, in the form of perceived minor irritations or demands, and pleasures have an impact on health outcomes as well. This view is in response to criticisms that life events theory ignores psychological mediators, such as the saliency of an event and the individual's coping resources for dealing with the event.

Given the relational view of stress and coping, it was argued that the effects of life events on health outcomes vary depending on the meaning of the events to the individual. For example, divorce for one individual might be a major loss, whereas for another individual it might be a relief and an opportunity to grow and move forward in life. It was argued that a difference in cognitive appraisal of the same event would likely lead to the event having different effects on health outcomes. In addition, the Hassles and Uplifts Model proposes that events that are perceived as negative versus those perceived as positive will have different effects on health, and that day-

to-day events that have positive tones or uplifts act as buffers for the negative effects of stressors on health. This is in contrast to the assumptions in life events theory that any change, no matter the emotional tone, would negatively affect health outcomes.

Another criticism of the life events theory is that research using this conceptualization explains relatively small amounts of the variance in health outcomes (Lazarus, 1984). Day-to-day events or microstressors are considered to be more proximal to health outcomes than life events, and therefore their cumulative effects can be greater than that of somewhat distant life events (DeLongis, Coyne, Dakof, Folkman, & Lazarus, 1982). Kanner, Coyne, Schaefer, and Lazarus (1981) suggested three possible explanations for how life events and daily microstressors relate to health outcomes. One explanation is that life events moderate the effect of microstressors on health outcomes. For example, a major life event such as divorce can change the relative stressfulness of an individual's daily routine and pattern, such as meal preparation and household management, thus moderating the effects of these day-to-day events on health. As a moderating variable, life events could have an effect on health even when all the effects of microstressors are statistically removed.

An alternative idea is that the effects of major life events are mediated by more proximal day-to-day events that then affect health outcomes. For example, divorce can lead to actual changes in daily routines that then can directly alter health outcomes. If microstressors mediate the effect of major life events, then the effects of life events on health outcomes could occur solely because of and through their effects on day-to-day occurrences. A third explanation is that life events and day-to-day hassles exert independent effects on health outcomes.

In addition to responding to theoretical criticism of the life events theory, the Hassles and Uplifts Model responded to concerns that research using scales measuring life events was psychometrically flawed by a lack of independence among the life events surveyed. Another concern is the lack of culturally appropriate life events for varying sociodemographic groups (DeLongis et al., 1982). Specifically, it was argued that life events such as divorce or death of a spouse often lead to other life events such as lower income or moving. Furthermore, items on the life events scales generally reflected white middle-class life situations that might be irrelevant or too narrow for other cultural and economic groups (DeLongis et al., 1982).

Congruent with the theoretical model of hassles and uplifts as day-to-day events that affect health and because of the saliency and potential threat or positive experience of the events, the original Hassles scales listed a wide variety of day-to-day events, such as too many things to do, yard work, and outside home maintenance. Uplifts included using skills well at work, the health of a family member, praying, or completing a task (Kanner et al., 1981). Day-to-day events on the measures were diverse and considered to reflect issues and experiences that spanned the daily life of individuals from a wide range of backgrounds (Kanner et al., 1981). The separate Hassles and Uplifts scales were later combined into a single scale on which respondents rated experiences as either a hassle or an uplift to better reflect the theoretical perspective that "perception" of events was central to their effect on health (DeLongis, 1985). Measurement of hassles and uplifts will be discussed later.

Empirical Examination of the Effects of Microstressors Versus Life Events on Health

Studies comparing the effects of hassles versus life events on health outcomes have consistently found hassles to be a better predictor of both psychological and somatic symptoms (DeLongis et al., 1982; Ivancevich, 1986; Jandorf, Deblinger, Neale, & Stone, 1986; Kanner et al., 1981; Monroe, 1983; Wagner, Compas, & Howell, 1988; Wein-

berger, Hiner, & Tierney, 1987; Wolf, Elston, & Kissling, 1989). A classic study (DeLongis et al., 1982) compared the effects of the two approaches to stress measurement using a repeated-measure, longitudinal design with 100 adults representing a probability sample of Alameda County residents. Subjects completed the Hassles and Uplifts scales monthly for 9 consecutive months, and a Life Events Questionnaire and Health Status Questionnaire were administered twice during the same period. This study, reported in two separate publications, found that hassles were better predictors of concurrent and later psychological symptoms (Kanner et al., 1981) and somatic symptoms (DeLongis et al., 1982) than were life events. Furthermore, when the effects of life events on health outcomes were statistically removed, hassles remained significantly related to both somatic and psychological symptoms (DeLongis et al., 1982; Kanner et al., 1981). The effect of hassles on psychological symptoms was also supported by Monroe's (1983) study with 73 adults who completed measures of hassles, uplifts, life events, and psychological symptoms at least three times in a 4-month period. He concluded that minor events were significantly better predictors of subsequent psychological symptoms than were life events.

Although the evidence that hassles were better predictors of health outcomes than life events was strong, two studies had different results. Zarski (1984) found that life experiences accounted for greater variance in somatic health than did hassles. A second study found that the number of life events directly affected hassles, which in turn affected perceived effects of life events and illness (Dykema, Bergbower, & Peterson, 1995). Zarski's descriptive study used a single cross-sectional measurement model with 397 subjects, and Dykema and colleagues used path analysis with cross-sectional data from a sample of 121 college students.

It is important to note that the Life Experience Survey used in Zarski's (1984) study asked subjects to rate on a 7-point scale the degree of the positive or negative life event, and Dykema et al.'s (1995) study found that it was the nature of the life events, not their frequency, that directly affected health outcomes. Thus, subjective saliency was included in both of these measures, unlike the more traditional measures of life events.

Results of studies examining the relative roles of hassles and life events on health outcomes have supported the explanation that hassles can act as mediators of life events. Studies have found bivariate relationships among hassles, life events, and health outcomes. When the effects of hassles on health outcomes are partialed out statistically, however, life events do not significantly contribute to explained variance in health outcomes (DeLongis et al., 1982; Ivancevick, 1986; Jandorf et al., 1986; Kanner et al., 1981; Wagner et al., 1988; Weinberger et al., 1987). One exception is the findings by Williams, Zyzanski, and Wright (1992). They reported that there was an additive effect for life events and hassles on the risk of inpatient admission among 444 Navajo Indians. The dependent variable in this study was not a continuous measure of somatic or psychological symptoms as it was in most of the other studies. A relative risk model for predicting likelihood of admission, given high or low scores on life events and hassles measures, was used. This study found that daily hassle scores were associated with increased outpatient use, whereas life events were not related to use of health care services.

In general, although numerous studies have found significant effects for hassles on health outcomes, most studies have found very limited support for uplifts (DeLongis et al., 1982; Jandorf et al., 1986; Kanner et al., 1981; Monroe, 1983; Wolf et al., 1989). Uplifts have been found to be related to reported higher energy levels (Zarski, 1984), variation in job performance and low absenteeism (Ivancevick, 1986), and fewer hospital admissions (Williams et al., 1992).

Although the life event measures have been challenged with regard to interdependence among the items, Hassles and Uplifts scales are not without problems. They have been particularly challenged in relation to the potential confounding of measures and health outcomes. Measurement of hassles and uplifts will be addressed later, but it is worth noting that part of the argument regarding the potential confounding of hassles and symptoms concerns the question of whether day-to-day stressors can be validly measured without including a subjective component. This challenge strikes at the very core of the theoretical underpinnings of the Hassles and Uplifts Model because saliency and the subjective nature of perceived threat are basic elements in defining day-to-day events as hassles.

➤ USE AND TESTING OF
THE HASSLES AND UPLIFT
MODEL ACROSS LIFE SPAN
AND CULTURE

Empirical Studies of the Effects of Hassles and Uplifts on Health Outcomes

The Hassles and Uplifts Model has been tested in relation to a wide variety of health-related outcomes, among several cultures, and across the life span. A significant relationship has consistently been found between psychological symptoms and daily hassles, whether the studies have used measures developed by Lazarus and colleagues (Kanner et al., 1981; Ravindran, Griffiths, Merali, & Anisman, 1996; Zarski, 1984) or other measures (Monroe, 1983; Wagner et al., 1988; Wolf et al., 1989). Similarly, daily hassles have been found to be predictors of physical symptoms using either an investigator-developed measure (Jandorf et al., 1986) or the measures developed by Lazarus's group (DeLongis et al., 1982; Zarski, 1984).

In addition to predicting physical symptoms, the timing and changes in hassles and uplifts have been examined in relation to episodes of physical symptoms (Stone, Reed, & Neale, 1987) and in relation to the common cold (Evans, Pitts, & Smith, 1988; Evans & Edgerton, 1991). In each study, desirable events (uplifts) decreased and undesirable events (hassles) increased three or four days before illness occurred. Interestingly, frequency of undesirable events (hassles) failed to be significantly related to an episode of upper respiratory infection in one of the studies (Evans et al., 1988) and was less strongly related to onset of cold symptoms than was frequency of desirable events in the other two studies (Evans & Edgerton, 1991; Stone et al., 1987). These studies provide strong support for the role of microstressors on health outcomes because they used prospective designs with repeated measures analysis. They also suggested a role for uplifts in health outcomes, whereas earlier retrospective studies did not.

Other health-related outcomes that have been examined as dependent measures and found to be related to hassles or uplifts or both include episodes of hospitalization and outpatient visits (Williams et al., 1992), symptoms of irritable bowel syndrome (Dancey, Whitehouse, Painter, & Backhouse, 1995), and quality of sleep (Weller & Avinir, 1993). The results of Williams and colleagues' study with Navajo Indians were described earlier. Dancey et al. used a prospective design to examine the relationship between daily symptoms of irritable bowel syndrome and hassles and uplifts. They found that total symptoms were associated with hassles in the following week; hassles in any week, however, were not associated with symptoms in the following week. There was no association between uplifts and irritable bowel symptoms. In contrast, Weller and Avinir (1993) found that hassles alone, uplifts alone, and a combined hassles and uplifts score were each correlated with quality of sleep in a sample of 41 people without sleeping disorders.

Hassles have also been found to be related to role change and the number of health problems among parents and partners of individuals with traumatic brain injury (Leathem, Heath, & Woolley, 1996) and to be greater in Type A college students compared to Type B students (Margiotta, Davilla, & Hicks, 1990). Thus, there is significant empirical evidence

that negative day-to-day events impact many aspects of health, whereas the role of positive day-to-day events remains unclear.

Effects of Hassles and Uplifts on Health Across the Age Continuum

Early studies examining the effects of hassles and uplifts on health outcomes were carried out with adults between the ages of 18 and 64 (DeLongis et al., 1982; Jandorf et al., 1986; Kanner et al., 1981; Monroe, 1983; Zarski, 1984). The hassles and uplifts measures used in these studies reflected items that were expected to be relevant to the working adult population. Theoretically, the Hassles and Uplifts Model is applicable for populations across the age continuum. Several studies were undertaken to examine whether or not hassles had an impact on health outcomes for both older and younger populations and, if so, whether the impact of hassles was the same or different for individuals at different developmental stages. Implicit in most of these studies is the assumption that the actual day-to-day events relevant to different age groups differ. Some of these studies will be reviewed.

Hassles and Older Adults

Two studies were implemented with the explicit purpose of comparing hassles and uplifts in older and younger adults. Folkman, Lazarus, Pimley, and Novacek (1987) used a retrospective, repeated measures longitudinal design with a revised version of the original Hassles and Uplifts scales. The sample consisted of 150 adults in their early forties and 141 adults in their late sixties. This study found a significant effect for age on the types of hassles endorsed by younger versus older adults. Younger adults reported significantly more hassles in the domains of work, finance, home maintenance, family, friends, and personal life, whereas older adults reported more hassles in the domains of environmental, social issues, and health.

Folkman et al. (1987) concluded that these differences logically reflected differences in developmental tasks, with younger adults concerned with work, home, and family and older adults concerned with health and the broader environmental and social issues. This study did not examine the effects of hassles on health outcomes, nor did it include examination of uplifts.

Ewedemi and Linn (1987) examined the differences in hassles between younger and older adults who were outpatients at a Veterans Medical Center. This study used a descriptive cross-sectional design with 25 younger and 25 older adults with chronic disease who completed study measures on only one occasion. The hassles and uplifts measures for this study consisted of 40 of the original 117 hassles items and 40 of the 135 original uplifts. The authors indicated that these items were selected because they were applicable to men who were in the age ranges being studied. Subjects in the study were categorized as being in "good" or "poor" health depending on self-rating of their health on a 5-point scale. Study findings indicated that hassles were greater for those who rated their health as poor, but this did not differ by age group. The results became nonsignificant when 11 items (that were considered to confound health outcomes) were eliminated from the scale. This study did not find any associations between uplift scores and age or perceived health.

In contrast, Weinberger and colleagues (1987) implemented their study using a sample of 134 older adults with arthritis and a mean age of 66 years. These authors also modified the original Hassles and Uplifts scales based on responses from 44 pretest telephone interviews. Seventy-three items were retained for this study; the omitted items were related to work, sexual relationships, and raising children. The authors stated that these items were probably not relevant to an elderly population that was not working. In addition, this study examined the effects of life events on arthritis-specific functional status. Uplifts

were excluded from the study because pretest data suggested respondents had a difficult time responding to the uplifts items. The authors stated that respondents were unwilling to estimate or were uncomfortable estimating the frequency of experiencing uplifts. The study found that hassles were better predictors of arthritis functional status than life events, and that hassles were strongly related to health status. Thus, findings in earlier studies with adults in their middle years were replicated in this study with older adults.

Similarly, several studies have been implemented with caregivers of family members with dementia and stroke (Kinney & Stephens, 1989a; Kinney, Stephens, Franks, & Norris, 1995). The samples in these studies have generally been late middle-aged adults with average ages from 57 to 60 years. These studies used a scale specifically targeting the unique hassles that would be faced by caregivers of family members (Kinney & Stephens, 1989b) and found that hassles were associated with caregivers' well-being (Kinney & Stephens, 1989a; Kinney et al., 1995). Uplifts were not directly associated with well-being, but when caregivers' uplifts outnumbered their hassles the net effect was lower levels of caregiver distress (Kinney et al., 1995).

Hassles and Children and Adolescents

Studies have also been implemented to examine the effects of hassles on health outcomes among children and adolescents. Kanner and Feldman (1991) studied the effects of perceived control over daily hassles and uplifts in a sample of 140 sixth graders. This cross-sectional study used a 50-item Children's Hassles and Uplifts Scale that consisted of 25 items reflecting hassles and 25 items reflecting uplifts in areas such as school, family, or friends. Hassles and uplifts were rated with regard to whether they had occurred in the past month and also rated on a 3-point scale with regard to their relative effect. Results of this study indicated that the number of hassles and the number of uplifts were significantly related to depression scores for both boys and girls. In addition, perceived control over uplifts was associated with better functioning, and lower control over hassles was associated with poorer functioning, in which functioning reflected both depression scores and levels of restraint.

Several studies of "day-to-day" events have been completed with adolescents. Miller, Tobacyk, and Wilcox (1985) examined which of the 117 hassles items and 135 uplifts items from the original scale (Kanner et al., 1981) were most frequently endorsed by 38 high school students. Subjects in this convenience sample had a mean age of 17 years and were found to endorse hassles that seemed developmentally appropriate, such as troublesome thoughts about one's future, concerns about weight, misplacing or losing things, social obligations, and fear of rejection. In addition, a significant bivariate relationship was found between adolescent hassles scores and their self-rating of their physical and psychological health on 9-point semantic differential scales. Uplifts were not significantly related to either physical or psychological health.

Wagner et al. (1988) also studied the impact of negative daily events on psychological health. Their study of 58 adolescents with a mean age of 18 years measured daily negative events, major negative events, and psychological symptoms at three time points: (a) 1 month before high school graduation, (b) 2 weeks after starting college, and (c) 3 months after the semester began. There was a single measure of daily and major events for this study, the Adolescent Perceived Events Scale. Causal modeling analysis using LISREL confirmed significant path coefficients between major events and daily events and between daily events and psychological symptoms, with no significant direct path relationship between major events and symptoms. The study supported the role of daily events in psychological health for adolescents and the effect of major life events on psychological symptoms mediated by daily events.

A related study (Wolf et al., 1989) researched the effect of hassles, uplifts, and life events on the psychological well-being of freshman medical students. This young adult sample of 55 students had a mean age of 24 years. The students completed the Medical Education Hassles/Uplifts Scale and other scales at least six times during a 9-month period. As in other studies, hassles were a better predictor of both concurrent and subsequent negative mood when compared to life events. This study, however, found that life events contributed to subsequent positive moods. Uplifts were found to be unrelated to psychological well-being.

The results of studies of hassles across the life span confirm that although specific hassles differ depending on age and development, day-to-day microstressors that are relevant to the individuals have a negative effect on health outcomes. This was demonstrated when the Hassles Scale was a broad and general measure, such as the original Hassles and Uplifts scales (Kanner et al., 1981), or with investigator-developed scales that addressed specific populations, such as caregivers or medical students (Kinney & Stephens, 1989a; Wolf et al., 1989). Furthermore, the relative strength of hassles as a predictor of health state and the mediating effect of hassles have been supported in samples across the age continuum (Wagner et al., 1988; Weinberger et al., 1987).

Effects of Hassles and Uplifts Across Different Cultural Groups

Research examining the effects of hassles and uplifts has been implemented in many countries throughout the world, and a few studies in the United States have used samples from diverse ethnic and racial groups. In England, several studies of hassles as predictors of specific illness symptoms, upper respiratory infections, and irritable bowel syndrome have been implemented (Dancey et al., 1995; Evans & Edgerton, 1991; Evans et al., 1988). Studies have also been conducted in New Zealand (Leathem et al., 1996), Canada (Ravindran et al., 1996), and Israel (Weller & Avinir, 1993). In the study by Weller and Avinir, the Hassles and Uplifts Scale was translated into Hebrew. In general, studies in different countries have found hassles to be related to the health outcome measures being studied.

The majority of studies examining the effects of hassles and uplifts on health outcomes have used samples composed of people that were predominantly white, well educated, and middle or upper middle class. Three exceptions are Williams et al.'s (1992) study with Navajo Indian subjects, Weinberger et al.'s (1987) study with older, black women, and Ivancevich's (1986) study with hourly assembly-line employees. Both Williams et al. and Weinberger et al. used revised versions of the original Hassles and Uplifts scales (Kanner et al., 1981) to make the scale more culturally and developmentally appropriate to their samples. In the study with Navajo Indians, the authors deleted selected items and also added many items that they describe as culturally relevant (Williams et al., 1992). The tool used with older black women omitted 44 of the original 117 items that were considered inappropriate for this population based on pretest telephone interviews (Weinberger et al., 1987). Ivancevich's study with assembly-line workers used the original tool developed by Kanner and colleagues (1981) and found that hassles most frequently cited were health of a family member, too many things to do, trouble relaxing, misplacing or losing things, too many interruptions, and unchallenging work. Furthermore, Ivancevich reported that test-retest correlations for both the Uplifts and Hassles scales were similar to those found in earlier studies with more upper-middle-class samples. More studies are needed before the role of day-to-day events in predicting health outcomes can be generalized across cultures and socioeconomic groups. Research to date, however, supports the applicability of the Hassles and Uplifts Model across diverse populations.

Summary

Empirical support for the Hassles and Uplifts Model has been provided using a variety of samples, study designs, measurement approaches for hassles, and health-related outcomes measures. In particular, the breadth of health-related outcomes that have been examined and found to be associated with microstressors is impressive and provides strong empirical support for the model. Study samples reported in the literature have varied from as small as 30 (Dancey et al., 1995) to several hundred subjects (Folkman et al., 1987; Weinberger et al., 1987). In general, sample sizes have been adequate and appropriate to the study designs and analyses used. Many of the studies found in the literature, however, have used a one-time administration of a measure asking for retrospective identification of hassles and have correlated this score with a variety of self-identified health outcomes also measured on one occasion only (Ewedemi & Linn, 1987; Kanner & Feldman, 1991; Kinney & Stephens, 1989; Kinney et al., 1995; Leathem et al., 1996; Miller, Wilcox, & Soper, 1985; Ravindran et al., 1996; Weller & Avinir, 1993; Williams et al., 1992; Zarski, 1984). Although contributing to the literature, these studies are limited in their ability to demonstrate causal relationships between ongoing daily microstressors and health outcomes, and they are not congruent with the process focus of the TTSC.

In contrast, many studies of the Hassles and Uplifts Model have been longitudinal, using repeated administrations of the Hassles and Uplifts scales to describe negative and positive day-to-day events that have occurred during the previous month (DeLongis et al., 1982; Folkman et al., 1987; Ivancevich, 1986; Kanner et al., 1981; Monroe, 1983; Weinberger et al., 1987; Wolf et al., 1989). Study periods have varied from 4 to 9 months, and repeated measures have allowed analyses that have examined both concurrent relationships between hassles and outcomes and the predictive effects of hassles on health outcomes.

One of the criticisms of some of the earlier studies of the Hassles and Uplifts Model was that retrospective measurement of hassles by asking individuals to recall experiences during an entire month may not be very reliable. DeLongis et al. (1987) responded to this criticism in part by having subjects in their later study of younger and older adults complete a revised Hassles and Uplifts measure for 4 consecutive days each month immediately before they were interviewed about their coping. Mean scores for hassles were calculated, thus providing a more consistent and therefore reliable measure of actual day-to-day stressors.

Alternately, many studies used a day-to-day approach to measuring stress of daily events. These studies also were longitudinal, used repeated measures that generally extended 9 to 12 weeks, and used a daily diary completed by subjects at the end of each day to measure day-to-day stressors (Evans & Edgerton, 1991; Evans et al., 1988; Jandorf et al., 1986; Stone et al., 1987; Wagner et al., 1988). The day-to-day measurement of hassles in a longitudinal design could be considered more prospective and is the most congruent with the TTSC, and results from these studies provide strong empirical support for the Hassles and Uplifts Model.

➤ HASSLES AND UPLIFTS AND NURSING KNOWLEDGE

Overview of Studies

The Hassles and Uplift Model has been empirically examined by researchers in the disciplines of nursing, psychology, medicine, organizational behavior, and behavioral health. Nurse scientists have been particularly attracted to the model as a possible explanation and predictor of health outcomes. Studies have examined the Hassles and Uplifts Model applied to such diverse health outcomes as perimenstrual symptoms (Woods, Most, &

Longenecker, 1985), rheumatoid arthritis (Crosby, 1988), perceptions of health in adolescent females (De Maio-Esteves, 1990), and depression in female nursing students (Williams, Hagerty, Murphy-Weinberg, & Wan, 1995). In addition, hassles and uplifts have been examined in relationship to symptoms of genital herpes (Swanson, Dibble, & Chenitz, 1995), as a covariate in understanding perceived health among subjects quitting smoking (Macnee, 1991), and as a predictor of exercise behavior in perimenopausal women (Evans & Nies, 1997).

The empirical use of the Hassles and Uplifts Model in nursing has centered on examination of common negative daily stressful events, or hassles, and the link between symptom expression and underlying illness state. Consistent with other empirical uses of the model, nurse researchers have focused mainly on examining the impact of hassles on health states and have not investigated uplifts as protective factors in health. Nursing studies, like those in other disciplines, have consistently found a significant relationship between a person's psychological perception of microstressors and the individual's subsequent perceptions of health or symptom expression or both.

Appropriateness and Use of the Model for Nursing

The process nature of the Hassles and Uplifts Model has made it particularly appropriate to nursing studies. One of the first nursing studies to use the Hassles and Uplift Model applied it to the examination of the experience of perimenstrual symptoms and the relationship of symptom level to stress (Woods et al., 1985). In this study, the Hassles and Uplifts Model was used as the conceptual basis for attempting to explain the influence of a women's psychosocial context on their experience of perimenstrual symptoms. Nursing studies using the Hassles and Uplift Model share a basic premise identified in

Woods et al.'s (1985) study: Individuals who perceive life as more stressful, experience and act on symptoms of illness more than those whose environment is individually perceived as less stressful. Stress, coping, and the subsequent impact of these variables on health has historically been considered integral to the practice of nursing. From this perspective, the Hassles and Uplift Model is both relevant and appropriate to nursing studies.

Most of the nursing research using the Hassles and Uplifts Model as the conceptual basis of study is predicated on the assumption that daily, common, continuous stressor events, referred to as hassles, have more and different impact than major stress events on individual perceptions of health. Only Woods et al.'s (1985) study does not make this assumption, instead trying to contrast the impact of major stress events with the impact of daily hassles.

There is consistency in the conceptual definitions for hassles and uplifts in most nursing studies using the Hassles and Uplifts Model. The researchers directly link their studies to the work of Lazarus (1966), drawing direct connections from the nursing studies to the larger body of stress and coping literature. All definitions have used language from Lazarus and others that describes hassles as irritating, frustrating, and distressing demands of everyday transactions with the environment, with the Swanson et al. (1995) and Williams et al. (1995) studies having the least explicit definitions. Although all the nursing studies provided conceptual definitions of the hassles variable, less consistent evidence was found regarding definitions of health and stress.

De Maio-Esteves (1990) and Macnee (1991) provided specific conceptual definitions of stress and health. Both authors used definitions derived from the Hassles and Uplift Model, citing stress as the relationship between person and environment that is perceived as taxing resources or endangering wellness. Health is viewed as the outcome of this dynamic relationship.

With the exception of the study by Woods and colleagues (1985), most of the studies used established measures of hassles, such as the Daily Hassles Scale (Kanner et al., 1981) or the Hassles and Uplift Scale (DeLongis et al., 1982). These research instruments rely on subjective determinants and patient self-reports of the impact of daily experiences, and it is this subjectivity of the measures that has been consistently identified as one of the criticisms of the use of the Hassles and Uplift Model. The subjectivity of measurement of hassles will be discussed later.

In all the studies in which the Hassles and Uplift Model is identified as a basis for the research, both the model and the subsequent measurement instrument are only one of numerous measures used to identify both levels of stress and the sequella impacts on perceived health. Many of the studies used measures specific to the illness state of interest, such as the Genital Herpes Questionnaire (Swanson et al., 1995), the Rheumatoid Arthritis Disease Activity instrument (Crosby, 1988), the Measurement of Exercise subscale (Evans & Nies, 1997), and the Menstrual Distress Questionnaire (Woods et al., 1985). Other studies used instruments measuring more generalized concepts of health, coping, or stress, such as the Bradburn Morale Scale (Macnee, 1991), the General Health Rating Index (De Maio-Esteves, 1990), and the Coping Scale (Williams et al., 1995).

Studies applying the Hassles and Uplift Model to nursing have used small to moderate sample sizes. Attempts have been made to reflect diversity in subjects, but most study samples were composed of predominantly white females. Samples for studies using the Hassles and Uplifts Model commonly employed convenience sampling strategies, and their sizes ranged from 35 (Evans & Nies, 1997) to 408 subjects (Williams et al., 1995). Woods et al. (1985) used a sample of 100 women who were drawn from different neighborhoods and who represented a mix of racial and socioeconomic backgrounds. In the sample, there was an average age of 27 years, and it comprised 63% white and 37% black women.

Crosby (1988) used a sample of 101 subjects—68 women and 33 men who had a mean age of 46 years. No information was provided about race in this study. De Maio-Esteves (1985) used a sample size of 159 adolescents between the ages of 14 and 16, all of whom were female and 86% of whom were white. Williams et al.'s (1995) study had the largest sample size, with 408 female nursing students. Swanson et al. (1995) and Evans and Nies (1997) both used samples that were composed of predominantly white women, and Macnee's (1991) sample of 240 subjects consisted of 114 men and 126 women, 70% of whom were white.

The Hassles and Uplifts Model has been empirically tested in nursing using a variety of methodologies. One study was longitudinal (Woods et al., 1985), and two studies used path analysis to examine both direct and indirect effects of hassles and uplifts on health (De Maio-Esteves, 1990; Williams et al., 1995). Cross-sectional designs, however, were the most common method used by nurse scientists.

Results from studies using the Hassles and Uplifts Model have contributed to the development of nursing knowledge. These findings are consistent with results discussed earlier from the larger body of research testing the Hassles and Uplifts Model. Like many of the nonnursing studies, Woods et al.'s (1985) study found that daily hassles were more influential in symptom expression of perimenstrual symptoms than were cumulative major life events. Also consistent with the greater body of research, the two studies that examined uplifts found them to have much lower correlation with symptom expression (either perimenstrual or depression) than hassles (Williams et al., 1995; Woods et al., 1985).

Findings from nursing studies have repeatedly supported the impact of hassles on specific symptom expression. Williams et al. (1985) reported that hassles were directly and indirectly related to depression. Macnee (1991) revealed that scores for the intensity of daily hassles were significantly higher and well-being scores lower for persons quitting smoking when compared to those of smokers and nonsmokers. Crosby (1988) found a posi-

tive significant correlation between the number of stress factors experienced in arthritis patients, the severity of factors experienced, and the patients' negative emotional stress levels. No direct relationship was found, however, between hassles and symptoms of rheumatoid arthritis.

Crosby's (1988) findings seemed to be supported by the finding of DeMaio-Esteves (1990) that there was a significant negative relationship between hassles and perceived health status, and that this relationship was mediated by introspective and problem-focused coping. Swanson et al. (1995) reported that young adults with genital herpes had greater hassles and lower perceived health scores when compared to those of young adults without herpes. Findings of nursing studies have been used to deductively conclude that the frequency and severity of hassles relate to emotional stress and perceived health. Swanson et al.'s (1995) study, however, raises an interesting point: the issue of direction of causality between perceived health and hassles. Given the process nature of the Hassles and Uplifts Model, causality may be appropriately examined only using longitudinal repeated measures designs.

➤ FIT OF HASSLES AND UPLIFTS MODEL TO NURSING SCIENCE

The process focus of the Hassles and Uplifts Model seems to have a natural fit with nursing studies. Expanding philosophical positions within nursing's meta-theoretical development have increasingly focused interest on the more subjective, less quantitative aspects of health and illness. Rethinking ontological and epistemological assumptions regarding the meta-theoretical basis of nursing practice has provided the opportunity for development of nursing science through methods of inquiry grounded increasingly less in logical empiricism. Central to the changing philosophical paradigms of nursing's meta-theory is the increased acceptance of the importance and richness of data obtained through what

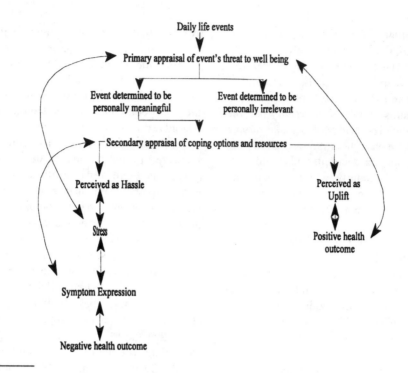

Figure 6.1. Schematic Representation of the Hassles and Uplifts Model as Described by Lazarus and Colleagues

were previously considered subjective data sources.

The Hassles and Uplifts Model (Figure 6.1) relies heavily on the transactional process of perceptions regarding stress impacting the ontological experiences of health. The Hassles and Uplifts Model requires acceptance of the importance of perceptions in the construction of reality and of the potential existence of multiple realities. Subjective data sources are critical and appropriate avenues for understanding the potential realities of health that exist in patients.

The fit of the Hassles and Uplifts Model goes beyond the metatheoretical level to the grand theory level as well. Walker and Avant (1995) clearly show that grand theories of nursing have been instrumental in establishing nursing as different from the practice of medicine. One of the common elements in all the grand nursing theories is health (Chinn & Kramer, 1995), which is almost always de-

fined as the goal of the practice of nursing (Chinn & Kramer, 1995; Walker & Avant, 1995). Although grand theories differ in conceptual definitions and semantics of expression of health, it remains a crucial aspect of the profession of nursing, and models that have research capability to test the notion of health are essential to continued nursing knowledge development.

The fit between the Hassles and Uplifts Model and nursing grand theory can be seen in the use of a cognitive perceptual approach to health in both the model and King's theory of goal attainment. Perception is one of 11 major concepts in King's theory of goal attainment, although it is not operationally defined. In addition, perception is included as part of the operationalization of the concept of interaction. Specifically, King proposes that both nurse's and client's perceptions lead to judgments and actions to accomplish the goal or outcome of care (George, 1995).

The Hassles and Uplifts Model can best be considered as a midrange theory from another discipline that has usefulness for nursing science. The model has a limited number of variables and limited scope, but it is testable and sufficiently broad to be of interest to the profession of nursing (Walker & Avant, 1995). Its specificity, usefulness, and empirical adequacy are evident in the number of nursing research studies that have been based on the model.

One of the puzzles in the literature regarding Hassles and Uplift theory is Lazarus's (1984) reference to his model as recursive followed by a narrative description of the transactional and process-focused nature of the model. The use of the Hassles and Uplifts Model in nursing knowledge development has consistently ignored this issue and has applied the model as a fully nonrecursive conceptual basis for research studies, consistent with postpositivistic methods of inquiry. For example, Crosby (1988) applied the Hassles and Uplifts Model to her study of the impact of stress factors on the disease expression of rheumatoid arthritis. This study interprets the Hassles and Uplifts Model as nonrecursive and specifies that interpretation of the model is analogous to "cybernetic" feedback loops (p. 453). Another example is De Maio-Esteves's (1990) discussion of her theoretical model that alludes to stress as affecting perceptions of health, which in turn affect appraisals of stress. Macnee (1991) discusses how the stress of quitting smoking can alter existing coping and states that this alteration of coping patterns could be perceived as stressful, thus clearly implying a nonrecursive use of the model.

Schematic of the Hassles and Uplifts Model

The Hassles and Uplifts Model was not presented in a schematic fashion by Lazarus (1966). Visual interpretation of the model is shown in Figure 6.1. The schematic begins with daily events and posits that these events are individually perceived as either a hassle or an uplift depending on the personal meaningfulness of the daily event and the relative perception of the potential for threat to well-being contained in the event. Both hassles and uplifts theoretically have equal influence on the health outcomes of an individual, with hassles having a negative impact and uplifts a positive impact. Hassles lead to stress, which is the intervening variable for negative health outcomes. Both stress and negative health outcomes relate to primary appraisal of daily events, as do positive health outcomes.

➤ INSTRUMENTS TO ASSESS HASSLES AND UPLIFTS

Hassles and uplifts were originally operationalized by Lazarus and his team (Kanner et al., 1981) by using two separate scales consisting of 117 items identified as daily stressors (hassles) and 135 items identified as positive daily events (uplifts). These items were generated by research staff and were considered to cover dimensions of work, health, family, friends, the environment, practical considerations, and chance occurrences. Initially, the scales were rated with regard to frequency and severity or strength; these two ratings, however, were found to be redundant. Therefore, participants were asked to rate hassles on a 3-point severity scale and to rate uplifts on a 3-point frequency of occurrence scale. Hassles scores were calculated to reflect the raw number of hassles checked, a summed severity score for all the hassles checked, or an intensity score by dividing the severity score by the number of hassles rated. Uplifts scores were computed for raw frequency, summed scores for the frequency of occurrence of the uplifts, and intensity.

This original scale was used in a variety of studies (DeLongis et al., 1982; Kanner et al., 1981; Miller et al., 1985; Ravindran et al., 1996; Weinberger et al., 1987) with supporting validity and stability through moderate to high test-retest correlations (Ivancevich,

1986; Kanner et al., 1981). The scale was later revised so that it consisted of only 53 single words or phrases that reflected aspects of daily life that could be evaluated as positive or negative. This was done to create a shorter scale that combined hassles and uplifts in response to criticism that the original scales did not allow for the subject experience of events as either positive (an uplift) or negative (a hassle) (Lazarus, 1990). Items on the shorter scale were rated on separate 4-point Likert-type scales for how much each item was a hassle or an uplift (DeLongis, 1985). This scale and its eight subscales have been shown to have both test-retest and internal consistency reliability (DeLongis, 1985), and this scale was used in a prospective study to demonstrate concurrent validity (DeLongis, Folkman, & Lazarus, 1988).

There are two major concerns regarding the hassles and uplifts measures: the subjective nature of the items included on the scale and the confounding of hassle measures with health outcomes. The first concern reflects an epistemological issue that is at the core of the Hassles and Uplifts Model, namely, whether microstressors should be viewed as objective environmental inputs or as products of subjective appraisals of threat in relation to environmental demands and personal resources (Lazarus, 1990; Lazarus, DeLongis, Folkman, & Gruen, 1985). Lazarus and colleagues have consistently responded to the criticism that their scale is too subjective by confirming that this is exactly what they intend and reflects what they believe to be theoretically sound.

The issue of confounds between the hassles and uplifts measures and health outcomes has received more attention and has generally been more difficult to resolve. Both the original and the revised hassles scales include items that directly address health concerns. In general, researchers have chosen to delete these items from their analysis to avoid the potential for obvious confounding between subjective ratings of health concerns as hassles and outcome measures of somatic or psychological symptoms. This reduces the stability of the measures, however.

There is concern that items on the Hassles Scale reflect psychopathology or distress and therefore are redundant of outcome measures of health (particularly psychological health). Lazarus and colleagues (1985) responded to this concern empirically and theoretically, and they confirmed that there is some confounding between measures of stress and those of illness that is inevitable given their relational theory of stress. They argue, however, that the confounding is limited and that the strength of the relationships found between hassles and health or well-being is too significant and extensive to reflect confounding alone. This argument is supported by studies of the effects of microstressors on health that have used measures other than the hassles and uplifts measures (Jandorf et al., 1986; Monroe, 1983; Stone et al., 1987).

As mentioned previously, another criticism of the hassles and uplifts measures has been the retrospective nature of the measurement. That is, subjects are asked to recall hassles or uplifts or both over long periods of time (Kanner et al., 1991). An approach to the measurement of daily events to address this concern has been the use of a daily diary with a list of events that are related to work, leisure, family and friends, and other events (Evans et al., 1988; Jandorf et al., 1986; Stone et al., 1987). These events are rated daily regarding their desirability and meaningfulness. Thus, subjects can determine whether a particular event is desirable or undesirable soon after it occurs, and events are rated daily (avoiding problems with retrospective recall) (Jandorf et al., 1986). The difficulty with this method of measurement is that it is very demanding of subjects' time and requires much effort; thus, subject retention may become an issue.

A final concern regarding measurement of day-to-day microstressors relates to the cultural or developmental relevance of specific measures. No studies have explicitly determined whether Hassles and Uplifts measures are culturally or developmentally appropriate. Folkman et al. (1987) and Miller and colleagues (1985), however, noted that selected hassles are endorsed more or less frequently depending on age. Several researchers have addressed this concern about cultural or developmental relevance by adapting established measures to the unique populations being studied (Ivancevich, 1986; Weinberger et al., 1987) or by developing their own measures (Kinney et al., 1995; Wagner et al., 1988). Additional studies are needed to more thoroughly examine the cultural and developmental relevance of selected measures of microstressors.

➤ IMPLICATIONS OF HASSLES AND UPLIFTS FOR NURSING THEORY, PRACTICE, AND RESEARCH

The Hassles and Uplifts Model takes stress and coping theory beyond the linear perspective of inputs and outputs that are reflected in the physiological models of stress and coping (Selye, 1950) and life events theory (Holmes & Rahe, 1967). It is a well-developed and tested model, clearly grounded and conceptualized within the larger TTSC. Relationships within the model are explicitly stated, and the concepts are theoretically and operationally defined. These relationships and concepts have received considerable testing and, at least for the hassles' portion of the model, have been repeatedly supported in a wide range of studies in both the field of nursing and others. The use of the model for developing and testing knowledge about the relationships between stress and health is evident given the large number of publications and studies based on the model.

The Hassles and Uplifts Model is very consistent with nursing's holistic view of persons and health and is congruent with most nursing theories. The model not only has use for theoretical knowledge development but also has been applied and tested in clinical nursing studies that have direct implications for practice. Research has supported the relationship of hassles to symptoms from rheumatoid arthritis, perimenstrual symptoms, genital herpes symptoms, and depression. These results suggest and assist the development of

nursing practice models that address the need to direct nursing care toward understanding and perhaps modifying clients' perceptions and coping approaches to day-to-day events. Knowledge gained from studies using the Hassles and Uplifts Model suggests that a combination of increasing hassles with decreasing uplifts leads to the development of common illnesses such as the cold (Evans & Edgerton, 1991; Evans et al., 1988). These results suggest the possibility of assisting clients to identify high-risk periods in their lives and a need to increase their self-care in other ways to perhaps offset the potential effects of day-to-day stressors. Therefore, the Hassles and Uplifts Model, because of the level of theory it represents and the extensive testing it has received, has many implications for nursing practice that need to be explored and tested further.

Implications for future research using the Hassles and Uplifts Model are extensive. The model has significant potential to be used as a means for controlling statistically for the effects of day-to-day stresses and strains when researchers are seeking to explore other factors that impact health outcomes. The model has received only limited testing in diverse cultures; therefore, additional studies with different socioeconomic groups are also needed. Issues of measurement and study design need continued examination. Furthermore, although results of empirical studies have consistently supported the effects of day-to-day events (that are perceived as salient and threatening on health outcomes), findings regarding the effects of positively toned events are inconsistent and controversial. Lazarus and colleagues originally proposed equal and balancing effects for hassles and uplifts. Empirical studies, however, suggest that uplifts may act more as modifiers for the effects of hassles or may have only an interaction effect on health outcomes. A modified schematic of the model derived from existing empirical testing and viewing uplifts as modifiers might appear as shown in Figure 6.2. This type of interactional effect for uplifts deserves exploration to further develop nursing's under-

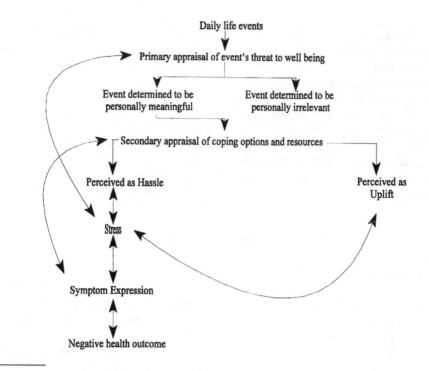

Figure 6.2. Modified Schematic of the Hassles and Uplifts Model Based on Results of Empirical Testing and Viewing Uplifts as Modifiers

standing of the role of perceptions and coping with daily events in stress and health.

In summary, the Hassles and Uplifts Model is a well-tested model that is congruent with nursing's perspective of health and has demonstrated utility for nursing practice. Future research is needed using samples from diverse cultures and socioeconomic backgrounds and to test the possible modifier effect of uplifts on the effects of hassles.

➤ REFERENCES

Chinn, P. L., & Kramer, M. K. (1995). *Theory and nursing: A systems approach* (4th ed.). St. Louis, MO: C. V. Mosby.

Crosby, L. J. (1988). Stress factors, emotional stress and rheumatoid arthritis disease activity. *Journal of Advanced Nursing, 13,* 452-461.

Dancey, C. P., Whitehouse, A., Painter, J., & Backhouse, S. (1995). The relationship between hassles, uplifts

and irritable bowel syndrome: A preliminary study. *Journal of Psychosomatic Research, 39*(7), 827-832.

DeLongis, A. (1985). *The relationship of everyday stress to health and well-being: Inter- and intraindividual approaches.* Unpublished doctoral dissertation, University of California, Berkeley.

DeLongis, A., Coyne, J. C., Dakof, G., Folkman, S., & Lazarus, R. S. (1982). Relationship of daily hassles, uplifts, and major life events to health status. *Health Psychology, 7*(2), 119-136.

DeLongis, A., Folkman, S., & Lazarus, R. S. (1988). The impact of daily stress on health and mood: Psychological and social resources as mediators. *Journal of Personality and Social Psychology, 54*(3), 486-495.

De Maio-Esteves, M. (1990). Mediators of daily stress and perceived health status in adolescent girls. *Nursing Research, 39*(6), 360-364.

Dykema, J., Bergbower, K., & Peterson, C. (1995). Pessimistic explanatory style, stress and illness. *Journal of Social and Clinical Psychology, 14*(4), 357-371.

Evans, M. S., & Nies, M. A. (1997). The effects of daily hassles on exercise participation in perimenopausal women. *Public Health Nursing, 14*(2), 129-133.

Evans, P. D., & Edgerton, N. (1991). Life-events and mood as predictors of the common cold. *British Journal of Medical Psychology, 64*, 35-44.

Evans, P. D., Pitts, M. K., & Smith, K. (1988). Minor infection, minor life events and the four day desirability dip. *Journal of Psychosomatic Research, 32*(4/5), 533-539.

Ewedemi, F., & Linn, M. W. (1987). Health and hassles in older and younger men. *Journal of Clinical Psychology, 43*(4), 347-353.

Folkman, S., Lazarus, R. S., Pimley, S., & Novacek, J. (1987). Age differences in stress and coping processes. *Psychology and Aging, 2*(2), 171-184.

George, J. B. (1995). Imogene M. King. In J. B. George (Ed.), *Nursing theories: The base for professional nursing practice* (pp. 209-228). Norwalk, CT: Appleton & Lange.

Holmes, T. H., & Rahe, R. (1967). The Social Readjustment Rating Scale. *Journal of Psychosomatic Research, 12*, 213-218.

Ivancevich, J. M. (1986). Life events and hassles as predictors of health, symptoms, job performance, and absenteeism. *Journal of Occupational Behavior, 7*, 39-51.

Jandorf, L., Deblinger, E., Neale, J. M., & Stone, A. A. (1986). Daily versus major life events as predictors of symptom frequency: A replication study. *Journal of General Psychology, 113*(3), 205-218.

Kanner, A. D., Coyne, J. C., Schaefer, C., & Lazarus, R. S. (1981). Comparison of two modes of stress measurement: Daily hassles and uplifts versus major life events. *Journal of Behavioral Medicine, 4*, 1-39.

Kanner, A. D., & Feldman, S. S. (1991). Control over uplifts and hassles and its relationship to adaptational outcomes. *Journal of Behavioral Medicine, 14*(2), 187-201.

Kinney, J. M., & Stephens, M. A. P. (1989a). Hassles and uplifts of giving care to a family member with dementia. *Psychology and Aging, 4*(4), 402-408.

Kinney, J. M., & Stephens, M. A. P. (1986b). Caregiving hassles scale: Assessing the daily hassles of family members with dementia. *The Gerontologist, 29*(3), 328-332.

Kinney, J. M., Stephens, M. A. P., Franks, M. M., & Norris, V. K. (1995). Stresses and satisfactions of family care givers to older stroke patients. *Journal of Applied Gerontology, 14*, 3-21.

Lazarus, R. S. (1966). *Psychological stress and coping process.* New York: McGraw-Hill.

Lazarus, R. S. (1984). Puzzles in the study of daily hassles. *Journal of Behavioral Medicine, 7*(4), 375-389.

Lazarus, R. S. (1990). Target article: Theory-based stress measurement. *Psychological Inquiry, 1*, 3-13.

Lazarus, R. S. (1993). Coping, theory and research: Past, present and future. *Psychosomatic Medicine, 55*, 234-247.

Lazarus, R. S., DeLongis, A., Folkman, S., & Gruen, R. (1985). Stress and adaptational outcomes: The problem of confounded measures. *American Psychologist, 40*(7), 770-779.

Leathem, J., Heath, E., & Woolley, C. (1996). Relatives perceptions of role change, social support and stress after traumatic brain injury. *Brain Injury, 10*, 27-38.

Lewin, K. A. (1951). Field theory and learning. In D. Cartwright (Ed.), *Field theory in social science: Selected theoretical papers by Kurt Lewin.* New York: Harper.

Macnee, C. L. (1991). Perceived well-being of persons quitting smoking. *Nursing Research, 40*(4), 200-203.

Margiotta, E. W., Davilla, D. A., & Hicks, R. A. (1990). Type A-B behavior and the self-report of daily hassles and uplifts. *Perceptual and Motor Skills, 70*, 777-778.

Miller, M. J., Tobacyk, J. J., & Wilcox, C. T. (1985). Daily hassles and uplifts as perceived by adolescents. *Psychological Reports, 56*, 221-222.

Miller, M. J., Wilcox, C. T., & Soper, B. (1985, November). Measuring hassles and uplifts among adolescents: A different approach to the study of stress. *The School Counselor*, 107-110.

Monroe, S. M. (1983). Major and minor life events as predictors of psychological distress: Further issues and findings. *Journal of Behavioral Medicine, 6*(2), 189-205.

Ravindran, A. V., Griffiths, J., Merali, Z., & Anisman, H. (1996). Primary dysthymia: A study of several psychosocial, endocrine and immune correlates. *Journal of Affective Disorder, 40*, 73-84.

Selye, H. (1950). Forty years of stress research: Principal remaining problems and misconceptions. *CMA Journal, 115*, 53-55.

Stone, A. A., Reed, B. R., & Neale, J. M. (1987, Summer). Changes in daily event frequency precede episodes of physical symptoms. *Journal of Human Stress*, 70-74.

Swanson, J. M., Dibble, S. L., & Chenitz, W. C. (1995). Clinical features and psychosocial factors in young adults with genital herpes. *Image: Journal of Nursing Scholarship, 27*, 16-22.

Wagner, B. M., Compas, B. E., & Howell, D. C. (1988). Daily and major life events: A test of an integrative model of psychosocial stress. *American Journal of Community Psychology, 16*(2), 189-205.

Walker, L. O., & Avant, K. C. (1995). *Strategies for theory construction in nursing* (3rd ed.). Norwalk CT: Appleton & Lange.

Weinberger, M., Hiner, S. L., & Tierney, W. M. (1987). In support of hassles as a measure of stress in predicting health outcomes. *Journal of Behavioral Medicine, 10*, 19-31.

Weller, L., & Avinir, O. (1993). Hassles, uplifts, and quality of sleep. *Perceptual and Motor Skills, 76,* 571-576.

Williams, R., Zyzanski, S., & Wright, A. L. (1992). Life events and daily hassles and uplifts as predictors of hospitalization and outpatient visitation. *Social Science Medicine, 34*(7), 763-768.

Williams, R. A., Hagerty, B. M., Murphy-Weinberg, V., & Wan, J.-Y. (1995). Symptoms of depression among female nursing students. *Archives of Psychiatric Nursing, 9*(5), 269-278.

Wolf, T. M., Elston, R. C., & Kissling, G. E. (1989, Spring). Relationship of hassles, uplifts, and life events to psychological well-being of freshman medical students. *Behavioral Medicine,* 37-45.

Woods, N. F., Most, A., & Longenecker, G. D. (1985). Major life events, daily stressors, and perimenstrual symptoms. *Nursing Research, 34*(5), 263-267.

Zarski, J. J. (1984). Hassles and health: A replication. *Health Psychology, 3*(3), 243-251.

CHAPTER 7

Stress, Psychosomatic Illness, and Health

Frances B. Wimbush and Margot L. Nelson

➤ STRESS AND PSYCHOSOMATIC HEALTH

For more than 300 years, Western culture has subscribed to a mechanistic model of health based on the philosophy of René Descartes (1596-1650) that the mind and body are separate and on the laws of physics created by Sir Isaac Newton (1642-1727) and inspired by the work of Descartes. This mechanistic paradigm (also called the "reductionist" model) compares the universe and all its components to a large mechanical clock in which everything operates in a sequential and predictable form. Influenced by Newtonian physics, the field of medicine applied this mechanistic model to the human organism. This era of medicine focused on signs and symptoms of dysfunction, and physicians were taught to "fix" or repair the parts that were not operating properly, primarily through medications and surgery.

In the mechanistic world of medicine, the responsibility for recovery was removed almost completely from the patient and placed with the physician. This model failed to include the multiple dimensions of the human

organism that contributed to both the development of the disease and the healing process (Seaward, 1997). These dimensions of mind, emotion, and spirit became "connected" to the body with the evolution of concepts such as stress and psychosomatic illness.

It has been estimated that as many as 70% to 80% of all patient visits to internists and family practice physicians are made by individuals with psychophysiologic conditions (Corbin, Hanson, Happ, & Whitby, 1988). Historically, the term *psychosomatic* was used to describe physical health problems that were the consequence of excessive emotional arousal, maladaptive coping, and chronic stress. The premise of psychosomatic illness is that the mind and emotions play important roles in the origins or progression of disease or both. All such illnesses affect the function and structure of the human body in some way as well. The term was first introduced in 1927 by Felix Deutsch, and the first major publication on the topic was by Helen Dunbar in 1935.

Dubos (1965) noted that even infectious organic diseases did not necessarily occur just because pathogenic (disease-causing) microbes entered the body. People are constantly exposed to pathogenic organisms because they are always present in the environment. Dubos contended that emotional states, such as anxiety, anger, fear, and frustration, reduce the body's resistance to these ever-present microorganisms, increasing the likelihood of disease. On the basis of the works of Cannon (1929), Selye (1936), and Bernard (1957), Dubos concluded that "stress" was the underlying factor that contributed to lowered resistance and consequent infection.

Although the term psychosomatic illness has been widely used by a variety of disciplines, the underlying assumption of linear relationships between behavioral and physiological processes is contradicted by the unitary conception of health espoused by nursing (Newman, 1994; Parse, 1992; Rogers, 1970). All health events and states are more accurately a reflection of the undivided multidimensional wholeness of the individual. Every aspect of one's health and being interacts with all others as a unitary pattern. Nonetheless, there are important interactions between stressors of various kinds and the development and progression of certain health conditions.

Stress-related illnesses range from the common cold to cancer. Clearly, psychological states involve physiological functions that cannot be separated from each other. Both must be addressed by the health professions, including nursing, when attempting to resolve patients' complaints. Health care professionals, especially nurses, who tend to have more consistent contact with patients with psychosomatic conditions, must use a holistic approach. Clients need care that addresses their physical, psychological, cognitive, emotional, spiritual, and social concerns; anything less is only partial care.

In this chapter, we discuss theory and research that support the psychophysiological basis for specific health conditions and the more common psychophysiological (psychosomatic) problems that health care providers encounter. These conditions include heart disease, hypertension, cancer, migraines, tem-

poromandibular joint disorder (TMJ), adult-onset allergic reactions, pain, and somatoform disorders. The latter, which have a stronger psychological basis, include body dysmorphic disorder, conversion disorder, hypochondriasis, somatization disorder, pain disorder, undifferentiated somatoform disorder, and somatoform disorder not otherwise specified. Each of the previously mentioned health states, whether physical or psychological in origin, will be examined in terms of its epidemiology, etiology, and contributing psychophysiological factors. Research, measurement, and nursing intervention and treatment will also be discussed.

➢ STRESS PATHWAYS

Physiology of Stress

To understand the relationship of stress to development of illness, it is necessary for the reader to have a thorough understanding of the physiology of stress. This includes an understanding of the sensory input into the brain, the role of the sympathetic and parasympathetic nervous systems, and the effects of neurochemical mediators (cortisol and catecholamines) and their role in mediating the stress response. It is also important to understand the roles of vasopressin and thyroxine and the role of the immune system in the development of possible illnesses. All of these are discussed in other chapters in this book, or the reader may wish to consult a physiology text such as Guyton's (1996) for a more in-depth review.

There is also a large body of research that discusses the mediating or buffering effects of social connections on the physiological stress response. These mediating factors include social and family relationships, the effects of social isolation and friendships, and the stress response. These are also addressed in other chapters in this book.

In summary, neuroendocrine levels and social context are affirmed by research as significant elements in mediating the physiological effects of stress. Findings strongly support the role of cortisol and catecholamines as significant mechanisms by which chronic effects of stress are mediated. Perceptions of social status, connectedness, and support clearly influence the physiological effects of chronic stress, particularly with respect to hypertension, coronary artery disease, and immune function.

➤ PSYCHOPHYSIOLOGICAL MODELS OF STRESS

There have been several research efforts to explain the relationship between stress and disease. Although there is currently not enough scientific information to create a substantiated stress and disease model, there are theoretical frameworks that are useful in attempting to understand portions of these very complex interrelationships. Some of the most prominent theories are the Borysenko Model, Pelletier's Premodel, and the Allostatic Load Model as frameworks for the health impact of stress.

Borysenko (1987, 1991) speculates that when the immune system is functioning normally, it is precisely regulated. When it is not in homeostasis, the result can be overcorrection or underreaction of the immune function or perhaps both. Disease can occur in either case. The causes of overreactions can be exogenous (e.g., allergic reaction to a foreign substance) or endogenous (e.g., lymphocytes attack and destroy healthy tissue, resulting in diseases such as arthritis or lupus). Borysenko suggests that an abundance of stress hormones produced by exaggerated autonomic responses can result in migraines, ulcers, hypertension, irritable bowel syndrome, coronary heart disease, and asthma. When an exogenous underreaction occurs, foreign substances undermine the ability of the B cells to prevent infection, resulting in, for example, colds, flu infections, or herpes. In endogenous underreactions, antigens are not attacked by T cells and may develop in neoplasms (cancerous tumors).

Borysenko (1987, 1991) suggests that psychological stress can disrupt the precise homeostasis of the immune system. Stress is the catalyst that causes the over- or underreaction that leads to harmful physiological effects. A relaxation intervention or regular use of a technique such as meditation or mental imagery may counteract the effects of stress, returning the immune system to its homeostatic balance. The connection between the mind's ability to perceive a situation as stressful and the resulting changes in the immune system has not been identified as clearly as have the other aspects of the body's response to stress.

In discussing the Pelletier Premodel, Pelletier and Herzing (1988) noted that controlled studies have not demonstrated that positive emotions can enhance immune function. They thought that parapsychology and metaphysics needed to be examined more carefully when developing a stress-disease model. Areas to be considered in this arena include multiple personality disorder (MPD), spontaneous remissions, hypnosis, placebos, subtle energy, and immunity enhancement. Often, persons with MPD have different personalities with different diseases or with no disease. In most cases, the person has experienced a major traumatic event as a child. Stress is strongly associated with the etiology of the disease, but its disappearance and reappearance with various personalities is confusing. Even more confusing is the sudden disappearance of a diagnosed illness. Often, these persons were thought to be terminally ill. Most have been cancer sufferers, but it has been documented in other diseases as well, including HIV. Such cases are often ignored because they are anecdotal and cannot be duplicated in controlled studies. When the unconscious mind is accessed via hypnosis, physiological changes are observed that are also often difficult to understand. Biochemical changes partly responsible for healing have occurred under hypnosis. Diseases that have been "cured" when a person undergoes hypnosis include asthma, hay fever, and contact dermatitis. Adrenocorticotropic hormone is reduced in very relaxed states, but this is not enough to account for these changes.

Pelletier and Herzing (1988) support the use of magnetic resonance imaging, which is based on the concept of subtle energy, for clinical diagnosis of health and illness. They also suggest that researchers in psychoneuro-immunology examine the relationship between the principles of physics and health. Pelletier suggests that immunoenhancement should be examined in relation to the use of mental imagery, meditation, and cognitive restructuring to enhance the immune system to create an environment that is conducive to spontaneous remission and other aspects of healing. If the immune system can be suppressed through conscious thought, the result of growth of tumors and other diseases, then it should be possible to enhance the immune system.

The Allostatic Load framework was developed by McEwen and Stellar (1993) (Figure 7.1). They proposed the concept as a framework for understanding the long-term effects of physiologic responses to stress. Allostasis, as previously defined by Sterling and Eyer (1988), is the ability to achieve stability (or balance) in response to stress. Allostatic load is the "wear and tear" resulting from chronic neural and neuroendocrine activity with repeated exposure to stress. An allostatic load is imposed by recurrent activation of the sympathetic nervous system (SNS) and the HPA axis, laying a physiological foundation for disease. Within this framework, it is not only important to one's health that responses to stress occur in a timely fashion but also that they are inactivated when they are no longer needed.

Individual interpretations, social context, genetic makeup, stage of development, gender, past learning and social history, and perception of threat are all incorporated into McEwen and Stellar's (1993) Allostatic Load Model. When one perceives a situation, such as taking a final examination, as stressful, catecholamines are released from sympathetic nerve endings and from the adrenal medulla. Cortisol is released from the adrenal cortex at the same time, providing energy and increased blood flow to deal with the anticipated crisis. When the stressful circumstance no longer exists (e.g., one completes—and, it is hoped, passes—the exam), the stress response is normally inactivated, allowing for a return to baseline levels of catecholamines and cortisol. If inactivation does not occur or is incomplete, one's organs are exposed to continued excessive amounts of these neuromediators.

McEwen (1998) cited the following circumstances in which allostatic load may predispose an individual to pathology and illness: (a) frequent exposure to stressful stimuli, (b) lack of adaptation (or habituation) to a stressful situation that occurs repeatedly (Kirschbaum, Prussner, & Stone, 1995), (c) failure to terminate allostatic responses when the stressor is removed (Lowy, Wittenberg, & Yamamoto, 1995), and (d) excessive levels of one element due to lack of another (e.g., secretion of excessive inflammatory cytokines due to inadequate cortisol secretion) (Munck, & Guyre, 1991).

Virtually any source of physical or emotional stress can impose an allostatic load, depending largely on its chronicity. McEwen and Stellar (1993) cited alcohol consumption as an example of the linkage between behavioral processes and allostatic load. Alcohol may be used initially as a way to cope with stress (Sher, 1987), but new stressors are introduced by the use and abuse of alcohol, including negative reactions of family and friends, feelings of guilt and anxiety, and adverse physical health reactions (Kushner, Shen, & Beltman, 1990). Drinking behaviors then increase as a way to cope with the escalating stress, and allostatic load continues to increase in cyclical fashion.

Investigators in the MacArthur Studies of Successful Aging (McEwen, Albeck, & Cameron, 1995; Seeman, McEwen, Singer, Albert, & Rowe, 1997) quantified allostatic load through urinary cortisol measurement and discovered that subjects with lower allostatic load scores had higher levels of physical and mental functioning. These subjects also had a lower incidence of cardiovas-

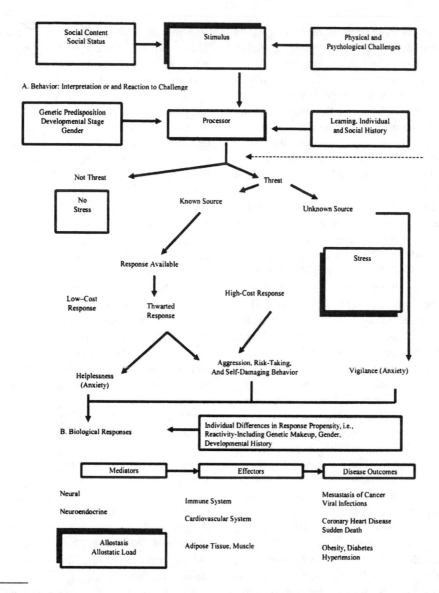

Figure 7.1. Allostatic load. Conceptual model of biology and behavior in which responses that are stressful result from the interpretation of, and behavioral and physiologic responses to, environmental challenges that may be stressful to some individuals and less or not stressful to others. (A) Physical and psychologic challenges operate within social context that includes individual social status. The processing of this information by the nervous system is biased by factors such as genetic predisposition that are operated on by developmental history, learning, and socioeconomic status; developmental age and gender are also important factors. Interpretation of a stimulus as threatening results in behavioral responses that vary in degree and cost to the individual and that are therefore stressful to varying degrees. Nonthreatening situations and low-cost responses are not considered stressful because they do not elevate physiologic responses. Stress refers to responses that are costly in terms of arousal of physiologic systems and elicitation of behaviors that are harmful. Thwarted responses may lead to aggression or result in helplessness that is similar to a response being unavailable. High-cost responses, which may include aggression, are ones that consume energy and that further increase risk to additionally challenge. All these responses, including vigilance and helplessness, have biological counterparts, and they feed back to influence additional stimulation and processing of that stimulation. (B) Behavioral responses are accompanied by neural and neuroendocrine responses that act on effectors, such as the immune and cardiovascular systems and adipose tissue and muscle. Chronic or repeated stimulation of these effectors may be due to thwarted or high-cost responses or to anxiety associated with vigilance or helplessness and may lead to allostatic load that, over time, increases risk for pathology and disease. Acute stress more readily precipitates disease when chronic stress has laid a pathophysiologic foundation (McEwen & Stellar, 1993).

cular disease, hypertension, and diabetes. In the 3-year follow-up, subjects with higher allostatic load scores at baseline were more likely to have decreased cognitive and physical functioning as well as evidence of cardiovascular disease. Although these findings lend support to the potential influence of allostatic load on specific health conditions, the use of urinary cortisol excretion as a unidimensional representation of allostatic load oversimplifies the concept.

McEwen and Stellar (1993) suggest that posttraumatic stress disorder (PTSD) provides an example of increased allostatic load. Persons with PTSD are hypervigilant and often angry and hostile (McFall, Murburg, Ko, & Veith, 1990). They have elevated catecholamine:cortisol ratios (Yehuda, Giller, Southwick, & Lowy, 1991), indicating the dominance of increased SNS activity. Hypervigilance may be both cause and result of increased SNS activity (McFall et al., 1990).

The allostatic model proposed by McEwen and colleagues offers a useful interactive and multidimensional framework for studying the relationships among physiological stress responses and the development of disease. Its primary limitation is in the recursive nature of the model, which does not allow for ongoing mutual interaction among the various elements. Although logically and empirically adequate, none of the models presented takes into account social factors and unique appraisals that are part of the whole of one's experience of stress. Perceptions of social status, connectedness, and support clearly influence the physiological effects of chronic stress, particularly with respect to health conditions such as hypertension, coronary artery disease, and immune function. Although these models may contribute to the further development of nursing frameworks, they are not by themselves adequate for nursing's holistic view of the human health experience.

Additional research needs to be conducted that addresses the immunological responses and the healing power of the mind. The roles of beliefs, positive emotions, and spiritual values should be incorporated into research related to stress, health, and illness. These spiritual aspects have largely been ignored by clinical medicine. There have been enough documented cases, however, so it is important to include these topics in future studies. Research should include the whole system approach to understand the stress-disease/mind-body phenomenon. Until a more complete model is available to examine the relationship between stress and disease, however, researchers must work with the models available. What is known about the current medical model is that physical symptoms do occur from stress and attack the health of specific regions of the body (Seaward, 1997).

It is also known that personal characteristics of the individual (age, gender, socioeconomic status, occupation, education, and fitness) all interact to either decrease or increase the person's response to stressful stimuli. Behaviors of the individual (smoking, alcohol and drug use and abuse, eating habits, and exercise) also influence the stress response either positively or negatively. Mediating factors such as coping ability, social support, economic resources, and types of relationships (conflict and supportive) either diminish or attenuate the person's responsiveness. The patients ability to cope, their spiritual resources, and "people" resources, such as family and friends, modify reactivity. Conflict and abusive relationships intensify reactivity (Thomas & Wimbush, 1999). Figure 7.2 provides an overview of the mediating factors of stress and illness.

➣ TARGET ORGANS AND THEIR DISORDERS

Psychosomatic illness can result from either an overresponsive autonomic nervous system or a suppressed immune system. It is important to understand how these physiological systems work and the pathways leading to the disease to understand the healing process. Some healing methods use a multifaceted approach, combining Western medicine with

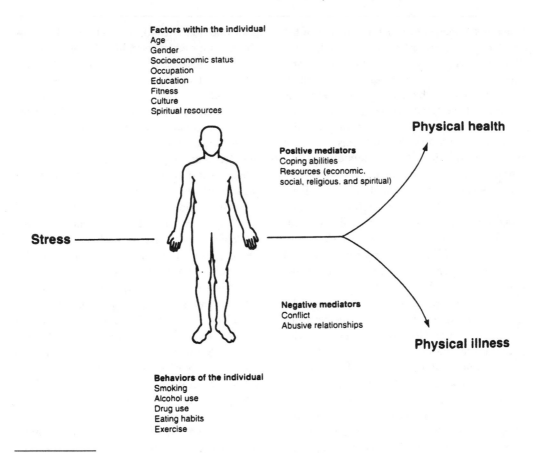

Figure 7.2. Factors within the individual
Age
Gender
Socioeconomic status
Occupation
Education
Fitness
Culture
Spiritual resources

Positive mediators
Coping abilities
Resources (economic,
social, religious, and spiritual)

Stress

Physical health

Negative mediators
Conflict
Abusive relationships

Physical illness

Behaviors of the individual
Smoking
Alcohol use
Drug use
Eating habits
Exercise

Figure 7.2. Overview of Factors Within and Around the Individual That Lead to Health and Illness

healing methods and using the power of the mind. Many physicians are reluctant to use this combination partly because they have had no formal training, and others consider a dual approach as a threat. This is compounded when there has been little or no demonstration of a relationship between specific stressors and a specific disease process.

During experiences of stress, specific target organs manifest more frequent physiological changes and may therefore be more susceptible to the neurochemical mediators of stress. These target organs vary with the individual. Any organ can be a target organ. Some people may have only one target organ (e.g., the gastrointestinal tract or the respiratory system), whereas others may have several target organs. Genetics, emotions, personality,

and environmental factors have all been suggested as explanations for target organs. Using Borysenko's model, the more common disorders and their target organs are discussed in the following sections based on two categories: nervous system-related and immune system-related disorders. A review of the role of stress in the development of the pathophysiology is followed by current research examples.

➤ DISORDERS MEDIATED BY THE AUTONOMIC NERVOUS SYSTEM

When a threat is perceived, organs that are innervated by nervous tissue are acted on by excessive secretions of the stress hormones.

These hormones stimulate the function of the target organ and increase the metabolic rate. When the organs do not have the opportunity to rest (relax), they may begin to dysfunction. Several illnesses have as initial symptoms factors that are stress related. If these are not recognized or remain untreated, they can develop into serious health problems. Some of the more common nervous system-related conditions are discussed here.

Bronchial asthma is an illness in which a pronounced secretion of bronchial fluids and constriction of the smooth muscle surrounding the bronchi restrict air movement. These effects produce a suffocating sensation, and the work of breathing increases dramatically. Asthmatic attacks can result in the need for emergency treatment and can sometimes be fatal. Some studies have linked the onset of asthmatic attacks with anxiety and others with an overprotective childhood.

Currently, β-adrenergic drugs are the first line of treatment. Relaxation techniques, such as mental imagery, autogenic training, and meditation, may be as effective as medications in delaying the onset and reducing the severity of the attacks (Henri-Benitez et al., 1990).

Tension headaches are produced by sympathetically mediated contractions of muscles of the forehead, eyes, neck, and jaw. Tension builds as the parasympathetic inhibition of muscle contraction is overpowered by sympathetic activity that increases contraction of the muscles and subsequent pain. Lower back pain can result from the same process. Over-the-counter medications such as aspirin and acetaminophen are the most common treatments. Tension headaches and low back pain have also been shown to be relieved through the use of meditation, mental imagery, and biofeedback (Blanchard et al., 1985).

Unlike tension headaches, which are produced by nervous tension in the facial muscles, a migraine headache is a vascular headache. Approximately 16 to 18 million people suffer from this type of pain. Migraines usually begin in adolescence and rarely develop after the age of 40. Four times as many women are treated for migraines as men. Migraines usually involve pain over either the left or right side of the head, usually not both, and headaches may last from 2 hours to days (Gallagher, 1990; Thomas & Wimbush, 1999). There are two types of migraine headaches: those with a prodrome, warning, or aura (classic migraine) and those without. Once the prodrome begins, the physiological pattern of the migraine is started (Saper, Silverstein, Gordon, & Hammel, 1993).

Migraines are thought to be the result of a sympathetic response to the baroreceptors of the carotid artery. Serotonin and norepinephrine are the mediators of neural transmission and vascular reactivity. The action of serotonin varies with the size of the blood vessel, causing constriction of large vessels in the external carotid tree and dilation of small vessels. Serotonin also promotes platelet aggregation. Norepinephrine levels increase during a migraine, causing vasoconstriction in the peripheral vascular bed (Thomas & Wimbush, 1999).

The response to the sympathetic stimulation involves a rapid constriction followed by a rapid dilation. The constriction is responsible for the prodrome and is often recognized by the client as a warning of an impending attack. During the dilation portion, blood moves quickly from the periphery to flood the cerebral vasculature. The change in vascular pressure, combined with humoral secretions, is thought to be the source for the intense pain often associated with migraines. Pain is usually inhibited during the vasoconstrictive phase of the aura until the aura fades and vasodilation occurs. This eliminates the pain inhibition and the migraine headache begins (Solomon & Lipton, 1990). Symptoms often described by clients include a flash of light followed by intense throbbing, dizziness, and nausea.

Migraines do not usually occur during the stressful period but rather hours later. This may account for the association of migraines with weekends and vacations (Benedittis, Lorenzetti, & Pieri, 1990). It has been speculated that migraines are related to the inability to express frustration and anger. The personality of migraine patients has been described as hardworking, hard driving, and perfectionistic. Symptoms of depression with insomnia, anorexia, constipation, lack of libido, and feelings of hopelessness are often reported (Thomas & Wimbush, 1999). Foods and beverages that cause vasoconstriction, such as alcoholic beverages and processed foods with nitrates, are associated with migraine headaches. Other foods that are high in tyramine (hard cheeses, beer, and red wine) and caffeine can precipitate a migraine as well (Saper et al., 1993).

Several medications are available for migraine treatment; current research, however, indicates that biofeedback and mental imagery can be equally effective and have fewer side effects. An effective strategy to avoid migraines is to avoid foods and beverages that may trigger a migraine and participate in daily exercise. Exercise increases vasodilation, which reduces the risk for developing a migraine.

Skeletal Muscle Conditions

Excessive contraction of the jaw muscles can lead to temporomandibular (TMJ). Often, persons are not aware that they have this problem. It is usually discovered during a dental exam when signs of clenching and grinding of teeth are noted. Other symptoms include jaw muscle pain, clicking or popping sounds when chewing, grinding of teeth during sleep, tension headaches, and earaches. Often, TMJ is so severe that the client cannot open his or her mouth wide enough to eat. Like migraines, TMJ is often associated with the inability to express feelings of anger. Other behaviors are also associated with TMJ symptoms, including activities such as resting the chin on the hand, chewing gum excessively, and nail biting. Severe cases require that a mouth brace be worn at night while sleeping. Exercises are

available, and surgery may be required. Relaxation techniques, including biofeedback and progressive muscle relaxation, have been shown to be effective in decreasing the muscle tension associated with TMJ (Eskola, Ylipaavalniemi, & Turtola, 1985; Thomas & Wimbush, 1999).

Gastrointestinal Disorders

Irritable bowel syndrome (IBS) is characterized by bouts of abdominal pain or tenderness, cramps, diarrhea, nausea, constipation, and excessive flatulence. These may be associated with a change in either the frequency or the texture of the stool. Symptoms must be present for at least 3 months. Changes in bowel habits include diarrhea alternating with constipation, a feeling of bloating or abdominal distension, and passage of mucus. The physiological mechanism for IBS symptoms seems to be an abnormal pain perception. Patients with IBS report a low pain threshold (Whitehead, 1992).

Irritable bowel syndrome is considered to be the result of excessive sympathetic neural stimulation to one or more areas of the gastrointestinal tract, with symptoms varying among individuals. This stress-related physical illness is most commonly associated with anxiety and depression. The hypothalamus is closely associated with emotional regulation and appetite regulation and may be part of the mind-body link for this condition (Mitchell & Drossman, 1997).

Data suggest that childhood trauma may be related to IBS later in life. Loss of parents, through death or divorce, has been reported more frequently by IBS patients than by healthy control subjects. It has also been reported that more than 50% of medical clinic patients with gastrointestinal disorders describe being abused sexually as children compared with 37% of medical clinic patients with other organic diseases (Whitehead, 1992).

Numerous controlled studies have demonstrated that a combination of psychological treatment approaches with standard medical therapy provides more benefits for IBS patients than medical treatment alone (Rowingson, 1993). Diets and medications are often prescribed, depending on the presenting symptoms. Several studies have incorporated relaxation and cognitive skills. Interventions include thermal biofeedback, progressive muscle relaxation, mental imagery, cognitive reappraisal, and behavior modification to reduce anxiety with good results (Guthrie, Creed, Dawson, & Tomenson, 1991). The events that result in ulcers and colitis begin with excessive sympathetic activity. Increased secretions of norepinephrine cause constriction of the vasculature in the lining of the stomach, leading to a decrease in the production of mucus by the inner lining of the stomach wall. The purpose of the mucus is to protect the stomach from the strong digestive enzymes in the stomach. If the ratio of mucus to digestive enzymes is disrupted, the inner lining becomes susceptible to the damage of the digestive enzymes. The stomach may actually begin to digest itself, resulting in a hole in the stomach wall. Ulcers were one of the first conditions that Selye associated with undue stress. Physicians have noted a strong association between anxiety and the symptoms of ulcers (most notably sharp stomach pains) (Mitchell & Drossman, 1997).

The colon is also prone to ulceration, with similar etiology resulting in colitis (inflammation of the inner lining of the colon). Relaxation techniques are often recommended along with a special diet to control the symptoms of this disease (Mitchell & Drossman, 1997).

For years it was thought that stress was the primary cause for stomach ulcers. Marshall, however, demonstrated that 75% of ulcers are caused by the bacteria Helicobacter, a carcinogen (Ubell, 1995). This bacterium can settle in the lining of the stomach, creating an open wound that is further irritated by digestive acids, resulting in moderate to severe ulceration. Antibiotics constitute the treatment of choice and have been effective for many people with ulcers. The following questions remain: What makes some people more susceptible to the bacteria than others, and why are antibiotics effective in only 75% of the people with ulcers?

Cardiovascular Conditions

The cardiovascular system as the target organ of stress is possibly the most researched area. There are two major links between the stress response and coronary heart disease. The first link is through hypertension and the second is related to atherosclerosis. The American Heart Association (AHA, 1991) estimates that cardiovascular disease is responsible for the death of one person every 32 seconds. The primary direct pathologic mechanisms of coronary artery disease are atherosclerosis and chronic injury to the coronary arterial endothelium (Manuck, Marsland, Kaplan, & Williams, 1995). The risk of atherosclerosis is closely linked to periodic or sustained elevations in blood pressure (Kaplan, Petersson, & Manuck, 1991; Muller, Tofler, & Stone, 1989), and both conditions have been linked to increased sympathetic nervous system (SNS) reactivity (Kaplan et al., 1991; Manuck, Olsson, & Hjemdahl, 1992; Potempa, 1994).

Hypertension

The most consistent and profound response during stress is elevation of blood pressure (Boone, 1991). More than 16 million Americans have elevated blood pressure. Hypertension is twice as frequent among African Americans than among Caucasians (Calhoun, 1992). In addition, the incidence of hypertension in African American women is four times that of Caucasian women. The incidence of hypertension is higher in men than in women until women reach menopause (AHA, 1999). Hypertension is defined by the World Health Organization as chronically elevated blood pressure exceeding 160/95 mmHg. Borderline hypertension is defined as blood pressure higher than 140/90 mmHg. The risk of developing fatal or nonfatal end organ damage is correlated with the amount of increase in blood pressure higher than 160/95 mmHg (AHA, 1999).

High blood pressure can result from increased cardiac output, increased peripheral resistance, and increased blood volume due to decreased sodium and water excretion. Vasopressin (ADH) also increases blood volume. The overall effect of these stress hormones is to elevate blood pressure considerably above an individual's resting levels to transport blood to areas where it is needed. Stress produces the same response, even when there is no conscious attempt to move from a stressor (Guyton, 1996).

Hypertension has been shown to be strongly linked to stressful lifestyles and to patterns of exaggerated response to stress. Genetically hypertensive animals show evidence of increased responses, such as greatly elevated levels of plasma norepinephrine and epinephrine, to acute stressors such as footshock (Chiueh & McCarty, 1981), anticipation of footshock (McCarty, Chiueh, & Kopin, 1978), and immobilization (Kvetnansky, McCarty, & Thoa, 1979) when compared to age-matched normotensives. As further evidence of the influential role of catecholamines in the development of hypertension, perinatal sympathectomy and treatment with adrenergic antagonists have been shown to prevent the development of hypertension in spontaneously hypertensive rats (Lee, Triggle, & Cheung, 1987; O'Sullivan & Harrap, 1995; Wu & Berecel, 1993).

In humans, strong links have been demonstrated between SNS and cardiovascular reactivity and the risk of hypertension (Nebjesm, Matthews, & Krantz, 1989). From a social environmental perspective, associations have been found between job strain, defined as high psychological demands and lack of control, and elevated ambulatory blood pressure (Schnall, Schwartz, Landsbergis, Warren, & Pickering, 1992). Because of the strong evidence that hypertension and job stress are correlated, high blood pressure has sometimes been used as an index of job stress (Pickering, Devereux, & James, 1996).

Cardiovascular reactivity has been proposed as a hypothetical mechanism contributing to the development of both coronary artery disease and hypertension. High cardiovascular reactivity has been described by Obrist (1981) and Potempa (1994) as a response to psychological stressors that exceeds the metabolic demand, resulting in a proportionately greater oxygen consumption for behavioral versus physical stimuli (Turner, Carroll, Hanson, & Sims, 1988). Whereas exercise tasks are associated with increased cardiac output and decreased peripheral resistance (Sherwood, Allen, Obrist, & Langer, 1986), psychological stressors are associated with slight reductions in cardiac output and increases in peripheral resistance. In the latter instance, there is preparation for "fight or flight." When the physical exertion does not occur, the increase in cardiac output is inappropriate, resulting in a compensatory vasoconstriction and elevation in blood pressure (Light, 1987; Sherwood & Turner, 1992).

Increased systolic blood pressure reactivity has been found both in borderline and in established hypertensives compared to control subjects for active coping tasks and for physical challenges such as exercise and cold pressor stimuli, although the reactivity to the coping tasks is greater (Pickering & Gerin, 1990). Exaggerated heart rate and blood pressure responses have also been found in individuals with a family history of hypertension (Matthews & Rakaczky, 1986).

Increased α-adrenergic tone and reactivity are reflected in increased peripheral vascular resistance (Weidmann, Grimm, & Meier, 1980), setting in motion a positive feedback pathway to facilitate the development of sustained hypertension. Because the vessels have higher resistance to flow, there is higher pressure, which in turn results in an increase in arterial wall thickness and remodeling (Egan, 1992). Enhanced reactivity to all vasoconstrictors has been a consistent finding in established hypertension (Egan, 1992).

Several factors have been postulated to affect cardiovascular reactivity through SNS channels. Nuclei in the brain stem and medulla are involved in cardiovascular regulation, and the medulla integrates autonomic responses and input from the limbic, cortical, cerebellar, and reticular areas of the brain (Holaday, 1983). The SNS and opiate systems interact through cortical-limbic modulation of emotional responses through adrenergic pathways (McCubbin, Cheung, Montgomery, Bulbulian, & Wilson, 1992). Light (1987) suggested that both high and low reactors begin each day at the same level, but high reactors have greater background (anticipatory) sympathetic activation and exaggerated responses to some stressors.

Endorphins and enkephalins have been proposed as inhibitory to central sympathetic activity. Their deficiency may result in greater adrenergic cardiovascular responses to stress through the absence of the normal inhibition (McCubbin et al., 1992).

Hyperinsulinemia is frequently observed in both animals and humans with hypertension (Reaven, 1991). Insulin resistance, occurring in diabetics, results in compensatory high levels of insulin production, high triglyceride levels, and glucose intolerance (Stern, Morales, Haffner, & Valdez, 1992). Increased SNS activity results, along with proliferation of arteriolar smooth muscle cells, in response to the high levels of insulin (DeFronzo & Ferrannini, 1991). Again, the increase in sympathetic tone is proposed as the link between stress, hyperinsulinemia, and hypertension development (Skyler, Donahue, Marks, Thompson, & Schneiderman, 1992).

The medical management of hypertension includes a variety of medications used in several ways. Several other mechanisms, however, may also contribute to the resolution of uncontrolled blood pressure. More conservative mechanisms to control blood pressure include dietary interventions to control weight; limited use of alcohol and caffeine; low-salt, low-cholesterol, and low-fat diets; and exercise (Boone, 1991).

Behavioral and psychological treatments of hypertension include psychotherapy, relaxation, and biofeedback. Biofeedback seems to be most effective when combined with pharmacology. Medications have been reduced be-cause of behavioral interventions and may decrease end organ damage (Thomas & Wimbush, 1999).

In summary, exaggerated sympathetic responses have been found consistently in people with hypertension or borderline hypertension and who have family histories of hypertension. In many instances, this SNS hyperactivity is correlated with a high level of job stress, high psychological demands, and lack of control. The balance of catecholamines and the inhibitory endorphins and enkephalins and hyperinsulinemia as a mediator of increased SNS activity has been proposed as a meaningful link to the development of hypertension.

Coronary Artery Disease

Coronary artery disease also has been thought to have a psychosomatic component. The three stages of coronary artery disease are atherogenesis, atherosclerosis, and arteriosclerosis. With atherogenesis, the initial stage of a fatty streak appears on the inner lining of the artery wall. There is evidence that this can occur as early as ages 3 to 5 years. As the fatty streak continues to develop around the perimeter of the artery and grow in length, a buildup of plaque occurs. This plaque results in a narrowing of the inside of the artery and is referred to as atherosclerosis. As the plaque accumulates, other constituents in the blood are attracted to the site, including calcium, resulting in an increased resistance in blood flow and increased blood pressure. As the individual ages, plaque hardens, resulting in rigid artery walls that no longer can constrict or dilate. This compounds the effect of high blood pressure and is one reason why resting pressure increases with age. At the third stage, arteriosclerosis, the arteries become hard and possibly occluded from the flow of blood. When the blood flow to any organ is impeded, signs of ischemia develop, resulting in pain (angina) or death of tissue (infarction). The degree of coronary artery blockage and the location of the affected artery determine the severity of the heart attack. The most extreme result is death. Similar etiology occurs in the carotid arteries that lead to the brain and arteries within the brain that provide oxygen to this major organ. Strokes, like coronary heart disease, are the end result of blocked arteries, creating an inadequate oxygen supply to the brain (Guyton, 1996).

Persistent stress, low social class, lack of control in one's job, job strain (defined by high psychological demands and lack of control), and certain enduring dispositional attributes are believed to affect arterial lesion progression and the development of coronary artery disease over time (Bosma et al., 1997; Cohen, Kaplan, & Manuck, 1994; Everson, Lynch, & Chesney, 1997). Although current thinking is equivocal regarding the legitimacy of the Type A behavior concept, a considerable body of research supports the association between competitiveness, time urgency, hostility, and drivenness and the development of coronary heart disease (Matthews, 1982, 1988; Review Panel, 1981).

Community-based prospective studies have suggested that higher hostility, as measured by questionnaire (Barefoot, Dodge, & Peterson, 1989) or interview, predicts both the severity (Seaward, 1997) and the progression (Dembroski, MacDougall, & Costa, 1989; Hecker, Chesney, & Black, 1988; Helmers, Krantz, & Howell, 1993; Julkunen, Salonen, & Kaplan, 1994) of coronary artery disease. Hostile individuals have shown excessive cardiovascular reactivity in the form of heart rate and sustained blood pressure responses to interpersonal laboratory stressors. Laboratory stressors producing this finding were conflict discussion tasks (Hardy & Smith, 1988; Smith & Allred, 1989), unsolvable anagrams with misleading instructions (Weidner, Friend, & Ficarrotto, 1989), and anagram tasks accompanied by harassment (Suarez, Harlan, & Peoples, 1993; Suarez, Kuhn, Schanberg, Williams, & Zimmerman, 1998; Suarez & Williams, 1990).

In summary, chronic elevations in cortisol and sympathomimetic neuromediators appear to facilitate the development of coronary artery disease and atherosclerosis. Stressors in the social environment, recurrent hostility, and a hard-driving disposition are additional influences for which there is strong research support.

➤ IMMUNE SYSTEM-RELATED DISORDERS

Emotional stress seems to change the molecular structure of biochemical agents or neuropeptides and to suppress the number and functions of several important leukocytes. Stress hormones (cortisol) may also decrease the effectiveness of leukocytes. During this process, the efficiency of protective mechanisms is decreased and the body mechanisms become more vulnerable to exogenous and endogenous antigens. Diseases that are the result of immune system disorders can be classified as exogenous (overactive or underactive) or endogenous (overactive or underactive).

Cohen, Tyrrell, and Smith (1991) found that the common cold is related to excessive stress. As B lymphocyte cells decrease, the body becomes more vulnerable to the influences of the viruses that produce the common cold. Colds and influenza are classified into the category of exogenous underreaction in Borysenko's model because there are not enough B lymphocytes to fight off the exogenous antigen (Cohen & Williamson, 1991).

An allergic reaction is initiated when a foreign substance (antigen), such as pollen, bee spores, dust, or mold, enters the body. When an antigen is present, granulocytes secrete histamines, which interact with the antigen. When there is an overactive immune response to exogenous antigens, the excess histamines cause swelling of mucus membrane tissue if the antigen is inhaled or of skin tissue in the case of infection. Some case studies have demonstrated that an actual contact with the allergen (an antigen capable of initiating this kind of reaction in an allergic individual) is not necessary to trigger the allergic response. In some individuals, allergic reactions can occur by merely thinking about or visualizing the stimulus that precipitated a previous attack. Allergic reactions seem to be more prevalent and severe in persons who are prone to anxiety. Over-the-counter medications containing antihistamine and a desensitization regime ("allergy shots") are the most common treatments that deal with allergies. Data also suggest that relaxation techniques may decrease the effects of external allergens (Seaward, 1997).

Tissue inflammation may also occur as a result of an immune response to normal cells (endogenous) that are perceived to be foreign antigens. In this situation, components of the immune system begin to attack healthy tissue, mistaking it for a foreign substance, or the healthy tissue may be damaged by the products of the immune response.

Rheumatoid arthritis, a joint and connective tissue disease, occurs when synovial membrane tissue becomes inflamed and swells, causing the joint to become inflamed. A substance known as the rheumatoid factor, a protein found in the blood, is thought to be associated with this disease. There is evidence that rheumatoid arthritis has a genetic link, and it also has an association with stress. The severity of arthritis pain is often related to episodes of stress, especially suppressed anger. Treatment ranges from pain relievers (aspirin) to steroid injections (cortisone), depending on the severity of the pain and rate of joint deterioration. Relaxation techniques are recommended as a complementary intervention to help reduce symptoms (Moran, 1991).

Cancer

Cancer is one of the most bewildering diseases of the modern day, affecting one in four Americans. Currently, the most effective treatment is prevention and early detection. The American Cancer Society (1994) defines cancer as a "large group of diseases all characterized by uncontrolled growth and spread of abnormal cells" (p. 4). There are many different types of cancer, and etiologies of each are not completely understood. There are also many theories regarding the development of cancer. The most prevalent theory is that there is a gene in the DNA that produces an abnormal cell. Such genes may be inherited, and some may be taken into the body from external sources (carcinogens). The production of an abnormal cell in the body is not uncommon. The body routinely produces mutant cells, and this process is kept in check by a normally functioning immune system, primarily through T cells and natural killer (NK) cells (Levenson & Bemis, 1991).

When a cell's genetic structure deviates from the normal cell structure, it is recognized by the immune system as an endogenous antigen and is typically destroyed by the cytotoxic T lymphocytes and NK cells. If these immune responses are depressed, the possibility of a cancerous growth is increased. If the mutant cell is not recognized, it multiplies much more quickly than a normal cell, resulting in a progressively enlarging tumor. In addition, because of the inability of the mutant cells to produce the enzymes necessary to perform normal cellular function, they take nutrients from healthy cells. Unlike normal tissue, cancer cells are not self-contained and are able to detach from their original site (cell type) and move to other areas throughout the body (metastasis) (Seaward, 1997; Temoshak, 1997).

Carcinogens have produced tumors in both laboratory animals and humans. Researchers are searching for endogenous factors, such as personality characteristics, that may play a role in the disease process. Although one can certainly not claim that one fourth of the population has similar personality traits that put them at risk for cancer, certain traits have been found to be common among individuals who develop cancer. The incidence of cancer appears to be higher among those who have difficulty expressing their emotions, have low self-esteem, and experience feelings of rejection. Interestingly, these same traits appear in persons with codependent or addictive personalities (Temoshak, 1997).

Traditional treatments for cancer include cytotoxic drugs, radiation, and surgery. Several studies (Siegel, 1986) have demonstrated that coping skills, cognitive restructuring, art therapy, and relaxation techniques such as mental imagery and meditation may be effectively used as complementary healing approaches. These methods are not thought to be a cure for cancer, but they have had a significant effect when used with traditional treatment modalities.

➤ DIAGNOSIS OF PSYCHOSOMATIC ILLNESS

Diagnosis begins with a multifocal assessment. The clinical history must be focused on the whole person—on the patient's story as told by him or her and not just on the presenting physical symptoms. A careful social, cultural, educational, occupational, cognitive, emotional, and family history can clarify potential relationships between the person's presenting problem and other contributing (stressful and nonstressful) factors in his or her life. The use of psychometric instruments can answer specific questions regarding the psychological status of the individual. There are a wide variety of instruments available for use in the clinical area. These were discussed in detail in Chapter 4, which focused on this group of diagnostic tools.

In addition to the use of psychometric measures in the assessment and diagnosis of psychosomatic illness, it is equally important to assess the physiological aspects of the stress response. The measurement of temperature, heart rate, blood pressure, and electrocardiogram pattern, in addition to a diary of events, contributes to a complete overview of the patient's holistic status (Thomas & Wimbush, 1999).

➤ SOMATOFORM DISORDERS

Somatoform disorders are defined as a group of disorders in which there are physical symptoms suggesting a physiological etiology, but no organic disease or physiological abnormalities are found. Because no evidence of physical disease is identified, the presumption is made that the physical problems are psychological in origin. This group of disorders, primarily classified as psychiatric disorders, is so widespread that it may involve as many as 30% to 40% of the medical clients seen in general and family practice settings (Fava, 1992).

The fourth edition of *Diagnostic and Statistical Manual of Mental Disorders* (*DSM-IV;* American Psychiatric Association [APA], 1994) lists several distinct and possibly related disorders. They differ from the category Psychological Factors Affecting Medical Conditions because no medical abnormalities are found in a somatoform disorder. The new *DSM-IV* category of Psychological Factors Affecting Medical Conditions may be useful with clients experiencing psychophysiological disorders. The primary feature of this condition is the presence of one or more specific psychological or behavioral features that negatively affect a general medical condition. The seven disorders are body dysmorphic disorder, conversion disorder, hypochondriasis, somatization disorder, pain disorder, undifferentiated somatoform disorder, and somatoform disorder not otherwise specified. The client diagnosed with one of these disorders often has physical symptoms that worsen during a life crisis but is not aware of the relationships between the symptom and stressful events. There is evidence of "doctor shopping" and of strained doctor-patient relationships in this population. This group of clients may submit to unnecessary surgical procedures. In addition, because health care providers are searching for the organic cause of specific symptoms, existing pathophysiology may be overlooked. Members of this group of clients may abuse psychoactive substances because of overuse of prescribed medications.

Many of these clients report a history of avoiding social or occupational activities. An obsessive-compulsive personality trait or depression are not uncommon in this group. These clients experience spiritual distress and are likely to resist referral to mental health professionals. The intensity of the physical symptoms often decreases with support from a concerned health care provider (APA, 1994).

Body Dysmorphic Disorder (Dysmorphophobia)

Body dysmorphic disorder is the preoccupation with an imagined flaw in appearance in a normal-appearing person. Clients with this disorder most frequently focus on a facial defect. They often are not concerned about physical deformity in other parts of the body. The client may focus on this defect for hours each day, and this thought may dominate his or her life with resulting impairment in social and work roles and in other important areas of functioning. The preoccupation is not better accounted for by another mental disorder (e.g., dissatisfaction with body shape and size in anorexia nervosa). The social isolation and depression related to their physical appearance may lead to repeated hospitalizations, suicide attempts, and even completed suicides. The key to diagnosis is the client's excessive concern regarding the perceived physical defect. Persons may present with this problem as early as the teen years through the twenties. They often seek plastic surgery, which will not correct their distorted ideation. No familial pattern or predisposing factors have been identified, and it is reported equally in males and females. It is a chronic condition that usually continues for several years (APA, 1994; Thomas & Wimbush, 1999).

Conversion Disorder

Conversion disorder is the presentation of an alteration or loss of a sensory motor function that is not the result of a physiological disorder. Conversion disorders present in response to a catastrophic event such as a threat of loss or harm, which results in the development of physical symptoms. These symptoms lead to serious deficits in functioning. Although conversion disorders are not often reported today, this was a common diagnosis 20 years ago. The most common conversion symptoms include paralysis, seizure, and disturbance in coordination or blindness. Psychological factors are thought to be associated with the symptom or deficit because the initiation or exacerbation of the symptom is preceded by conflict or other stressors. This group of clients may present with the complete array or neurological symptoms (APA, 1994).

The symptoms experienced by the client are serious but not intentionally produced (as in factitious disorder or malingering). The symptom cannot, after appropriate investigation, be fully explained by a general medical condition, by the direct effect of a substance, or as a culturally sanctioned behavior or experience. The symptom or experience causes clinically significant distress or impairment in social, occupational, or other important areas of functioning. The symptom is not limited to pain or sexual dysfunction, does not occur exclusively during the course of somatization disorder, and is not better accounted for by another mental disorder. The type of symptom or deficit is specified (motor, sensory, seizures or convulsions, or mixed presentation). The key to identification of a conversion disorder is that the person appears calm although the symptoms are serious. The calmness and apparent lack of concern are referred to as la belle indifference (APA, 1994; Thomas & Wimbush, 1999).

Onset occurs most commonly during adolescence and early adulthood, although it may appear at any age. Conversion disorder is more common in women than in men, and there is evidence of a familial pattern. Often, a predisposing physical illness with similar symptoms has been present either in the client or in a person close to the client (APA, 1994). Conversion disorder has been reported more frequently in rural populations and in clients with lower socioeconomic and educational status.

Clients who experience a conversion disorder derive primary gain in that the stress that they experienced from the trauma is no longer felt; secondary gain also is obtained in that, because of the conversion symptoms, the client no longer has to participate in stressful activities (e.g., a soldier who develops paralysis can no longer hold a gun and is removed from a combat situation) (APA, 1994; Thomas & Wimbush, 1999).

Hypochondriasis

Hypochondriasis has five major diagnostic criteria. First, the patient has a preoccupation with bodily functions (focusing on heartbeat, breathing, digestion, or a minor physical ailment such as a small scratch or cough). Second, the patient interprets the symptoms as a serious illness, despite appropriate medical evaluation and reassurances. Third, the preoccupation is not a delusional intensity (as in delusional disorder, somatic type) and is not restricted to a particular concern about appearance (as in body dysmorphic disorder). The client can acknowledge the possibility that he or she is exaggerating the extent of the disease or that the disease may not be present. Fourth, the preoccupation causes clinically significant distress and impairment in social, occupational, and other important areas of functioning. Finally, the preoccupation lasts at least 6 months. This preoccupation is not better accounted for by generalized anxiety disorder, obsessive-compulsive disorder, panic, a major depressive episode, separation anxiety, or another somatoform disorder (APA, 1994; Thomas & Wimbush, 1999).

Hypochondria most commonly occurs between 20 and 30 years of age; it may appear at any age. It is seen equally in males and females, and no familial pattern exists. Predisposing factors include stress and past experience with the presenting symptoms. Usually, the condition is chronic, with remission and exacerbation of the symptoms. It is most important in the diagnosis that an early stage of a medical condition is not overlooked. Doctor shopping is common with this group of clients because they cannot get the answers they want. These clients resist referral to mental health practitioners (APA, 1994; Thomas & Wimbush, 1999).

Somatization Disorder

The client with somatization disorder has many physical complaints that occur with no identified organic basis. If a medical condition is present, the physical complaints or resulting social or occupational impairment are in excess of what would be expected from the history, physical exam, or laboratory findings. The identification of somatization must include four pain symptoms in differing sites or functions (e.g., head, abdomen, back, joints, extremities, chest, rectum, during menstruation, during sexual intercourse, or during urination). It also includes a history of two gastrointestinal symptoms other than pain (e.g., nausea, bloating, vomiting other than during pregnancy, diarrhea, or intolerance of several different foods). The diagnostic criteria also includes one sexual or reproductive symptom other than pain (e.g., sexual indifference, erectile or ejaculatory dysfunction, irregular menses, excessive menstrual bleeding, or vomiting throughout pregnancy). The final criteria for this diagnostic category is a history of one pseudoneurological symptom suggesting a neurological condition but not limited to pain (e.g., conversion symptoms such as impaired coordination or balance, paralysis or localized weakness, difficulty swallowing or complaints of a lump in the throat, aphonia, urinary retention, hallucinations, loss of touch or pain sensation, double vision, blindness, deafness, and seizures; dissociative symptoms such as amnesia; or loss of consciousness other than fainting). The symptoms are not intentionally produced or feigned (as in factitious disorder or malingering) (APA, 1994; Thomas & Wimbush, 1999).

The difference between somatization and conversion disorders is based mainly on the number of signs and symptoms; somatization disorder includes multiple physical symptoms in several body systems. The most common complaints are pseudoneurological, gastrointestinal, female reproductive, psychosexual, pain, and cardiopulmonary. Many clients in this diagnostic group are anxious or depressed (APA, 1994).

Somatization disorder symptoms begin during the teen years and sometimes in the twenties and include physical symptoms that have occurred for several years. The client seeks treatment and has significant impairment in social, occupational, or other areas of functioning. Menstrual difficulties are often one of the earliest complaints in females. Younger clients may present with a variety of initial complaints, such as abdominal pain, depression, headaches, or seizures. The diagnosis is not often seen in males. A familial tendency is seen with somatization disorders. Somatization disorder is a chronic problem. The client's symptoms vary in seriousness, but it is unusual for a year to pass without the client seeing a health care provider (APA, 1994; Thomas & Wimbush, 1999).

Pain Disorder

The client with pain disorder is preoccupied with complaints of pain in one or more anatomical sites, and the pain is of sufficient severity to warrant clinical attention. The pain is intense enough to cause clinically significant distress or impairment in social, occupational, or other important areas of functioning. Psychological factors are thought to have an important role in the onset, severity, exacerbation, or maintenance of the pain. The pain is not voluntarily produced, and the diagnosis is not appropriate if the pain is better accounted for by another mental or physical disorder. The diagnosis is specified as either acute (duration of less than 6 months) or chronic (duration of 6 months or longer). Pain disorder usually begins during the third or fourth decade and occurs more frequently in women. The more common complaints include headache and musculoskeletal pain. Some evidence of a familial pattern has been noted (APA, 1994; Thomas & Wimbush, 1999).

Clients in this diagnostic category report a history of excessive analgesic use with no pain relief and frequently request surgery. It is not unusual for the client to have adopted a lifestyle of an invalid. Clients who are depressed or who have pain related to a terminal illness are at increased risk for suicide attempts. The clients in this diagnostic category resist the possibility that psychological factors may be involved. They spend considerable time and energy searching for care. In many clients, the diagnosis of major depression is also appropriate (APA, 1994; Thomas & Wimbush, 1999).

Somatoform Disorder Not Otherwise Specified

This category includes disorders with somatoform symptoms that do not meet the criteria for any specific somatoform disorder. For example, pseudocyesis is a false belief accompanied by physical signs of pregnancy and may include abdominal enlargement, reduced menstrual flow, amenorrhea, subjective sensation of fetal movement, nausea, breast engorgement and secretions, and labor pains at the expected date of delivery. Endocrine changes may be present, but there is no evidence of a medical condition that causes endocrine changes (a hormone-secreting tumor). A second complaint in this category is nonpsychotic hypochondriacal symptoms of less than 6 months' duration. A third example of a disorder in this category is that involving unexplained physical complaints, such as fatigue or body weakness, of less than 6 months' duration that are not due to another mental disorder (APA, 1994).

Undifferentiated Somatoform Disorder

This diagnostic category is used when the client's symptoms and physical findings do not meet the description of somatoform disorder. The client has fewer physical complaints or symptoms (e.g., fatigue, loss of appetite, and gastrointestinal or urinary complaints), and the symptoms are not voluntarily produced and last at least 6 months. The symptoms are not like the multiple exaggerated complaints seen in somatoform disorders. As in many of the somatoform disorders, the symptoms cannot be explained by physical abnormalities after medical examination and are thought to be psychological in origin. In addition, the client's complaints occur without the diagnosis of another somatoform or psychotic disorder. There are no data to support that this diagnosis is more common in one gender or has common predisposing factors or familial tendencies. Many clients with this diagnosis are anxious and depressed, but they have fewer physical and social limitations than those with somatoform disorder. The course of the disease is variable (APA, 1994; Thomas & Wimbush, 1999).

➤ TREATMENT OF SOMATOFORM DISORDERS

Treatment of clients in this diagnostic category has traditionally been limited to insight-oriented psychotherapy. The success of this approach has been limited. A holistic framework is more appropriate in situations in which it is difficult to determine a physiological basis for the client's symptoms. The clinician must take into account physical, psychosocial, and spiritual sources for the behavior that is being demonstrated. Although clients usually resist suggestions that they may have psychological reasons for these disorders, they do respond to a caring environment in which their symptoms are respected and they are not dismissed as "crazy" or "neurotic." When the clinician seriously considers the client's expressions of pain and other symptoms (the client's whole story of illness), the clinician is providing holistic care. When this occurs, the client and the health care provider are more likely to become mutually engaged in a meaningful plan for recovery (Thomas & Wimbush, 1999).

➤ REVIEW OF NURSING RESEARCH

Very little nursing research has focused on theory building in the area of stress and so-called psychosomatic diseases. Exceptions are the work of Page and colleagues in the area of pain and its immune-suppressive effects (Page & Ben-Eliyahu, 1997; Page, Ben-Eliyahu, & Liebeskind, 1994; Page, Ben-Eliyahu, & Yirmiya, 1993) and that of Zeller and colleagues in psychoneuroimmunology (Swanson, Cronin-Stubbs, Zeller, Kessler, & Bieliauskas, 1993a, 1993b; Swanson, Zeller, & Spear, 1994; Zeller, McCain, & Swanson, 1996). Although impairment of immune function in association with exposure to a variety of stressful stimuli is thoroughly discussed elsewhere in this volume (see Chapter 3), this relationship is an important illustration of how stress interacts with physiological function (Cohen, Kaplan, Cunnick, Manuck, & Rabin, 1992; Cohen, Koyle, Skoner, Rabin, & Baltney, 1997). The only example that will be discussed here in detail is that of pain as a stressful experience that can lead to immune suppression (Kusnecov & Rabin, 1994; Page & Ben-Eliyahu, 1997).

Pain generally produces activation of the HPA axis and the SNS, increasing the levels of epinephrine, norepinephrine, and cortisol. Cortisol elevations in conjunction with surgical trauma are related to immune suppression (Pollock, Babcock, & Romsdahl, 1984; Pollock, Lotova, & Stanford, 1991). Surgery-induced immune suppression is of particular clinical concern because of the increased risks of infection and metastatic disease in cancer patients (Page & Ben-Eliyahu, 1997).

Analgesic and anesthetic interventions have been shown to reduce both the neuroendocrine response to surgical pain (Anand, Sippel, & Aynsley-Green, 1987) and the immune effects (Salomaki, Leppaluoto, & Laitinen, 1993; Tonnesen, 1989). In a comparison study of animal responses to surgery and morphine, retention and metastasis of tumor cells were evaluated. A substantial increase in the number of retained radiolabeled tumor cells followed the surgical experience (Page et al., 1994). The number of metastases that developed was significantly greater in animals that did not receive morphine (Page et al., 1993). Conversely, serum cortisol levels and numbers of metastases were reduced in animals given morphine.

A search of the Cumulative Index for Nursing and Allied Health Literature database revealed 40 research citations related to stress and health between 1985 and 1998. Sixteen of these could be clearly identified as nursing studies. Of 182 stress citations relating to cardiovascular conditions, including hypertension, 61 were clearly identifiable as research conducted by nurses. Of 25 research citations relating immune function to stress, at least 9 were nursing studies. Examples of nursing research topics included quality of life, predictors of recovery from acute conditions, health and illness experiences, stress-modulating interventions (e.g., imagery, relaxation, meditation, hypnosis, and massage), and the effects of various care models for people living with various health conditions. In addition, nursing research studies have addressed the outcome of pain relief, stabilized or improved immune function, and cardiovascular response. Table 7.1 provides a summary of nursing intervention studies published between 1987 and 1998 that used physiological outcomes.

➤ CONCLUSIONS

Much attention is currently being given to the relationship between stress and disease. As lifestyles become more stressful, the incidence of several illnesses that have demonstrated close links to stress also increases. Although stress is not a direct cause of disease and illness, the relationship is too significant to be only a coincidence. As researchers continue to examine the association between stress and disease, more explanations will be forthcoming.

Psychophysiological disorders are the underlying cause of the majority of client visits to internists and family practice physicians. Because psychological and spiritual components affect clients' physical symptoms, it is important that this group of people be treated in a holistic manner. Many illnesses belong in this diagnostic category, and this chapter presented only the most prevalent. The health care provider needs to remember that there are multiple causes for the presenting symptoms, and many of them are directly or indirectly related to stress in the client's life.

TABLE 7.1 Published Nursing Intervention Studies Using Physiological Outcome Variables, 1987-1998

Intervention	Reference	Participants	Outcomes	Theoretical Framework
Touch				
Gentle human touch	Modicin-McCarty (1992)	Medically fragile preterm infants ($n = 20$)	Less active sleep and motor activity; more quiet sleep	
Touch	Routasalo and Lauri (1998)	Cancer patients in palliative care	80% "improvement"	
Touch and relaxation	Markut (1989)	Patients undergoing cardiac catheterization ($n = 90$)	Reduced anxiety with relaxation; decreased heart rate and diastolic blood pressure with both; decreased systolic blood pressure with relaxation	
Therapeutic touch	Mersmann (1993)	Mothers of nonnursing preterm infants ($n = 18$)	Greater quantity of milk letdown with TT ($p < .05$)	Rogers's Science of Unitary Human Beings
Therapeutic touch	Hughes, Meize-Grochowski, and Harris (1996)	Hospitalized adolescent psychiatric patients	Description of therapeutic relationship and body-mind connection for participants	
Therapeutic touch, pain control, trust	Messenger and Roberts (1994)	Persons dying	Nursing interventions used; serenity increased (inner peace)	
Therapeutic touch and relaxation	Gagne and Toye (1994)	Veterans Administration psychiatric inpatients ($n = 31$)	Decreased anxiety with both interventions	
Sensory stimulation (auditory, tactile, and visual)	Cummins (1992)	Female nursing home patients in persistent vegetative state ($n = 10$)	Increased Glasgow Coma Scale scores ($p = .02$); increased responses ($p = .05$)	
Massage				
Nursing back rub	Groer et al. (1994)	Well elderly adults ($n = 32$)	Decreased anxiety; increased s-IgA in experimental group	
Back rub	Tyler, Winslow, Clark, and White (1989)	Critically ill patients ($n = 173$)	Variable changes in venous O_2 saturation and heart rate	
Back massage and relaxation	Richards (1998)	Critically ill older men ($n = 69$)	Increased sleep efficiency	

(continued)

TABLE 7.1 Continued

Intervention	Reference	Participants	Outcomes	Theoretical Framework
Massage (preop)	van der Riet (1993)	General surgical and gynecological patients in rural hospital (n = 60)	Decreased preop anxiety	
Massage	Ferrell-Tarry and Glick (1993)	Hospitalized males with cancer pain (n = 9)	Less pain perception (60%); less anxiety (24%); increased feeling of relaxation (58%); decreased heart rate, respirations, and blood pressure	
Massage	Nixon, Teschendorff, Finney, and Karnilowicz (1997)	Surgical patients (n = 39)	Decreased postop pain perception	
Massage	Weinrich and Weinrich (1990)	Cancer patients experiencing pain (n = 28)	Decreased pain in males immediately after massage	
Massage	Strong (1989)	Preterm infants	Decreased pulse and increased respiration; increased stress-releasing and self-comforting behavior; increased time in quiet sleep	
Massage and aromatherapy	Evans (1995)	Cancer patients in palliative care	80% improved in some way	
Imagery				
Guided imagery	Cise (1994)	Middle-aged obese women	Stories and description of issues and emotions; transformation	Rogers' Science of Unitary Human Beings and Lazarus's theory of emotion
Guided imagery	Troesch, Rodehaver, Delaney, and Yanes (1993)	Cancer patients receiving cisplatin chemotherapy (n = 28)	More positive experience with chemotherapy (p < .001)	
Imagery and relaxation	Sloman, Brown, Aldana, and Chee (1994)	New oncology admissions (n = 67)	Decrease in subjective pain rating with relaxation; decreased nonopiate PRN analgesia with both	Orem's theory

Intervention	Reference	Participants	Outcomes	Theoretical Framework
Guided imagery and muscle relaxation	Eller (1994)	Asymptomatic HIV-infected individuals ($n = 69$)	Less depression with relaxation ($p < .04$); less fatigue with imagery ($p < .04$); increased CD4+ count with relaxation ($p < .02$)	
Imagery and relaxation	Aubuchon (1990)	Congestive obstructive pulmonary disease patients in the community ($n = 83$)	Increased hope with both; decreased dyspnea and increased respiratory function with imagery	
Visualization and relaxation versus visualization and cognitive coping skills training	Arathuzik (1994)	Persons with metastatic breast cancer, experiencing pain ($n = 24$)	Increased ability to decrease pain with both interventions	
Imagery, relaxation, and distraction	Broome, Lillis, McGahee, and Bates (1994)	Children with cancer, having lumbar punctures	Decreased report of pain	
Guided imagery versus maximal inspiratory muscle training versus both	Moody, Fraser, and Yarandi (1993)	Adults with moderate chronic bronchitis and emphysema ($n = 19$)	Increased quality of life perception with imagery	
Relaxation				
Relaxation (progressive muscle relaxation [PMR])	Arakawa (1997)	Cancer chemotherapy patients ($n = 60$)	Decreased nausea, vomiting, and anxiety	
Relaxation	Moye and Hanlon (1996)	Nursing home residents ($n = 13$)	Decreased pain; increased morale	
Relaxation versus control	Hase and Douglas (1987)	Myocardial infarction patients ($n = 30$)	Less psychological stress and pain; greater ambulation postdischarge with relaxation	
Relaxation (PMR) and guided imagery	Sloman (1995)	Patients with cancer pain	Decreased sensory pain intensity and severity with both	
Muscle relaxation, imagery, and relaxing music versus back massage	Richards (1993)	Elderly men with chronic illness ($n = 69$)	Decreased anxiety with both; increased sleep efficiency and increased REM sleep with massage	

(continued)

TABLE 7.1 Continued

Intervention	Reference	Participants	Outcomes	Theoretical Framework
Jaw relaxation versus sedating music versus both	Good (1992)	Postop abdominal surgery patients ($n = 84$)	Decreased anxiety and decreased sensation and distress of pain for all	Orem and Gate control pain theory
Music				
Relaxing music	Goddaer and Abraham (1994)	Nursing home residents with severe cognitive deficit ($n = 29$)	Decreased agitated behavior, physically nonaggressive behavior, and verbal agitation	Hall and Buckwalter model of decreased stress threshold with dementia
Music versus music and informational video versus rest		Postop coronary artery bypass surgery ($n = 96$)	Increased mood with music; decreased heart rate and blood pressure with all interventions	
Meditation				
Meditation	Gibson (1996)	Meditators ($n = 18$)	Description of personal experience of meditation	
Aromatherapy				
Aromatherapy	Cannard (1996)	Patients in acute coronary care	Relaxation; stress reduction; decreased sleep disturbance	
Lavender essential oil	Hudson (1996)	Acutely ill elderly	Trend of improved sleep	

➢ REFERENCES

American Cancer Society. (1994). *Cancer facts.* Atlanta, GA: Author.

American Heart Association. (1991). *Heart and stroke facts.* Dallas: Author.

American Heart Association. (1999). *1993 heart and stroke facts and statistics.* Dallas: Author.

American Psychiatric Association. (1994). *Diagnosis and statistical manual of mental disorders* (4th ed.). Washington, DC: Author.

Anand, K. J. S., Sippel, W. G., & Aynsley-Gren, A. (1987). Randomized trial of fentanyl anaesthesia in preterm babies undergoing surgery: Effects on the stress response. *Lancet, 1,* 243-247.

Arakawa, S. (1997). Relaxation to reduce nausea, vomiting, and anxiety induced by chemotherapy in Japanese patients. *Cancer Nursing, 20,* 342-349.

Arathuzik, D. (1994). Effects of cognitive behaviour strategies on pain in cancer patients. *Cancer Nurse, 17,* 3.

Aubuchon, B. L. (1990). *The effects of positive mental imagery on hope, coping, anxiety, dyspnea and pulmonary function in persons with chronic obstructive pulmonary disease: Tests of a nursing intervention and a theoretical model.* Unpublished doctoral dissertation, University of Texas at Austin.

Barefoot, J. C., Dodge, K. A., & Peterson, B. L. (1989). The Cook-Medley hostility scale: Item content and ability to predict survival. *Psychosomatic Medicine, 51,* 46-57.

Benedittis, G., Lorenzetti, A., & Pieri, A. (1990). The role of stressful life events in the onset of chronic primary headache. *Pain, 40,* 65-75.

Bernard, C. (1957). *An introduction to the study of experimental medicine.* New York: Dover. (Original work published 1865)

Blanchard, E., Andrasik, F., Evans, D., & Hillhouse, J. (1985). Biofeedback & relaxation techniques for headaches. *Biofeedback & Self-Regulation, 10*(1), 69-73.

Boone, J. (1991). Stress & hypertension. *Primary Care, 18,* 623-649.

Borysenko, M. (1987). Psychoneuroimmunology. *Annals of Behavioral Medicine, 9,* 3-10.

Borysenko, M. (1991, October 25-26). *Stress and the immune system.* Paper presented at the Stress and Immune System conference, Washington, DC.

Bosma, H., Marmot, M. G., Hemingway, H., Nicholson, A. C., Brunner, E., & Stansfield, S. A. (1997). Low job control and risk of coronary heart disease in Whitehall II study. *British Medical Journal, 314,* 558-565.

Broome, M. E., Lillis, P. P., McGahee, T. W., & Bates, T. H. E. (1994). The use of distraction and imagery with children during painful procedures. *European Journal of Cancer Care, 3,* 26-30.

Calhoun, D. (1992). Hypertension in blacks: Socioeconomic stressors and sympathetic nervous system activity. *American Journal of Medical Sociology, 304,* 306-311.

Cannard, G. (1996). The effect of aromatherapy in promoting relaxation and stress reduction in a general hospital. *Complementary Therapies in Nursing & Midwifery, 2,* 38-40.

Cannon, W. (1929). *Bodily changes in pain, hunger, fear, and rage: An account of recent research into the function of emotional excitement* (2nd ed.). New York: Appleton.

Chiueh, C. C., & McCarty, R. (1981). Sympathoadrenal medullary hyperreactivity to footshock but not to cold stress in spontaneously hypertensive rats. *Physiological Behavior, 26* 85-89.

Cise, J. C. S. (1994). *Self-reflective guided imagery among middle aged obese women in a support group setting.* Unpublished doctoral dissertation, Indiana University, Bloomington.

Cohen, S., Kaplan, J. R., Cunnick, J. E., Manuck, S. B., & Rabin, B. S. (1992). Chronic social stress, affiliation and cellular immune response in nonhuman primates. *Psychological Science, 3,* 301-304.

Cohen, S., Kaplan, J., & Manuck, S. (1994). Social support & coronary heart disease: Underlying psychological and biological mechanisms. In S. Shumaker and S. Czajkowsi (Eds.), *Social support and cardiovascular disease* (pp. 195-221). New York: Plenum.

Cohen, S., Koyle, W. J., Skoner, D. P., Rabin, B. S., & Baltney, J. M., Jr. (1997). Social ties and susceptibility to the common cold. *Journal of the American Medical Association, 277,* 1940-1944.

Cohen, S., Tyrrell, D., & Smith, A. (1991). Psychological stress and susceptibility to the common cold. *New England Journal of Medicine, 325,* 606-612.

Cohen, S., & Williamson, G. (1991). Stress and infectious disease in humans. *Psychological Bulletin, 109,* 5-24.

Corbin, L., Hanson, R., Happ, S., & Whitby, A. (1988). Somatoform disorders. *Journal of Psychosocial Nursing & Mental Health Services, 26*(9), 31-34.

Cummins, J. J. (1992). *A nursing intervention study of auditory, tactile, and visual stimulation of elderly female patients in the persistent vegetative state.* Unpublished doctoral dissertation, University of Texas at Austin.

DeFronzo, R., & Ferrannini, E. (1991). Insulin resistance: A multifaceted syndrome responsible for NIDDM, obesity, hypertension, dyslipidemia, and atherosclerotic cardiovascular disease. *Diabetes Care, 14,* 173-194.

Dembroski, T. M., MacDougall, J. M., & Costa, P. T. (1989). Components of hostility as predictors of sudden death and MI in the multiple risk factor intervention trial. *Psychosomatic Medicine, 51,* 514-522.

Diamond, S., & Dalessio, D. (1986). *The practicing physician's approach to headache* (4th ed.). Baltimore, MD: Williams & Wilkins.

Dubos, R. (1965). *Man adapting.* New Haven, CT: Yale University Press.

Dunbar, H. (1935). *Emotions and bodily changes.* New York: Columbia University Press.

Egan, B. (1992). Vascular reactivity, sympathetic tone, and stress. In E. Johnson, W. Gentry, & S. Julius (Eds.), *Personality, elevated blood pressure, and essential hypertension.* Washington, DC: Hemisphere.

Eller, L. S. (1994). *Guided imagery: A nursing intervention for symptoms related to infection with human immunodeficiency virus.* Unpublished doctoral dissertation, Case Western Reserve University, Cleveland, OH.

Eskala, S., Ylipaavalniemi, P., & Turtola, L. (1985). TMJ-dysfunction symptoms among Finnish University students. *Journal of American College Health, 33*(4), 172-174.

Evans, B. (1995). Nursing an audit into the effects of aromatherapy massage and the cancer patient in palliative and terminal care. *Complementary Therapies in Medicine, 3,* 239-241.

Everson, S. A., Lynch, J. W., & Chesney, M. A. (1997). Interaction of workplace demands and cardiovascular reactivity in progression of carotid atherosclerosis: Population based study. *British Medical Journal, 314,* 553-558.

Fava, G. (1992). The concept of psychosomatic disorder. *Psychotherapy Psychosomatic, 58,* 1-12.

Ferrell-Tarry, A. T., & Glick, O. J. (1993). The use of therapeutic massage as a nursing intervention to modify anxiety and the perception of cancer pain. *Cancer Nursing, 16,* 93-101.

Gagne, D., & Toye, R. C. (1994). The effects of therapeutic touch and relaxation therapy in reducing anxiety. *Archives of Psychiatry Nursing, 8,* 184-189.

Gallagher, R. (1990). Precipitating causes of migraine. In S. Diamond (Ed.), *Migraine headache prevention and management* (pp. 1-30). New York: Dekker.

Gibson, A. (1996). Personal experiences of individuals using meditations from a metaphysical source. *Visions: The Journal of Rogerian Nursing Science, 4,* 12-23.

Goddaer, J., & Abrahamn, I. L. (1994). Effects of relaxing music on agitation during meals among nursing home residents with severe cognitive impairment. *Archives of Psychiatric Nursing, 8,* 150-158.

Good, M. P. L. (1992). *Comparison of the effects of relaxation and music on postoperative pain.* Unpublished doctoral dissertation, Case Western Reserve University, Cleveland, OH.

Groer, M., Mozingo, J., Droppleman, P., Davis, M., Jolly, M. L., Boynton, M., Davis, K., & Kay, S. (1994). Measures of salivary secretory immunoglobin A and state anxiety after a nursing back rub. *Applied Nursing Research, 7,* 2-6.

Guthrie, E., Creed, F., Dawson, D., & Tomenson, B. (1991). A controlled trial of psychological treatment for the irritable bound syndrome. *Gastroenterology, 100,* 450-457.

Guyton, A. (1996). *Textbook of medical physiology* (9th ed.). Philadelphia: W. B. Saunders.

Hardy, J. H., & Smith, T. W. (1988). Cynical hostility and vulnerability to disease: Social support, life stress, and physiological response to conflict. *Health Psychology, 7,* 447-459.

Hase, S., & Douglas, A. (1987). Effects of relaxation training on recovery from myocardial infarction. *Australian Journal of Advanced Nursing, 5,* 18-27.

Hecker, M. H. L., Chesney, M. A., & Black, G. W. (1988). Coronary-prone behaviors in the Western Collaborative Group Study. *Psychosomatic Medicine, 50,* 153-164.

Helmers, K. F., Krantz, D. S., & Howell, B. A. (1993). Hostility and MI in CAD patients: Evaluation by gender and ischemia index. *Psychomatic Medicine, 55,* 29-36.

Henri-Benitez, M., Castresana, C., Gonzales-de-Rivera, J., & Marco, R. (1990). Autogenic psychotherapy for bronchial asthma. *Psychology Psychosomatica, 11*(6), 11-16.

Holaday, J. (1983). Cardiovascular effects of endogenous opiate systems. *Annual Review of Pharmacology & Toxicology, 23,* 541-594.

Hudson, R. (1996). Nursing. The value of lavender for rest and activity in the elderly patient. *Complementary Therapies in Medicine, 4,* 52-57.

Hughes, P. P., Meize-Grochowski, R., & Harris, C. N. D. (1996). Therapeutic tough with adolescent psychiatric patients. *Journal of Holistic Nursing, 14,* 6-23.

Julkunen, J., Salonen, R., & Kaplan, G. A. (1994). Hostility and the progression of carotid atherosclerosis. *Psychosomatic Medicine, 56,* 519-526.

Kaplan, J. R., Petersson, K., & Manuck, S. B. (1991). Role of sympathoadrenal medullary activation in the initiation and progression of atherosclerosis. *Circulation, 84*(Suppl. 6), V123-V132.

Kirschbaum, C., Prussner, J. C., & Stone, A. A. (1995). Persistent high cortisol responses to repeated psychological stress in a subpopulation of healthy men. *Psychosomatic Medicine, 57,* 468-474.

Kushner, M., Shen, J., & Beltman, B. D. (1990). The relation between alcohol problems and the anxiety disorders. *American Journal of Psychiatry, 147,* 685-695.

Kusnecov, A. W., & Rabin, B. S. (1994). Stressor-induced alterations of immune function: Mechanisms and issues. *International Archives of Allergy and Immunology, 105,* 107-121.

Kvetnansky, R., McCarty, R., & Thoa, N. B. (1979). Sympatho-adrenal responses of spontaneously hypertensive rats to immobilization stress. *American Journal of Physiology, 236,* H457-H462.

Lee, R. M. K. W., Triggle, C. R., & Cheung, D. W. T. (1987). Structural and functional consequence of neonatal sympathectomy on the blood vessels of spontaneously hypertensive rats. *Hypertension, 10,* 328-337.

Levenson, J., & Bemis, C. (1991). The role of psychological factors in cancer onset & progression. *Psychosomatica, 32*(2), 124-132.

Light, K. (1987). Psychosocial precursors of hypertension: Experimental evidence. *Circulation, 76*(Suppl.), 167-175.

Lowy, M. T., Wittenberg, L., & Yamamoto, B. K. (1995). Effect of acute stress on hippocampal glutamate levels and spectrin proteolysis in young and aged rats. *Journal of Neurochemistry, 65,* 268-274.

Manuck, S. B., Marsland, A. L., Kaplan, J. R., & Williams, J. K. (1995). The pathogenicity of behavior and its neuroendocrine mediation: An example from coronary artery disease. *Psychosomatic Medicine, 57,* 275-283.

Manuck, S. B., Olsson, G., & Hjemdahl, P. (1992). Does cardiovascular reactivity to mental stress have prognostic value in postinfarction patients? A pilot study. *Psychosomatic Medicine, 54,* 102-108.

Markut, C. F. (1989). *Effects of nonprocedural touch and relaxation training on the psychophysiological stress level of patients undergoing cardiac catherization.* Unpublished doctoral dissertation, Catholic University of America, Washington, DC.

Matthews, K., & Rakaczky, C. (1986). Familial aspects of the type A behavior pattern and physiologic reactivity to stress: In T. Schmidt, T. Dembroski, & G. Blumchen (Eds.), *Biological and psychological factors in cardiovascular diseases.* New York: Springer-Verlag.

Matthews, K. A. (1982). Psychological perspectives on the type A behavior pattern. *Psychological Bulletin, 91,* 292-323.

Matthews, K. A. (1988). Coronary heart disease and type A behaviors: Update on and alternative to the Booth-Kewley and Friedman quantitative review. *Psychological Bulletin, 104,* 373-380.

McCarty, R., Chiueh, C. C., & Kopin, I. J. (1978). Spontaneously hypertensive rats: Adrenergic hyperresponsivity to anticipation of electric shock. *Behavioral Biology, 23,* 180-188.

McCubbin, J., Cheung, R., Montgomery, T., Bulbulian, R., & Wilson, J. (1992). Endogenous opioids and stress reactivity in the development of essential hypertension. In E. Johnson, W. Gentry, & S. Julius (Eds.), *Personality elevated blood pressure, and essential hypertension.* Washington, DC: Hemisphere.

McEwen, B. (1998). Protective and damaging effects of stress mediators. *New England Journal of Medicine, 338*(3), 171-179.

McEwen, B. S., Albeck, D., & Cameron, H. (1995). Stress and the brain: A paradoxical role for adrenal steroids. *Vitamins and Hormones, 51,* 371-402.

McEwen, B. S., & Stellar, E. (1993). Stress and the individual: Mechanisms leading to disease. *Archives of Internal Medicine, 153,* 2093-2101.

McFall, M., Murburg, M., Ko, G., & Veith, R. (1990). Autonomic responses to stress in Vietnam combat veterans with posttraumatic stress disorder. *Biological Psychiatry, 27,* 1165-1175.

Mersmann, C. A. (1993). *Therapeutic touch and milk letdown in mothers of non-nursing preterm infants.* Unpublished doctoral dissertation, New York University, New York.

Messenger, T. H. E., & Roberts, K. T. (1994). The terminally ill: Serenity nursing interventions for hospice clients. *Journal of Gerontological Nursing, 20,* 17-22.

Mitchell, M., & Drossman, D. (1997). Irritable bowel syndrome: Understanding & treating a biopsychosocial disorder. *Annals of Behavioral Medicine, 9*(3), 13-18.

Modicin-McCarty, M. A. J. (1992). *The physiological and behavioral effects of a gentle human touch nursing intervention on preterm infants.* Unpublished doctoral dissertation, University of Tennessee, Knoxville.

Moody, L. E., Fraser, M., & Yarandi, H. (1993). Effects of guided imagery in patients with chronic bronchitis and emphysema. *Clinical Nursing Research, 2,* 478-486.

Moran, M. (1991). Psychological factors affecting pulmonary & rheumatological diseases. *Psychosamatics, 32*(1), 13-18.

Moye, J., & Hanlon, S. (1996). Clinical comments. Relaxation training for nursing home patients: Suggestions for simplifying and individualizing treatment. *Clinical Gerontologist, 16,* 37-48.

Muller, J. E., Tofler, G. H., & Stone, P. H. (1989). Circadian variation and triggers of onset of acute cardiovascular disease. *Circulation, 79,* 733-743.

Munck, A., & Guyre, P. M. (1991). Glucocorticoids and immune function. In R. Ader, D. L. Felten, & N. Cohen (Eds.), *Psychoneuroimmunology* (2nd ed., pp. 447-474). New York: Academic Press.

Nebjesm, N. S., Matthews, K. A., & Krantz, D. S. (1989). Cardiovascular reactivity to the cold pressor tests as a predictor of hypertension. *Hypertension, 14,* 524-536.

Newman, M. (1994). *Health as expanding consciousness* (2nd ed.). New York: NLN Press.

Nixon, M., Teschendorff, J., Finney, J., & Karnilowicz, W. (1997). Expanding the nursing repertoire: The effect of massage on post-operative pain. *Australian Journal of Advanced Nursing, 14,* 21-26.

Obrist, P. (1981). *Cardiovascular psychophysiology: A perspective.* New York: Plenum.

O'Sullivan, J. B., & Harrap, S. B. (1995). Resetting blood pressure in spontaneously hypertensive rats: The role of bradykinin. *Hypertension, 25,* 162-165.

Page, G. G., & Ben-Eliyahu, S. (1997). The immune-suppressive nature of pain. *Seminars in Oncology Nursing, 13,* 10-15.

Page, G. G., Ben-Eliyahu, S., & Liebeskind, J. C. (1994). The role of LGL/NK cells in surgery-induced promotion of metastasis and its attenuation by morphine. *Brain, Behavior & Immunology, 8,* 241-250.

Page, G. G., Ben-Eliyahu, S., & Yirmiya, R. (1993). Morphine attenuates surgery-induced enhancement of metastatic colonization in rats. *Pain, 54,* 21-28.

Parse, R. R. (1992). Human becoming: Parse's theory of nursing. *Nursing Science Quarterly, 5,* 35-41.

Pelletier, K., & Herzing, D. (1988). Psychoneuroimmunology: Toward a mind body model. *Advances, 5,* 27-56.

Pickering, T., & Gerin, W. (1990). Cardiovascular reactivity in the laboratory and the role of behavioral factors in hypertension: A critical review. *Annals of Behavioral Medicine, 12,* 3-16.

Pickering, T. B., Devereux, R. B., & James, G. D. (1996). Environmental influences on blood pressure and the role of job strain. *Journal of Hypertension, 14*(Suppl.), S179-S185.

Pollock, R. E., Babcock, G. F., & Romsdahl, M. M. (1984). Surgical stress-mediated suppression of murine natural killer cell cytotoxicity. *Cancer Research, 44,* 3888-3891.

Pollock, R. E., Lotzova, E., & Stanford, S. D. (1987). Effect of surgical stress on murine natural killer cell cytotoxicity. *Journal of Immunology, 138,* 171-178.

Pollock, R. E., Lotova, E., & Stanford, S. D. (1991). Mechanism of surgical stress on murine natural killer cell cytotoxicity. *Journal of Immunology, 138,* 171-178.

Potempa, K. (1994). An overview of the role of cardiovascular reactivity to stressful challenges in the etiology of hypertension. *Journal of Cardiovascular Nursing, 8,* 27-38.

Reaven, G. M. (1991). Insulin resistance, hyperinsulinemia, hypertriglyceridemia, and hypertension. Parallels between human disease and rodent models. *Diabetes Care, 14*(3), 195-202.

Review Panel. (1981). Coronary-prone behavior and coronary heart disease: A critical review. *Circulation, 19,* 583-589.

Richards, K. C. (1993). *The effect of a muscle relaxation, imagery, and relaxing music intervention and a back massage on the sleep and psychophysiological arousal of elderly males hospitalized in the critical care environment.* Unpublished doctoral dissertation, University of Texas at Austin.

Richards, K. C. (1998). Effect of a back massage and relaxation intervention on sleep in critically ill patients. *American Journal of Critical Care, 7,* 288-299.

Rogers, M. E. (1970). *An introduction to the theoretical basis of nursing.* Philadelphia: Davis.

Routasalo, P., & Lauri, S. (1998). Expressions of touch in nursing older people. *European Nurse, 3,* 95-104.

Rowingson, J. (1993). Low back pain. In C. Warfield (Ed.), *The principles and practices of pain management* (pp. 129-140). New York: McGraw-Hill.

Salomaki, T. E., Leppaluoto, J., & Laitinen, J. O. (1993). Epidural versus intravenous fentanyl, for reducing hormonal, metabolic, and physiologic responses after thoracotomy. *Anesthesiology, 79,* 672-679.

Saper, J., Silverstein, S., Gordon, C., & Hammel, R. (1993). *The handbook of headache management.* Baltimore, MD: Williams & Wilkins.

Schnall, P. L., Schwartz, J. E., Landsbergis, P. A., Warren, K., & Pickering, T. G. (1992). Relation between job strain, alcohol, and ambulatory blood pressure. *Hypertension, 19,* 488-494.

Seaward, B. (1997). *Managing stress: Principles and strategies for health and well-being* (2nd ed.). Boston: Jones & Bartlett.

Seeman, T. E., McEwen, B. S., Singer, B. H., Albert, M. S., & Rowe, J. W. (1997). Increase in urinary cortisol excretion and memory declines: MacArthur studies of successful aging. *Journal of Clinical Endocrinology and Metabolism, 82,* 2458-2465.

Selye, H. (1936). Syndrome produced by diverse nocuous agents. *Nature, 138,* 32.

Sher, K. J. (1987). Stress response dampening. In H. T. Bland & K. E. Leonard (Eds.), *Psychological theories of drinking and alcoholism* (pp. 227-271). New York: Guilford.

Sherwood, A., Allen, M. T., Obrist, P. A., & Langer, A. W. (1986). Evaluation of beta-adrenergic influences on cardiovascular and metabolic adjustments to physical and psychological stress. *Psychophysiology, 23,* 89-104.

Sherwood, A., & Turner, J. (1992). A conceptual and methodological overview of cardiovascular reactivity research. In J. Turner, A. Sherwood, & K. Light (Eds.), *Individual differences in cardiovascular responses to stress.* New York: Plenum.

Siegel, B. (1986). *Love, medicine, and miracles.* New York: Perennial Library.

Skyler, J., Donahue, R., Marks, J., Thompson, N., & Schneiderman, N. (1992). Insulin: A determinant of blood pressure? In E. Johnson, W. Gentry, & S. Julius (Eds.), *Personality, elevated blood pressure, and essential hypertension.* Washington, DC: Hemisphere.

Sloman, R. (1995). Relaxation and the relief of cancer pain. *Nursing Clinics of North America, 30,* 697-709.

Sloman, R., Brown, P., Aldana, E., & Chee, E. (1994). The use of relaxation for the promotion of comfort and pain relief in persons with advanced cancer. *Contemporary Nurse: A Journal for the Australian Nursing Profession, 3,* 6-12.

Smith, T. W., & Allred, K. B. (1989). Blood pressure reactivity during social interaction in high and low cynical hostile men. *Journal of Behavioral Medicine, 11,* 135-143.

Solomon, S., & Lipton, R. (1990). Diagnosis and pathophysiology of migraine. In S. Diamond (Ed.), *Migraine headache prevention and management.* New York: Dekker.

Sterling, P., & Eyer, J. (1988). Allostasis: A new paradigm to explain arousal pathology. In S. Fisher & J. Reason (Eds.), *Handbook of life stress, cognition and health* (pp. 629-649). New York: John Wiley.

Stern, M., Morales, P., Haffner, S., & Valdez, R. (1992). Hyperdynamic circulation and the insulin resistance syndrome. *Hypertension, 20,* 802-808.

Strong, C. B. (1989). *The effect of massage on premature infants.* Unpublished doctoral dissertation, University of Arizona, Tucson.

Suarez, E. C., Harlan, E. S., & Peoples, M. C. (1993). Cardiovascular and emotional responses in women: The role of hostility and harassment. *Health Psychology, 12,* 459-468.

Suarez, E. C., Kuhn, C. M., Schanberg, S. M., Williams, R. B., & Zimmerman, E. A. (1998). Neuroendocrine, cardiovascular, and emotional responses of hostile men: The role of interpersonal challenge. *Psychosomatic Medicine, 60,* 78-88.

Suarez, E. C., & Williams, R. B. (1990). The relationships between dimensions of hostility and cardiovascular reactivity as a function of task characteristics. *Psychosomatic Medicine, 52,* 558-570.

Swanson, B., Cronin-Stubbs, D., Zeller, J., Kessler, H., & Bieliauskas, L. (1993a). Characterizing the neuropsychological functioning of persons with HIV infection: AIDS dementia complex: A review. *Archives of Psychiatric Nursing, 7,* 74-81.

Swanson, B., Cronin-Stubbs, D., Zeller, J., Kessler, H., & Bieliauskas, L. (1993b). Characterizing the neuropsychological functioning of persons with HIV infection: Neuropsychological functioning of persons at different stages of HIV infection. *Archives of Psychiatric Nursing, 7,* 82-90.

Swanson, B., Zeller, J., & Spear, G. (1994, April). The effects of cortisol on HIV production by human macrophages [abstract]. In *Proceedings of the Midwest Nursing Research Society Meeting* (p. 204). Indianapolis, IN: Midwest Nursing Research Society.

Temoshak, L. (1997). Personality, coping style, emotion & cancer. *Cancer Surveys, 6,* 545-567.

Thomas, S., & Wimbush, F. (1999). The journey embedded in psychophysiological disorders. In V. Carson (Ed.), *Mental health nursing.* Philadelphia: Saunders.

Tonnesen, E. (1989). Immunological aspects of anaesthesia and surgery—with special reference to NK cells. *Danish Medical Bulletin, 36,* 263-281.

Troesch, L. M., Rodehaver, C. B., Delaney, E. A., & Yanes, B. (1993). The influence of guided imagery on chemotherapy-related nausea and vomiting. *Oncology Nursing Forum, 20,* 1179-1185.

Turner, J., Carroll, D., Hanson, J., & Sims, J. (1988). A comparison of additional heart rate during active psychological challenge calculated from upper and lower body dynamic exercise. *Psychophysiology, 25,* 89-104.

Tyler, D. O., Winslow, E. H., Clark, A. P., & White, K. M. (1989). Effects of a 1-minute back rub on mixed venous oxygen saturation and heart rate in critically ill patients. *Heart & Lung: Journal of Critical Care, 19,* 562-565.

Ubell, E. (1995, April 2). Soon, we won't have to worry about ulcers. *Parade Magazine,* pp. 8-19.

Van der Riet, P. (1993). Effects of therapeutic massage on pre-operative anxiety in a rural hospital, Part 1. *Australian Journal of Rural Health, 1,* 11-16.

Weidmann, P., Grimm, M., & Meier, A. (1980). Pathogenic and therapeutic significance of cardiovascular pressor activity as related to plasma catecholamines in borderline and established essential hypertension. *Clinical and Experimental Hypertension, 2,* 427-449.

Weidner, G., Friend, R., & Ficarrotto, T. J. (1989). Hostility and cardiovascular reactivity to stress in women and men. *Psychosomatic Medicine, 51,* 36-45.

Weinrich, S. P., & Weinrich, M. C. (1990). The effect of massage on pain in cancer patients. *Applied Nursing Research, 3,* 140-145.

Whitehead, W. (1992). Behavioral medicine approaches to gastrointestinal disorders. *Journal of Consulting and Clinical Psychology, 60,* 605-612.

Wu, J. N., & Berecel, K. H. (1993). Prevention of genetic hypertension by early treatment of spontaneously hypertensive rats with the angiotensin converting enzyme inhibitor captopril. *Hypertension, 22,* 139-146.

Yehuda, R., Giller, E., Southwick, S., & Lowy, M. (1991). Hypothalamic-pituitary-adrenal dysfunction in posttraumatic stress disorder. *Biological Psychiatry, 30,* 1031-1048.

Zeller, J. M., McCain, N. L., & Swanson, B. (1996). Psychoneuroimmunology: An emerging framework for nursing research. *Journal of Advanced Nursing, 23,* 657-664.

PART IV

Interactional and
Transactional
Models

CHAPTER 8

Salutogenesis

"Origins of Health" and Sense of Coherence

Martha E. Horsburgh

➤ **THE SALUTOGENESIS MODEL**

Recalling an event that occurred toward the end of his incarceration in the concentration camps of Nazi Germany, Victor Frankl (1959) wrote,

> Not only our experiences, but all we have done, whatever great thoughts we may have had, and all we have suffered, all this is not lost, though it is past; we have brought it into being. Having been is also a kind of being, and perhaps the surest kind. Then I spoke of the many opportunities of giving life a meaning. I told my comrades (who lay motionless, although occasionally a sigh could be heard) that human life, under any circumstances, never ceases to have a meaning, and that this infinite meaning of life includes suffering and dying, privation and death. I asked the poor creatures who listened to me attentively in the darkness of the hut to face up to the seriousness of our position. They must not lose hope but should keep their courage in the certainty that the hopelessness of our struggle did not detract from its dignity and its meaning. (p. 104)

Dr. Frankl and many others lost family members and friends to World War II concentration camps, were stripped of their possessions, and suffered from hunger, cold, and brutality. The threat of extermination faced them every hour of every day. What facilitated their survival in the face of such horrific adversity? This question stimulated medical sociologist Aaron Antonovsky's life's work—the scientific search for factors that facilitate human health and well-being in the face of pathogens, stresses, and strains that are endemic in the human condition. It is the question of "salutogenesis," the origins of health, and "good beginnings" (Antonovsky, 1979).

➤ **DEVELOPMENT OF THE SALUTOGENESIS MODEL**

Born in Brooklyn in 1923, Aaron Antonovsky studied history and economics as an undergraduate. He served in the United States Army during World War II and later studied at Yale University, receiving both master's and doctoral degrees in sociology. He emigrated with his wife to Israel in 1960 and served as professor and chair of the Department of Sociology of Health, Faculty of Health Services, Ben Gurion University, Beersheba (Antonovsky, 1987).

Influenced by Selye's (1956) work on the "generalized adaptation syndrome," Dubos's (1960, 1968) contributions on psychosocial and cultural influences on human adaptation, and the work of many other scientists of his time, Antonovsky (1972) published the first of his formulations in the area of individual stress coping and health. Antonovsky argued that it was time to move beyond consideration of individual diseases and their unique etiologies to search for common phenomena that enhance individuals' abilities to adapt to threats in general. Antonovsky posited that (a) serious consideration be given to a common etiology of disease, (b) health be operationalized using a "breakdown" continuum with "no breakdown" at one extreme and "life-threatening breakdown" at the other, and (c) persons use "generalized resistance resources" to resolve tensions that occur from a variety of internal and external stressors and demands.

In his book *Health, Stress and Coping* (1979), Antonovsky developed the salutogenesis orientation. Research with menopausal women suggested to him that cultural stability exerted positive benefits for individual health. Additional work with a subsample of these women, who were concentration camp survivors of World War II, led Antonovsky to ask "the revolutionary question and the origin of my concern with what I only later began to call salutogenesis (pp. 6-7): "How do some of these people manage to stay reasonably healthy?" (p. 8). He argued that salutogenesis could provide an important addition to "pathogenesis," or the traditional medical model, and advocated allocation of resources to study the origins of health.

Analyzing United States's epidemiological data, Antonovsky (1979) concluded that at any one time "at least one third and quite possibly a majority of the population of any modern industrial society is characterized by some morbid condition" (p. 15). He noted that pathogenesis, which focuses on individual diseases, categorizes persons in an artificially dichotomous way as either "nonpatients" or "patients." Nonpatients are further classified as "healthy" or "sick" (self-diagnosed or diagnosed by another layperson), whereas patients are further classified as "diseased," with clear or unclear medical diagnosis, or "not diseased" (e.g., hypochondriac and malingerer). The question of pathogenesis, "Why do people get this or that disease?", reinforces the categorization of individuals in this dichotomous manner.

In contrast to the pathogenic approach, Antonovsky (1979) stressed that it is only when we ask the question of salutogenesis, "Why do people stay healthy?" (p. 35), that we begin to search for factors that promote health despite the "ubiquity of pathogens—microbiological, chemical, physical, psychological, social, and cultural" (p. 13). The question of salutogenesis offers three advantages compared to the question of pathogenesis. It focuses attention on the common denominators of health, including individuals' subjective interpretations. Second, it embraces the notion of multiple causation and encourages a broad approach consistent with the field of health promotion. Finally, salutogenesis seeks to describe and explain factors that move individuals toward the healthy end of a health continuum. Health and illness are no longer viewed as dichotomies. Rather, a multidimensional health-illness continuum is posited, with "two poles that are useful only as heuristic devices and are never found in reality: absolute health and absolute illness" (p. 37).

This health-illness continuum, or "ease/dis-ease continuum" (Antonovsky, 1979, p. 65), is composed of two subjective dimensions as perceived by the individual and two objective dimension as perceived by the health professional. The former includes four pain categories ranging from "none" to "severe" and four categories of functional limitations ranging from none to "severely limiting." The latter includes six prognostic implications ranging from "not acute or chronic" to "serious, acute, and life-threatening" and four action implications ranging from "no particular health-related action needed" to "active therapeutic intervention required" (p. 65). This offers the possibility of 384 individual combinations that may be used to describe an individual's location on the ease/dis-ease continuum. This mapping of ease/dis-ease profiles, and the search for factors that place an individual somewhere on the continuum, culminated in the development of the model of salutogenesis (Figure 8.1).

➤ **THE SALUTOGENESIS MODEL: CONCEPTS AND RELATIONS**

The major substantive elements of the salutogenesis model were elucidated by Antonovsky in 1979 and further refined in his subsequent book, *Unraveling the Mystery of Health: How People Manage Stress and Stay Well* (1987). The model seeks to describe the process of staying healthy despite exposure to stress. It is a cognitive model of human responses to stress that, over time and within a sociocultural and historical context, influence health. The following are the main conceptual elements of the salutogenesis model: (a) stressors; (b) tension, tension management, and stress; (c) generalized resistance resources-resistance deficits; (d) sense of coherence; and (e) individual placement on the health ease/dis-ease continuum, the outcome of interest. Each of these is briefly described followed by a discussion of the relations purported among them.

Stressors

Stressors are viewed within the model of salutogenesis (Antonovsky, 1979, 1987) as endemic to the human condition. Indeed, Antonovsky suggests that human existence is characterized by moderate to severe levels of stressors. In 1979, he differentiated stressors from other stimuli, noting that stressors upset the individual's homeostasis and present "demands to which there are no readily available or automatic responses" (p. 72). Stressors are viewed as human and environmental, occurring from within the individual or from without, and imposed or freely chosen or both. Stressors, when recognized as such by the individual, engender a state of "tension."

Tension, Tension Management, and Stress

Tension, tension management, and stress are differentiated within the model of salutogenesis (Antonovsky, 1979, 1987). A state of tension is viewed as the response to a stressor and is both an emotional and physiological phenomenon—"the recognition in the brain that some need one has is unfulfilled, that a demand on one has to be met, that one must do something if one is to realize a goal" (1987, p. 130). Outcomes associated with tension can be salutary, neutral, or negative with respect to health. The nature of the outcome depends on the ability of the individual to manage tension. Tension management is defined as "the rapidity and completeness with which problems are resolved and tension dissipated" (1979, p. 96). If tension management is effective, stress does not ensue and the impact on health may be neutral or even salutary. If tension is not managed effectively, the individual enters a state of stress (the state of the organism in response to the failure to manage tension well and to overcome stressors). The ability of the individual to manage tension, and avoid or manage stress or both, is influenced by factors known as generalized resistance resources.

Generalized Resistance Resources-Resistance Deficits and Stressors

In 1979, Antonovsky defined a *generalized resistance resource* (GRR) as "any characteristic of the person, group, or environment

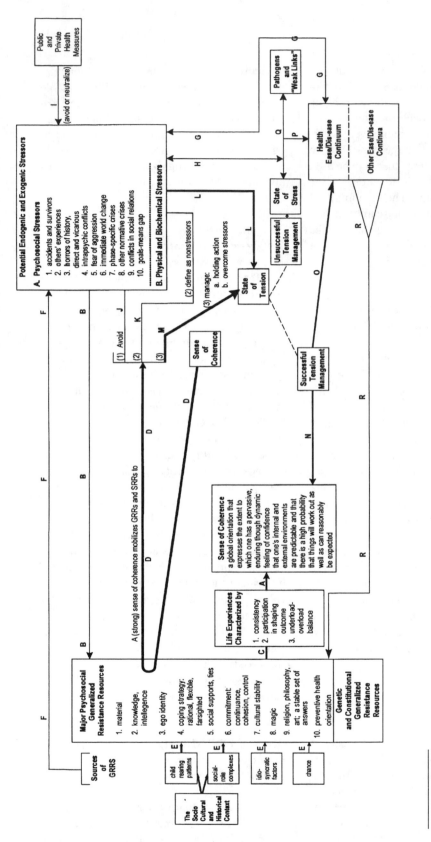

Figure 8.1. Health, stress, and coping: The salutogenic model of health. A, life experiences shape the sense of coherence; B, stressors affect the generalized resistance resources (GRRs) at one's disposal; C, by definition, a GRR provides one with sets of meaningful, coherent life experiences; D, a strong sense of coherence mobilizes the GRRs and specific resistance resources (SRRs) at one's disposal; E, child-rearing patterns, social role complexes, idiosyncratic factors, and chance build up GRRs; F, the sources of GRRs also create stressors; G, traumatic physical and biochemical stressors affect health status directly, and health status affects the extent of exposure to psychosocial stressors; H, physical and biochemical stressors interact with endogenic pathogens and "weak links" and with stress to affect health status; I, public and private health measures avoid or neutralize stressors; J, a strong sense of coherence, mobilizing GRRs and SRRs, avoids stressors; K, a strong sense of coherence, mobilizing GRRs and SRRs, defines stimuli as nonstressors; L, ubiquitous stressors create a state of tension; M, the mobilized GRRs (and SRRs) interact with the state of tension and manage a holding action and the overcoming of stressors; N, successful tension management strengthens the sense of coherence; O, successful tension management maintains one's place on the health ease/dis-ease continuum; P, interaction between the state of stress and pathogens and weak links negatively affects health status; Q, stress is a general precursor that interacts with the existing potential endogenic and exogenic pathogens and weak links; R, good health status facilitates the acquisition of other GRRs. Note that A, C–E, and L–O represent the core of the salutogenic model. Reproduced with permission from Antonovsky (1979, pp. 184-185).

178

that can facilitate effective tension management" (p. 99). Later, GRRs were defined as "phenomena that provide one with sets of life experiences characterized by consistency, participation in shaping outcome, and an underload-overload balance" (Antonovsky, 1987, p. 19). GRRs include (a) material resources, such as money, shelter, and food; (b) knowledge and intelligence—a means to know the real world and to acquire skills; (c) ego identity—a sense of inner self that is integrated but flexible; (d) a coping strategy that is rational, flexible, and farsighted; (e) social supports—ties or deep interpersonal roots and commitment; (f) commitment and cohesion with one's cultural roots; (g) cultural stability; (h) ritualistic activities and answers provided by one's culture that anthropology labels collectively as magic (e.g., ceremony for crop failure and ceremony for accession of leaders); (i) religion and philosophy—a stable set of answers to life's perplexities; (j) preventive health orientation; (k) genetic and constitutional GRRs; and (l) an individual's state of health (Antonovsky, 1979, 1987).

It is important to briefly discuss the GRR coping strategy. Antonovsky (1979, 1987) distinguishes coping strategies from coping behaviors that individuals may employ to deal with stress. The former refers to an "overall plan of action for overcoming stressors" (1979, p. 112)—a plan that is rational, flexible, and farsighted. It is rational in that it is fairly accurate and objective, flexible in that there is a willingness to consider and use alternative strategies, and farsighted in that the individual anticipates the response of the environment to his or her action plan. Antonovsky uses the latter term, coping behaviors or "coping," in a generic way to indicate actions taken by individuals to deal with stress. Used in this broad way, coping is not depicted within the model of salutogenesis.

To enhance the parsimony of the salutogenesis model, Antonovsky (1987) merged GRRs and his earlier notions of stressors (discussed previously) into one concept, generalized resistance resources-resistance deficits (GRR-RDs). He ranked each GRR on a continuum: The higher a person is on the continuum, the more likely he or she is to have consistent, balanced life experiences and high participation in decision making. Conversely, the lower the person is on the continuum, the more likely he or she will have inconsistent, poorly balanced life experiences with low participation in decision making. In the first instance, the phenomena are viewed as GRRs (e.g., high material resources and good state of health). In the second instance, they are viewed as generalized resistance deficits (GRDs) (e.g., low material resources and poor state of health). Both GRRs and GRDs contribute to the development of one's "sense of coherence," a central concept of the salutogenesis model.

The Sense of Coherence

Antonovsky (1979) introduced a central concept of the model of salutogenesis—the sense of coherence (SOC). Sense of coherence is an abstract phenomenon descriptive of individuals. It is an enduring view of the world, and "a crucial element in the basic personality structure of an individual and in the ambiance of a subculture, culture, or historical period" (p. 124). From birth, the model of salutogenesis (Antonovsky, 1979, 1987) views individuals as constantly in situations of challenge, response, tension, stress, and resolution. The more these experiences are characterized by "consistency, participation in shaping outcome, and an underload-overload balance of stimuli" (1979, p. 187), the more an individual will begin to view the world as coherent and predictable. Childhood and adolescence are viewed as crucial points in the development of a person's SOC. By young adulthood, individuals are viewed as having acquired a tentative SOC that then becomes relatively stable throughout adulthood.

Antonovsky (1987) defined SOC as follows:

> A global orientation that expresses the extent to which one has a pervasive, enduring though dynamic feeling of confidence that (1) the stimuli deriving from one's internal and external environments in the course of living are structured, predictable, and explicable; (2) the resources are available to one to meet the demands posed by these stimuli; and (3) these demands are challenges, worthy of investment and engagement. (p. 19)

The SOC is an individual disposition characterized by the degree to which individuals expect their world to be comprehensible, manageable, and meaningful. *Comprehensibility* refers to the extent to which stimuli make cognitive sense and are relatively orderly, consistent, structured, and clear. *Manageability* is the perception that resources are at one's disposal that are adequate to meet the demands posed, whereas *meaningfulness* refers to the extent to which "one feels that life makes sense emotionally" (p. 18), that at least some of the demands posed by life are worth engagement, and these are viewed as challenges rather than burdens.

Although the three components of SOC are viewed as highly related to one another, they are discussed in terms of relative importance. Meaningfulness is viewed as the motivational component of the SOC, and it is the most central of the three components. Antonovsky (1987) stresses that a meaningful commitment must underlie the effort to comprehend and manage over the long term. Comprehensibility is viewed as second in importance because manageability is largely dependent on how one perceives stimuli. Antonovsky stresses, however, that this does not mean that manageability is unimportant. If people do not believe that they can manage, they are less likely to find meaning or to strive to comprehend. Antonovsky noted that it is SOC viewed as a whole that is the major determinant of an individual's placement on the health ease/dis-ease continuum.

Individual Placement on the Health Ease/Dis-Ease Continuum

As described earlier, an individual's placement on the health ease/dis-ease continuum ("breakdown" continuum is another term used to refer to this concept) is indicated by pain, functional limitation, prognostic implications, and action implications. It is both an objective and subjective phenomenon, and it embraces the notion of multicausality.

Relations Among the Concepts of the Salutogenesis Model

The salutogenesis model proposes a recursive relation between SOC and GRR-RDs. These factors help to shape the SOC, whereas a strong SOC helps to mobilize GRRs for the purpose of tension management. Poorly managed stressors lead to a state of tension, and poorly managed tension leads to stress and negative placement on the health ease/dis-ease continuum. In both situations, in which GRRs or GRDs are chronic and built into the life situation of the person, they are viewed as the primary determinants of the strength of an individual's SOC (Antonovsky, 1987, p. 29).

As noted previously, the salutogenesis model proposes to answer the following question: Why do persons stay healthy despite experiencing high stress? Within the salutogenesis model, SOC is viewed as a "very major determinant of maintaining one's position on the health ease/dis-ease continuum and of movement toward the healthy end" (Antonovsky, 1987, p. 15). Antonovsky poses both cognitive and physiologic mechanisms through which the SOC exerts salutary benefits. In explaining cognitive mechanisms, Antonovsky used the work of Lazarus and Folkman (1984) regarding cognitive appraisals. He drew on research conducted in the basic sciences that had linked chronic stress with immune suppression as early evidence for a physiologic mechanism(s).

Antonovsky wrote that a strong SOC mobilizes persons' abilities to use resources toward both avoiding and managing stress. Upon initial confrontation with a stimuli, a person with a strong SOC is more likely to define that stimuli as a nonstressor. Even if the stimuli is initially appraised as a stressor, the person with a strong SOC is likely to view the stressor as having low relevance (less danger) and to feel less or shorter lived tension. When an individual with a strong SOC perceives that he or she is confronted with a formidable stressor, the individual is more likely to feel a sense of engagement, commitment, and willingness to cope. Furthermore, he or she is likely to have developed a rich repertoire of GRRs on which to draw to deal with the stressor, both the behavioral aspects (coping) and the emotive aspects (emotional regulation). Tension is resolved relatively quickly and does not become stress, or stress is resolved relatively quickly. Finally, the person with a strong SOC is better able to judge the efficacy of his or her behaviors to manage tension or cope with stress or both and is more likely to discern the need for, and make use of, alternative actions.

➤ LEVEL OF DEVELOPMENT OF THE SALUTOGENESIS MODEL

The model of salutogenesis has relatively wide but clearly demarcated boundaries. It is purported to transcend culture and historical period. It is a cognitive model, however, and as such does not apply to individuals who lack the ability to perceive stressors. Application of the model for children is unclear, although research to examine the development of sense of coherence in children and adolescence is important because these periods of human growth and development are viewed as integral to promoting the development of a strong SOC in adults.

The salutogenesis model is highly abstract and encompasses a relatively large number of concepts (e.g., sense of coherence, ease/dis-ease continuum, the GRR-RDs coping strategy, and magic). Direction is provided, however, for operationalization of some of the main model concepts (e.g., sense of coherence, ease/dis-ease continuum).

➤ MEASUREMENT: THE ORIENTATION TO LIFE QUESTIONNAIRE

A 29-item Sense of Coherence Questionnaire (SOC-29) was developed by Antonovsky (1987) to measure an individual's sense of coherence. A shorter version, the 13-item SOC-13, is composed of a subset of items from the SOC-29. Published as an appendix in Antonovsky's 1987 book, the measures were developed based on the theoretical definition of SOC and its subconstructs, comprehensibility, manageability, and meaningfulness. Both the SOC-29 and SOC-13 are 7-point, semantic differential scales. Scores on the SOC-29 may range from 29 to 203, and those on the SOC-13 from 13 to 91. The SOC-29 has 11 comprehensibility, 10 manageability, and 8 meaningfulness items. The SOC-13 is composed of 5 comprehensibility, 4 manageability, and 4 meaningfulness items. To minimize response bias, almost half of the items have negatively worded stems that are reverse coded so that a higher score indicates a stronger SOC.

To date, the SOC-29 or SOC-13 or both have been used by more than 113 researchers or research teams and in 14 languages representing predominantly Western, Judeo-Christian cultures. More than half of the respondents have been women and include adults of all ages, although a few studies examined adolescents and older children (Antonovsky, 1993). Furthermore, both measures have been examined with healthy, community-based and "clinical" samples. Despite diagnosed illness, clinical subjects have reported a strong SOC. This finding is consistent with Antonovsky's (1987) contention that the SOC is fairly stable in adulthood.

Most research has examined the SOC in individuals; Smith (1997), however, used the SOC-13 to examine family worldviews. She provided a theoretical rationale for using the

TABLE 8.1 Normative Data From Nursing Research Using the SOC-29

Population	N	M	SD	Cronbach's Alpha	Reference
Canadian men receiving chronic ambulatory peritoneal dialysis and their spouses	56	143.5	28.1	.92	Horsburgh, Rice, and Matuk (1998)
Swedish women with fibromyalgia[a]	30	143.5	Not reported	.89 combined subjects	Soderberg, Lundman, and Norberg (1997)
Swedish healthy women[a]	30	147.5	Not reported		
Female, American, nephrology nurses	49	148.7	24.2	Not reported	Lewis, Bonner, Campbell, Cooper, and Willard (1994)
Swedish adults with insulin-dependent diabetes[a]	20	143.0	19.0	Not reported	Lundman and Norberg (1993)
American women and men with rheumatic disorders	1,333	148.0	29.7	.95	Hawley, Wolfe, and Cathey (1992)
Osteoarthritis	$n = 403$	154.9	26.7	Not reported	
Rheumatoid arthritis	$n = 572$	149.9	27.9	Not reported	
Fibromyalgia	$n = 358$	137.5	32.4	Not reported	
American nephrology nurses	238	143.1	23.0	Not reported	Lewis et al. (1992)

a. The questionnaires were translated into Swedish and adapted to Swedish culture by Langius, Bjorvell, and Antonovsky (1991).

higher score of two family members to determine family score (p. 210).

Normative data were originally reported for the SOC-29 using Israeli and American samples (Antonovsky, 1987); means ranged from 132.4 ($SD = 22.0$) to 160.4 ($SD = 16.7$). In 1993, Antonovsky listed normative data from an additional 21 studies that had examined a broader variety of Western, Judeo-Christian populations. Normative data recently reported in nursing research are consistent with those published by Antonovsky (1987, 1993) (Table 8.1).

Normative data for the SOC-13 were not reported by Antonovsky in 1987. In 1993, he reported data from nine individual studies of Western, Judeo-Christian populations, and means ranged from 55 ($SD = 0.7$) to 68.7 (SD = 10.0). Again, these data are consistent with means recently reported in nursing research (Table 8.2).

Reliability

Despite the fact that the SOC measures were designed to include comprehensibility, manageability, and meaningfulness, Cronbach's alpha internal consistency coefficients reported for the SOC-29 meet Nunnally's (1978) criterion of .80 for established measures (Table 8.1). Coefficients for the SOC-29 are higher than those reported for the SOC-13. This may be related to the sensitivity of Cronbach's alpha to the number of tool items—the SOC-29 has more than double the

TABLE 8.2 Normative Data From Nursing Research Using the SOC-13

Population	N	M	SD	Cronbach's Alpha	Reference
American female and male family members	368	Not reported	Not reported	.78	Smith (1997)
American elderly women and men	152	62.0	9.8	.87	Coward (1996)
American female and male health workers employed in community settings	653	Not reported	Not reported	.82	George (1996)
Home health aides	$n = 158$	65.1	12.8	Not reported	
Licensed practical nurses	$n = 55$	70.2	11.8	Not reported	
Registered nurses	$n = 400$	70.0	10.1	Not reported	
Social workers	$n = 40$	73.8	8.9	Not reported	
Swedish women and men with uremia[a]	38	66.8	11.2	.76	Klang, Bjorvell, and Clyne (1996)
American men and women with coronary artery disease who survived cardiac arrest	149	69.2	13.0	.87	Motzer and Stewart (1996)
American men and women with cancer	32	68.4	11.7	.84	Post-White et al. (1996)
American black and Hispanic women at risk for HIV infection[b]	581	Not reported	Not reported	.76	Nyamathi (1993)
Swedish women and men with cancer[a]	46	Not reported	Not reported	.78	Tishelman, Taube, and Sachs (1991)

a. The questionnaires were translated into Swedish and adapted to Swedish culture by Langius, Bjorvell, and Antonovsky (1991).

b. Wording was simplified, and a 5-point question format was used.

number of items. Cronbach's alphas reported for the Swedish translation of the SOC-13 were low. Furthermore, Nyamathi (1993) reported a low Cronbach's alpha for the modified SOC-13 used with 581 black and Hispanic women. These findings may reflect limitations due to translation and modification of the SOC-13. Additional testing of SOC-29 and SOC-13 is warranted with non-Western, non-white populations.

Because the salutogenesis model proposes that SOC is relatively stable in adulthood, it is reasonable to examine test-retest reliability of SOC-29 and SOC-13 in adult populations. Several test-retest correlations have been reported for the measures. Correlations have ranged from $r = .41$ after 2 years to $r = .97$ after 5 weeks (Antonovsky, 1993). Overall, test-retest scores appear satisfactory and are consistent with measurement of a relatively stable construct.

In summary, the SOC-29 has stronger empirical support for internal consistency than does the SOC-13. Because the SOC-29 is not a particularly lengthy measure, researchers might wish to give it preference over the SOC-13. Furthermore, researchers who plan to use either SOC measure in non-Western cultures should consider pretesting it with their population of interest.

Validity

The SOC is an abstract and relatively "young" construct, having first appeared in the published literature approximately 20 years ago. A relatively large amount of empirical work, however, has examined whether the SOC-29 and, to a much lesser extent, the SOC-13 measure what they purport to measure. As stressed by Antonovsky (1993), there is no "gold standard" measure of the SOC construct.

Content validity of the measures is strong because they were developed by the theorist (Antonovsky, 1987) with input from three colleagues familiar with the theory of salutogenesis. Individual items were selected on the basis that each "referred cleanly to one and only one of the three SOC components" (Antonovsky, 1993, p. 727). This approach might be expected to produce a measure with three identifiable subscales. Factor analyses carried out by Antonovsky (1993) and others (Hawley, Wolfe, & Cathey, 1992; Sandell, Blomberg, & Lazar, 1998), however, have failed to demonstrate support for individual subscales. Rather, a single dominant factor explaining a modest 30% to 36% of the variance in participants' scores is evident, in addition to a few weaker factors. Therefore, use of the total SOC score is recommended, and use of the three subscale scores is discouraged because individual items typically load on more than one factor. Of concern is the relatively low amount of variance accounted for by factor solutions reported for the SOC-29; a substantial percentage of the variance remains unexplained.

Construct validity of the SOC measures has been examined using both convergent and discriminant approaches. Support for convergent validity has been hindered by the fact that little psychometric work has been carried out to develop alternative measures of the SOC, and these are unpublished (Antonovsky,

1993). Empirical support for convergent validity of the SOC-13 was published in a study by Yeheskel (1995) that was conducted with 10 female and 10 male Holocaust survivors living in Israel. Using individual structured interviews, participants recalled their recent experiences, their experiences during the war, and experiences when they were 6, 15, 24, and 45 years of age. Quality of experience and biographical scores at each age and in each of the three components of the SOC were assessed and summed to provide an overall score for each individual. Participants completed the SOC-29 following interview. Convergent validity of the SOC-29 was supported with a high positive correlation between participants' biographical scores and the SOC-29. Furthermore, Yeheskel reported that meaningful activity was the strongest contributor to overall participants' experiences, a finding consistent with Antonovsky's (1987) view that meaningfulness is the central component of the SOC.

Empirical support for discriminant validity of the SOC measures has proved problematic. Motzer and Stewart (1996) noted a high positive correlation between quality of life and the SOC-13 for 149 men and women who survived cardiac arrest, raising concern that the two measures were not empirically distinct. Similarly, Horsburgh, Rice, and Matuk (1998) reported high positive correlations between the SOC-29 paired with three independent life satisfaction measures examined with 48 dialysis patients and their spouses. Bivariate correlations among the three life satisfaction measures were essentially identical to the former correlations, raising concern that the SOC-29 was not empirically distinct from life satisfaction measures. Unfortunately, sample sizes in both studies were too small to support factor analyses of the combined life satisfaction and SOC measures.

Hawley et al. (1992) noted with concern strong correlations among psychological scores (depression and anxiety) and the SOC, and they suggested that the SOC may "measure the other side of psychological distress" (p. 1916). They concluded, "One attractive aspect of the SOC concept is that it measures intrinsic strengths of an individual rather than weaknesses, but whether such strength is different from the absence of weakness begs the question" (p. 1917). Mlonzi and Strumpfer (1998) examined personality correlates of the SOC-29 with 100 black university undergraduates. Stepwise multiple regression showed sustained relations for emotional stability, independence, tough poise, and extroversion (control excluded), explaining 49% of the variance on the SOC-29. They concluded that the SOC-29 measured a mixture of personality domains that may be interpreted as support for construct validity and raised a concern that it may be assessing the absence of psychological distress and neuroticism.

Marshall, Wortman, Vickers, Kusulas, and Hervig (1994) offered a particularly cogent perspective on the issue of validity of personality constructs. They noted that the apparent proliferation of constructs, both salutary (e.g., hardiness, dispositional optimism, self-efficacy, and SOC) and nonsalutary (e.g., neuroticism, depression, and anxiety), poses barriers to the progression of health-related personality research. It becomes difficult to decide which concept(s) should be examined and impedes aggregation of findings across studies. Most important, researchers are compelled to ask if a given personality construct possesses "unique explanatory power . . . or is it essentially redundant with existing constructs" (pp. 278-279). Empirical examination of the SOC measures has not answered this question (nor indeed has it been answered for many other constructs).

As noted earlier, there is no gold standard for the SOC. Hence, criterion validity may be examined by consideration of the extent to which the SOC scale correlates with other phenomena using a hypothesis testing approach. In the following section, the empirical adequacy of the salutogenesis theory is examined, and the reader will find support for criterion validity within the discussion of the SOC.

Validity testing of the SOC measures with "known groups" has generally been supportive. Differences on mean scores among samples that would be expected to differ (according to the theory) have been demonstrated. Although not always statistically significant, or from the same studies, normative data vary in predictable ways (Antonovsky, 1993). George (1996) reported the lowest mean score on the SOC-13 with home health aides. In contrast, social workers (those with the most education and, likely, the most material possessions) scored the highest (Table 8.2).

In conclusion, the SOC-29 holds promise as a measure of SOC, but additional development is warranted (Antonovsky, 1993), and additional psychometric work remains to be done. Future studies should include both self-report and objective measures as well as controls for possible confounding variables (Flannery & Flannery, 1990). Most of the completed work has been cross-sectional; there is an urgent need for longitudinal and quasi-experimental work. Studies that discriminate among an increasing number of similar constructs, such as hardiness, locus of control, meaning in life, and self-efficacy, should receive high priority (Flannery & Flannery, 1990; Hawley et al., 1992; Marshall et al., 1994). Furthermore, because the SOC concept is purported to transcend culture (Antonovsky, 1993), psychometric examination of the measures should be carried out in non-Western populations. Nunnally (1978) suggests that garnering support for the validity of an abstract concept, such as the SOC, is an important and ongoing process. Additional investigation of the reliability and validity of the SOC measures is necessary to support future research to examine the SOC and its hypothesized salutary benefits for outcomes of interest to nursing.

➤ LOGICAL AND EMPIRICAL ADEQUACY OF THE SALUTOGENESIS MODEL

The structure of the model of salutogenesis (Antonovsky, 1979, 1987) appears to meet criteria proposed by Walker and Avant (1995) for logical adequacy of a model or theory. The salutogenesis model appears logical and has been used in a variety of health-related disciplines, including nursing, to generate relatively precise research questions and hypotheses. The content of the model intuitively "makes sense" and is consistent with or draws on related theory and research of other highly regarded scientists and social scientists.

An increasing number of health researchers have empirically examined relations derived from the model of salutogenesis. Overall, empirical support for the model reflects an early stage of development.

Published empirical findings from psychological research, and studies conducted by other nonnursing allied health disciplines, offer modest support for the salutogenesis model (Antonovsky, 1979, 1987). These studies differ from work reported by nurse researchers in the following ways: (a) Samples were more often drawn from nonclinical samples (often psychology students); (b) research designs featured more control and internal validity (quasi-experimental and longitudinal designs were more common); and (c) measurement issues received more attention. Despite these differences, empirical results of these studies are generally supportive of, and often complimentary to, those reported in the nursing literature.

For example, psychiatrists Flannery and Flannery (1990) conducted a prospective, longitudinal study of 95 college students. Consistent with the salutogenesis model, negative relations were supported between the SOC and life stress and psychological symptomatology. A quasi-experimental, time-series design was used by psychologists McSherry and Holm (1994) to compare low, medium, and high SOC undergraduate students (20 students in each group) on a variety of psychological and physiological measures prior to, during, and after a stressful encounter. Consistent with the salutogenesis model, low SOC subjects reported more psychological distress or arousal and less favorable cognitive appraisal and coping.

Measurement issues have received much attention in nonnursing research. Psychometric work has focused on the SOC-29/13 (Antonovsky, 1987). Led in many cases by psychologists, results of these studies suggest that the SOC measures, although moderately related to basic personality traits, do measure something beyond traits such as neuroticism and extroversion. Disagreement persists, however, regarding what is the "something extra" and its clinical relevance in comparison to similar constructs (Flannery & Flannery, 1990; Gibson & Cook, 1996; Mlonzi & Strumpfer, 1998; Sandell et al., 1998).

► EMPIRICAL ADEQUACY OF THE SALUTOGENESIS MODEL IN NURSING RESEARCH

The preponderance of the empirical evidence garnered through nursing research is supportive of the model of salutogenesis with some limitations, and results are generally consistent with those of other health-related disciplines. In general, nursing studies have used more clinical samples and have relied more on cross-sectional designs that preclude causal interpretation of observed relations. Measurement issues have not been well addressed.

Generalized Resistance Resources and Deficits and the Sense of Coherence

Relations among the following GRR-RDs and the sense of coherence have been examined in nursing research: health state, material resources, knowledge and intelligence, and religion and philosophy.

Three cross-sectional, correlational nursing studies have examined the hypothesized relation between health state and the SOC. Viewed together, empirical evidence for this relation is inconclusive. Coward (1996) reported a moderate positive relation between self-reported health and SOC scores of 152 well adults. Participants rated their health using four categories that ranged from "very good" to "poor." The high degree of subjectivity of participants' self-rated health may have inflated the reported relation.

Soderberg, Lundman, and Norberg (1997) reported no difference on SOC scores for 30 Swedish women with fibromyalgia and 30 healthy Swedish women. Subjects' SOC scores, however, did vary in the hypothesized direction (Table 8.1), and results were prone to Type II error because the two subsamples were small.

In contrast, Hawley et al. (1992) used both bivariate and multivariate approaches. They reported significant differences among three groups of adults with rheumatic disease. Adults with the least intrusive disease (osteoarthritis) reported the strongest SOCs. Adults with rheumatoid arthritis reported the next highest SOC scores, whereas participants with the most intrusive disease (fibromyalgia) reported the weakest SOCs. With age and depression controlled, however, differences among the groups were eliminated. The multivariate findings underscore the importance of viewing bivariate relations with caution because they are more prone to the confounding influence of other factors. One could argue that in controlling for depression (which has been strongly associated with SOC) Hawley et al. may have partialled out much of the relationship between health state and SOC in their participants. Additional research is needed to examine the relationship between health state and SOC. Longitudinal research that examines SOC across a period of change in health state would be particularly helpful.

Three cross-sectional, correlational nursing studies have examined the hypothesized positive relation between material resources and SOC (Coward, 1996; Horsburgh et al., 1998; Nyamathi, 1993). Viewed together, empirical evidence for this relation is also inconclusive. It is difficult to aggregate findings across these studies because each used a different measure of material resources, and it could be argued that none captured the complexity of the construct.

Nyamathi (1993) reported no relation between homelessness and SOC in 398 black and Hispanic homeless women compared to 183 black and Hispanic women who were in drug rehabilitation treatment programs. Horsburgh et al. (1998) also found no relation between the socioeconomic status and SOC in adults with end stage renal disease and their spouses; the sample was small, however, and the statistic was prone to Type II error. The measure of socioeconomic status measured both social class (material resources) and education (knowledge and intelligence). In contrast, Coward (1996) reported a moderate, positive, bivariate relation between adults' self-rated financial status and their SOC. Participants rated their finances on a 5-point, single-item scale (1 = "quite secure" and 5 = "poor"). The high degree of subjectivity of participants' self-rated finances could have been particularly prone to confounding factors, such as mood and response bias.

Additional research is needed to examine the relationship between material resources and SOC. Samples should be deliberately stratified to maximize variance on material resources to ensure that adequate numbers of participants with extremely low material resources are represented. Scatterplots should be examined to detect nonlinear relationships, and linear statistics should be used only if warranted. A multimeasurement approach that captures the full breadth of the construct should be employed.

Four cross-sectional, correlational nursing studies have examined the hypothesized positive relation between knowledge and intelligence and SOC (George, 1996; Hawley et al., 1992; Klang, Bjorvell, & Clyne, 1996; Nyamathi, 1993). Viewed together, empirical evidence is supportive, although again it is difficult to aggregate findings across studies because the researchers used different measures and different approaches. The salutogenesis theory views knowledge and intelligence as including information about the world and skills that facilitate knowledge acquisition. In most societies, the GRR/RD is contingent on literacy and formal education and includes knowledge about opportunities and one's rights within society (Antonovsky, 1979).

Klang and colleagues (1996) reported higher SOCs in participants with university education, but the statistic was not reported. Nyamathi (1993) found no relation between education and the SOC. It is unclear, however, how the construct was measured, and a description of participants' educational profile was not provided. The degree of heterogeneity of this sample on education is not clear.

Hawley et al. (1992) measured the number of years of formal education of their subjects. Although the positive correlation between education and SOC was nonsignificant, when subjects were grouped according to years of education those with less than a Grade 8 education scored significantly lower than other groups. Findings suggest that the relation between education and the SOC may be most pronounced at lower levels of education.

George's (1996) participants were quite diverse with regard to education. George reported a slight positive relation between education and SOC. Furthermore, a one-way analysis of variance showed that licensed practical nurses, registered nurses, and social workers all had stronger SOCs than home health aides (participants without college or university education).

More research is needed to examine the hypothesized positive relationship between knowledge and intelligence and SOC because Antonovsky (1979) views it as the "decisive GRR" in coping with stressors (p. 108). Samples should be deliberately stratified to maximize variance on knowledge and intelligence, and adequate numbers of participants with lower levels need to be included. Again, the relationship with SOC should be examined using scatterplots to detect nonlinear patterns. A multimeasurement approach that captures the full breadth of the construct should be used.

One nursing study found no relationship between the GRR-RD, religion and spirituality, and SOC (Post-White et al., 1996); statistical power was low, however. The salutogenesis model proposes that a strong sense of religion and spirituality contributes to the SOC by providing ready answers to human events such as death and pain (Antonovsky, 1979). This relationship requires additional study because Antonovsky views the answers provided by one's culture and religion as "probably the most powerful GRR of all" (p. 119).

In conclusion, empirical examination of relations between GRR-RDs and the SOC has just begun. In general, GRR-RDs are rich, complex constructs, and operationalization is challenging. Furthermore, the salutogenesis model proposes recursive relations between the GRRs and SOC that limit the utility of linear approaches to analysis. Structural equation modeling may be more helpful to future research because it permits examination of recursive relations. Finally, the salutogenesis model proposes interrelations among the GRR-RDs as these influence the SOC. Empirical work has not begun to examine these, although a synthesis of related empirical findings may provide direction for future research.

Relations Between the Sense of Coherence and Symptoms and Distress

The salutogenesis model proposes a positive relation between SOC and an individual's perception of symptoms and distress. Antonovsky (1987) noted that "the person with a strong SOC is more likely to define stimuli as nonstressors" (p. 132). Furthermore, when a stimulus is appraised as a stressor, it is likely to be viewed as less burdensome by persons with a strong SOC.

This beneficial influence has been the focus of seven nursing studies conducted with both clinical and nonclinical samples. The empirical findings are largely supportive of the hypothesized relation; in general, individuals with stronger SOCs have reported lower distress. It is difficult to aggregate findings across studies, however, because all studies used different outcome measures and reliability and validity with study samples were reported in only three (George, 1996; Nyamathi, 1993; Tishelman, Taube, & Sachs, 1991).

Three Swedish studies, each conducted with a unique clinical population, have examined the relationship between SOC and perceived symptoms and distress. Lundman and Norberg (1993) found no relation between SOC and "worries" of adults with diabetes. Individuals with a strong SOC, however, were less worried about insulin reactions and how the disease affected their relatives and friends. Tishelman et al. (1991) reported a moderate, negative relation between SOC and cancer-related symptom distress (e.g., nausea, appetite, fatigue, pain, mood, and outlook). Similarly, Klang et al. (1996) found a moderate correlation between SOC and uremia-related symptoms (fatigue, energy, sleep, mobility, mood, loneliness, and general health).

Two studies examined the relationship between SOC and distress with nonclinical samples. Lewis, Bonner, Campbell, Cooper, and Willard (1994) reported a large, negative relation between 49 female dialysis nurses' SOC and their personal stress and a moderate, negative relation with their work stress. Moderate and small negative relations were found with emotional exhaustion and depersonalization, respectively. George (1996) studied the relationship between SOC and community health workers' appraisals of risk in making home visits ($N = 653$). A small negative relation was reported between SOC and reported frequency of encounters with risk. None was found between SOC, paired with appraised risk associated with characteristics of the home visit, and the percentage of home visits appraised as involving personal risk.

Two studies evaluated SOC and symptoms and distress using multivariate approaches. Hawley et al. (1992) examined SOC and perceived impact of arthritis. They reported large negative relations between SOC,

paired with depression and anxiety, and small, negative relations with disease severity, pain, and functional disability (activities of daily living). To examine the relation between SOC and demographic, clinical, and psychological variables, they used stepwise multiple regression. Their results showed that "psychological variables explain essentially all of the measurable difference between patients in their SOC scores" (p. 1917). Hawley and colleagues questioned if the SOC-29 was not measuring the "other side" of psychological distress. Their concern is supported by results of Coward (1996), who reported large, bivariate relationships between SOC and two independent measures of mood and affect. Individuals reporting stronger SOCs reported lower levels of psychological distress.

Nyamathi (1993) studied hypothesized benefits of SOC on appraisal of threat, emotional distress (mood), and personal and environmental concerns (e.g., survival, hopelessness, despondency, drug addiction, parenting, and safety) of 581 black and Hispanic women at risk for contacting HIV. She found a large negative relationship between SOC and emotional distress. Moderate, negative relations were reported with concerns and appraisal of threat. The stronger the SOC, the fewer the concerns, appraisal of threat, and emotional distress. These findings were reconfirmed with multivariate analyses comparing women with a strong SOC to women with a weak SOC. Nyamathi concluded that her findings supported the view that women with a stronger SOC appraised their environments as less threatening to their well-being than did women with a weaker SOC.

In conclusion, empirical nursing research supports the hypothesized benefit of a strong SOC on individuals' perceptions of their symptoms and distress. Longitudinal work is needed to examine time sequencing of variables and to increase understanding of the processes whereby SOC and other personal resources may benefit one's appraisal of stimuli. To address the issue of construct validity of the SOC raised by Hawley et al. (1992), the relative contributions of related psychological constructs of interest (e.g., depression, mood, and affect) need to be examined.

Relation Between the Sense of Coherence and Tension Management and Coping Behaviors

The salutogenesis model proposes a positive relation between the SOC and individual coping behavior. When confronted with an acute or chronic stressor, a person with a stronger SOC "is more likely to respond behaviorally with adaptive health behavior" (Antonovsky, 1987, p. 153). The benefit of a stronger SOC on coping has been examined in two nursing studies, and results are supportive. In general, individuals with a stronger SOC reported "better" coping behavior.

George (1996) reported a small positive relation between SOC and the ability of community health professionals to refuse high-risk visits. Nyamathi (1993) reported a small negative relation between SOC and the high-risk behaviors of black and Hispanic women; women with a stronger SOC were less likely to report high-risk behaviors, including intravenous drug use, nonintravenous drug use, frequency of unprotected sexual activity, history of sexually transmitted disease, and having a partner who used intravenous drugs. Nyamathi generated a path model to further examine these relations. Her schematic depicts a direct-effects relationship between SOC and risk behavior in addition to an indirect effect through appraisal. Nyamathi did not report the percentage of variance in risk behavior explained by SOC and appraisal.

Clearly, additional research is needed to examine SOC and coping behaviors, especially in relation to health-related behaviors of interest to nursing (e.g., self-care, adherence, and risk taking). Longitudinal cohort designs that consider these relationships across adolescence and young adulthood may permit examination of the development of SOC as it relates to both healthy and high-risk behavior.

Relations Between the Sense of Coherence and Subjective and Objective Health and Well-Being

The salutogenesis model states that by managing tension and coping well with stress, the person with a strong SOC will "reinforce or improve his or her health status" (Antonovsky, 1987, p. 152). Hence, a positive relation between the SOC and health and well-being is posited that is mediated or moderated or both by tension management and coping.

Five studies examined hypothesized, positive relationships between SOC and subjective health and well-being (Horsburgh et al., 1998; Motzer & Stewart, 1996; Post-White et al., 1996; Soderberg et al., 1997), one studied a hypothesized positive relation between SOC and an objective health indicator (Lundman & Norberg, 1993), and one examined SOC and family and individual adaptation (Smith, 1997).

Horsburgh et al. (1998) reported large, positive, bi-variate relations between SOC, paired with three independent measures of life satisfaction. Participants who reported a stronger SOC were more likely to report higher life satisfaction. The size of these relations, however, was as large as the inter-correlations among the three life satisfaction measures, raising concern that the SOC-29 may have been measuring life satisfaction.

Noting a large, positive, bivariate relationship between SOC and self-reported quality of life, Motzer and Stewart (1996) also raised concerns regarding conceptual overlap. To examine this, they deleted items on both research measures that they judged as redundant and recomputed the correlation. A significant positive relationship remained, and they concluded that this was not merely "the result of measurement artifact" (p. 295).

Soderberg and colleagues (1997) and Coward (1996) also reported large, positive, bivariate relationships between SOC and self-reported well-being. The issue of conceptual overlap, however, was neither raised nor examined. Post-White and colleagues (1996) reported a moderate, positive relation between SOC and quality of life for 32 adults with cancer. Reliability of the quality of life measure was reportedly low.

Both Horsburgh et al. (1998) and Motzer and Stewart (1996) used hierarchical multiple regression to further examine the size of the relationship between SOC and well-being and quality of life, controlling for other variables. The former reported SOC as the strongest individual predictor of life satisfaction, with 41% to 55% of the variance explained by three predictors. Motzer and Stewart reported SOC as the strongest individual predictor of quality of life, with 64% of the variance explained by 17 predictors. This seemed to be too many predictor variables for a sample size of 149.

Lundman and Norberg (1993) reported no relationship between SOC and glycated hemoglobin levels of 20 Swedish adults with diabetes. The correlation (−.26), however, was in the predicted direction: Participants with a stronger SOC had lower glycated hemoglobin levels, suggesting better metabolic control. The small sample size predisposed for a Type II error.

Smith (1997) examined behavioral aspects (family problem-solving communication style) and SOC as these contributed to both family and individual adaptation. Controlling for social desirability, stepwise multiple regression showed that family problem-solving communication style and SOC explained 38% of family adaptation and 29% of individual adaptation. Family problem-solving communication style was the strongest individual predictor of family adaptation, whereas SOC was the strongest predictor of individual adaptation. Smith did not report tests for mediating or moderating effects or both of family problem-solving communication style on the relation between SOC and adaptation.

In summary, although empirical support for the relationship between SOC and self-re-

ported life satisfaction and well-being is encouraging, additional research is needed. Psychometric work is warranted to examine conceptual overlap among the SOC-29/13 and self-report measures of life satisfaction and well-being. Longitudinal and experimental approaches are required to provide insight into causal sequencing of variables, and future work must strive to incorporate objective health indicators among the dependent variables of interest. Finally, future nursing research should place higher priority on examination of the relation between SOC and health and the mediating or moderating influences or both of tension management and behavior because nursing interventions aimed at facilitating tension management and positive health behavior are a strong focus of contemporary nursing (McCloskey & Bulechek, 1996).

➤ USEFULNESS OF THE SALUTOGENESIS MODEL IN NURSING

All nurses have encountered clients who have reached higher levels of health and well-being despite severe adversity (e.g., chronic illness, poverty, and war). The salutogenesis model (Antonovsky, 1979, 1987), which is based on human strengths rather than weaknesses, frames a revolutionary perspective and possesses intuitive appeal. It is not surprising that it has received increasing attention within nursing.

The GRR-RDs support a multicausal perspective that recognizes contributions of cultural, historical, psychosocial, spiritual, and biological factors to health. This broad perspective reminds nurses that issues of war, unemployment, education, cultural instability, and poverty are integral to health promotion and disease prevention and supports a renewed impetus for social activism within the nursing profession.

The salutogenesis model (Antonovsky, 1979, 1987) stresses the importance of fostering a strong sense of coherence during childhood and adolescence and supports efforts to eradicate social ills such as child poverty. It supports health-promotion programs as diverse as parenting programs and efforts to preserve and reestablish the language and culture of aboriginal young people. Although the model suggests that nursing interventions to facilitate a strong SOC in adults are limited, it urges the identification of adults who are at risk for poor tension management, stress, and negative health outcomes. Individuals with a weak SOC may be identified and offered more supportive nursing interventions (e.g., counseling, behavior management, and emotional support) maintained over longer periods of time. Furthermore, although originally designed to explain individual health, Smith's (1997) work suggests that the salutogenesis model offers direction for the investigation of family health and well-being.

The current and future usefulness of the salutogenesis model is limited primarily by issues of empirical validity and measurement. There is an urgent need to differentiate the central construct of the model, the sense of coherence, from similar phenomena, such as hardiness, self-efficacy, self-transcendence, hope, and life satisfaction. Comparative studies that examine the relative contribution of these constructs to outcomes of interest for nursing are imperative because it makes little sense to fund two or more research programs if the central constructs of these programs cannot be empirically distinguished from one another. Rigorous comparative research will require measures with high levels of empirical support for reliability and validity.

➤ GENERALIZABILITY OF THE SALUTOGENESIS MODEL IN NURSING

Overall, generalizability of the salutogenesis model in nursing includes primarily sentient adults of Western, Judeo-Christian background, inclusive of women and men, both well and diagnosed with chronic illness. With a few noteworthy exceptions (Nyamathi, 1993), little research has been devoted to examination of the model with populations evidencing low levels of generalized resistance resources (e.g., material resources and knowledge and intelligence). This is an important gap because GRR-RDs may negatively influence SOC and placement on the ease/dis-ease continuum primarily when they are manifested at low levels.

Because the salutogenesis model was developed from a predominantly Western, Judeo-Christian tradition and is purported to transcend culture, future research should examine the model with aboriginal, Middle and Far-Eastern populations. This is especially important as the North American health care systems strive to promote the health of aboriginal and increasing immigrant populations. Indeed, these populations present unique opportunities to examine cultural commitment and cohesion, cultural stability, and religion and philosophy because these GRRs contribute to the development of a strong sense of coherence, positive tension and stress management, and positive health outcomes.

There is an urgent need for longitudinal research to examine childhood levels of GRR-RDs because these contribute to a strong SOC in adolescence and young adulthood. Furthermore, these studies should encompass tension and stress management processes because these develop and impact both subjective and objective health and placement on the ease/dis-ease continuum. The model of salutogenesis suggests that nursing and allied health interventions, targeted toward enhancing childhood exposure to positive GRRs, may be particularly useful in promoting healthy lifestyles and healthy populations.

➤ PARSIMONY OF THE SALUTOGENESIS MODEL

The salutogenesis model (Antonovsky, 1979, 1987), as depicted in Figure 8.1, is not parsimonious. Because the model seeks to explain complex and abstract human phenomena, however, a high degree of complexity is not surprising. Antonovsky's work yields many testable hypotheses with a high degree of relevance for nursing. As noted previously, the major barrier to the determination of the heuristic relevance of the model, and its further development, is the empirical adequacy of model constructs. It can be anticipated that research and theoretical efforts devoted to this issue will yield high dividends for nursing practice and health promotion as the nursing profession, and other health professions, seek to understand factors that facilitate human health and well-being in the face of severe life stress.

➤ REFERENCES

Antonovsky, A. (1972). Breakdown: A needed fourth step in the conceptual armamentarium of modern medicine. *Social Science and Medicine, 6,* 537-544.

Antonovsky, A. (1979). *Health, stress and coping.* San Francisco: Jossey-Bass.

Antonovsky, A. (1987). *Unraveling the mystery of health: How people manage stress and stay well.* San Francisco: Jossey-Bass.

Antonovsky, A. (1993). The structure and properties of the sense of coherence scale. *Social Science Medicine, 36,* 725-733.

Coward, D. D. (1996). Self-transcendence and correlates in a healthy population. *Nursing Research, 45,* 116-121.

Dubos, R. J. (1960). *The mirage of health.* London: Allen & Unwin.

Dubos, R. J. (1968). *Man, medicine and environment.* New York: Praeger.

Flannery, R. B., & Flannery, G. J. (1990). Sense of coherence, life stress, and psychological distress: A prospective methodological inquiry. *Journal of Clinical Psychology, 46,* 415-420.

Frankl, V. E. (1959). *Man's search for meaning.* New York: Washington Square Press.

George, V. D. (1996). Field-workers sense of coherence and perception of risk when making home visits. *Public Health Nursing, 13,* 244-252.

Gibson, L. M., & Cook, M. J. (1996). Neuroticism and sense of coherence. *Psychological Reports, 79,* 343-349.

Hawley, D. J., Wolfe, F., & Cathey, M. A. (1992). The Sense of Coherence Questionnaire in patients with rheumatic disorders. *Journal of Rheumatology, 19,* 1912-1918.

Horsburgh, M. E., Rice, V. H., & Matuk, L. (1998). Sense of coherence and life satisfaction: Patient and spousal adaptation to home dialysis. *ANNA Journal, 25,* 219-228.

Klang, B., Bjorvell, H., & Clyne, N. (1996). Perceived well-being in predialysis uremic patients. *ANNA Journal, 23,* 223-229, 260.

Langius, A., Bjorvell, H., & Antonovsky, A. (1991). The sense of coherence concept and its relation to personality traits in Swedish samples. *Scandinavian Journal of Caring Sciences, 5,* 41-57.

Lazarus, R. S., & Folkman, S. (1984). *Stress, appraisal, and coping.* New York: Springer.

Lewis, S. L., Campbell, M. A., Becktell, P. J., Cooper, C. L., Bonner, P. N., & Hunt, W. C. (1992). Work stress, burnout, and sense of coherence among dialysis nurses. *ANNA Journal, 19,* 545-554.

Lewis, S. L., Bonner, P. N., Campbell, M. A., Cooper, C. L., & Willard, A. (1994). Personality, stress, coping, and sense of coherence among nephrology nurses in dialysis settings. *ANNA Journal, 21,* 325-336.

Lundman, B., & Norberg, A. (1993). The significance of a sense of coherence for subjective health in persons with insulin-dependent diabetes. *Journal of Advanced Nursing, 18,* 381-386.

Marshall, G. N., Wortman, C. B., Vickers, R. R., Kusulas, J. W., & Hervig, L. K. (1994). The Five-Factor Model of Personality as a framework for personality-health research. *Journal of Personality and Social Psychology, 67,* 278-285.

McCloskey, J. C., & Bulechek, G. M. (Eds.). (1996). *Nursing interventions classification (NIC)* (2nd ed.). New York: C. V. Mosby.

McSherry, W. C., & Holm, J. E. (1994). Sense of coherence: Its effects on psychological and physiological processes prior to, during, and after a stressful situation. *Journal of Clinical Psychology, 50,* 476-487.

Mlonzi, E. N., & Strumpfer, D. J. (1998). Antonovsky's sense of coherence scale and 16PF second-order factors. *Social Behavior and Personality, 26,* 39-50.

Motzer, S. U., & Stewart, B. J. (1996). Sense of coherence as a predictor of quality of life in persons with coronary heart disease surviving cardiac arrest. *Research in Nursing & Health, 19,* 287-298.

Nunnally, J. C. (1978). *Psychometric theory.* New York: McGraw-Hill.

Nyamathi, A. M. (1993). Sense of coherence in minority women at risk for HIV infection. *Public Health Nursing, 10,* 151-158.

Post-White, J., Ceronsky, C., Kreitzer, M. J., Nickelson, K., Drew, D., Mackey, K. W., Koopmeiners, L., & Gutknecht, S. (1996). Hope, spirituality, sense of coherence, and quality of life in patients with cancer. *Oncology Nursing Forum, 23,* 1571-1579.

Sandell, R., Blomberg, J., & Lazar, A. (1998). The factor structure of Antonovsky's Sense of Coherence scale in Swedish clinical and non-clinical samples. *Personality and Individual Differences, 24,* 710-711.

Selye, H. (1956). *The stress of life.* New York: McGraw-Hill.

Smith, S. (1997). The retirement transition and the later life family unit. *Public Health Nursing, 14,* 207-216.

Soderberg, L., Lundman, B., & Norberg, A. (1997). Living with fibromyalgia: Sense of coherence, perception of well-being, and stress in daily life. *Research in Nursing and Health, 20,* 495-503.

Tishelman, C., Taube, A., & Sachs, L. (1991). Self-reported symptom distress in cancer patients: Reflections of disease, illness or sickness. *Social Science and Medicine, 33,* 1229-1240.

Walker, L. O., & Avant, K. C. (1995). *Strategies for theory construction in nursing* (3rd ed.). Norwalk, CT: Appleton & Lange.

Yeheskel, A. (1995). The intimate environment and the sense of coherence among Holocaust survivors. *Social Work in Health Care, 20,* 25-35.

CHAPTER 9

Evolution of a Model of Stress, Coping, and Discrete Emotions

Richard S. Lazarus

ecause I am writing for two kinds of readers in nursing, those who are familiar with my work and ideas and those who are not, what I present in this chapter follows a historical perspective of the emergence over the years of my basic ideas about psychosocial stress and emotion. Both these topics also include the coping process as an essential component. The content of this chapter is divided into my early work and ideas (beginning in the 1950s), transitional views in the 1960s and 1970s (some of which occurred again quite recently), and present themes in the 1980s and 1990s (that flow from my increasing recognition that stress and emotion are two interdependent themes that should be combined as one).

A fundamental theme of my approach is that stress and emotion can no longer be divided into two separate research and theoreti-

cal literatures (Lazarus, 1993). Readers interested in my latest views about stress and emotion, including my espousal of a narrative approach to research and theory in contrast to a system theory approach, should review my latest book (Lazarus, 1999).

Although first proposed in ancient Greece, cognitive-mediational approaches to the mind, and my own views too, were greatly influenced by the work of a substantial number of distinguished modern psychologists. Largely oriented to personality, social, and clinical issues, two generations of psychological scholars deviated sharply from the radical behaviorist stance that had dominated and severely limited psychological theory and research for more than 50 years.

One generation, which included Gordon Allport, Kurt Lewin, Henry Murray, and Edward Tolman, articulated their main theoreti-

AUTHOR'S NOTE: Aspects of this chapter have been adapted from Lazarus (in press).

cal and metatheoretical outlooks in the 1930s. The second generation, which included Solomon Asch, Jerome Bruner, Harry Harlow, Fritz Heider, George Kelly, David McClelland, Gardner Murphy, Julian Rotter, Mutzafer Sherif, and Robert White, published their main work in the late 1940s and 1950s.

Both generations were enormously influential in moving many scientific scholars toward an approach to mind and behavior that was epistemologically more open and congenial to theory and inference and a wide variety of methodological approaches to obtaining knowledge. This also led to a more modern definition of psychology as the science of mind, which broke away from the severely constricting radical behavioristic-positivist tradition of defining it as the science of behavior.

Even this distinguished list of psychological mavericks is substantially incomplete because there were also many frankly phenomenological psychologists who had considerable influence in personality and clinical psychology in those days. Along with members of many deviant movements of European origin, such as the gestaltists and existentialists, these mavericks set the stage for renewed interest in cognitive mediation and value-expectancy theory.

➤ MY EARLY WORK AND IDEAS

In this section, I discuss the origins and terminology of the appraisal construct and my version of appraisal and coping theory as applied to psychological stress. I will later show that these concepts—and that of relational meaning—are also central concepts in my motivational-cognitive-relational approach to the emotions, within which stress is properly encompassed.

In my earliest monograph dealing with stress and coping theory and research (Lazarus, 1966), appraisal was the centerpiece of my approach. At that time, stress had little if any cachet in social science; this was to change greatly, however, during the 1970s.

Selye's (1956/1976) approach to physiological stress helped greatly to influence this change. Janis's (1951, 1958) works on the stress experienced by surgical patients had not yet achieved much notice but were to be treated later as classics. Mechanic's (1962/1978) monograph about students under stress also gained major attention in the 1970s. Although there had been important theoretical contributions even before the 1960s, such as those of Leeper (1948) and McReynolds (1956), emotion as a topic of research and theory burgeoned mainly during the 1980s and 1990s.

Origins and Terminology of the Appraisal Construct

How did appraisal first emerge as the main mediational construct of psychological stress and emotion? Because I am one of the earliest contributors, I first portray my role in this topic. I first began to think programmatically about individual differences in psychological stress in the early 1950s when my research was sponsored by the military and focused on the effects of stress on skilled performance. Early on, and based on research data, it seemed obvious that the arousal and effects of stress depended on how different individuals evaluated and coped with the personal significance of what was occurring.

I was greatly impressed by a World War II monograph written by two research-oriented psychiatrists, Grinker and Spiegel (1945), about how flight crews managed the constant stress of air battles and flak from antiaircraft guns on the ground. These authors were among the first to refer to "appraisal," although the term was employed only casually. They wrote,

> The emotional reaction aroused by a threat of loss is at first an undifferentiated combination of fear and anger, subjectively felt as increased tension, alertness, or awareness of danger. The whole organism is keyed up for trouble, a process whose physiological

components have been well studied. Fear and anger are still undifferentiated, or at least mixed, as long as it is not known what action can be taken in the face of the threatened loss. If the loss can be averted, or the threat dealt with in active ways by being driven off or destroyed, aggressive activity accompanied by anger is called forth. This *appraisal* [italics added] of the situation requires mental activity involving judgment, discrimination, and choice of activity, based largely on past experience. (p. 122)

Appraisal aside, Grinker and Spiegel's (1945) monograph contains most of the important basic themes of a theory of stress and emotion. Their work is centered mainly on anger and fear, the characteristics of which are not typical of all emotions. Their approach centered on how soldiers construe what is happening to them, thereby adopting a phenomenological or subjective outlook. The authors' reference to actions that can be taken in the face of threat, and defense mechanisms, implies the important role of coping.

One can see in the Grinker and Spiegel (1945) work that stress and emotion concern the personal meaning of what was happening, which in military combat was the imminent danger of being killed or maimed. In addition, what a soldier could do to cope with this danger was severely constrained by debilitating guilt or shame about letting one's buddies down, the potential accusation of cowardice for refusing voluntarily to commit to battle, and the threat of punishment. Because this was an intractable conflict, the only viable way to escape was to depend on intrapsychic forms of coping, such as denial, avoidance, detachment, and magical thinking, which in those days were considered both pathological and pathogenic.

In a published review that emphasized the individual differences observed in stress research, Lazarus, Deese, and Osler (1952, p. 294) wrote that "the situation will be more or less stressful for the individual members of the group, and it is likely that differences in the *meaning* of the situation will appear in [their] performance." My concern with indi-

vidual differences in motives, beliefs, coping, and relational meaning in the stress process was articulated often in those days and thereafter.

Lazarus, Deese, and Osler (1952, p. 295), for example, wrote that "stress occurs when a particular situation threatens the *attainment of some goal* [italics added]." Lazarus and Baker (1956a, p. 23) stated that stress and emotion depend on "the degree of *relevance of the situation to the motive state* [italics added]," which is a statement about the person-environment relationship. In another article, Lazarus and Baker (1956b, p. 267) wrote that "relatively few studies have attempted to define stress in terms of internal psychological processes which may vary from *individual to individual* [italics added] and which determine the *subjects' definition of the situation* [italics added]."

In those days, I made the same mistake that William James (1890) made in his discussion of the relationship of emotion to action—that is, I used the term "perception" instead of appraisal. Thus, Lazarus and Baker (1956a, p. 22) wrote that "psychological stress occurs when a situation is perceived as thwarting or potentially thwarting to some motive state, thus resulting in affective arousal and in the elicitation of *regulative processes* aimed at the management of the affect" (italics added). The expression "regulative processes" refers to coping.

The word *perception* is ambiguous because it does not explicitly indicate an evaluation of the personal significance of what is happening for well-being. *Apperception* would have been more apt because it implies thinking through the implications of an event. John Dewey (1894) was quite clear on this score, but William James failed to indicate that perception meant more than the mere registration of what is occurring.

One reason for the terminological lapse was the influence of the New Look movement. In its usage, the term perception was given much broader connotations than it had in classical perception psychology. When New Look psychologists spoke of perception, it also encompassed the personal meaning of what was being perceived. In other words, how people construe events was said to depend on variations in motivation and beliefs. Much more clearly than perception, the term *appraisal* connotes an evaluation of the significance to the individual of what is happening for well-being.

Influenced by Magda Arnold's (1960) monograph on emotion and personality, I first began to use appraisal for this evaluation in Lazarus (1964) and Speisman, Lazarus, Mordkoff, and Davison (1964). Arnold had developed an impressive programmatic case for a cognitive-mediational approach to the emotions, with appraisal being her central construct. Tolman's (1932) book—courageous in those days because it spoke of purposive behavior—preceded all other work in turning attention from a past-directed mind (centered on what had been learned) to a future-directed focus on the possible outcomes of motivated action.

Those who favor a cognitive-mediational approach must also recognize that Aristotle's (1941) *Rhetoric* more than 2,000 years ago applied this approach to many emotions in terms that seem remarkably modern. More than a century ago, Robertson (1877) also put the same basic ingredients together—namely, evaluative thought, motivation (or a personal stake), beliefs (or knowledge), and degree of excitement—in a *Rashomon*-like[1] description of individual differences in emotion. Robertson wrote,

Four persons of much the same age and temperament are traveling in the same vehicle. At a particular stopping place it is intimated to them that a certain person has just died suddenly and unexpectedly. One of the company looks perfectly stolid. A second comprehends what has taken place, but is in no way affected. The third looks and evidently feels sad. The fourth is overwhelmed with grief which finds expression in tears, sobs, and exclamations. Whence the difference of the four individuals before us? In one respect they are all alike: An announcement has been made to them. The first is a foreigner, and has not understood the communication. The second has never met with the deceased, and could have no special regard for him. The third had often met with him in social intercourse and business transactions, and been led to cherish a great esteem for him. The fourth was the brother of the departed, and was bound to him by native affection and a thousand ties earlier and later. From such a case we may notice that [to experience an emotion] there is need first of some understanding or apprehension; the foreigner had no feeling because he had no idea or belief. We may observe further that there must secondly be an affection of some kind; for the stranger was not interested in the occurrence. The emotion flows forth from a well, and is strong in proportion to the waters; it is stronger in the brother than in the friend. It is evident, thirdly, that the persons affected are in a moved or excited state. A fourth peculiarity has appeared in the sadness of the countenance and the agitations of the bodily frame. Four elements have thus come forth to view. (p. 413)

The premise of appraisal theory is that people (and infrahuman animals) are constantly evaluating relationships with the environment with respect to their implications for personal well-being (Lazarus, 1981; Lazarus & Folkman, 1984; Lazarus & Launier, 1978). Although my theory is subjective in outlook, it is not classical phenomenology but a modified subjectivism. In my view of appraisal, people negotiate between two complementary frames of reference: First, wanting to view what is happening as realistically as possible to cope with it and, second, wanting to put the best possible light on events so as not to lose hope or sanguinity. In effect, appraisal is a compromise between life as it is and what one wishes it to be, and efficacious coping depends on both.

Dissident voices still argue against the scientific adequacy of a cognitive-mediational approach to stress and the emotions, thereby demonstrating what might be regarded as residual behaviorism. For example, Hobfoll (1998) has regularly expressed scientific disdain about a subjective epistemology and metatheory, even when it is only partial as in my version noted previously. This is evident in his emphasis on loss as an objective antecedent condition of stress and his principle of conservation of resources as the basis of stress. What is a loss, however, or a threat of loss is not adequately defined before the fact of the emotional reaction without reference to a person's values, goal hierarchy, beliefs, resources, and coping styles and processes. What individuals consider important or unimportant to their well-being influences how emotionally devastating any loss will be and what coping choices must be made to manage it—therefore affecting the details of the observed emotional reaction and subjective experience. This is true even when loss is normatively defined, which refers, of course, to a collective average. With regard to any given individual rather than some epidemiological (probabilistic) estimate, an average value is of little predictive utility. The concept of loss without detailed specification of its personal significance for various individuals or types of individuals offers less precision than when personality is taken into account. Therefore, Hobfoll's (and anyone else's) claim that an analysis of stress in terms of objective stimulus conditions is more scientific than a cognitive-mediational analysis is specious.

About my own work with Folkman, and that of Bandura, Meichenbaum, and Seligman, Hobfoll (1998) writes,

> I argue against a strictly cognitive view of stress. I suggest from the outset that the cognitive revolution has misled us in our understanding of the stress process. But this should not be construed to mean that elements of the stress phenomenon are not cognitive, or that cognitive psychology does not provide valuable insights into our understanding of stress. Rather, I will argue that cognitive notions have colonized too much of inquiry into stress, have misinterpreted elements of the stress process that are environmental as being a matter of appraisal (as opposed to objective reality that is perceived), and have served a Western view of the world that emphasizes control, freedom, and individual determinism. I suggest that resources, not cognitions, are the *primum mobile* on which stress is hinged. . . . Cognition is the player not the play. (pp. 21-22)

Unfortunately, what Hobfoll (1998) says about cognitive mediation is a red herring, suggesting that he has not read carefully what I and other cognitive mediationists have written, so he ends up co-opting what has already been said and passing it off as his own. Nor does he seem to understand what it means to speak of relational meaning, or that the theory is cognitive, motivational, and relational. He presents a stereotypical and erroneous view of what such a theory is about, despite the vagueness and internal inconsistency of his own position. What he proposes is no substitute at all because, in the main, it remains just as circular as traditional stimulus-response psychology.

This circularity stems from the fact that what makes a so-called stressor stressful is not adequately spelled out before the fact but depends on the quality, intensity, and duration of the stressor stimulus, which varies greatly from person to person even in very similar environmental circumstances. (For more detail, see Lazarus and Folkman, 1984, and Lazarus, 1999; also see Parkinson and Manstead, 1992, for another critique of appraisal theory.) In general, most epistemically focused criticisms of appraisal theory seem to be a case of the pot, which has historically been overzealous of the need to demonstrate its scientific credentials, calling the kettle black.

Appraising in Stress Theory

Early on (Lazarus, 1966), my theorizing about stress drew on concepts of appraisal and coping. Before proceeding with the role of appraisal in stress theory, however, it is useful to distinguish linguistically between the verb form, *appraising,* which refers to the act of making an evaluation, and the noun form, *appraisal,* which stands for the evaluative product. The former usage offers the advantage of emphasizing the appraisal process as a set of cognitive actions, and I use this convention here. I first suggested this in Lazarus and commentators (1995). McAdams (1996) also employed it with respect to the concept of self. He referred to the process by which a person constructs selfhood developmentally with the accurate but awkward verb form "selfing" and the product of this construction with the noun "self."

In my treatment of psychological stress, I emphasize two kinds of appraising, primary and secondary. Figure 9.1 presents a schematization of the main variables of the system that were originally presented by Lazarus and Folkman (1984).

Primary Appraising

This process has to do with whether or not what is happening is relevant to one's values, goal commitments, beliefs about self and world, and situational intentions and, if so, in what way. Because we do not always act on them, values and beliefs are apt to be weaker factors in mobilizing action and emotion than goal commitments. Thus, one may think it is good to have wealth but not worth making a major sacrifice to obtain it. The term *goal commitment* implies that a person will strive hard to attain the goal despite discouragement and adversity.

I have always stood by the widely acknowledged principle that if there is no goal commitment, there is nothing of adaptational importance at stake in an encounter to arouse emotions. The person goes about dealing with routine matters until there is an indication that something of greater adaptational importance is taking place, which will interrupt the routine because it has more potential for harm, threat, or challenge (Mandler, 1984).

What questions does one ask in primary appraising in any transaction? Fundamental is whether anything is at stake—in effect, one asks "Are any of my goals, important personal relationships, or core beliefs and values repre-

sented here?" and "If I do have a stake, what might the expected outcome be?" If the answer to the fundamental primary appraisal question is "no stake"—in other words, the transaction is not relevant to one's well-being—there is nothing further to consider.

Secondary Appraising

This process focuses on what can be done about a troubled person-environment relationship—that is, the coping options and the social and intrapsychic constraints against acting them out. Such an evaluation and the personal meanings a person constructs from the relationship are the essential cognitive underpinnings of coping actions.

In any stressful transaction, one must evaluate coping options, decide which ones to choose, and decide how to set them in motion (Lazarus & Launier, 1978). This is the function of secondary appraising. The questions addressed vary with the circumstances, but they concern diverse issues, such as the following: Do I need to act? What can be done? Is it feasible? Which option is best? Am I capable of carrying it out? What are the costs and benefits of each option? Is it better not to act? What might be the consequences of acting or not acting? When should I act? Decisions about coping actions are not usually etched in stone. They must often be changed in accordance with the flow of events, although they may be unchangeable once matters go beyond a given point. I shall address coping after concluding the discussion of appraisal.

The qualifying adjective, secondary, does not connote a process of less importance than primary, but it suggests only that primary appraising is a judgment about whether what is happening is worthy of attention and, perhaps, mobilization. Primary appraising never operates independently of secondary appraising, which is needed to attain an understanding of one's total plight. In effect, there is always an active interplay of both. The distinctly different contents of each type of appraisal justify treating them separately, but each should be

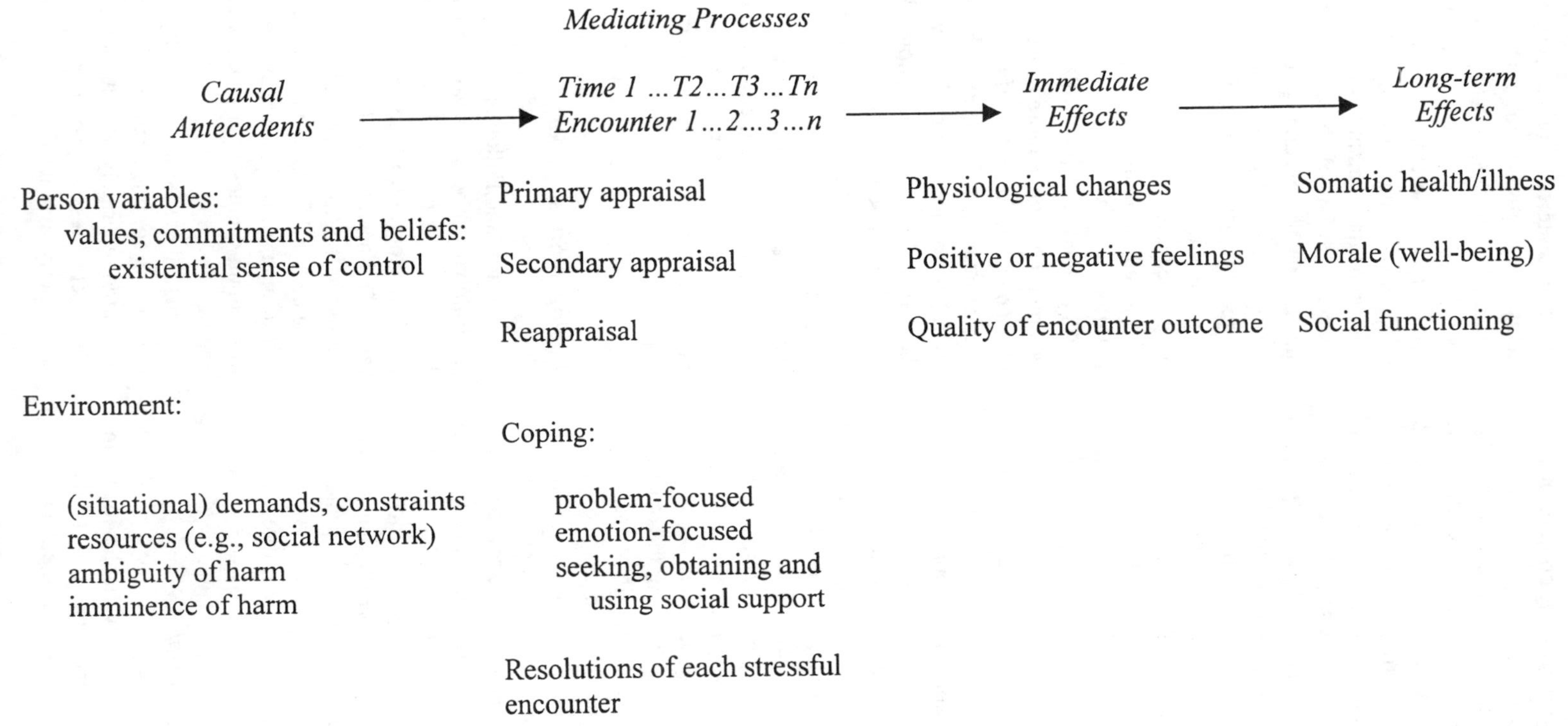

Mediating Processes

Causal Antecedents → *Time 1 ...T2...T3...Tn Encounter 1 ...2...3....n* → *Immediate Effects* → *Long-term Effects*

Person variables:
values, commitments and beliefs:
existential sense of control

Environment:

(situational) demands, constraints
resources (e.g., social network)
ambiguity of harm
imminence of harm

Primary appraisal
Secondary appraisal

Reappraisal

Coping:

    problem-focused
    emotion-focused
    seeking, obtaining and
      using social support

Resolutions of each stressful
    encounter

Physiological changes

Positive or negative feelings

Quality of encounter outcome

Somatic health/illness

Morale (well-being)

Social functioning

Figure 9.1. A Systems Theoretical Schematization of Stress, Coping, and Adaptation (reproduced with permission from Lazarus & Folkman, 1984, p. 305)

201

regarded as integral meaning components of a more complex process.

The main appraisal variants of psychological stress are harm and loss, threat, or challenge (Lazarus, 1966, 1981; Lazarus & Launier, 1978). Harm and loss consists of damage that has already occurred. Threat consists of the possibility of such damage in the future. Challenge is similar to Selye's (1974) eustress in that people who feel challenged pit themselves enthusiastically against obstacles and feel expansive—even joyous—about the struggle that will ensue. Performers of all sorts, whether musicians, entertainers, actors, or public speakers, love the liberating effects of challenge and hate the constricting effects of threat.

These three types of stress reaction should be separated only for convenience of analysis. For example, harm appraisals, which concern the past, also have implications for the future. Therefore, they usually contain components of threat; challenge appraisals do too. Threat and challenge are mostly focused on the future, and we are usually in a state of uncertainty because we have no clear idea about what will actually happen.

Threat and challenge can occur in the same situation, although one or the other usually predominates. In some situations, we are more threatened than challenged, and in other situations the reverse may be true. Although threat appraisals may be subordinated to challenge in a particular situation, favorable personal resources capable of producing a desired outcome may reverse the balance between the two appraisals, which could quickly change in the face of shifting fortunes or the need to cope. Thus, threat and challenge are not immutable states of mind. As a result of appraising and reappraising, threat can be transformed into challenge and vice versa.

Antecedents of Appraisal

The two main sets of variables jointly influencing whether the appraisal is that of threat or challenge are environmental and per-sonality centered. Some environmental circumstances impose too great a demand on a person's resources, whereas others provide considerable latitude for available skills and persistence, thereby influencing whether threat or challenge will occur. The substantive environmental content variables having an influence consist of diverse situational demands, constraints, and opportunities. Formal environmental variables consist of situational dimensions, such as novelty versus familiarity, predictability versus unpredictability, clarity of meaning versus ambiguity, and temporal factors such as imminence, timing, and duration.

Personality dispositions influencing whether a person is more prone to threat or to challenge include self-confidence or self-efficacy (Bandura, 1977, 1989, 1997). The more confident we are of our capacity to overcome dangers and obstacles, the more likely we are to be challenged rather than threatened; a sense of inadequacy, however, promotes threat. Nevertheless, and consistent with a relational analysis of stress, in any transaction both the environmental circumstances and the personality dispositions combine in determining whether there will be a threat or challenge appraisal.

Coping in Stress Theory

Lazarus and Folkman (1984, p. 141) offer the following process view of coping: "We define coping as constantly changing cognitive and behavioral efforts to manage specific external and/or internal demands that are appraised as taxing or exceeding the resources of the person." Simply stated, coping is the effort to manage psychological stress. I present three main themes of a process approach to coping.

First, there is no universally effective or ineffective coping strategy. Coping must be measured separately from its outcomes so that the effectiveness of each coping strategy can be properly evaluated. Efficacy depends on the type of person, the type of threat, the stage of the stressful encounter, and the outcome modality—that is, subjective well-being, social functioning, or somatic health. Because the focus is on flux or change over time and diverse life conditions, a process formulation is also inherently contextual.

Thus, denial, which was once thought to be harmful and signify pathology, can be quite beneficial in certain circumstances but harmful in others. I illustrate this using diseases of several kinds, which are especially stressful when life threatening or handicapping. (See Maes, Leventhal, and de Ridder, 1996, for a recent review of research on coping with chronic diseases.)

In a heart attack, denial is dangerous if it occurs while the person is deciding whether or not to seek medical help. This is a period in the attack in which the person is most vulnerable, and delay in treatment as a result of denial can be deadly. Denial is useful during hospitalization, however, because it is an antidote to so-called cardiac neuroses, a syndrome in which the patient is inordinately fearful of dying suddenly. This fear prevents the patient from engaging in activity that would facilitate recovery. Denial again becomes dangerous when the patient returns home and must reestablish normal life activities. The danger at this clinical stage is that denial will lead the patient to take on too much, including stressful work and too much recreational pressure, which may have contributed to the cardiovascular disease in the first place.

There is also much research (Lazarus, 1983) suggesting that denial is useful in elective surgery (Cohen & Lazarus, 1973) but counterproductive in other diseases such as asthma, in which being vigilant has value (Staudenmeyer et al., 1979). Hospitals infantalize patients, so vigilance is not very useful, whereas denial is just what the doctor ordered: "Depend on me or my nurses and you will be fine." The danger in asthma is that a person who begins to experience an asthmatic attack must be vigilant enough to take medication or seek medical help. Denial defeats any effort to ward off the attack, so deniers often wind up in a hospitalized asthmatic crisis compared with more vigilant asthmatics.

All this suggests that we need to understand when denial, and other forms of coping, are beneficial or harmful. The explanatory principle I favor is that, when nothing can be done to alter the condition or prevent further harm, denial can be beneficial. When denial or any other defense or illusion prevents necessary adaptive action, however, it will be harmful (Lazarus, 1983, 1985).

Consider another illness, prostate cancer, which is very common in older men. The idea that one has a dangerous cancer provides an ever-present stressful background of life and death concerns, which potentiate many specific threats. For example, there is the threat posed by having to make a decision about how to treat the disease—especially in light of the conflicting judgments about what to do by physicians.

Another threat concerns the periodic need after surgery to determine whether cancer cells are still present or have spread to other organs. After surgery, there may be a period of low anxiety until the patient is again examined for medical evidence about the current status of the cancer. This period of low anxiety is the result of having survived surgery and, perhaps, good news from the pathology report. It could also be the result of coping by avoidance or distancing since all the patient can really do at this stage is wait, and vigilance and high anxiety would serve no useful purpose at such a time. As the time for the diagnostic examination nears, however, avoidance or distancing are no longer likely to be effective, and anxiety will increase. If there is evidence of a recurrence or spread of the cancer, the patient is forced to cope in new ways to deal with the changed set of life-threatening options. Life now may depend on radiation treatment.

Another threat is uncertainty about what to tell others, such as acquaintances, friends, and loved ones, about one's situation. Avoidance and silence are frequent coping strategies. A contrasting strategy is to tell everyone, or selected persons, such as acquaintances, friends, and loved ones, the truth about what is happening in an effort to gain social support and to be honest and open. Collective coping in the United States has for a long time involved the maintenance of silence about a disease that, like breast cancer, was considered a social embarrassment. The result was that few men and their loved ones knew much about the disease, and most were ill prepared to deal with it. This secrecy is rapidly diminishing, with the useful result that increasingly more men and their loved ones now have the necessary understanding, which enables them to deal more effectively with the serious threats that the disease imposes.

The threats previously mentioned, and the coping processes they generate, apply to any potentially fatal or disabling disease. Consider the following examples, which involve two other diseases. In the first, an unmarried, 35-year-old woman with multiple sclerosis must decide whether or not to announce to the men she is dating that she has a progressive, debilitating ailment. Not to do so would be unfair to them, but being open about it might chase them away. Also, in the case of breast cancer, men with whom a woman might be intimate might, without forewarning, discover with distress that the woman has lost one or both breasts. What is the woman's best coping strategy? Should she tell them in advance? How should this be evaluated? These are difficult questions for patients who must face these decisions and for coping researchers.

It is not valid to assume that the way an individual copes with one threat will be the same as that chosen for a different threat. The evidence, in fact, indicates otherwise. A key principle is that the choice of coping strategy will usually vary with the adaptational significance and requirements of each threat and its status as a disease, which will change over time.

Let me assure you that what I am saying about coping with a health crisis, such as cancer, is not solely a dispassionate intellectual analysis. I have an intimate personal knowledge about it, having recently been a patient with prostate cancer. The disease was discovered more than 4 years ago, and I had to decide what to do about it. I had major surgery and am now fine, free of this cancer I hope permanently.

The second theme is that to study the coping process requires that we describe in detail what the person is thinking and doing at each stage with each specific threat. In the late 1970s and 1980s, I, as well as many others in the United States and Europe, developed measurement scales and research designs for this purpose (Folkman & Lazarus, 1988a).

Research on the coping process requires an intraindividual research design, nested within interindividual comparisons in which the same individuals are studied in different contexts and at different times. Many individuals must be compared to avoid dependence on a single case. This is the only way to observe change and stability in what is happening within any individual across conditions and over time. The best generic research design for this kind of research is longitudinal.

The following is the third theme of a process approach to coping: There are at least two major functions of coping, which I refer to as problem focused and emotion focused. With respect to the problem-focused function, a person obtains information on which to act and mobilizes actions for the purpose of changing the reality of the troubled person-environment relationship. The coping actions may be directed at either the self or the environment. To illustrate using my own health crisis, when I sought the opinions of different medical specialists about what treatment to select, and which surgeon was the best available, I was engaging in what seems to be problem-focused coping.

The emotion-focused function is aimed at regulating the emotions tied to the stress situation—for example, by avoiding thinking about the threat or reappraising it without changing the realities of the stressful situation. To again illustrate, I first approached my prostate problem vigilantly rather than with avoidance. After the decision had been made to have surgery, however, because there was nothing further I could do I made an effort to distance myself from the potential dangers that lay ahead. I also reassured myself that I had chosen the right course and secured the best surgeon available. These efforts constitute a pattern of emotion-focused coping.

When we reappraise a threat, we are altering our emotions by constructing a new relational meaning of the stressful encounter. Although at first I was very anxious at the discovery of the disease (my father died of it), I reassured myself that all the medical tests pointed to a cancer that was localized within the prostate gland and had not yet spread, so I was a good candidate for surgery. I was convinced—or more accurately, I tried to convince myself—that my surgeon was one of the best in the area, and that much more was now known about the surgical procedure than in the past so that my chances were very good. Also, as I mentioned previously, I distanced myself from threats I could not do anything about, so the initial anxiety was lessened.

Reappraisal is an extremely effective way to cope with a stressful situation. It is often difficult, however, to distinguish it from an ego defense, such as denial. When the personal meaning of what is happening fits the evidence, it is not an ego defense but rather one of the most durable and powerful ways of controlling destructive emotions.

An example of reappraisal that serves as a form of coping and involves important interpersonal relationships can be seen in efforts to manage the emotion of anger. If one's spouse or lover has managed to offend by what he or she has said and done, instead of retaliating to repair one's wounded self-esteem, one might be able to recognize that, being under great stress, the spouse or lover could not realistically be held responsible; in effect, he or she was not in control of himself or herself, and it would be advantageous to assume that the basic intention was not malevolent.

This reappraisal of another's intentions makes it possible to empathize with the loved one's plight and excuse the outburst. This should defuse or prevent the anger that would ordinarily have been felt in response to the assault. Also, it is hoped that the other person would do the same if one behaves badly under pressure. To construct a benign reappraisal is easier said than done. This example, however, illustrates the power of this form of cognitive coping to lessen or turn negative emotions into positive ones by changing the relational meaning of the encounter.

At the risk of adding further complications, I offer an important qualification to what I have just said about the two most important coping functions. The way I have spoken about them invites certain errors, or bad habits of thought, about the distinction between problem-focused and emotion-focused coping. This distinction, which has been widely endorsed in the field of coping measurement and research, leads to their treatment as distinctive coping action types, which is an oversimple and too literal conception of how coping works.

One error is that when we allow ourselves to slip into the language of action types, we often end up speaking as if it is easy to decide which thought or action belongs in the problem-focused or emotion-focused category. On the surface, some coping factors, such as confrontive coping and planful problem solving, seem to represent the problem-focused function, whereas others, such as distancing, escape avoidance, and positive reappraisal, seem to represent emotion-focused coping.

This way of thinking is too simple, however. For example, if a person takes a Valium before an exam because of distressing and disabling test anxiety, we could be convinced that this act serves both functions, not just one. Although the emotion and its physiological sequelae, such as excessive arousal, dry mouth, trembling, and intrusive thoughts about failing, can be reduced by the drug, performance is also likely to improve because these symptoms will now interfere less with the performance. We should have learned by now that the same act may have more than one function and usually does.

A second error is that we contrast the two functions, and even try to determine which is more useful. In a culture centered on control over the environment, it is easy to come to the erroneous conclusion, which is common in the research literature, that problem-focused coping is always or usually a more useful strategy. There is evidence, however, that in certain circumstances problem-focused coping can be detrimental to health and well-being (Collins, Baum, & Singer, 1983). In the study by Collins et al., people who continued to struggle to change conditions that could not be changed, thus relying rigidly on problem-focused coping, were far more troubled over the long haul than those who accepted the reality and relied more on emotion-focused coping.

Although it is legitimate to ask which coping strategies produce the best adaptational outcomes under different sets of conditions, this way of thinking fails to recognize that in virtually all stressful encounters the person draws on both functions. In nature, the two functions of coping are never separated. Both are essential parts of the total coping effort, and ideally each facilitates the other.

It is the fit between thinking, wanting, emotion, action, and the environmental realities that determines whether coping is efficacious or not. However seductive it is to think of the two functions as separate and distinct, coping should never be thought of in either-or terms but as a complex of thoughts and actions aimed at improving the troubled relationship with the environment—in other words, a process of seeking the most serviceable meaning available in the situation, one that supports realistic actions while also viewing the situation in the most favorable way possible.

➣ TRANSITIONAL VIEWS

What I refer to as transitional views grew gradually out of my analysis of stress and coping, and these do not represent positions that, strictly speaking, I have reached very recently. These positions deal with two awkward and unresolved conceptual and methodological issues about the difference between appraising and coping and how appraisal works. My thoughts about them, which I discuss in the following sections, span the period between the 1980s and the mid-1990s and reflect my efforts to think through problems of appraisal theory.

Confusions About Appraising and Coping

Conceptually, appraising and coping go hand in hand and overlap, which results in uncertainty about whether, in any given instance, a stress-related thought or action is an appraisal, a coping process, or both. The uncertainty stems from the fact that cognitive coping (like an ego defense) is basically a reappraisal, which is difficult to distinguish from the original appraisal except for its history. The answer about which process is taking place—secondary appraisal or coping—must always be based on a full exploration of what is going on in the mind of a particular individual and the context in which the person-environment transaction occurs. My solution is to say an appraisal is the result of a coping process when it constitutes a motivated search for information and the constructed meanings on which to act under stress.

When thinking of appraisal decisions, it is important to recognize that the traditional appraisal questions I listed previously have been posed in very general terms, and additional details about the transaction are usually required to make a decision about what to do (Janis & Mann, 1977). Because conditions vary greatly with respect to a harm or loss, threat, challenge, and benefit, to make decisions and take action we need to ask more detailed questions. In effect, these broad types of stress reactions must be narrowed to much more specific ones.

For example, on the negative affective side, the harm or loss might be bereavement, a rejection, or a minor or serious slight; the

threat may be a life-threatening or terminal illness; and challenge could arise from an uncertain job opportunity. On the positive affective
side, the relevant decisions and actions might
have to do with an achievement, reward, or
honor that justifies, for example, joy or pride.

Even these more narrowly defined damaging, threatening, challenging, and beneficial subconditions might have to be broken
down further to identify the requirements for
making coping decisions. For example, it is
likely that different versions of bereavement,
such as how the person died or the quality of
the relationship before the death, influence the
emotional state to be experienced and what
can or must be done to cope effectively. Also,
if the source of pride could be seen by an important other as a competitive putdown, one
might decide to soft-pedal it to preserve the
interpersonal relationship. Just as individuals
take these small but significant details into account in their own coping efforts, the scientific study of appraising and coping, and clinical efforts to help people cope more
effectively, must consider them in the search
for workable principles.

How Appraisals Are Constructed

The issue of how appraisal works is important if we are to make a thorough examination of the validity and utility of appraisal theory. Magda Arnold (1960) viewed appraising
as instantaneous rather than deliberate. She
wrote,

> The appraisal that arouses an emotion is not
> abstract; it is not the result of reflection. It is
> immediate and undeliberate. If we see
> somebody stab at our eye with his finger,
> we avoid the threat instantly, even though
> we may know that he does not intend to hurt
> or even to touch us. Before we can make
> such an instant response, we must have esti-
> mated somehow that the stabbing finger
> could hurt. Since the movement is immedi-
> ate, unwitting, or even contrary to our better
> knowledge, this appraisal of possible harm
> must be similarly immediate. (p. 172)

Originally (Lazarus, 1966), I thought that
Arnold had underemphasized the complexity
of evaluative judgments that are often called
for in garden-variety stress emotions, and I
still do. I am now more impressed with the in-
stantaneity of much appraising, however, even
in complex and abstract cases. Appraisals are
usually dependent on many subtle cues in the
environment, previous experience, and a host
of personality variables, such as goals, situational intentions, personal resources, and lia-
bilities.

All these sources of input, and probably
additional ones, are involved in the decision
about how to evaluate adaptational demands,
constraints, and opportunities and how to
cope, which makes the speed of many or most
appraisals seem quite remarkable. Little is
known about how the process works. I am inclined to believe the necessary information is
often at the tips of our fingers, operating as
tacit knowledge (Polanyi, 1966) about ourselves and our environment (see Merleau-
Ponty, 1962, for the concept of embodied
thought). Therefore, scanning inputs in an
analogy to a digital computer is probably not
the way appraisal actually works.

When Arnold (1960) wrote her monograph, psychology was just beginning to think
in terms of stepwise information processing.
This is one reason why my own treatment of
appraising was considerably more abstract
than Arnold's and also more conscious and
deliberate. Despite the redundancy of the expression, I used the term "cognitive appraisal"
to emphasize the complex, judgmental, and
conscious process that must often be involved
in appraising (Lazarus, 1966).

There is considerable agreement about
the two main ways in which an appraisal
might be made. First, the process of appraising can be deliberate and largely conscious.
Second, it can be intuitive, automatic, and unconscious. Under some conditions, a slow, deliberate search for information is required on
which to predicate a judgment about what is at
stake and what should be done to cope with
the situation. At other times, a very rapid appraisal is more adaptive.

Most of the scenarios resulting in an emotion are recurrences of basic human dilemmas of living, including triumph, attainment of a goal, loss, disappointment, uncertain threat, violating a moral stricture, and being insulted or subtly demeaned. Most of us, especially if we have lived long enough, have already experienced these more than once, an example of the wisdom of the ages (Lazarus, 1991). A recurrence can never be identical in detail, but its personal significance can remain the same.

I have referred to this latter principle as the short-circuiting of threat (Lazarus & Alfert, 1964; Lazarus & Launier, 1978; Opton, Rankin, Nomikos, & Lazarus, 1965). The metaphor is the electrical short circuit in which the original route to the end of the wire is shortened by something that cuts the circuit at a much earlier point. At the psychological level, in contrast to having always to deliberate and learn anew about the import of threatening events, which would be a very inefficient way of monitoring our relationships with the environment, we are enabled to respond quickly and automatically to an adaptational crisis, even without awareness of the process, as a result of what we have already learned.

There is widespread acceptance of the idea that many of our appraisals are the result of unconscious processes. One of the most remarkable changes in outlook that has taken place since the 1950s is the attitude of psychologists toward unconscious processes. In earlier times, psychology was mostly nihilistic about the ability of the science to deal with the unconscious mind (Eriksen, 1960, 1962). The question at that time mainly concerned whether an appraisal can be unconscious rather than about the dynamics of unconscious psychological processes.

In addition to their influence on social actions, present-day thinking asks about how unconscious processes work—for example, whether they are smart or dumb. This is an allusion to the primitive and wishful thinking that Freud suggested characterizes unconscious (id) processes. This issue, among others, is still being debated (see a special section of *American Psychologist* edited by Loftus, 1992, that included brief articles by Bruner; Erdelyi; Greenwald; Jacoby, Lindsay, & Toth; Kihlstrom, Barnhardt, & Tataryn; Lewicki, Hill, & Czyzewska; Loftus & Klinger; and Merikle).

The 1980s and 1990s produced an explosion of interest in the unconscious (Lazarus & commentators, 1995). This interest and research centers mainly on what might be called the cognitive unconscious— that is, what we fail to attend to and how unconscious processes influence our thoughts, feelings, and actions. Articles and books by Bargh (1990), Bowers (1987), Brewin (1989), Brody (1987), Buck (1985), Epstein (1990), Kihlstrom (1987, 1990), LeDoux (1989), Leventhal (1984), Shepard (1984), Uleman and Bargh (1989), and others attest to this interest.

Another kind of unconsciousness, which is the result of ego-defense processes, is usually referred to as the dynamic unconscious (Erdelyi, 1985). It receives far less attention compared to the cognitive unconscious, especially in nonclinical circles. Unconscious appraising based on casual inattentiveness should be distinguished from defensive reappraisal, which involves motivated self-deception (Lazarus, 1991; Lazarus & commentators, 1995; Lazarus & Folkman, 1984).

Does an unconscious appraisal based on ego defense differ from appraisals that are based on inattention? The answer to this question is not known for sure, but the main theoretical difference is that, compared with the dynamic unconscious, the contents of the cognitive unconscious should be relatively easy to make conscious by drawing attention to the conditions under which they have occurred. Making the dynamic unconscious conscious, however, is another matter. Because, presumably, the person does not wish to confront threatening thoughts, especially those related to socially proscribed goals, their exclusion from consciousness must be intentional—that is, they are a means of coping with threat. In such a case, awareness would defeat the function of the defensive maneuver.

Mental contents that result from ego defense pose another serious problem. They distort what a person can tell us about the relational meaning of an encounter with the environment. This makes the task of assessing how the person is appraising the encounter very difficult because what is reported about the inner mental life cannot be accepted at face value. It is difficult to identify the truth, but the solution need not be completely refractory. Skilled clinicians, and even laypersons, are often able to make reasonable and, it is hoped, accurate inferences about defenses and what is being concealed by them. They draw on observed contradictions of three kinds to alert themselves to defensive distortions in self-reported appraisals (Lazarus & commentators, 1995).

One such contradiction is between what a person says at one moment and what he or she says at another moment. A second is the contrast between what is said and contrary behavioral and physiological evidence—for example, voice quality and gestures that give evidence of discomfort, physical flushing or paling, and willful acts that belie what is being said. A third contradiction is between what is said and the normative response to the same provocative situation. If most people would be angered or made fearful in the same situation, we can use this knowledge clinically to second-guess the person who denies one or another of these emotions. We need to be wary of this strategy, however, because in many cases individuals have different motives and perspectives on the events of interest, so we could be wrong in any particular instance. A comparable strategy in research is the use of multiple levels of observation, such as self-reports, actions, and bodily changes.

The problem with depending on contradictions among different response measures to second-guess the truth is that we do not know the natural correlation among these measures. Because each has somewhat different causal antecedents—physiological measures being captive of energy mobilization; verbal reports depending on knowledge, willingness, and ability to expose the truth; and

actions being influenced by social opportunities and constraints—the correlations among the measures are usually low, even when intraindividual analysis is employed. Thus, response discrepancies are a somewhat unreliable source of evidence about defense.

This correlation problem should also indicate why no single response measure, such as facial expressions or physiological arousal, can be regarded as criterial about a person's inner emotional state. There is a need for evidence to confirm one or another interpretation when we observe a discrepancy as well as basic research on how response measures are correlated under diverse conditions, which has not been undertaken programmatically.

In my judgment, introspective or self-report data about subjective experience tend to be viewed too negatively by psychologically oriented scientists. Under certain conditions, this kind of data can certainly be seriously flawed as a source of information about personal meanings. The negative general opinion about the validity of such data, however, is not fully justified for two reasons. First, little or no effort is usually made to maximize accuracy and minimize the sources of error. Second, problems of validity and how to interpret what is observed are no less daunting for behavioral and psychophysiological data compared with introspection. Despite the claim that they are more objective response measures than self-report, both have their own validity problems, which must be taken just as seriously as those involved in self-report. There is no simple, guaranteed route to the truth of what is in our minds—only fragmentary clues that we must investigate carefully through hard work.

Casually constructed questionnaires, such as those used in survey research, are particularly vulnerable to error when we want to examine accurately and in-depth what people want, think, and feel and the contexts in which they do so. This has led me to propose that in-depth studies of individuals over time and across circumstances, which is an adaptation of the clinical method, must be employed in the study of appraisal and coping in the emotions (Lazarus & commentators, 1990, 1995).

➤ PRESENT THEMES

The analysis of appraising in the context of stress and coping can be readily applied to the emotions by making some modifications (Lazarus, 1966, 1968, 1981, 1999; Lazarus, Averill, & Opton, 1970). Also, as noted previously, the concepts of stress and emotion need to be conjoined, with emotion being the more inclusive concept. To understand positively toned emotional states, the analysis must be expanded from a focus solely on harm, threat, and challenge to a focus on a variety of benefits—each associated with its own emotion. Each of the negatively toned emotions also has its own special pattern of appraisal and relational meaning.

As in the case of stress, emotions are tied jointly or interactively to social and physical conditions of importance and person variables, such as goals, goal hierarchies, personal values, belief systems, and personal resources. What changes as we shift our attention from stress to the emotions are the primary and secondary appraisal judgments and relational meanings that must be added to accommodate each of the emotions we wish to understand.

In this section, which covers the 1990s, I discuss my cognitive-motivational-relational theory of the emotions (Lazarus, 1991), focusing especially on the distinctive features of the approach. Most of the ideas expressed here are more recent than those previously discussed, although they are not inconsistent with the earlier positions I took when my main focus was stress and coping. I refer to this theory as cognitive-motivational-relational because motivation and cognition and the meanings constructed about the person-environment relationship are conjoined in the emotion process and serve as crucial concepts.

Despite some important differences in detail, there is remarkable agreement among theorists about what a person is supposed to think to react with many of the diverse emotions. In the 1980s and 1990s, many emotion theorists with a cognitive-mediational perspective sought to analyze what a person must want and think to feel one or another of the various emotions. In addition to my own work, some of the most active and visible theorists and researchers include Conway and Bekerian (1987), Dalkvist and Rollenhagen (1989), de Rivera (1977), de Sousa (1987), Frijda (1986), Oatley and Johnson-Laird (1987), Ortony, Clore, and Collins (1988), Reisenzein (1995), Roseman (1984), Scherer (1984), Smith and Ellsworth (1985), Solomon (1976), and Weiner (1985, 1986).

The main appraisal variables common to cognitive-mediational theories include having a goal at stake, whether the goal is facilitated or thwarted, and locus of control or responsibility for what happened, typically referred to as accountability, legitimacy, and controllability. Pleasantness is also viewed by some as an appraisal variable, but I consider it to be a response to, rather than an antecedent of, appraisal. Figure 9.2 provides an updated schematization of the psychosocial system of the discrete emotions, with stress integrated within it, which is discussed in Lazarus (1999). The reader might want to compare it with the earlier schematization, emphasizing stress from Lazarus and Folkman (1994).

Distinctive Features of My Theoretical Approach

Despite substantial agreement, my current view of appraisal processes differs from other theoretical positions in at least six main ways: (a) I point to a motivational basis of the choice of a discrete emotion—that is, its quality in addition to its intensity; (b) I treat appraisals as hot rather than cold cognitions; (c) more than most others, I emphasize coping as an integral feature of the emotion process; (d) I assume that emotions have an implacable logic and reject the widespread penchant for thinking of emotions as irrational; (e) I be-

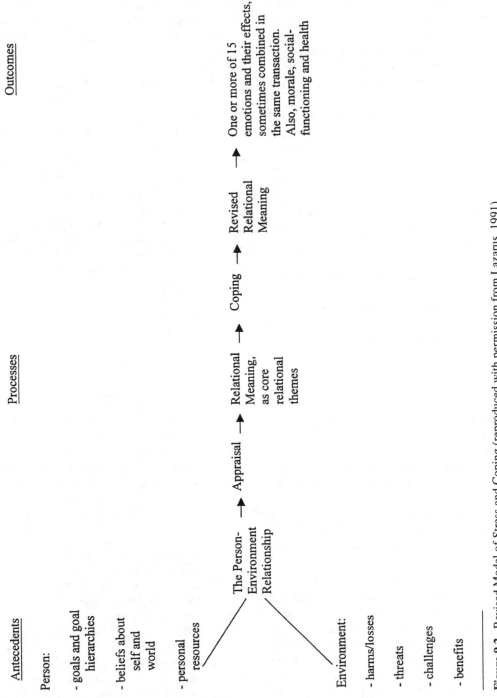

Figure 9.2. Revised Model of Stress and Coping (reproduced with permission from Lazarus, 1991)

lieve that the division of emotions into positive and negative can be misleading—positively toned and negatively toned emotional states are interdependent; and (f) perhaps most important, I treat relational meanings as core relational themes that are derived from the process of appraising. In effect, I view appraisal in holistic terms as a synthesis, in contrast with the dominant reductive science outlook seeking to separate causes of phenomena, each of which constitutes only a part of the whole.

The differences between my views and those of other appraisal theorists are reprised throughout the following sections. I also interweave my theoretical stance about the appraisals involved in each of the emotions, thereby outlining my theoretical approach along with discussions of the distinctions between my approach and other appraisal-based approaches.

The Motivational Basis of Emotion Quality

Few appraisal theorists advocate a major role for diverse personal goals in shaping the quality of an emotion, although they all recognize the importance of the fate of antecedent goals in emotional intensity and the new goals that each emotion generates. I take the position that many ego involvements—that is, goal commitments focused on one's ego identity or self—influence the quality of an emotional experience. These ego involvements include self- or social esteem, moral values, ego ideals, important meanings and ideas, the well-being of other persons, and life goals.

For example, shame, pride, and anger are the result of the fate of our desire to preserve or enhance self- or social esteem; guilt is about moral issues; and anxiety, which is par excellence an existential emotion having to do with one's being in the world and personal fate (e.g., life and death), and so forth. Table 9.1 presents a list of ego involvements and some of the discrete emotions they help shape. For a developmental analysis of emergent goals in the shaping of the self-conscious emotions, namely, shame, guilt, embarrass-

ment, and pride, see Mascolo & Fischer, 1995.

One can see the role of goals in the emotions in the following analysis of the main appraisal components I propose for each emotion. For a fuller account, see Lazarus (1991). The following are the main appraisal components of the discrete emotions I tend to examine:

Primary appraising: The three primary appraisal components are goal relevance, goal congruence, and type of ego involvement.

Goal relevance is fundamental to whether an encounter is viewed by a person as relevant to well-being. In effect, there is no emotion without a goal at stake.

Goal congruence or incongruence refer to whether the conditions of an encounter facilitate or thwart what the person wants. If conditions are favorable, a positively toned emotion is likely to be aroused. If unfavorable, a negatively toned emotion follows.

Types of ego involvement. See Table 9.1.

Secondary appraising: As in the case of stress emotions, this has to do with options for coping with emotional encounters. Three basic judgments are involved: blame or credit for an outcome, coping potential, and future expectations. They complete the primary appraisal decisions leading to each of the positive and negative emotions.

Both blame and credit require a judgment about who or what is responsible for a harm, threat, challenge, or benefit. Two kinds of information influence this judgment. The first is that the outcome of the transaction is the result of an action that was under the control of the provocateur or perpetrator. If what occurred could not have been avoided, it is more difficult to attribute blame or credit. The second is the attribution of a malevolent or benign intention to the other person, which increases the odds of blame or credit being attributed.

Coping potential arises from the personal conviction that we can or cannot act successfully to ameliorate or eliminate a

TABLE 9.1 Types of Ego Involvement and the Emotions They Influence[a]

Ego Involvement		Emotions
Self- and social esteem	_____	Anger, pride
Moral values	_____	Guilt
Ego ideals	_____	Shame
Meanings and ideas	_____	Anxiety
Other persons and their well-being	_____	All emotions
Life goals	_____	All emotions

SOURCE: From Lazarus (1991).

a. Ego involvements refer to commitments, which might be thought of as goals that fall within the rubric of what we usually mean by ego identity.

harm or threat or bring to fruition a challenge or benefit.

Future expectations may be positive or negative—that is, the troubled person-environment relationship will change for better or worse.

Hot Versus Cold Cognitions

I consider appraisals as hot or emotional cognitions (Lazarus & Smith, 1988) and attributions as cold and abstract (Smith, Haynes, Lazarus, & Pope, 1993). The attributional dimensions explored by Weiner (1985, 1986), such as locus of causality, stability, controllability, intentionality, and globality, represent what I consider cold information rather than hot or emotional appraisals.

The important point for cognitive psychology is that information is not meaning. Meaning or, more precisely, relational meaning refers to the personal significance of information that is constructed by the person. Meaning or personal significance is what gives an appraisal its emotional quality. Thus, whereas locus of causality (or responsibility) is a factor in blaming someone, which depends on the situational context, responsibility is neutral or coolly distanced. Attributing blame or credit to someone rather than responsibility carries the immediate relational

heat, which of course is a metaphor for emotion.

Coping Is an Integral Feature of the Emotion Process

Coping is central to my approach to the emotions, just as it originally was for stress. Unfortunately, the importance of coping is often understated and sometimes ignored in appraisal theories of emotion. It is as if coping is conceived as having been brought about through an entirely separate process only after an emotion has occurred rather than, as I see it, being an integral part of the emotion-generating process. It also plays a role at the earliest possible moments of the emotion process. In other words, the cognitive and motivational underpinnings of coping—that is, secondary appraising of coping options—originate with the first recognition of one's trouble or good fortune. The resulting coping thoughts and actions serve as bridges between the relational meaning of the encounter and how the person acts and feels. In effect, appraisal unites coping with the emotion process.

We cannot properly understand an emotion without reference to coping thoughts and actions. If the transaction is appraised as posing a great danger—for example, the person believes he or she could not safely cope with retaliation for attack on another—anxiety or fright is a more likely emotional reaction than anger, or the aroused anger will be suffused with anxiety. In effect, coping prospects and coping consequences have a strong influence on which emotion will be experienced; they serve as mediators of subsequent emotions (Folkman & Lazarus, 1988a, 1988b).

The Implacable Logic of Emotion: Rationality and Irrationality

People in Western society, including many of its scholars, regard emotions as irrational. Typically, we think of emotions as a form of craziness and believe they do not follow logical rules. We constantly pit emotion against reason, as if they are inevitably in opposition. Our culture says that it was emotions that made us act foolishly and that emotions make us abandon reason.

In writing about the public attitude toward the death penalty, columnist Anthony Lewis (1998), whom I respect and admire for his consistently thoughtful analyses of human fashions and foibles, nevertheless wrote the following sentence that epitomizes this tendency: "People want the death penalty, I am convinced, for emotional rather than rational reasons" (p. A15). I would change this sentence to say "for reasons that are not thoughtful or wise."

I acknowledge that sometimes emotions interfere with the thoughtful examination of an issue, but it is the quality of thought that should usually be blamed, not our emotions. Even when we suspect direct emotional interference, this does not allow us to predict the direction of the reasoning, as in the previous example about the death penalty. It is no more irrational to desire the death penalty than to rue the penalty, as many people do. Rather, it is the reasoning that Lewis should castigate, not the emotions involved in the issue. This is a very common type of reasoning error in today's media.

Another example appeared in a psychology best-seller, *Emotional Intelligence*, in which Daniel Goleman (1995), previously the science writer for the *New York Times*, speaks of two separate minds—one devoted to emotions and the other to reason. He states, "In a very real sense we have two minds, one that thinks and one that feels" (p. 8). He also says, "Our emotions have a mind of their own, one which can hold views quite independently of our rational mind" (p. 20). I am sure that this was written to appeal to the untutored layperson. It is bad science and misleading, however, especially as applied to what is known about the brain, which Goleman continuously refers to as the arbiter of our actions. It is the mind that is the arbiter; the brain is the organ that merely makes reason and emotion possible.

My argument is a hard sell in that it is difficult to shake off more than 2,000 years of Western habits of thought, with its roots in ancient Greece. Plato's views about cognition, motivation, and emotion were taken over in the Middle Ages by the Catholic Church, which emphasized the antithesis between reason and emotion and the need to regulate its parishioner's emotions and animal instincts by reason and an act of will. Despite the fact that such a struggle implies conflict between thought, motivation, and reason, this is no reason to perpetuate an outlook in which emotion is reified as always separate from reason. The position taken by Aristotle (1941) in the *Rhetoric,* which the Church and Western civilization largely ignored, is a wiser but less familiar view—namely, that although conflict can take place between these two agencies of mind, emotion depends on reason.

Integration Versus Disconnection in the Mind. A mentally healthy person may suffer from conflicts, but the mind is, in the main, integrated and its parts work in harmony if we are to function well. Otherwise, we could not engage in coordinated planning and make decisions about what we want and what is good for us. We have one mind, not three, and when this is not so we are dysfunctional or mentally ill. Only when we are at war with ourselves do thought, motivation, and emotion diverge importantly, but this dissociation is pathological rather than a healthy state of mind (Lazarus, 1989). Cognition, motivation, and emotion are parts of a larger, integrated subsystem (the mind), which in turn is embedded in even larger systems—for example, the family, social group, society, nation, or ecosystem.

To the extent that the emotion process is individualized—that is, dependent on a person's goals, beliefs, and personal resources—we would have no hope of understanding it without detailed knowledge of the person. Emotions would be unpredictable. Although it is correct to say that we employ reason to keep destructive emotions from getting out of control, the arousal of emotion depends on reason, as Aristotle maintained, although it might be bad reasoning. Our emotions follow clear, normative cognitive rules, as does their regulation, although the variables we need to consider depend on the individual being considered.

The key principle here is that emotions flow from the way we appraise what is happening in our lives. Despite the great appeal that blaming human folly on our emotions has had in much of Western thought, emotions follow an implacable logic, as long as we view them from the standpoint of an individual's premises about self and world, even when they are not realistic. It is this logic that we need to understand.

Economists think of rationality as making decisions that maximize self-interest in any transaction. One problem with this presumption is that to do so requires that we know what our self-interests are, and often we cannot say or are incorrect about these. Another problem is that economists venerate self-interest compared with other important human values, such as sharing our bounty with the community, sacrificing for our children, manifesting loyalty even when it could place us in jeopardy, and being concerned with fairness, justice, and compassion—in other words, the very values we call idealistic (often as a putdown), which should be hallmarks of a civilized society. Self-interest as a value can be greatly overdone, and it has consistently produced extensive worldwide mis-

ery along with great wealth for a limited segment of the population.

Of course, it is foolish to act constantly against one's best interests, although people often do so. In a fit of anger, for example, we attack powerful and threatening others or, worse, alienate those whom we love with angry and cutting assaults. It is also unwise and counterproductive not to appraise danger when it is present or to appraise it when it is not present, although people often do both. This is not so much because we think illogically but because we have appraised events in a particular way, based perhaps on unwise or inaccurate assumptions and goals. Inappropriate assumptions result in emotions that present a poor fit with the realities of the situation being faced. It is reason, which depends on the confluence of our ancestral and ontogenetic past and present realities, that has failed us and not our emotions. The main occasions in which emotions get in the way of reason are when they distract or misdirect our attention.

Emotions reflect the fate of our goal striving. We have many goals, however, not just one, and actions seeking attainment of one goal often end up, perforce, defeating other goals. This is what it means to speak of conflict, which adds greatly to emotional distress because it complicates finding a maximally desirable solution. If we are convinced people are out to harm us, it is reasonable to feel frightened or angry. Diagnosing this as paranoia—that is, as delusions of persecution or grandeur—does not help us understand these feelings but rather the lack of realism in our thoughts and feelings. It is necessary to identify the operating assumptions that the paranoid person is making about self and world, and the reasons, to understand the fear and anger; in other words, the delusions must be examined from the individual's personal perspective.

We all live by making many foolish assumptions about the world, which program us to experience inappropriate emotions in our daily lives. We do this for many reasons, which I will discuss later. Once it is clear that we have made the wrong assumption, our feelings can readily be explained because they follow from what we have assumed, however erroneous that assumption might be. There is a sensible logic to the emotions that flows from the erroneous premise, and this logic provides an opportunity to understand and even predict emotions. Calling them irrational or an indication of mental illness merely denigrates someone else's reasoning without helping us understand the assumptive basis on which it rests and how it came into being.

Main Causes of Poor Reasoning. My wife Bernice and I (Lazarus & Lazarus, 1994) noted five common causes of erroneous judgments that influence our emotions. The first consists of physical ailments, such as damage to the brain, mental retardation, and psychosis. Such persons are unable to think normally, so their emotions are likely to have inadequate foundations. Pointing to these ailments is not enough to understand why they think and feel as they do. Despite their ailments, we need to identify the beliefs, motives, and thoughts about the life situation to which they are displaying inappropriate emotions. For example, why do they feel anger rather than anxiety or shame? Suggesting merely that there is brain damage does not provide the answer; one needs to understand the individual's psychosocial dynamics and perhaps developmental history.

The second cause of judgmental error is a lack of knowledge about the situation in which we have a stake. With an opaqueness similar to the distortion that results from ego defense, ignorance can distort our relationship with the environment, leading to actions and emotions that make sense only from the standpoint of what we think to be true.

For example, knowing nothing about microorganisms as causes of disease, physicians in the 19th century carried germs from cadavers they had recently dissected to the wombs of women delivering babies, thereby spreading a deadly disease called childbed fever. It was ignorance, not emotion or irrationality, that led them to engage in actions that today

we would abhor from the standpoint of our improved knowledge. Ironically, physicians today, who tend to blame germs that have become resistant to antibiotics instead of thinking preventively, still spread infection in modern hospitals by failing to wash their hands often enough. Also, antibiotics are still being overprescribed, thereby adding to the problem.

The third cause of inappropriate emotion and action is that we have not paid attention to the correct aspects in our social relationships. In most social relationships, there is too much to take into account, and we must decide what is useful and important and what is not. Often, we make a bad guess. Our attention can also be intentionally misdirected. For example, magicians create their magic by misdirecting the audience's attention. Also, we may judge that the other person is lying on the basis of faulty assumptions about how to tell (Ekman, 1985/1992), and we put our trust in people who are skillfully concealing their real motives and exhibiting false ones.

Fourth, when we are dealing with a personal crisis, such as a life-threatening disease, we may be unable to face the truth so we cope using ego defenses, such as denial. We should feel threatened and anxious and act accordingly, but because of our need to believe otherwise we sell ourselves on the idea that we are well or that the illness is temporary and minor and we will get better. This kind of self-deception is not always harmful because when we are not able to change the situation there may be nothing better to think and do about our plight than what is needed to preserve our morale. Defenses can be dangerous, however, when they prevent us from doing what is necessary to save our lives or well-being (Lazarus, 1983).

Fifth, when we make errors in judgment, it is often the result of ambiguity about what is going on. Our social relationships are filled with uncertainty about what other people are thinking, wanting, intending, and feeling, and it is easy to make the wrong guess. We see malevolence where it does not exist or good intentions where there is venality or evil, so we react with an inappropriate emotion. The cause lies in faulty reasoning and not emotion, which merely reflects that reasoning.

In summary, the theory of appraising and appraisal provides a set of propositions about what one must think to feel a given emotion. This is the implacable logic of which I previously spoke. If the theory is sound, we should to some degree be able to tell what a person has been thinking, assuming we know what that person is feeling. Also, we should be modestly able to predict the emotional reaction if we know beforehand what is thought by the person about the encounter or the life situation. This principle gives us considerable power over our emotions because it states the cognitive principles that lie behind each emotion. Knowledge, when it is sound, is power; when it is unsound, it results in foolishness, not only in actions but also in the emotions we experience.

The Interdependence of the Emotions

It is common in the psychology of emotion to distinguish sharply between negative and positively toned emotions and to treat them as if they were opposites. I consider this trend to be unfortunate. Dividing emotions into two types, negative and positive, distorts their individual substantive qualities and the complex meanings inherent in each discrete emotion.

Occasionally, even positively toned emotions involve harms and threats and sometimes originate in negative life conditions. For example, relief occurs when we are dealing with a threat that has abated or disappeared. Hope commonly occurs in a situation in which we are threatened but hope for the best. Consider, for example, what happens when we are awaiting a biopsy for a suspected cancer or when we fear we will do poorly on an exam or interview for an important job. In both instances, we hope our fear has been misguided.

The same reasoning also applies to happiness and pride. For example, although happy about something, we may fear that the favor-able conditions provoking our happiness will soon end, so we engage in anticipatory coping to prevent this from happening. We may also fear that when conditions of life are favorable, others will resent our good fortune and try to undermine our well-being. In addition, when pride is viewed by another as the result of having taken too much credit for our success or that of our child or student protegé, or when our pride is viewed by others as a competitive putdown, we may be wise to keep it to ourselves. Biblical language expresses this in the aphorisms "pride goeth before a fall" and "overweening pride."

Love is commonly viewed as a positive emotional experience, but it can be very negative when unrequited or when we have reason to believe our lover is losing interest. When gratitude violates our beliefs and values, the social necessity of displaying it even when it is grudging can be quite negative. Finally, compassion is aversive when we fail to control our emotional reaction to the suffering of others. In effect, we should avoid the tendency to keep the emotions separate and inviolate when, in reality, they are interdependent.

This theme emphasizes the close relationships among emotions and not just their separateness. This is often not recognized in appraisal-centered theoretical approaches because these theorists are mainly concerned with distinguishing the cognitive-motivational-relational antecedents of each discrete emotion, which is a valid concern that should not blind us to their interdependence. It might be wiser not to study a single emotion by itself but rather to examine closely related clusters of emotion—that is, those emotions that are readily transformed into others by virtue of a change in the appraised relational meaning.

For example, pride and shame are closely related because they have cognate relational meanings; their meanings are opposite—that is, being credited with a socially valued outcome versus being slighted or demeaned. Furthermore, anger can also be a way of coping with shame, which is often an extremely distressing emotion because it requires accepting the blame for a serious failing that impugns one's character. In the context of shame, anger involves shifting the blame to another, which helps one feel more in command of oneself and one's relationships. The important point here is that a sudden change in what has been happening or self-generated reappraisal can transform one emotion into another. If we study the emotions separately, we will miss this interdependence.

The Core Relational Themes for Each Emotion

One of my major metatheoretical positions is that the standard examination of appraisal components is conducted at too elemental a level of analysis to be adequate for thorough understanding. In searching for psychological causes, we run the risk of losing the forest for the trees—that is, we ignore the phenomenon as it occurs in nature in favor of its component parts (Lazarus, 1998a, 1998b).

Most appraisal theories are good at distinguishing the separate components of meaning on which the emotion rests, but they do not address how they are organized into the basic relational meaning for each emotion, as in the six primary and secondary appraisals I noted earlier. The partial meanings must be combined to produce the final, integrated gestalt, which characterizes emotional phenomena in nature and defines their overall meanings. In other words, the process of appraising must be examined at a higher level of abstraction, to which I refer as the core relational theme for each emotion. This theme is a terse synthesis of the separate appraisal components into a complex meaning-centered whole. It is one of the features that make my appraisal theory distinctive.

There is no contradiction between the two levels of abstraction—namely, the separate appraisal components and the core relational themes. The same ideas are dealt with as partial meanings and as synthesized wholes. Table 9.2 presents what I think is a plausible list of core relational themes for each of the 15 emotions with which I deal,

which is not an exhaustive list of all the emotions of interest.

I conclude the presentation of my appraisal theory by asking whether appraisal theory makes the emotions too cognitive and cold to be realistic. The best answer depends on what a person who had no emotions would be like. Dreikurs (1967) provided the following interesting and revealing answer, which addresses only one side of the matter. In dichotomizing reason and emotion, and by emphasizing Dionysian-like commitment, enthusiasm, and excitement in contrast with Appollonian reasonableness, Dreikurs seems to forget that both excitement and reason are conjoined in most emotions. He writes,

> We may easily discover the purpose of emotions when we try to visualize a person who has no emotions. His thinking ability could provide him with much information. He could figure out what he should do, but never would be certain as to what is right and wrong in a complicated situation. He would not be able to take a definite stand, to act with force, with conviction, because complete objectivity is not inducive to forceful actions. This requires a strong personal bias, an elimination of certain factors which logically may contradict opposing factors. Such a person would be cold, almost inhuman. He could not experience any association which would make him biased and one-sided in his perspectives. He could not want anything very much and could not go after it. In short, he would be completely ineffectual as a human being. (p. 207)

Such a person would not be a flesh-and-blood biological creature but a machine like Lieutenant Commander Data on *Star Trek, the Next Generation* or the nonhuman Vulcan, Mr. Spock, in the original television series. They are creatures that are incapable of responding emotionally. We should, however, reject the idea that an ideal human would be one who only thinks rather than feels, although I believe thought can occur without

TABLE 9.2 Core Relational Themes for Each Emotion

Emotion	Relational Theme
Anger	A demeaning offense against me and mine
Anxiety	Facing uncertain, existential threat
Fright	An immediate, concrete, and overwhelming physical danger
Guilt	Having transgressed a moral imperative
Shame	Failing to live up to an ego ideal
Sadness	Having experienced an irrevocable loss
Envy	Wanting what someone else has
Jealousy	Resenting a third party for loss or threat to another's affection or favor
Disgust	Taking in or being too close to an indigestible object or idea
Happiness	Making reasonable progress toward the realization of a goal
Pride	Enhancement of one's ego identity by taking credit for a valued object or achievement—either one's own or that of someone or a group with which we identify
Belief	A distressing goal-incongruent condition that has changed for the better or gone away
Hope	Fearing the worst but yearning for better and believing a favorable outcome is possible
Love	Desiring or participating in affection, usually but not necessarily reciprocated
Gratitude	Appreciation for an altruistic gift that provides personal benefit
Compassion	Being moved by another's suffering and wanting to help
Aesthetic experiences	Emotions aroused by these experiences can be any of those previously mentioned; there is no specific plot

significant emotion but not vice versa. Emotions are complex, organized subsystems consisting of thoughts, beliefs, motives, meanings, subjective experiences, and physiological states. They depend on appraisals, which arise from and facilitate our struggles to survive and flourish in the world.

I am confident that appraisal as a psychological construct, especially as applied to our emotional life, will continue to be a productive idea. Nevertheless, much more must be learned about how appraisals work and affect social relationships. Although the concept makes some psychologists uneasy, I believe it is central to an understanding of how we survive and flourish during the course of our lives.

➤ NOTE

1. *Rashomon* was a Japanese movie that became a classic. It viewed the same major emotional altercation from the disparate viewpoints of four different persons. The movie highlighted the distinctive experience and outlook of these individuals.

➤ REFERENCES

Aristotle. (1941). *Rhetoric*. In R. McKeon (Ed.), *The basic works of Aristotle*. New York: Random House.

Arnold, M. B. (1960). *Emotion and personality* (Vols. 1 & 2). New York: Columbia University Press.

Bandura, A. (1977). Self-efficacy: Toward a unifying theory of behavioral change. *Psychological Review, 84*, 191-215.

Bandura, A. (1989). Human agency in social cognitive theory. *American Psychologist, 44,* 1175-1184.

Bandura, A. (1997). *Self-efficacy: The exercise of control.* New York: Freeman.

Bargh, J. A. (1990). Auto-motives: Preconscious determinants of social interaction. In E. T. Higgins & R. M. Sorrentino (Eds.), *Handbook of motivation and cognition* (Vol. 2, pp. 93-130). New York: Guilford.

Bowers, K. S. (1987). Revisioning the unconscious. *Canadian Psychology/Psychologie Canadienne, 28,* 93-132.

Brewin, C. R. (1989). Cognitive change processes in psychotherapy. *Psychological Review, 96,* 379-394.

Brody, N. (Ed.). (1987). The unconscious [Special issue]. *Personality and Social Psychology Bulletin, 13.*

Bruner, J. (1992). Another look at New Look 1. *American Psychologist, 47,* 780-783.

Buck, R. (1985). Prime theory: An integrated view of motivation and emotion. *Psychological Review, 92,* 389-413.

Cohen, F., & Lazarus, R. S. (1973). Active coping processes, coping dispositions, and recovery from surgery. *Psychosomatic Medicine, 35,* 375-398.

Collins, D. L., Baum, A., & Singer, J. E. (1983). Coping with chronic stress at Three Mile Island. *Health Psychology, 2,* 149-166.

Conway, M. A., & Bekerian, D. A. (1987). Situational knowledge and emotions. *Cognition and Emotion, 1,* 145-188.

Dalkvist, J., & Rollenhagen, C. (1989, September). On the cognitive aspect of emotions: A review and model. *Reports from the Department of Psychology, University of Stockholm,* No. 703.

de Rivera, J. (1977). A structural theory of the emotions. *Psychological Issues, 10,* 9-169.

de Sousa, R. (1987). *The rationality of emotion.* Cambridge: MIT Press/Bradford.

Dewey, J. (1894). The theory of emotion. *Psychological Review, 1,* 553-569.

Dreikurs, R. (1967). *Psychodynamics and counseling.* Chicago: Adler School of Professional Psychology.

Ekman, P. (1992). *Telling lies: Clues to deceit in the marketplace, politics, and marriage.* New York: Norton. (Original work published 1985)

Epstein, S. (1990). Cognitive experiential self-theory. In L. A. Pervin (Ed.), *Handbook of personality theory and research* (pp. 165-192). New York: Guilford.

Erdelyi, M. H. (1985). *Psychoanalysis: Freud's cognitive psychology.* New York: Freeman.

Erdelyi, M. H. (1992). Psychodynamics and the unconscious. *American Psychologist, 47,* 784-787.

Eriksen, C. W. (1960). Discrimination and learning without awareness: A methodological survey and evaluation. *Psychological Review, 67,* 379-400.

Eriksen, C. W. (Ed.). (1962). *Behavior and awareness— A symposium of research and interpretation* (pp. 3-26). Durham, NC: Duke University Press.

Folkman, S., & Lazarus, R. S. (1988a). *Manual for the Ways of Coping Questionnaire.* Palo Alto, CA: Consulting Psychologists Press.

Folkman, S., & Lazarus, R. S. (1988b). Coping as a mediator of emotion. *Journal of Personality and Social Psychology, 54,* 466-475.

Frijda, N. H. (1986). *The emotions.* Cambridge, UK: Cambridge University Press.

Goleman, D. (1995). *Emotional intelligence: Why it can matter more than IQ.* New York: Bantam.

Greenwald, A. G. (1992). New Look 3: Unconscious cognition reclaimed. *American Psychologist, 47,* 766-779.

Grinker, R. R., & Spiegel, J. P. (1945). *Men under stress.* New York: McGraw-Hill.

Hobfoll, S. E. (1998). *Stress, culture, and community: The psychology and philosophy of stress.* New York: Plenum.

Jacoby, L. L., Lindsay, D. S., & Toth, J. P. (1992). Unconscious influences revealed: Attention, awareness, and control. *American Psychologist, 47,* 802-809.

James, W. (1890). *Principles of psychology.* New York: Holt.

Janis, I. L. (1951). *Air war and emotional stress.* New York: McGraw-Hill.

Janis, I. L. (1958). *Psychological stress: Psychoanalytic and behavioral studies of surgical patients.* New York: John Wiley.

Janis, I. L., & Mann, L. (1977). *Decision making.* New York: Free Press.

Kihlstrom, J. F. (1987). The cognitive unconscious. *Science, 237,* 1445-1452.

Kihlstrom, J. F. (1990). The psychological unconscious. In L. A. Pervin (Ed.), *Handbook of personality: Theory and research* (pp. 445-464). New York: Guilford.

Kihlstrom, J. F., Barnhardt, T. M., & Tataryn, D. J. (1992). The psychological unconscious: Found, lost, regained. *American Psychologist, 47,* 788-791.

Lazarus, R. S. (1964). A laboratory approach to the dynamics of psychological stress. *American Psychologist, 19,* 400-411.

Lazarus, R. S. (1966). *Psychological stress and the coping process.* New York: McGraw-Hill.

Lazarus, R. S. (1968). Emotions and adaptation: Conceptual and empirical relations. In W. J. Arnold (Ed.), *Nebraska Symposium on Motivation* (pp. 175-266). Lincoln: University of Nebraska Press.

Lazarus, R. S. (1981). The stress and coping paradigm. In C. Eisdorfer, D. Cohen, A. Kleinman, & P. Maxim (Eds.), *Models for clinical psychopathology* (pp. 177-214). New York: Spectrum.

Lazarus, R. S. (1983). The costs and benefits of denial. In S. Breznitz (Ed.), *The denial of stress* (pp. 1-30). New York: International Universities Press.

Lazarus, R. S. (1985). The trivialization of distress. In J. C. Rosen & L. J. Solomon (Eds.), *Preventing health risk behaviors and promoting coping with illness* (Vol. 8, Vermont conference on the primary prevention of psychopathology, pp. 279-298). Hanover, NH: University Press of New England. (Reprinted from *The master lecture series,* Vol. 3, pp. 121-144, by B. L. Hammonds & C. J. Scheier, Eds., 1983, Washington, DC: American Psychological Association)

Lazarus, R. S. (1989). Constructs of the mind in mental health and psychotherapy. In A. Freeman, K. M. Simon, L. E. Beuktler, & H. Arkowitz (Eds.), *Comprehensive handbook of cognitive therapy* (pp. 99-121). New York: Plenum.

Lazarus, R. S. (1991). *Emotion and adaptation.* New York: Oxford University Press.

Lazarus, R. S. (1993). From psychological stress to the emotions: A history of changing outlooks. In *Annual review of psychology* (pp. 1-21). Palo Alto, CA: Annual Reviews, Inc.

Lazarus, R. S. (1998a). *Fifty years of the research and theory of R. S. Lazarus: An analysis of historical and perennial issues.* Mahway, NJ: Lawrence Erlbaum.

Lazarus, R. S. (1998b). The cognition-emotion debate: A bit of history. In T. Dalgleish & M. Power (Eds.), *The handbook of cognition and emotion* (pp. 3-19). Cambridge, UK: Wiley.

Lazarus, R. S. (1999). *Stress and emotion: A new synthesis.* New York: Springer.

Lazarus, R. S. (in press). Relational meaning and discrete emotions. In K. R. Scherer, A. Schorr, & T. Johnstone (Eds.), *Appraisal processes in emotion: Theory, methods, research.* New York: Oxford University Press.

Lazarus, R. S., & Alfert, E. (1964). The short-circuiting of threat by experimentally altering cognitive appraisal. *Journal of Abnormal and Social Psychology, 69,* 195-205.

Lazarus, R. S., Averill, J. R., & Opton, E. M., Jr. (1970). Towards a cognitive theory of emotion. In M. Arnold (Ed.), *Feelings and emotions* (pp. 207-232). New York: Academic Press.

Lazarus, R. S., & Baker, R. W. (1956a). Personality and psychological stress—A theoretical and methodological framework. *Psychological Newsletter, 8,* 21-32.

Lazarus, R. S., & Baker, R. W. (1956b). Psychology. *Progress in Neurology and Psychiatry, 11,* 253-271.

Lazarus, R. S., & commentators. (1990). Theory based stress measurement. *Psychological Inquiry, 1,* 3-51.

Lazarus, R. S., & commentators. (1995). Vexing research problems inherent in cognitive-mediational theories of emotion, and some solutions. *Psychological Inquiry, 6,* 183-265.

Lazarus, R. S., Deese, J., & Osler, S. F. (1952). The effects of psychological stress upon performance. *Psychological Bulletin, 49,* 293-317.

Lazarus, R. S., & Folkman, S. (1984). *Stress, appraisal, and coping.* New York: Springer.

Lazarus, R. S., & Launier, R. (1978). Stress related transactions between person and environment. In L.

A. Pervin & M. Lewis (Eds.), *Perspectives in interactional psychology* (pp. 287-327). New York: Plenum.

Lazarus, R. S., & Lazarus, B. N. (1994). *Passion and reason: Making sense of our emotions.* New York: Oxford University Press.

Lazarus, R. S., & Smith, C. A. (1988). Knowledge and appraisal in the cognition-emotion relationship. *Cognition and Emotion, 2,* 281-300.

LeDoux, J. W. (1989). Cognitive-emotional interactions in the brain. *Cognition and Emotion, 3,* 267-289.

Leeper, R. W. (1948). A motivational theory of emotion to replace "emotion as a disorganized response." *Psychological Review, 55,* 5-21.

Leventhal, H. (1984). *A perceptual motor theory of emotion* (pp. 271-291). Hillsdale, NJ: Lawrence Erlbaum.

Lewicki, P., Hill, T., & Czyzewska, M. (1992). Nonconscious acquisition of information. *American Psychologist, 47,* 796-801.

Lewis, A. (1998, January 2). *New York Times,* p. A15.

Loftus, E. F. (Guest Ed.). (1992). Science watch. *American Psychologist, 47,* 761-809.

Loftus, E. F., & Klinger, M. R. (1992). Is the unconscious smart or dumb? *American Psychologist, 47,* 761-765.

Maes, S., Leventhal, H., & de Ridder, D. T. D. (1996). Coping with chronic diseases. In M. Zeidner & N. S. Endler (Eds.), *Handbook of coping: Theory, research, applications* (pp. 221-252). New York: John Wiley.

Mandler, G. (1984). *Mind and body: Psychology of emotion and stress.* New York: Norton.

Mascolo, M. F., & Fischer, K. W. (1995). Developmental transformations in appraisals for pride, shame, and guilt. In J. P. Tangney & I. W. Fischer (Eds.), *Self-conscious emotions: The psychology of shame, guilt, embarrassment, and pride* (pp. 64-113). New York: Guilford.

McAdams, D. P. (1996). Personality, modernity, and the storied self: A contemporary framework for studying persons. *Psychological Inquiry, 7,* 295-321.

McReynolds, P. (1956). A restricted conceptualization of human anxiety and motivation. *Psychological Reports, Monograph Supplements, 6,* 293-312.

Mechanic, D. (1978). *Students under stress: A study in the social psychology of adaptation.* New York: Free Press. (Original work published 1962)

Merikle, P. M. (1992). Perception without awareness: Critical issues. *American Psychologist, 47,* 792-795.

Merleau-Ponty, M. (1962). *Phenomenology of perception* (C. Smith, Trans.). London: Routledge & Kegan Paul.

Oatley, K., & Johnson-Laird, P. N. (1987). Towards a cognitive theory of emotions. *Cognition and Emotion, 1,* 29-50.

Opton, E. M., Jr., Rankin, N., Nomikos, M., & Lazarus, R. S. (1965). The principle of short-circuiting of threat: Further evidence. *Journal of Personality, 33,* 622-635.

Ortony, A., Clore, G. L., & Collins, A. (1988). *The cognitive structure of emotions.* New York: Cambridge University Press.

Parkinson, B., & Manstead, A. S. R. (1992). Appraisal as a cause of emotion. *Review of Personality and Social Psychology, 13,* 122-149.

Polanyi, M. (1966). *The tacit dimension.* Garden City, NY: Doubleday.

Reisenzein, R. (1995). On appraisal as causes of emotions. *Psychological Inquiry, 6,* 233-237.

Robertson, G. C. (1877). Notes. *Mind: A Quarterly Review, 2,* 413-415.

Roseman, I. J. (1984). Cognitive determinants of emotion: A structural theory. In P. Shaver (Ed.), *Review of personality and social psychology: Vol. 5. Emotions, relationships, and health* (pp. 11-36). Beverly Hills, CA: Sage.

Scherer, K. R. (1984). On the nature and function of emotion: A component process approach. In K. R. Scherer & P. Ekman (Eds.), *Approaches to emotion* (pp. 293-317). Hillsdale, NJ: Lawrence Erlbaum.

Selye, H. (1974). *Stress without distress.* Philadelphia: J. B. Lippincott.

Selye, H. (1976). *The stress of life.* New York: McGraw-Hill. (Original work published 1956)

Shepard, R. N. (1984). Ecological constraints on internal representation: Resonant kinematics of perceiving, imagining, thinking, and dreaming. *Psychological Review, 91,* 417-447.

Smith, C. A., & Ellsworth, P. C. (1985). Patterns of cognitive appraisal in emotion. *Journal of Personality and Social Psychology, 48,* 813-838.

Smith, C. A., Haynes, K. N., Lazarus, R. S., & Pope, L. K. (1993). In search of the "hot" cognitions: Attributions, appraisals, and their relation to emotion. *Journal of Personality and Social Psychology, 65,* 916-929.

Solomon, R. C. (1976). *The passions: The myth and nature of human emotion.* Garden City, NY: Doubleday.

Speisman, J. C., Lazarus, R. S., Mordkoff, A. M., & Davison, L. A. (1964). The experimental reduction of stress based on ego-defense theory. *Journal of Abnormal and Social Psychology, 68,* 367-380.

Staudenmeyer, H., Kinsman, R. S., Dirks, J. F., Spector, S. L., & Wangaard, C. (1979). Medical outcome in asthmatic patients. Effects of airways hyperactivity and symptom-focused anxiety. *Psychosomatic Medicine, 41,* 109-118.

Tolman, E. C. (1932). *Purposive behavior in animals and man.* New York: Appleton.

Uleman, J. S., & Bargh, J. A. (Eds.). (1989). *Unintended thought.* New York: Guilford.

Weiner, B. (1985). An attributional theory of motivation, achievement, and emotion. *Psychological Review, 92,* 548-573. New York: Springer.

Weiner, B. (1986). *An attributional theory of motivation and emotion.* New York: Springer-Verlag.

CHAPTER 10

Coping With Stress

Programs of Nursing Research

Jane H. Backer, Tamilyn Bakas,
Susan J. Bennett, and Patricia K. Pierce

 he purpose of this chapter is to examine stress, coping, and health with a focus on the phenomenon of coping and nursing research. Previous chapters in this volume addressed stress and stressors. With Darwin's evolutionary theory emphasizing the "struggle for survival" and an increasing emphasis on behavioral problem-solving activities, the foundation for "coping" was laid. Other perspectives that have contributed to its evolution have been Freud's (1917/1946) psychoanalytic theory (which identified elements of appraisal), Erickson's (1963) notion that healthy human development was predicated on successful negotiation of life's challenges and crises, and case studies of the process of managing life demands (Moos, 1986). Key psychologists who have contributed to the increasing conceptualization of coping include Janis (1958), Pearlin and Schooler (1978), and Lazarus

(1966, 1978, 1991, 1998). According to Lazarus (1998), "stress itself as a concept pales in significance for adaptation compared with coping" (p. 202). Coping is viewed as an essential construct in both of Lazarus's interactional and transactional models of stress, coping, and adaptation (health outcomes) (Lazarus, 1966; Lazarus & Folkman, 1984). See Chapter 9 for a comprehensive description of the evolution of Lazarus's theory of stress and coping.

Although definitions of coping have varied from what it is that people do (action only) to what they are, in terms of a personality trait (e.g., hypervigilant), the conceptualization most often used in nursing research has been the one proposed by Lazarus. He defined coping as the "constantly changing cognitive and behavioral efforts to manage specific external and/or internal demands that are appraised as taxing or exceeding the resources of the person" (Lazarus & Folkman, 1984, p. 141). Coping is viewed as (a) process-oriented rather than trait-oriented, (b) nonautomated adaptive behavior, (c) effort rather than outcome, and (d) managing rather than mastery of life stressors.

Lazarus (1966) was particularly interested in examining the relationship between coping and adaptation (including somatic health and illness, well-being, and social functioning). It was this work that drew the attention of nurse researchers and clinicians alike. Prior to the development of Lazarus's theory, the literature tended to focus on stress as a stimulus (Holmes & Rahe, 1967) or as a response (Selye, 1936). The critical variables of "appraisal" and coping were missing. Without these theoretical concepts, directions for intervention to reduce stress were vague and unspecified (Rice, 1990). For example, relaxation therapy prescribed to reduce anxiety during a threatening event without attention to or consideration of the patient's appraisal of the experience was found to be ineffective (Rice, Caldwell, Butler, & Robinson, 1986). When these factors were attended to, the association between stress and coping was more evident (Rice, Mullin, & Jarosz, 1992). Lazarus's notions of appraisal and coping as important factors for experienced stress are significant contributions to the development of nursing science. Nurse researchers have viewed Lazarus's theory of stress and coping as appropriate for model development (Scott, Oberst, & Dropkin, 1980), framing nursing studies (Rice et al., 1986), deriving midrange theories for practice (Baldree, Murphy, & Powers, 1982), and creating instruments to assess the phenomenon of coping (Jalowiec, 1991).

In time, nursing science has derived its own theoretical structures and an increasing knowledge base of the relationships among stress and coping and health. A search of the Cumulative Index for Nursing and Allied Health Literature (CINAHL) revealed more than 5,000 citations for "coping" since 1982. The keyword "stress" generated more than 10,000 references, and the combination of stress, coping, and health resulted in more than 800 references. Numerous nurse scientists have examined the phenomena of stress, coping, and health during the past 40 years or more. Because it is impossible to review all their work in the space available, three exemplar research programs have been selected and will be explicated to give the reader a sense of the creative work in this area.

Research initiated in the 1960s by Jean Johnson examined stress reduction and nursing interventions to facilitate coping in adults and children experiencing threatening health care events (see Johnson, 1999, for a summary). A second program established by Scott et al. (1980) developed and tested a stress-coping model to study adaptation in an acute care cancer center. A third research agenda, directed by Anne Jalowiec (Jalowiec & Powers, 1981), examined relationships among the constructs of Lazarus's stress and coping theory in chronically ill adults, extended his work with additional constructs, and created a tool for the measurement of coping in patient populations.

➤ PROGRAMS OF RESEARCH

Nursing Intervention, Stress Reduction, and Coping (Jean E. Johnson)

From the beginning of her research career, Johnson based her research on information processing explanations of cognition and their application by Leventhal (1970) in his parallel response model of coping. The parallel response model proposed that deferent cognitive processes were involved in the control of danger from a threatening event and the control of emotional reactions. Research conducted in the laboratory and in clinical settings has shown that the effects of preparatory information on clients' coping outcomes differ with the content that is included in the information. Preparatory information for a threatening event that includes description of (a) physical sensations and symptoms, (b) temporal characteristics, (c) environmental features, and (d) cause of sensations, symptoms and experiences in concrete-objective terms results in a reduction in the amount of disruption by the event on clients usual activities and a reduction in emotional distress in clients who are prone to such reactions (e.g., Johnson, 1996; Johnson, Fieler, Wlasowicz, Mitchell, & Jones, 1997). Clients benefit most from instruction in coping technique and self-care activities when these are combined with descriptions of what they will experience in concrete-objective terms (e.g., Johnson, Rice, Fuller, & Andress, 1978; Johnson, Nail, Lauver, King, & Keys, 1988). Preparatory information that describes subjective responses, such as emotions, distress, and degree of difficulty, result in an increase in emotional reactions and distress (e.g., Ahes, Blanchard, & Leventhal, 1983; Suls & Fletcher, 1985). The self-regulation theory developed from and supported by this research provides an explanation of the cognitive processes that mediate the effects of the specific types of information on coping outcomes. These mediating processes include the composition of cognitive representations of events, the characteristics of events attended to, decisions about actions to initiate, and evaluation of affects of the actions taken. Concrete-objective descriptions of an impending event allows clients to make decisions about how they will cope with a health care event and to evaluate the affect of their coping on what they desire to achieve.

Empirical Adequacy

Replication and extension of Johnson's work can be found in studies with adult surgical patients (Hill, 1982; Johnson, Christman, & Stitt, 1985; Johnson, Fuller, Endress, & Rice, 1978; Johnson, Rice, et al., 1978), women undergoing pelvic examination (Fuller, Endress, & Johnson, 1978), children experiencing cast removal (Johnson, Kirchhoff, & Endress, 1975), adults having barium enemas (Hartfield & Cason, 1981), and patients on mechanical ventilation (Kim, Garvin, & Moser, 1999).

An assessment of the impact of Johnson's research was published in 1984 in *Current Contents* (Garfield, 1984). The study of citation patterns in nursing journals from 1966 to 1983 showed that Johnson was the most frequently cited author. She authored 5 of the 18 most cited articles in nursing journals and 3 of the 14 highly cited nursing articles published in non-nursing journals. Her research continues to be cited frequently. (See Table 10.1.)

Critical Examination

Dr. Johnson's research is exemplary for many reasons. She used theoretically based, randomized trial methodology that is essential for the growth of nursing science and nursing practice. Her work is patient based. Interventions that she, her colleagues, and other nurse scientists have designed and tested were derived from clinical data obtained from patients undergoing the specific procedures that were being studied. (One means for securing the needed sensory information about a health care event from patients is described by Rice, Sieggreen, Mullin, & Williams, 1988, in their study with arteriogram patients.) The focus of Johnson's work was on positive health outcomes; this has important implications for today's health care agenda of self-care and health promotion. When available, tools with established validity and reliability were used. Even though study sample sizes were frequently small and somewhat homogeneous in cultural identity, the findings were remarkably similar across populations in diverse settings undergoing a variety of health care procedures.

Implications

Johnson and her colleagues' results have widespread implications for research, theoretical model building, and clinical nursing practice. Because of the strengths of the research, the findings need to become a part of all nursing and health education curricula. As a standard of practice, nurses should be providing patients who are undergoing health

(text continued on page 231)

TABLE 10.1 Summary of Johnson and Colleagues' Research

Reference	Purpose	Design	Sample	Instruments	Key Findings	Relative Strengths and Weaknesses
Fuller, Endress, and Johnson (1978)	To examine the effects of cognitive control information and relaxation on coping with an aversive health exam	2×2 factorial design—four groups: sensory, sensory and relaxation, health education, and health education and relaxation	24 women undergoing a routine pelvic exam; mean age, 21 years; mean education level, 12.5; majority were black	Radial pulse, overt distress behaviors, and fear self-report	The sensory group had significantly fewer distress behaviors ($p <$ .02) and less pulse rate change ($p < .02$).	Volunteer sample, randomly assigned to groups; acceptable interrater agreement on use of distress behavior scale; limited generalizability to other populations
Hatfield and Cason (1981)	To test the effects of three types of information conditions on patients' anxiety proneness and thereby extend the applicability of Johnson's findings in a different group of patients	Quasi-experimental—three groups: sensation, procedure, and control	24 hospitalized patients undergoing barium enema	Spielberger's State-Trait Anxiety Inventory; Anxiety proneness measured by trait subscale and used as covariate	Sensations: Significantly less state anxiety was reported by sensation group than by the other two groups ($p <$ .05). Hypothesized differences in mean state anxiety between the three groups were not found, however.	Small volunteer sample; reliability and validity of the State-Trait Anxiety Inventory not reported for the sample; patients randomized to group; extended Johnson's results to a different population
Hill (1982)	To test the effects of four types of information conditions on patients' postoperative orientation, stimulus experiences, mood, and functional performance	Experimental—four groups: behavioral instructions (also called behavioral control), sensation information (also called cognitive control), behavioral and sensation information, and general information	40 hospitalized patients undergoing first-time cataract surgery	Postoperative orientation—confusion by the Profile of Mood States, cognitive orientation by the Pfeiffer Short Portable Mental Status Questionnaire; Stimulus experiences—structured patient interview that was tape-recorded	Behavioral and cognitive control interventions had no significant effect on dependent variables. Patients who received the combination of behavioral and cognitive control interventions, however, had significantly lower number of days after discharge when leaving their homes.	Small volunteer sample; reliability and validity of instruments not reported for the sample; Patients randomized to group; extended Johnson's results to a different population

Study	Purpose	Design	Sample	Measures	Results	Comments
				Mood (anxiety and depression)—Profile of Mood States		
				Performance—number of times out of bed during postoperative day, length of hospital stay, and number of days after discharge when patient first left home		
Johnson (1973)	To test the incongruency hypothesis by exposing subjects to ischemic pain in three experiments	1. Experimental—two groups: irrelevant and relevant information	1. 20 males, random selection, mean age 21.4 years	1. Mood adjective checklist, degree of sensation, and degree of distress	1. Relevant: There was significantly more congruence between expectations and actual experience ($p < .02$) and significantly less distress ($p < .05$).	1. Manipulation check for perception of sensory experience, random selection, and random assignment to groups; all subjects males, university students, and relatively young; no tool reliability or validity information included
		2. Experimental—four groups: relevant and irrelevant information; attention and distraction	2. 48 males, random selection and assignment to groups	2. Same as No. 1	2. Relevant: There was significantly less distress ($p < .05$). This supports the incongruity hypothesis.	2. Experimenter naive to subject group
		3. Experimental—two groups: relevant and irrelevant information	3. 24 males, randomly assigned to groups	3. Same as No. 1	3. There were no significant group differences.	3. Same as above

(continued)

TABLE 10.1 Continued

Reference	Purpose	Design	Sample	Instruments	Key Findings	Relative Strengths and Weaknesses
Johnson, Christman, and Stitt (1985)	To evaluate effects, both short term and long term, of personal control interventions on the postoperative experience	Experimental—2 × 3 × 2 factorial design 1. Description of postoperative experience in sensory terms 2. Instruction in cognitive-coping strategies, instructions in a coping strategy that was behaviorally focused, and no instruction 3. Experimental or control instruction about posthospital phase	168 hospitalized patients undergoing hysterectomy	1. Hospital phase: pain—number of medications, patient ratings during ambulation on Postoperative Day 3; mood—Profile of Mood States; physical activity—number of times out of bed; Physical Recovery Index; hospital length of stay 2. Posthospital phase: mood—Profile of Mood States; physical activity—date when patients first left their house after hospital discharge	Patients who received behavioral coping intervention had significantly fewer pain medications; patients who received cognitive coping intervention reported significantly better physical recovery but had longer lengths of stay. Posthospitalization recovery had different patterns of effects of effects than during hospitalization.	Volunteer sample; reliability and validity of instruments not reported for the sample; complex 2 × 3 × 2 factorial design makes results difficult to evaluate; patients randomized to group; extended some of Johnson's results to a different population
Johnson, Fuller, Endress, and Rice (1978)	To replicate the Johnson, Rice, Fuller, and Endress (1978) study, to explore the effects of sending patients preadmission information, and to evaluate the effects of reexposure to information and temporal information on post-op course	Experimental—five groups: preadmission (specific, nonspecific, and no information), sensory information, restatement of information	Persons undergoing either a cholecystectomy or herniorrhaphy randomly assigned to groups; stratified by age and physician	MACL; subjective pain report; number of parenteral analgesic doses; number of times ambulated; amount of bother to get up; length of post-op hospitalization; and posthospitalization recovery	Cholecystectomy sample: replicated findings ($F = 24.81$, $p < .001$). Sensory with temporal information significantly reduced helplessness ($p < .01$).	Hospital staff naïve to interventions; volunteer sample, randomly assigned to groups; herniorrhaphy sample hospital stay too brief for repeated data collection

Study	Purpose	Design	Sample	Variables	Findings	Comments
Johnson, Kirchhoff, and Endress (1975)	To test incongruency hypothesis with children	Experimental—three groups: sensations, procedure, control	89 children undergoing cast removal; ages 6 to 11 years; mostly males; mostly black	Radial pulse; minor distress; major distress	Sensation group had no significant pulse rate changes during procedure whether or not child had fear of procedure.	Used control group from original study for comparison; data collected at different points in time Medical and nursing staff naive to subject group; most subjects had arm casts removed; acceptable reliability of distress score observation; findings may not be generalizable to other populations
Johnson and Leventhal (1974)	To test the effects of behavioral instruction and sensation information during a noxious medical exam	Experimental—four groups: sensation description, behavioral instruction, combination, and control (none)	48 hospitalized patients undergoing endoscopic exam	Tranquilizer (mg); heart rate changes; hand and arm movements; gagging; number of seconds to pass tube	Sensation description: Subjects < 50 years of age had less tranquilizer ($p < .025$) and less gagging ($p < .025$). Combination: There was significantly more time to pass the tube ($p < .01$).	Volunteer sample; caregivers naive to subject group; stratified by gender
Johnson, Morrissey, and Leventhal (1973)	To test the effects of specific information on patients' tolerance of a threatening procedure	Quasi-experimental—three groups: sensations, procedure, control	99 in- and outpatients undergoing an endoscopic exam	Dose (mg) of sedation; heart rate changes; hand and arm movements; gagging; restlessness	Sensations: Significantly less sedation was used ($p < .05$), and there were fewer hand and arm movements ($p < .02$).	Volunteer sample; nonrandom assignment to groups; no tool reliability and validity information included

(continued)

TABLE 10.1 Continued

Reference	Purpose	Design	Sample	Instruments	Key Findings	Relative Strengths and Weaknesses
					Procedure: Significantly more restlessness than sensation ($p < .01$). Effects were similar for both genders.	
Johnson and Rice (1974)	To test the effect of giving sensory information that varied in degree of accurateness and completeness	Experimental—four groups: false sensory, partial sensory, full sensory, no sensory	61 male university students, 18 to 25 years old; no chronic or acute health problems	Mood adjective checklist; sensation and distress scale	Partial and full sensory groups had significantly less distress ($p < .05$).	Volunteer sample, but random assignment to groups; no tool reliability or validity information included; experimenter naive to subject group
Johnson, Rice, Fuller, and Endress (1978)	To determine the effects of sensory information, temporal information, coping behavior information, and combinations of these on subjective and objective indicators of recovery from a cholecystectomy (1) or herniorrhaphy (2)	(1 and 2) 2 × 3 experimental—six groups: procedure, sensation information, and coping instruction and control	1. 81 cholecystectomy patients, predominantly female; mean age 44 years 2. 68 herniorrhaphy patients, predominantly male	Number parenteral analgesics; subjective reports of pain; number of times ambulated; amount of bother to get up; MACL; length of hospitalization; posthospital recovery	1. Sensory group had significantly increased recovery. 2. There were no significant effects of interventions on outcomes.	Hospital staff naive to subject group; volunteer sample, randomly assigned to groups; limited evaluation and influence of situational factors (physicians' orders); limited generalizability to other populations

care procedures with detailed information about sensations they can expect to experience during the event along with additional information needed to anchor it in time and space and to understand their experience. Given the current health care agenda, it is essential that patients become active participants in their own care because they are discharged from hospital units increasingly earlier and are expected to resume their daily activities in their work world. Patients who have the information that they need will be in a position to become more involved and more positive health care partners.

Since the mid-1980s, Johnson has employed "self-regulation theory" to describe, explain, and predict the outcomes of her preparatory information research. This has built on the commonsense model of illness representation (Leventhal & Johnson, 1983). Cancer patients have been the focus of much of this work (Johnson, 1996; Johnson, Fieler, Jones, Wlasowicz, & Mitchell, 1997). A detailed description of Johnson's ongoing work with self-regulation theory can be found in Chapter 20 of this volume, in her own book (Johnson et al., 1997), and an article on the theory (Johnson, 1999).

A Stress-Coping Model (Scott, Oberst, & Dropkin)

A second body of nursing research concerns the development and testing of Scott, Oberst, and Dropkin's (SOD; 1980) stress-coping model. It was designed as a theoretical base to study adaptation to stress in an acute care cancer center. The model was deductive in origin because it was derived from several theories. Although a large portion of the model was taken from Lazarus's (1966, 1981) theory of stress and coping, the creators also incorporated the works of Izard (1979), Plutchik, Kellerman, and Conte (1979), Weisman (1979), Frankenhauser (1975), Mason (1975), and Sigg (1975). This allowed for further specification of the model's compo-

nents and provided new direction for nursing diagnoses and intervention.

Oberst and colleagues later extended their model to include the concepts "caregiver burden" and "self-care burden" (derived from Orem's theory of self-care) as major antecedents of appraisal and further specified antecedents (person factors, illness factors, and resources) of caregiver burden and self-care burden (Carey, Oberst, McCubbin, & Hughes, 1991; Oberst, Hughes, Chang, & McCubbin, 1991). Oberst and colleagues focused on mood state as the major health outcome of their research (Carey et al., 1991; Oberst et al., 1991). Although Scott et al. (1980) did not identify specific underlying theoretical assumptions, the following assumptions, which are quite similar to those foundational to Lazarus and Folkman's (1984) model, are inferred:

1. The stress-coping process is dynamic in nature, continually changing over time.
2. Everyone experiences anxiety when initially encountering a stressor.
3. To experience stress, a person must have some level of cognitive activity.
4. For stress-related emotions to occur, there must be a cognitive appraisal of demands exceeding resources.
5. Individuals differ in their perception of environmental stimuli that can be interpreted as stressful or nonstressful.
6. Neurotransmission occurs simultaneously with emotional response.

An assumption of the SOD model that is quite different from the Lazarus theory is that every individual under stress initially experiences anxiety (Scott et al., 1980). Then, as the process unfolds, anxiety develops into more specific emotions, such as fear, anger, and sadness. In contrast, Lazarus and Folkman (1984) proposed that appraisal determines the type of emotion(s) the person initially experiences. One individual may feel anxious whereas another may have anger and depression depending on their respective appraisals of the situation. Lazarus (1991) suggests core

TABLE 10.2 Concepts and Conceptual Definitions of Scott, Oberst, and Dropkin's (1980) Stress-Coping Model

Concept	Definition
Stress	A situation in which environmental demands, internal demands, or both tax or exceed the adaptive resources of an individual, social, or tissue system.
Coping	A process that includes use of goal-directed strategies that are initiated and maintained over time and across encounters by means of cognitive appraisal and regulation of emotion and physiologic response. Modes of coping include motor and expressive behaviors aimed at changing the stressor and regulation of emotional and physiologic response aimed at preservation of integrity.
Appraisal	The total stress and coping process, including primary and secondary appraisals, coping strategies, neurocognitive activity, affective and physiologic responses, and behavioral outcomes. Primary appraisal focuses on evaluation of the stressor array, whereas the secondary appraisal and later reappraisals focus on evaluating the effectiveness of coping responses and changes in the stress configuration.
Neurocognitive activation	Evaluation of a stimulus array using the neurocognitive apparatus for stress interpretation.
Affective response	Arousal of a feeling state as a consequence of neurocognitive activation. Feeling state is closely linked to simultaneously occurring biochemical and physiologic changes. Primary appraisal initiates a generalized global anxiety, and secondary appraisal refines the general response into more specific emotions associated with the stress situation. This can develop into mood states and attitudes.
Physiological response	Changes in secretion of substances and activation of sympathetic nervous system pathways in response to the cognitive "fight," "flight," or "freeze" command.
Behavioral response	All neurocognitive, affective, and physiologic responses to the stress situation measured by observable expressive and motor actions, self-report, and end organ response.
Adaptation	The presence of a balance between demands and the power to deal with them that occurs as a result of coping efforts. Desirable adaptational outcomes include "minimum impairment of functioning; economical balance among demands, power or resources, and cost; strengthening of assimilation and accommodation modes within the system; growth and learning; achievement of acceptable goals" (Scott et al., 1980, p. 17).

relational themes that determine the type of stress-related emotion(s) initially experienced (see Chapter 9, this volume).

Major concepts of the SOD model are stress, coping, appraisal, neurocognitive activation, affective response, physiological response, behavioral response, and adaptation. All of these are conceptually defined in Table 10.2.

Definitions of coping, adaptation, and affective response (emotion) proposed by Scott et al. (1980) are consistent with those of Lazarus and Folkman (1984); definitions of appraisal and secondary appraisal are not, however. The former incorporates all the stress concepts into a broad definition of appraisal that includes emotions and coping strategies. The latter defines appraisal as solely an evaluative process that determines whether a situation is perceived as stressful or not and what coping strategies, if any, will be used.

Scott et al. (1980) proposed two types of appraisal, primary and secondary. Their conceptual definitions of primary appraisal and reappraisal are consistent with those of Lazarus (Lazarus, 1966; Lazarus & Folkman, 1984), but the theorists differ in their thinking about secondary appraisal. They refer to secondary appraisal as the evaluation of the effectiveness of coping strategies used and changes in the stressful situation. In contrast, Lazarus and Folkman view secondary appraisal as the judgment about what coping strategies to use to alter or alleviate the stressful situation. Folkman (1997) extended the conceptualization of secondary appraisal to include the determination of emotions.

Some of the SOD model conceptual definitions are not mutually exclusive, and the labels assigned to the concepts are not consistently used in the model description. Definitions of "behavioral response" and coping include some of the same attributes. The schematic representation of the model indicates that behavioral response is a concept independent of neurocognitive activation (appraisal), affective response, and physiologic responses to a stress situation, whereas behavioral response is conceptually defined as incorporating all these elements. The terms "behavioral response" and "behavioral display" are used interchangeably, which leads to confusion about their meaning.

Some of the relationships among concepts of the SOD model are not explicitly stated but can be inferred from the schematic representation of the model. For example, primary appraisal directly impacts affective response (emotions) and physiologic responses, and both interact with one another and with behavioral display and response. Following primary appraisal, secondary appraisal or reappraisal occurs, during which the initial stressor is considered in terms of its relevance and meaning and the available coping resources. Then, coping resources are selected and evaluated for their effectiveness in reduc-

ing stress and negative emotion. The cycle begins again and continues repeatedly until adaptation occurs.

Although the SOD and Lazarus and Folkman's models share many similarities, a major difference between the two is the symmetry of the relationships. The former proposes linear relationships between appraisal and emotion and between emotion and behavioral response (coping), whereas Lazarus and Folkman (1984) depict bidirectional relationships.

Empirical Adequacy

A literature search was conducted to find evidence of empirical support for the SOD model by exploring the Social Sciences Index from 1980 to 1998 and by searching CINAHL and MEDLINE from 1980 to 1999. Sixteen articles and one dissertation (Dropkin, 1994) were located that cited the model. Table 10.3 contains a summary and critique of some of these studies.

Because the SOD model is based on broad assumptions and includes many concepts, it has been applicable across a wide variety of client populations. For example, the SOD model was used to study caregivers of cancer patients receiving chemotherapy (Carey et al., 1991), adults with chronic low back pain (Pellino & Oberst, 1992), and women with breast cancer (Kessler, 1998). Another example is Oberst et al.'s (1991) study of symptom distress among adults receiving radiation therapy for cancer.

Most studies based on the SOD model used operational definitions that were consistent with the conceptual definitions of the model concepts. All the studies used descriptive, correlational designs with two exceptions; one used a psychometric design (Kessler, 1998) and the other a quasi-experimental design (Roman et al., 1995). Eleven of the studies were cross-sectional, and 6 were longitudinal. Most of the studies employed measures that had evidence of established reliability and validity and had adequate sample sizes. Few samples were culturally or racially

(text continued on page 249)

TABLE 10.3 Studies Citing the Scott et al. (1980) Stress-Coping Model

Reference	Purpose	Design	Sample	Instruments	Key Findings	Relative Strengths and Weaknesses
Bramwell, MacKenzie, Laschinger, and Cameron (1995)	To assess primary caregiver's appraisal of the need for overnight respite and willingness to receive this support from trained laypersons; used SOD model as a context for secondary appraisal of sleep	Cross-sectional, descriptive correlational design	37 primary caregivers of community hospice patients	Three open-ended questions addressing (a) estimated hours of sleep (stress configuration), (b) perceived adequacy of sleep (coping effectiveness), and (c) willingness for overnight respite (coping resources)	Those with less hours of sleep were more likely to report less adequacy of sleep ($\chi^2 = 5.30$, $p < .05$). Those with less adequacy of sleep reported more willingness for overnight respite ($\chi^2 = 9.53$, $p < .001$). Those with less hours of sleep reported more willingness for overnight respite ($\chi^2 = 3.80$, $p < .05$). Findings were consistent with Scott et al.'s (1980) model.	All participants were interviewed by one investigator; therefore, interrater reliability was not a concern. Relatively small sample from one agency limits generalizability. Consistency of open-ended questions with conceptual definitions of the model can be questioned.
Carey, Oberst, McCubbin, and Hughes (1991)	To describe time and difficulty associated with caregiving tasks, examine caregiver's appraisals of their situations, and explore what variables are predictive of caregiver mood	Cross-sectional, descriptive correlational design	49 family caregivers of cancer patients receiving chemotherapy	Caregiving Burden Scale; Appraisal of Caregiving Scale; Profile of Mood States; Family Hardiness Index; single items for patient dependency, caregiver age, caregiver health, and others	Burden is predicted by patient dependency (47% variance accounted for). Burden, family hardiness, and caregiver health predicted 50% of variance in negative appraisal.	There was acceptable reliability and validity of instruments. Alphas for this study ranged from .73 to .97. The instrument was taken home to complete; thus, it cannot be ensured that responses were from caregivers.

	To investigate the relationship of anxiety and use of problem-focused coping strategies to self-care and resocialization	Longitudinal, descriptive correlational design	75 adults with moderate to severe disfiguring head or neck cancer surgery	State Trait Anxiety Inventory; Ways of Coping Questionnaire; Disfigurement/Dysfunction Scale; Coping Behaviors Score	Negative appraisal and age explained 49% of the variance in mood disturbance. Findings support appraisal as a mediator between effects of illness and contextual factors on caregiver outcomes. Level of post-op anxiety was negatively related to self-care ($p < .05$). Relationships among anxiety, problem-focused strategies, self-care, resocialization, degree of disfigurement and dysfunction, and post-op anxiety were all nonsignificant.	It was a small sample with lower-middle to upper-middle income, educated caregivers overrepresented. Minorities were not addressed. Means indicate high family hardiness and low mood disturbance in relation to the ranges.
Dropkin (1994)						
Dropkin (1997)	To determine if an individual's use of coping strategies prior to facial disfigurement or dysfunction is predictive of coping effectiveness after head and neck cancer surgery	Longitudinal, descriptive correlational design	117 adults about to undergo head or neck cancer surgery associated with disfigurement and dysfunction	Ways of Coping Checklist; Disfigurement/Dysfunction Scale; Coping Behaviors Score; Healing Process Checklist; length of post-op stay	There was 56% variance of length of stay predicted by 16 variables, with post-op complications being the best predictor (46%), followed by gender, pre-op radiation, and chemotherapy.	Sample was limited to Caucasian, moderate to high socioeconomic status patients with an unusually long length of stay in the hospital. Internal consistency reliability estimates were not provided for the scales based on the sample.

(continued)

TABLE 10.3 Continued

Reference	Purpose	Design	Sample	Instruments	Key Findings	Relative Strengths and Weaknesses
					There was 25% variance in postop coping predicted by 15 variables, with post-op complications being the best predictor, followed by pre-op coping.	
					Compromised physiologic postop healing provides support for the Scott et al. (1980) model regarding the simultaneous affective and physiologic responses to stress.	
Fedewa and Oberst (1996)	To gain insight into the caregiving tasks of family members caring for a child with a renal transplant and to examine the relationships between caregiver burden, appraisal, and mood state	Cross-sectional, descriptive correlational	20 family caregivers of pediatric renal transplant patients	Caregiving Burden Scale; Appraisal of Caregiving Scale; Profile of Mood States; demographic variables	Caregiving demand was unrelated to appraisal or mood.	Small, convenience sample of middle- to upper-middle-class caregivers was used.
					Caregiving difficulty was unrelated to appraisal.	There was a patient age range of 4 to 17 years, with a mean of 14 years.
					Caregiving difficulty was mildly related to mood ($r = .33$, $p < .05$).	There were acceptable reliability estimates for scales (.71 to .88)
					Relationships hypothesized by the model were not supported in this population.	There were relatively low scores with little variability for scales.
					Caregiver appraisal was unrelated to mood.	

Hart (1986/1987)	To identify similarities and differences in stressful events and coping behaviors among family and nonfamily significant others	Exploratory, cross-sectional design	25 family and 25 nonfamily caregivers of 25 cancer chemotherapy patients (triad sample)	Interview form to measure events perceived as stressful and coping behavior to reduce stressful events	No significant differences between family and nonfamily caregivers in stressfulness of events were found. The mean level of stress was higher for nonfamily when the patient lived with family caregivers ($p < .05$). The study did not test the theory.	Single items were used to measure the variables. A small convenience sample was used. Scoring of the level of stress ladder is unclear. There was high variability in relation to the means for levels of stress by event.
Kessler (1998)	To develop and evaluate the psychometric properties of the Cognitive Appraisal of Health Scale	Psychometric testing design	201 women with breast cancer	Cognitive Appraisal of Health Scale; 5 single-item secondary appraisal items	Intercorrelations among primary and secondary appraisals were consistent with the theory ($p < .01$). Internal consistency of subscales ranged from .76 to .88.	Moderate intercorrelations and high cross-loadings in the factor structure may indicate overlapping constructs. There was a high variability in time since diagnosis. Race was not reported.
Munkres, Oberst, and Hughes (1992)	To describe perceptions of symptom distress, self-care burden, appraisal of illness, and mood; to identify differences according to stage of illness; and to test a theoretical model of the mediating effects of appraisal	Descriptive correlational, cross-sectional design	60 cancer patients receiving chemotherapy for initial and recurrent cancer	Modified Symptom Distress Scale; Self-Care Burden Scale; Family Hardiness Index; Appraisal of Illness Scale; Profile of Mood States; personal and illness characteristics	Appraisal, symptom distress, and perceived seriousness predicted 36% of variance in affective mood, with appraisal partially mediating the effects of symptom distress. Somatic mood (36%) was best predicted by symptom distress and universal self-care burden.	Alpha coefficients were acceptable (.77 to .94), except for health deviation self-care burden difficulty (.63). The study used primarily a middle-class, well-educated, married sample from a single setting. Scores were low for mood, self-care burden, and appraisal.

(continued)

TABLE 10.3 Continued

Reference	Purpose	Design	Sample	Instruments	Key Findings	Relative Strengths and Weaknesses
					Symptom distress (21%) was predicted best by recurrence and symptom control.	
					Economic status, symptom distress, and recurrence status predicted 49% of appraisal variance.	
					Universal self-care burden (45%) was predicted best by economic status and perceived dependency.	
					Relationships supported were consistent with the theory.	
Nolan, Grant, and Ellis (1990)	To reconceptualize burden within a transactional stress framework, and to test such a model	Cross-sectional, descriptive correlational design	554 informal caregivers	Closed- and open-ended questions for environmental factors; Career Perceived Problem Checklist with two response scales (experience and stressfulness); Maliase Inventory with two subscales (psychological and physical)	Drawn from Lazarus's transactional theory, among other theorists including Scott et al. (1980), path analysis predicting 47% variance in psychological malaise supporting the mediating role of appraisal.	The study used a large, population-based sample.
					Path analysis predicting 20% variance in physical malaise did not support mediating role of appraisal.	Internal consistency reliability estimates for scales were not reported.

| Northouse, Templin, Mood, and Oberst (1998) | To compare stress, resources, appraisal, and patterns of adjustment in benign and malignant groups; compare psychosocial responses of patients verses spouses; and determine correspondence in levels of adjustment in patients and spouses | Longitudinal, mixed design analysis of covariance | Couples adjusting to benign ($n = 73$) and malignant ($n = 58$) breast disease | Smilkstein Stress Scale; Dyadic Adjustment Scale; Family APGAR; Social Support Questionnaire; Mishel Uncertainty in Illness Scale; Beck Hopelessness Scale; Brief Symptom Inventory; Psychosocial Adjustment to Illness Scale | This was a comparison study between benign and malignant groups over time. It cited Scott et al. (1980) but did not test theory.

Couples with malignancy reported greater decreases in marital and family functioning, uncertain appraisals, and more adjustment problems with illness compared to benign couples.

Levels of adjustment by women with malignancy corresponded with their those of their husbands over time.

Couples with high distress or increased role problems at diagnosis were more likely to remain highly distressed at 60 days and 1 year. | Women and their spouses were significantly older in the cancer group and were in early stages of cancer. Both groups were well educated. Race was not reported.

Quality instruments with alphas for the sample ranged from .70 to .95. |

(continued)

TABLE 10.3 Continued

Reference	Purpose	Design	Sample	Instruments	Key Findings	Relative Strengths and Weaknesses
Oberst, Hughes, Chang, and McCubbin (1991)	To describe the self-care demands of patients receiving ambulatory radiation therapy; to identify antecedent illness, personal, and resource factors that contribute to self-care burden; and to test a model of the effects of self-care burden and appraisal of the meaning of illness on patient's mood	Descriptive correlational cross-sectional design	72 adults receiving radiation therapy for cancer	Self-Care Burden Scale; Symptom Distress Scale; Family Hardiness Index; Appraisal of Illness Scale; Profile of Mood States; personal and illness characteristics	Symptom distress was the best predictor of universal self-care burden, whereas dependency was the best predictor of health deviation self-care burden.

Universal self-care burden, family hardiness, and symptom distress were significant predictors of stress appraisals. Health deviation self-care burden was not entered into the regression equations.

Appraisal mediated the effects of universal self-care burden and symptom distress on affective mood, partially supporting the model. Health deviation self-care burden was not mediated by appraisal.

Predictors of affective mood included stress appraisals (35%) followed by symptom distress, family hardiness, and health deviation self-care burden. Universal self-care burden was not entered. | Patients were primarily middle income with various types of cancer represented. No data on race were reported.

Alpha reliability estimates were acceptable (.75 to .96), except for the diet subscales, which were not used in subsequent analyses.

There was great variability in symptom distress and mood scores.

There were low means in relation to the ranges for self-care burden and mood scores. |

Oberst, Thomas, Gass & Ward (1989)	To test reliability of the newly developed Appraisal of Caregiving Scale; to describe demands of caregiving; to explore interrelationships between caregiver and situational characteristics, appraisal, and demands.	Crosssectional, descriptive correlational design	47 family caregivers of cancer radiotherapy patients	Appraisal of Caregiving Scale, Caregiver Load Scale	Predictors of somatic mood were symptom distress (50%) followed by appraisal. Family hardiness, universal and health deviation self-care burden were not entered.	Sample in lower middle to upper middle income range, no race reported.
					Caregiver load was positively correlated with patient dependency ($r = .53$, $p < .001$) and length of time on radiation ($r = .35$, $p < .05$).	Small convenience sample from a single site.
					Strong correlations between caregiver load and the harm/loss ($r = .48$) and threat ($r = .41$) appraisal subscales ($p < .001$).	Reliability alphas acceptable (.72 to .91).
						Measures in early stages of development.
					Harm/loss and threat appraisal subscales highly correlated ($r = .85$, $p < .001$).	There were high intercorrelations between threat and harm and loss subscales and between benign and challenge subscales, suggesting overlap.
					Challenge and benign correlated ($r = .64$, $p < .001$). Threat and benign correlated ($r = -.32$, $p < .05$).	

(continued)

TABLE 10.3 Continued

Reference	Purpose	Design	Sample	Instruments	Key Findings	Relative Strengths and Weaknesses
Pellino and Oberst (1992)	To describe how persons with chronic low back pain appraise or evaluate their illness and explore the relationships between this appraisal, pain level, mood, and personal control over pain.	Cross-sectional, descriptive correlational design	40 chronic low back pain patients	Appraisal of Illness Scale; Locus of Control Scales; modified Headache Locus of Control Scale; Survey of Pain Attitudes Solitude Subscale; Profile of Mood States; Visual Analog Scale for pain, patient, and illness characteristics	There was 29% variance in pain accounted for by internal control of pain, with challenge and negative appraisals not entered. There was 61% variance in mood accounted for by internal control of pain, challenge appraisal, and negative appraisal, with the pain rating not entered. A mediating role of appraisal on mood was supported. There was 41% variance of negative appraisal from lack of social support and internal control of pain. There was 28% variance of challenge appraisal from general powerful others locus of control and internal control of pain. There was 12% internal control of pain predicted by years of education.	The sample had a fairly high level of education and income. Race was not reported. There was a relatively small, convenience sample recruited from one site. Alpha reliability estimates for scales were between .80 and .90, except for internal pain control (.64). Subjects scored high on internal locus of pain control.

| Roman et al. (1995) | To explore differences in maternal mood states, self-esteem, family functioning, maternal-infant interaction, and home environment between mothers of preterm infants who participated in a nurse-managed program of parent-to-parent support and those who served as a comparison group | Longitudinal, quasi-experimental design | 58 mothers of preterm infants at discharge, 42 mothers at 1 and 4 months after discharge, and 47 mothers at 12 months after discharge | Rosenberg Self-Esteem Scale; Profile of Mood States; Feetham Family Functioning Scale; Barnard Nursing Child Assessment Scale; Caldwell's Home Observation for Measurement of the Environment Inventory | Intervention was based on a family ecological model that cited Scott et al. (1980), among other theorists. During the first 4 months, there was a group by time interaction. Mothers in the treatment group increased self-esteem, whereas mothers in the comparison group decreased self-esteem. Anxiety-tension was less in the treatment group during the first 4 months. Treatment group at 12 months scored higher on the Bernard measure and the Caldwell measure. The study did not test theory, just used it as rationale for intervention. | The study controlled for potential contamination of comparison families by enrolling them in the study first, with a phase lag before initiating the treatment group. Minorities were underrepresented. Alpha reliability estimates for the sample ranged from .76 to .96. The study provides a good description of intervention and training of volunteers. Of the 56 subjects, only 21 returned data for all four data collection points. A small, nonrandom convenience sample was used. |

(continued)

TABLE 10.3 Continued

Reference	Purpose	Design	Sample	Instruments	Key Findings	Relative Strengths and Weaknesses
Scott, Oberst, and Bookbinder (1984)	To evaluate anxiety level and problem-solving ability in men prior to cystoscopy and 6 to 8 weeks following cystoscopy and to determine the relations among these variable measures and concurrent stressors, coping methods, and degree of problem resolution following hospitalization	Longitudinal, descriptive correlational design	30 men with chronic genitourinary cancer	State-Trait Anxiety Inventory; Critical Thinking Appraisal; Social Readjustment Scale; COPE Interview	In support of Scott et al. (1980), the higher the problem-solving activity, the lower the state anxiety. Trait anxiety was not significantly related, however. Both state and trait anxiety, and concurrent major life changes, were associated with problem resolution. State and trait anxiety were correlated pre- and postcystoscopy.	The majority of the sample members were educated businessmen or professionals and actively employed. A small, nonrandom convenience sample was used. Race was not reported. Critical Thinking Ability scores were all in the 90th percentile. Alpha reliability estimates were not provided for the sample. Gender-linked responses may have influenced the responses.
Ward, Carlson-Dakes, Hughes, Kwekkeboom, and Donovan (1998)	To test a model of the relationships among concepts relevant to analgesic use	Cross-sectional, descriptive correlational	182 men and women with cancer	Barriers Questionnaire; Brief Pain Inventory; revised version of the Pain Management Index (coping); Medication Side Effect Checklist; Center for Epidemiological Studies Depression Inventory; single-item rating health	Drawn from Scott et al. (1980) and other theories is the proposition that beliefs drive coping. Findings supported this proposition in that beliefs (barriers) were significantly related to analgesic use (coping). All the relationships in the model for the study were supported, except analgesic use (coping) was unrelated to side effects.	The majority of patients were Caucasian, married, and had post-high school education. It is questionable whether coping should be operationalized as analgesic use. Reliability alphas ranged from .70 to .91. Mean scores were low for pain, barriers, side effects, depression, and interference with life activities.

| Wong and Bramwell (1992) | To determine the relationship between uncertainty and anxiety associated with mastectomy for breast cancer and to examine the responses of women to partial or complete mastectomy for breast cancer during the early rehabilitative phase | Longitudinal, descriptive correlational design | 25 women having their first partial or modified radical mastectomy | State-Trait Anxiety Inventory; Mishel Uncertainty Illness Scale; Semistructured Interview Schedule | There was a significant relationship between uncertainty and state anxiety postdischarge ($r = .42$, $p < .05$), consistent with Scott et al.'s (1980) model. The relationship, however, was not significant before discharge.

Descriptive findings indicated changes in appraisals over time, consistent with Scott et al.'s (1980) model. | A small, nonrandom convenience sample from two sites was used. Race was not reported.

Alpha reliabilities ranged from .71 to .92.

It is questionable whether frequencies of appraisal responses adequately capture the conceptual definition of appraisal.

It is uncertain whether all subjects were informed of their final pathology results and need for further treatment.

There was too little time between Time 1 and Time 2 to determine differences.

Subjects asked the researcher many questions about treatments, which may have influenced the findings. |

TABLE 10.4 Selected Measures for the Scott, Oberst, and Dropkin (1980) Concept of Stressors

Name of Measure (Developer)	Variables Measured	Brief Description	Reliability	Validity	Populations Studied
Caregiver Load Scale (Oberst, Thomas, Gass, & Ward, 1989)	Time and energy family caregivers expend in caregiving activities	10-item self-report tool rated on a 5-point response scale	Internal consistency alpha = .87.	There is content validity with caregivers and clinicians and construct validity by correlations with patient's dependency and length of time receiving treatment.	Family caregivers of cancer radiotherapy patients (Oberst et al., 1989) Family caregivers of hip fracture patients (Williams, Oberst, Bjorklund, & Hughes, 1996)
Caregiving Burden Scale (Carey, Oberst, McCubbin, & Hughes, 1991)	Time (demand) and difficulty associated with caregiving tasks; modified from the Caregiver Load Scale	14-item self-report tool rated on two separate 5-point response scales (demand and difficulty)	Internal consistency alphas = .83 for demand and .89 for difficulty.	Correlation between demand and difficulty = .73. Combined demand and difficulty score correlated with patient dependency and seriousness.	Family caregivers of outpatient chemotherapy patients (Carey et al., 1991) Family caregivers of pediatric renal transplant patients (Fedewa & Oberst, 1996) Family caregivers of stroke survivors (Bakas & Champion, 1999)
Self-Care Burden Scale (Oberst, Hughes, Chang, & McCubbin, 1991)	Self-care tasks representing demands related to health deviation and universal self-care	13-item self-report tool rated on two separate 5-point response scales (demand and difficulty) with three subscales (universal self-care, health deviation, and diet)	Internal consistency reliability alphas = .70 to .92, except for the diet demand subscale (.46).	Factor analysis supported three subscales. Health deviation and universal self-care correlated (r = .56); both are subscales predicted by symptom distress and dependency.	Cancer radiation therapy patients (Oberst et al., 1991) Cancer chemotherapy patients (Munkres, Oberst, & Hughes, 1992)

TABLE 10.5 Selected Measures for the Scott et al. (1980) Concept of Appraisal

Name of Measure (Developer)	Variables Measured	Brief Description	Reliability	Validity	Populations Studied
Appraisal of Caregiving Scale (Oberst, Thomas, Gass, & Ward, 1989)	Intensity of potential stress responses associated with caregiving tasks, relationships, interpersonal support, lifestyle, emotional and physical health, and overall personal impact	53-item self-report scale; four subscales (harm and loss, threat, challenge, and benign) rated on a 5-point Likert-type scale	Internal consistency alphas = .72 to .91 for the subscales.	Content was validated by six clinical experts. Each subscale was related to at least one other caregiver or illness variable. High intercorrelations among the subscales indicate overlapping constructs.	Family caregivers of cancer radiotherapy patients (Oberst et al., 1989)
Appraisal of Caregiving Scale (Carey, Oberst, McCubbin, & Hughes, 1991)	Same as the Appraisal of Caregiving Scale by Oberst et al. (1989), only 19 items added	72-item self-report scale; four subscales (harm and loss, threat, challenge, and benign) rated on a 5-point Likert-type scale	Internal consistency alphas = .74 to .91 for the subscales.	Harm and loss and threat were highly correlated (r = .90) so they were combined into negative appraisal. Negative appraisal and age predicted mood, lending support for construct validity.	Family caregivers of outpatient chemotherapy patients (Carey et al., 1991) Family caregivers of pediatric renal transplant patients (Fedewa & Oberst, 1996) Family caregivers of stroke survivors (Bakas & Champion, 1999)
Appraisal of Illness Scale (Oberst, Hughes, Chang, & McCubbin, 1991)	Possible appraisals in response to illness-related situations and concerns	27-item self-report total scale measuring threat, loss, financial strain, and overall stressfulness rated on a 5-point scale	Internal consistency reliability alpha = .95 for the total scale.	Appraisal was predicted by symptom distress and family hardiness. Appraisal mediated the relationship between self-care burden and mood.	Cancer radiation therapy patients (Oberst et al., 1991) Cancer chemotherapy patients (Munkres, Oberst, & Hughes, 1992) Chronic low back pain patients (Pellino & Oberst, 1992)

(continued)

TABLE 10.5 Continued

Name of Measure (Developer)	Variables Measured	Brief Description	Reliability	Validity	Populations Studied
The Cognitive Appraisal of Health Scale (Kessler, 1998)	Multiple dimensions of primary and secondary appraisals associated with potentially stressful health-related events	28-item self-report scale; four subscales (threat, challenge, harm and loss, and benign and irrelevant) and 5-item secondary appraisal scale; 5-point response scale for all items	Internal consistency reliability alphas = .72 to .88.	Content validity was determined by six experts. Construct validity was determined by factor analysis. There were correlations among subscales and correlations with secondary appraisal items.	Women with breast cancer (Kessler, 1998)

diverse or both. Tables 10.4 and 10.5 summarize selected instruments used to measure the SOD concepts of stressors and appraisal, respectively.

Studies have supported a relationship between appraisal and affective response as proposed in the SOD model and, for the most part, the proposed relationship between caregiver burden and appraisal. Results indicated that as the level of threat increased, persons experienced greater mood disturbance (Carey et al., 1991; Munkres, Oberst, & Hughes, 1992; Oberst et al., 1991; Pellino & Oberst, 1992). Greater caregiver burden was associated with higher levels of threat and harm (Carey et al., 1991; Oberst, Thomas, Gass, & Ward, 1989). Likewise, greater self-care burden was related to more stressful appraisals in illness situations (Oberst et al., 1991). Self-care burden was not found to be a significant predictor of stressful appraisals in illness situations (Munkres et al., 1992). Lower economic status was related to more stressful appraisals in illness situations and more self-care burden. This finding suggests that economic status may be a mediating variable between self-care burden and stressful appraisals.

Few researchers have examined coping using the SOD model as their theoretical framework, possibly due to the lack of clarity regarding how coping strategies fit into the model. Of the studies that were conducted, findings are mixed. Scott, Oberst, and Bookbinder (1984) found that greater use of problem-solving coping in stressful situations was associated with less state anxiety in men with genitourinary cancer. No significant association between coping and length of hospital stay was found in a study of patients who underwent head and neck surgery for cancer (Dropkin, 1997). Similarly, Ward, Carlson-Dakes, Hughes, Kwekkeboom, and Donovan (1998) found no significant relationship between coping defined as analgesic use and quality of life in patients with cancer after controlling for pain and analgesic side effect severity.

The measures of coping and the dependent variables differed among the studies, and problems with reliability and validity of the coping measures may have accounted for some of the mixed results. For example, Dropkin (1997) did not examine coping strategies individually but rather combined eight different types of efforts into one broad measure. Some coping strategies may be more important than others in contributing to a person's quality of life, and their use may change depending on appraisal.

Critical Examination

A weakness of the SOD model is the inconsistency in some of the relationship statements. For example, Scott et al. (1980) state that emotion, endocrine, and behavioral responses are dependent variables following the appraisal of the stress configuration. Later, however, the authors indicate that emotion is a powerful intervening variable between appraisal and behavioral response rather than a dependent variable. Also, schematic representations of the model fail to depict the direct relationship between appraisal and behavioral responses that is indicated in the narrative description of the model.

A second concern is that the model does not clearly indicate how coping strategies fit into the model. It is possible that the intent was to incorporate coping strategies within the behavioral display and response concept. This is not clear, however, because they were treated as different concepts when they were defined.

In summary, the SOD model shares many similarities with Lazarus and Folkman's (1984) model but differs in three ways: (a) the assumption that every individual under stress initially experiences anxiety, (b) conceptual definitions of appraisal and secondary appraisal, and (c) linear relationships among the concepts. Major weaknesses of the model include considerable overlap between the concepts of behavioral response and coping; inconsistencies in how some of the concepts are related;

and lack of clarity in terms of the relationship of coping to other concepts in the model.

Implications

A major contribution of Oberst and colleagues' work is that they extended the Lazarus model by the addition of two major antecedents to emotions: caregiver burden and self-care burden. The SOD model can also be used as a general framework from which midrange theories can be derived to guide nursing research studies. Future studies need to examine caregiver burden and self-care burden with longitudinal designs to determine the relationships among the various constructs over time. Use of reliable and valid measures of coping that are consistent with the SOD model conceptual definitions would be beneficial for comparing results across studies of caregiving. Little is known about the contribution of coping to specific health outcomes in caregivers.

Nursing implications that can be derived from the empirical findings include the importance of assessing caregiver burden (e.g., time and effort with caregiving tasks) when working with individuals who provide for family and significant others experiencing illness. Individuals with high caregiver burden may be more likely to appraise the caregiving situation as highly stressful and experience negative mood states. Thus, these individuals may benefit from nursing interventions designed to alleviate stress.

Coping Measurement (Anne Jalowiec)

A third program of research that has generated substantial nursing knowledge of stress, coping, and health relationships was directed by Anne Jalowiec and colleagues. Their major contributions have been made in two primary areas. They examined relationships among selected constructs in Lazarus's (1966) theory of stress and coping with cardiac transplantation patients, and they developed and evaluated the psychometric properties of the Jalowiec Coping Scale.

The research of Jalowiec and colleagues (Grady, Jalowiec, & White-Williams, 1996, 1999; Grady et al., 1993; Jalowiec & Powers, 1981; Jalowiec, Murphy, & Powers, 1984) built on the work of Lazarus's (1966) interaction model. She extended that model to incorporate additional constructs that were applicable to persons with chronic illnesses, such as cardiomyopathy. Particularly noteworthy is Jalowiec's addition of the constructs "symptoms" as an antecedent and "quality of life" as a health outcome of the stress and coping process. In addition, she employed a longitudinal research design to examine changes in patients undergoing transplanation. This methodological approach is consistent with Lazarus's assumption that stress and coping are dynamic processes that change over time and space. Jalowiec identified the need for measurement of psychosocial needs in patients undergoing transplantation in the early 1980s when transplants of any kind were uncommon.

Jalowiec Coping Scale

The Jalowiec Coping Scale (JCS) (Jalowiec et al., 1984) is the most frequently used measure of coping in nursing studies. The JCS was initially developed because existing instruments designed to measure coping did not adequately address coping behaviors used by individuals with health problems. Their simple "yes or no" checklists limited the variability of subjects' responses. The original 1977 JCS was based on Lazarus's stress and coping theoretical framework. It was revised in 1987 to assess a larger number of coping strategies and to include an appraisal of perceived coping effectiveness (Jalowiec, 1991).

The JCS assesses coping with numerous physical, emotional, and social stressors. Included are life, developmental, work, and illness stressors and stressors related to natural disasters. It measures use and effectiveness of 60 cognitive and behavioral coping strategies.

Items are categorized into eight coping sub-scales: confrontive, evasive, optimistic, fatal-istic, emotive, palliative, supportant, and self-reliant. Use and effectiveness are rated on a 0- to 3-point scale (never used to often used and not helpful to very helpful). The JCS can be used for adults of all ages in both well and ill populations. It has been used with both patient and family member populations (Jalowiec, Grady, & White-Williams, 1994; Jalowiec & Powers, 1981). It is either self- or interviewer-administered and takes 10 to 15 minutes to complete with a grade school reading level. The JCS has been translated into 18 languages and used cross-culturally worldwide.

The JCS has numerous strengths. For both the use and the effectiveness compo-nents, there are multidimensional subscales. Although situation-specific coping can be as-sessed, items are sufficiently broad to have relevance to a wide variety of encounters. The 4-point scaling allows for variability in re-sponses. The homogeneity reliabilities for to-tal use and total effectiveness scales have been consistently high, and content and predictive validity have been well established (Jalowiec, 1991).

Several psychometric limitations of the scale have been noted. A major weakness of the JCS is the low reliabilities of several of its subscales. Only two of the eight coping subscales (confrontive coping and evasive coping) have consistently reached acceptable reliability levels (i.e., αs = .70 or higher). Mean Cronbach coefficient alphas for the re-maining six coping subscales have been less than .60 with one exception—the mean alpha for "optimistic coping" subscale, which was .68 (Jalowiec, 1991). Additional studies are needed to identify the extent to which persons use only one or two strategies, in which case the internal consistency reliability would be low and there could be a "ceiling effect" due to the use of few strategies.

Another weakness of the JCS is that con-firmatory factor analysis has failed to support the eight-factor structure proposed for the scale (Jalowiec, 1988). Although this may have been due to the small sample sizes, the structure of the scale needs further evaluation. In addition, the coping effectiveness scale does not provide information about what a person considers when he or she determines the efficacy of a coping strategy. It is possible that a person views a particular coping strat-egy as helpful in reducing stress, but the cost for using that particular strategy may be too great. For example, a person who fails to take any action by avoiding thinking about his or her symptoms of illness may view this as an effective coping strategy because it reduces or eliminates stress-related emotions. By not taking appropriate action, however, the person could place his or her life in jeopardy, and thus the price for avoidance is too high to be considered effective.

Empirical Adequacy

Studies conducted by Anne Jalowiec were identified through CINAHL and MED-LINE searches. Research by other investiga-tors using the JCS or aspects of Jalowiec's work also were selected. Twenty-one citations were found. An overview of studies based on Jalowiec's work is presented in Table 10.6. Table 10.7 lists selected measures for coping, including the JCS.

Critical Evaluation

Anne Jalowiec's contributions to nursing science are substantial, particularly in the ar-eas of stress, coping, and health and the mea-surement of these constructs in persons under-going cardiac transplantation. The research conducted by Jalowiec and colleagues is clearly theoretically based and consistent with assumptions of Lazarus's theory of stress and coping. The longitudinal methodology used in many of the studies allows for careful exami-nation of relationships among important vari-ables (including stressors, social support, cop-ing, functioning, emotions, and quality of life) over time and provides empirical support for Lazarus's model in a chronically ill patient population. Jalowiec extended Lazarus's work by adding the constructs of "symptoms" and

(text continued on page 258)

TABLE 10.6 Selected Research Studies Based on Jaloweic's Work

Reference	Purpose	Design	Sample	Instruments	Key Findings	Relative Strengths and Weaknesses
Grady et al. (1993)	To examine the helpfulness of interventions by health care providers as perceived by persons awaiting heart transplants and to examine the relationship between interventions and quality of life	Descriptive correlational	Convenience sample of 175 adults awaiting heart transplantation; mean age = 52; majority were male, white, married, and not working; mean level of education, 13 years	Heart Transplant Intervention Scale, 89 items measure helpfulness of interventions (six subscales); Social Support Index, measures extent of social support; SIP, measures functional disability; Heart Transplant Symptom Checklist, measures bother from symptoms; Heart Transplant Stressor Index, measures how much each factor is a stressor; Jalowiec Coping Scale, measures coping use and effectiveness.	The 11 most helpful interventions were ranked—the 3 most helpful were provision of information, teaching self-care, and emotional support. Satisfaction with social support was significantly correlated with perceptions of helpfulness of intervention ($p < .0001$). Subjects with more functional disability perceived interventions to be more helpful ($p < .003$). Subjects with greater symptom distress perceived interventions as more helpful ($p < .006$).	The study had adequate tool reliability and validity. Findings may not apply to other samples and populations. Tools may not be valid with other populations.

Herth (1990)	To examine the relationship of supportive networks, concurrent losses, and coping skills to adaptation among elderly widow(er)s	Descriptive correlational	75 bereaved spouses obtained via stratified random sampling; mean age = 79; most were females, most Caucasian, and most had high school education or less; mean number of years married = 49	Herth Health Scale, measures hope as multidimensional concept; JCS, measures use and effectiveness of coping behaviors; GRI, measures grief resolution, the adaptation measure for this study	There were significant positive relationships between level of grief resolution and level of hope, the presence of one or fewer losses, and use of problem-focused coping ($p < .001$). There was a significant negative relationship between level of grief resolution and hope and use of emotion-focused coping ($p < .001$). Those whose spouse died in a hospice setting had significantly better grief resolution ($p < .001$).	The study had good tool reliability and validity. Findings may not apply to other samples and populations. There was a single measure of adaptation. No r or p values were given for correlation between hope and grief resolution.
Jalowiec, Grady, and White-Willliams (1994)	To examine transplant-related stressors of patients during the wait for a new heart and to examine psychometric properties of a tool that measures heart transplant stressors during the pre-op waiting period	Descriptive and methodological	Same as described in Grady et al. (1993)	Heart Transplant Stressor Scale, 78 transplant-related factors rated on the level of stressfulness	Cronbach alpha for total scale = .95 and for subscales was from .78 to .90. Three-month test-retest reliability = .73. Construct validity was determined with contrasted groups ($t = 7.76, p = .000$). Common stressors dealt with symptoms, medications, waiting for a donor, and dependency.	Items were developed by researchers and clinical experts—50% of items seen as relevant by the majority of sample. Findings may not apply to other transplant populations.

(continued)

TABLE 10.6 Continued

Reference	Purpose	Design	Sample	Instruments	Key Findings	Relative Strengths and Weaknesses
Killeen (1990)	To examine the relationship between stress, coping, and influence on health of caregivers	Correlational	Purposive sample of 126 family caregivers who provided care in the home of persons more than 65 years old	Perceived Stress Scale, measures perception of life situations as stressful; JCS, measures use of coping behaviors; Current Health Scale, measures perception of person's own health	There was a significant increase in the amount of stress as amount of free time decreased ($p < .006$). There was a significant positive relationship between perceived stress and use of emotion-focused coping behaviors ($p < .001$). Caregivers used significantly more problem-focused than emotion-focused coping behaviors ($p < .001$). Persons with higher levels of stress had significantly lower perceptions of health ($p < .05$).	There was good reliability and validity for all tools used, except for emotion-focused coping scale ($\alpha = .63$). Recipients of care were older persons, and findings may not apply when recipients are younger. Fifty percent of caregivers had a supportive role versus total care.
Murphy, Powers, and Jalowiec (1985)	To update the psychometric property information of the Hemodialysis Stressor Scale	Methodological— combined date from two samples	174 dialysis patients; mean age: Sample 1 = 48, Sample 2 = 45; sample 1 had more married subjects and more time on dialysis	Hemodialysis Stressor Scale, measured incidence and severity of stressors; 21 items with two dimensions (physiological and psychological); rated on 5-point Likert-type scale	Two- and three-factor analyses were performed. The three-factor solution was the most concise and interpretable: Factor I (psychobiological), $\alpha = .83$; Factor II (psychosocial), $\alpha = .79$; Factor III (dependency and restriction), $\alpha = .70$. These factors explained 31% of the variance	The study used a volunteer sample. Data were combined from two studies conducted in different circumstances. There was an even distribution on gender and good Cronbach alphas for three factors. The study provided additional evidence of reliability and validity for the tool.

Powers and Jalowiec (1987)	To identify predictors of physiological and psychosocial outcomes of care in hypertensive patients	Descriptive correlational	450 persons with hypertension randomly selected, mean age = 59 years; nearly equal distribution between genders; mostly white and unemployed	Psychological Adjustment to Illness Scale (PAIS), measures adjustment to chronic illness; MHLOCS, measures control over health; Quality of Life, measures quality of life; JCS, measures use of coping behaviors; Hypertension Knowledge Test, measures knowledge of hypertension; sodium, calcium, potassium, and caloric intake/day; Health History Questionnaire, measures general health information; hypertension control, physician evaluated	There were eight significant predictors of hypertension control (e.g., better PAIS score, more illness-related job problems, and greater satisfaction with health care). There were 19 significant predictors of adjustment to chronic illness (e.g., negative history of cardiac medications, fewer hypertension-related health problems, and hypertension under control). 42% of the variance was explained.	Random selection was used, but subjects were mostly white, unemployed, and middle-aged. Findings may not be applicable to other populations. There was evidence of reliability and validity for all tools, except for internal control dimension of MHLOCS. A large percentage of variance was explained with variables included in the study.
Wikoff and Miller (1989)	To further examine psychometric properties of JCS in a different population	Methodological	210 spouses of persons undergoing cardiac surgery; mean age = 60 years; mostly female and white	JCS, 34-item scale measuring use of coping behaviors	The three-factor solution was most interpretable (congruent with those previously found by Jalowiec): Factor I (confrontive), $\alpha = .84$; Factor II (palliative), $\alpha = .70$; and Factor III (emotive), $\alpha = .74$.	A wide geographic area was used to obtain subjects. The study used a volunteer sample, and findings may not apply to other populations. The study showed support for factors in JCS.

TABLE 10.7 Selected Measures for Coping

Name of Measure (Developer)	Variables Measured	Brief Description	Reliability	Validity	Populations Studied
Jalowiec Coping Scale (Jalowiec, Murphy, & Powers, 1984)	General or situation-specific coping behavior associated with stressful situations	40-item self-report tool rated a 5-point response scale (degree of use) with two subscales (problem oriented and affective oriented)	Evidence of stability was provided by a 2-week and a 1-month retest, with significant rhos ranging from .78 to .86. Alpha reliability estimates were .85 and .86 for two separate samples ($N = 141$ and $N = 150$).	Content validity was supported by 20 experts in stress and coping in which items were dichotomized into problem- and affective-oriented items with 85% consensus. Construct validity was supported by a two-factor solution in which 80% of the problem items loaded on Factor I, and 56% of the affective items loaded on Factor II. A four-factor solution, however, provided the most meaningful conceptual pattern (cognitive, tension-modulating, powerlessness, and other-directed).	Hypertensive and emergency room patients (Jalowiec & Powers, 1981) Dialysis patients (Baldree, Murphy, & Powers, 1982; Murphy, 1982; Swanson, 1982)
Jalowiec Coping Scale (Jalowiec, 1988)	Same as the Jalowiec Coping Scale (Jalowiec et al., 1984), only reanalyzed using 1,400 subjects	40-item self-report tool rated a 5-point response scale (degree of use) with two subscales (problem oriented and affective oriented)	Reliability estimates supported the trichotomous model (coefficient of determination = .95) and homogeneity of content within each factor ($\alpha = .85, .70,$ and .75).	Content validity was substantiated by the review of 20 experts, a literature base, a large number of items, and diverse coping behaviors. Confirmatory factor analyses using LISREL-IV yielded a trichotomous model as the best fit with the labels confrontive, emotive, and palliative for the three coping dimensions.	For this study, data were obtained from 22 different investigators from 10 states. Types of subjects were patients (56%), nurses (25%), family members of patients (10%), and graduate students (9%). Patients were from a wide variety of populations.

Instrument	Description	Tool	Reliability	Validity	Populations
Jalowiec Coping Scale (Jalowiec, 1991)	Jalowiec Coping Scale revised to include 20 more items, two response scales, and eight subscales based on 744 subjects	60-item self-report tool rated two 4-point response scales (use and effectiveness) with eight coping style subscales (confrontive, evasive, optimistic, fatalistic, emotive, palliative, supportant, and self-reliant)	Alpha reliability estimates for total use and effectiveness scales were .64 to .97. Mean alphas for use subscales were as follows: confrontive (.80), evasive (.72), optimistic (.68), fatalistic (.52), emotive (.58), palliative (.48), supportant (.52), and self-reliant (.59). Mean alphas for effectiveness subscales were as follows: confrontive (.80), evasive (.74), optimistic (.74), fatalistic (.47), emotive (.55), palliative (.50), supportant (.55), and self-reliant (.61). Retest correlations for total use and effectiveness scales were .56 to .72.	Content validity was supported by 25 experts in stress and coping. Agreement of the subscales ranged from 54% (emotive) to 94% (supportant). Additional support for validity provided was by Jaloweic data on pre-op cardiac transplant patients (N = 142). There were significant correlations of the subscales with a variety of illness, stress, health, social, and quality of life variables. Correlations among subscales ranged from .14 to .65. Factor analysis of the new scale was not provided.	Samples of 12 different investigators included elderly, family members of critically ill, preterm mothers, nurses, and patients with end stage renal disease, cardiac problems, cardiac transplant surgery, and back problems.
Ways of Coping Questionnaire (Folkman & Lazarus, 1988c)	Revised version of the Ways of Coping Checklist; assesses thoughts and actions individuals use to cope with stressful encounters of everyday living	66-item self-report tool with a 4-point response scale (use of strategy) and eight subscales (confrontive, distancing, self-controlling, social support, responsibility, escape-avoidance, planful problem solving, and positive reappraisal)	Alpha reliabilities for the 50 items in the eight subscales ranged from .61 (distancing) to .79 (positive reappraisal).	Factor analysis of the remaining 50 items yielded eight subscales. Sixteen items were eliminated from the analysis due to the nature of the loadings. Intercorrelations among subscales ranged from .01 to .39. Construct validity was based on results of studies reported by Folkman and Lazarus (1988). Findings were consistent with theoretical propositions.	The earlier version was based on community residents ages 45 to 64, married couples, and college students. This version was developed based on 150 community-residing married couples with at least one child living at home. This scale has been used with several different types of populations.

"quality of life," which are important outcomes for persons undergoing transplantation (Grady et al., 1995, 1999).

Overall, Jalowiec's work supports the relationships proposed in the Lazarus model with some exceptions. Jalowiec identified that symptoms were among the most common stressors experienced by patients undergoing cardiac transplantation. In addition, she found that symptoms and health status were significant predictors of quality of life among patients receiving heart transplants (Grady et al., 1995). Patients used a variety of coping strategies to deal with the stressors they experienced. Other investigators have built on the knowledge gained from Jalowiec's work by incorporating symptoms as an important stressor that can diminish quality of life in persons living with chronic illness (Murphy, Powers, & Jalowiec, 1985).

Because Jalowiec's work has been primarily descriptive and longitudinal, rather than experimental, there are gaps in knowledge regarding whether interventions directed at managing stressful symptoms can improve coping and enhance quality of life. Nursing investigators are currently focusing on symptom management as a primary way to improve quality of life, and it has become a priority funding area at the National Institute for Nursing Research (University of San Francisco School of Nursing Symptom Management Faculty Group, 1994).

The JCS is available for use in research. Additional psychometric testing is warranted to validate and strengthen the subscale structure. Also needed is the determination of the sensitivity of the JCS to focused nursing care. This sensitivity issue will be critical as nursing interventions are evaluated for effectiveness in improving health outcomes in chronically ill populations.

Other Stress and Coping Research

Other theories or models or both that have been derived from Lazarus's work are widely recognized in nursing and are discussed in-depth in other chapters of this volume. These include Mishel's uncertainty model (Mishel, 1981, 1984), social support theories and models (Norbeck & Tilden, 1983), Benner's (1984) and Benner and Wrubel's (1989) work on caring, and Roy's Adaptation Model (Andrews & Roy, 1991; Roy & Roberts, 1981), which was based on the conceptualizations of Selye (1936) and Lazarus (1966, 1978).

Summary

The contributions of the previously discussed nurse scientists to the extension of Lazarus's theory of stress and coping in promoting coping and health of patients are very important. Their research represents a continuous, concerted effort by nurse scientists to apply, adapt, and modify this psychological theory to situations that are stress producing and require effective coping to derive positive health benefits.

Nurse researchers have examined many aspects of the Lazarus model and, in general, the results have provided support for the relationships among the proposed stress, coping, and health concepts. Empirical support appears strongest for the relationship between specific stressors (particularly stress-inducing procedures) and symptoms and the outcomes of functional status and negatively toned emotions. There is less empirical support for coping as the major factor influencing health. This is inconsistent with Lazarus's studies that supported a strong relationship between coping strategies and positive outcomes (Folkman & Lazarus, 1980, 1985, 1986). This inconsistency may be due, at least in part, to the difficulties in the measurement of coping in illness populations and the primary use of descriptive, cross-sectional designs in nursing. It also may mean that individuals faced with health problems employ coping strategies that they do not usually use.

Johnson et al. (1985), Johnson, Fuller, et al. (1978), and Johnson, Rice, et al. (1978) did not incorporate an instrument to directly measure coping efforts in their studies; coping was inferred by postoperative recovery indicators, such as ambulation activity and venturing from the home. Jalowiec and Scott, Oberst, and Dropkin, for the most part, did not use experimental designs. Because little was specifically known about coping in heart transplantation and cancer populations when these investigations were conducted, use of longitudinal descriptive designs to examine phenomena was deemed more appropriate. Limited availability of questionaires to measure the constructs also may have contributed to the selection of the methodologies used.

A major contribution of these scientists is the extension of the stress and coping model to varying patient populations, including those experiencing diagnostic procedures and acute and chronic diseases. Lazarus's empirical studies were conducted mostly with community-residing and essentially healthy individuals (Folkman & Lazarus, 1980, 1985, 1986).

The breadth of the Lazarus model was extended for nursing by the addition of concepts from nursing research. Jalowiec's addition of quality of life to the model added another dimension to the coping process that has gained increasing importance in nursing and other health care research. Quality of life is now recognized as a critical construct for persons with chronic diseases, such as heart failure and cancer. There is also consensus among health care researchers that symptoms are an important component of quality of life (Wilson & Cleary, 1995).

In addition to contributions to theory development and extension, nursing researchers have made outstanding progress in the measurement of constructs within the stress and coping model. One of the primary problems in early stress-related research was the lack of valid, reliable instruments to measure complex and multidimensional psychosocial constructs, such as appraisal, coping, and functional status. Building on conceptual definitions when available, investigators such as Johnson, Scott, Oberst, Dropkin, and Jalowiec examined and modified instruments to measure these complex constructs in patient populations. These researchers also provided exemplars for employing methodologies that were appropriate for examining stress and coping in various patient populations. These methodologies, including experimentally designed studies, can be used with other populations to continue building the science of stress and coping in nursing.

➤ IMPLICATIONS FOR NURSING RESEARCH, THEORY, AND PRACTICE

Contributions of the previously discussed nurse scientists and other scientists in stress, coping, and health during the past 40 years have provided direction for future theory development, research, and practice. There now exists an increasing cadre of nurse scientists who are experts in this area. It is time for nursing to rapidly create its own models and theories, measurements, and interventions and to test them across diverse cultural, racial, and ethnic groups. Gaps in nursing knowledge need to be attended to as research seeks to improve patient outcomes.

Additional studies are needed to identify the effects of choice of selected coping strategies on specific health outcomes. Coping is a complex construct, and choice and personal control are key elements (see Chapter 19, this volume). General measures of coping do not appear to be adequate to assess specific nursing interventions. More situation-specific measures are needed. Longitudinal designs are requisite to determining the ebb and flow of coping patterns and to identifying appropriate predictors of long-term health outcome.

The implications for use of this research knowledge in nursing practice are widespread. It is imperative that nurse scientists disseminate the knowledge gained to nurse educators, nurses in practice, and other health providers. Coping knowledge needs to be incorporated into the daily work of nurses. For this to occur, scientists will need to publish their research in usable "language" that provides direction for clinicians. Publishing the information in traditional sources read by practicing nurses, such as standard medical-surgical nursing textbooks and practice journals, could enhance its use.

Johnson's results can be used to design patient education programs. Nursing needs to instruct patients about common sensations associated with procedures they are to experience, such as insulin injection, cardiac catheterization, and radiation oncology. Jalowiec's and Oberst's results can be integrated into practice by educating nurses about symptoms that impair overall quality of life and making symptom management a priority. Patients and their families must also learn about presenting symptoms and their management.

Research utilization is key to expanding the practicing nurse's knowledge base, leading to improved quality of care for patients and their families. For example, the Stetler-Marram (Stetler, 1994) model of research utilization could be used to frame a study for translating stress and coping knowledge into practice with selected groups of patients. Only with the translation of research into nursing practice can the true value of studying stress, coping, and health relationships be realized.

➤ REFERENCES

Ahles, T. A., Blanchard, E. G., & Leventhal, H. (1983). Cognitive control of pain: Attention to the sensory aspects of the cold pressor stimulus. *Cognitive Theory and Research, 7,* 159-178.

Andrews, H. A., & Roy, C. (1991). Essentials of the Roy Adaptation Model. In C. Roy & H. A. Andrews (Eds.), *The Roy Adaptation Model: The definitive statement* (pp. 3-25). Norwalk, CT: Appleton & Lange.

Bakas, T., & Champion, V. (1999). Development and psychometric testing of the Bakas Caregiving Outcomes Scale. *Nursing Research, 48*(5), 250-259.

Baldree, K., Murphy, S., & Powers, M. A. (1982). Stress identification and coping patterns in patients on hemodialysis. *Nursing Research, 31,* 107-112.

Benner, P. (1984). *From novice to expert.* Menlo Park, CA: Addison-Wesley.

Benner, P., & Wrubel, J. (1989). *The primacy of caring.* Menlo Park, CA: Addison-Wesley.

Bramwell, L., MacKenzie, J., Laschinger, H., & Cameron, N. (1995). Need for overnight respite of primary caregivers of hospice clients. *Cancer Nursing, 18*(5), 337-343.

Carey, P. J., Oberst, M. T., McCubbin, M. A., & Hughes, S. H. (1991). Appraisal and caregiving burden in family members caring for patients receiving chemotherapy. *Oncology Nursing Forum, 18*(8), 1341-1348.

Dropkin, M. J. (1994). Anxiety, problem-focused coping strategies, disfigurement/dysfunction and postoperative coping behaviors associated with head and neck cancer (Doctoral dissertation, New York University, 1994). *Dissertation Abstracts International, 56/03,* 1345.

Dropkin, M. J. (1997). Coping with disfigurement/dysfunction and length of hospital stay after head and neck cancer surgery. *ORL-Head and Neck Nursing, 15,* 22-26.

Erickson, E. H. (1963). *Childhood and society* (2nd ed.). New York: Norton.

Fedewa, M. M., & Oberst, M. T. (1996). Family caregiving in a pediatric renal transplant population. *Pediatric Nursing, 22*(5), 402-407, 417.

Folkman, S. (1997). Positive psychological states and coping with severe stress. *Social Science and Medicine, 45,* 1207-1221.

Folkman, S., & Lazarus, R. S. (1980). An analysis of coping in a middle-aged community sample. *Journal of Health and Social Behavior, 21,* 219-239.

Folkman, S., & Lazarus, R. S. (1985). If it changes it must be a process: Study of emotion and coping during three stages of a college examination. *Journal of Personality and Social Psychology, 48,* 150-170.

Folkman, S., & Lazarus, R. S. (1986). Stress processes and depressive symptomatology. *Journal of Abnormal Psychology, 95,* 107-113.

Folkman, S., & Lazarus, R. S. (1988). *Manual for the ways of coping questionnaire.* Palo Alto, CA: Consulting Psychologists Press.

Frankenhauser, M. (1975). Experimental approaches to the study of catecholamines and emotion. In I. Levi (Ed.), *Emotions—Their parameters and measurement* (pp. 209-234). New York: Raven Press.

Freud, S. (1946). Mourning and melancholia (J. Riviere, Trans.). In *Collected papers, 4.* London: Hogarth Press. (Original work published 1917)

Fuller, S. S., Endress, M. P., & Johnson, J. E. (1978). The effects of cognitive and behavioral control on coping with an aversive health examination. *Journal of Human Stress, 4,* 18-25.

Garfield, E. (1984). Citation patterns in nursing journals and their most-cited articles. *Current Contents, 43,* 3-12.

Grady, K. L., Jalowiec, A., & White-Williams, C. (1996). Improvement in quality of life in patients with heart failure who undergo transplantation. *Journal of Heart & Lung Transplantation, 15*(8), 749-757.

Grady, K. L., Jalowiec, A., & White-Williams, C. (1999). Predictors of quality of life in patients at one year after heart transplantation. *Journal of Heart & Lung Transplantation, 18*(3), 202-210.

Grady, K. L., Jalowiec, A., White-Williams, C., Hetfleisch, M., Penicook, J., & Blood, M. (1993). Heart transplant candidates' perception of helpfulness of health care provider interventions. *Cardiovascular Nursing, 29*(5), 33-37.

Grady, K. L., Jalowiec, A., White-Williams, C., Pifarre, R., Kirklin, J. K., Bourge, R. C., & Contanzo, M. R. (1995). Predictors of quality of life in patients with advanced heart failure awaiting transplantation. *Journal of Heart & Lung Transplantation, 14,* 2-10.

Hart, K. (1986/1987). Stress encountered by significant others of cancer patients receiving chemotherapy. *Omega, 17*(2), 151-167.

Hartfield, M. J., & Cason, C. L. (1981). Effect of information on emotional responses during barium enema. *Nursing Research, 30,* 151-155.

Herth, K. (1990). Relationship of hope, coping styles, concurrent losses, and setting to grief resolution in the elderly widow(er). *Research in Nursing and Health, 13,* 109-117.

Hill, B. J. (1982). Sensory information, behavioral instructions and coping with sensory alteration surgery. *Nursing Research, 31,* 17-21.

Holmes, T. H., & Rahe, R. H. (1967). The social readjustment rating scale. *Journal of Psychosomatic Research, 11,* 213-218.

Izard, C. E. (1979). Emotions in personality and psychopathology: An introduction. In C. E. Izard (Ed.), *Emotions in personality and psychopathology.* New York: Plenum Press.

Jalowiec, A. (1988). Confirmatory factor analysis of the Jalowiec Coping Scale. In C. F. Waltz & O. L. Strickland (Eds.), *Measurement of nursing outcomes: Vol. 1. Measuring client outcomes* (pp. 287-308). New York: Springer.

Jalowiec, A. (1991). *Psychometric results on the 1987 Jalowiec Coping Scale.* Unpublished manuscript, Loyola University of Chicago, Maywood, IL.

Jalowiec, A., Grady, K. L., & White-Williams, C. (1994). Stressors in patients awaiting a heart transplant. *Behavioral Medicine, 19,* 145-154.

Jalowiec, A., Murphy, S. P., & Powers, M. J. (1984). Psychometric assessment of the Jalowiec Coping Scale. *Nursing Research, 33*(3), 157-161.

Jalowiec, A., & Powers, M. J. (1981). Stress and coping in hypertensive and emergency room patients. *Nursing Research, 30,* 10-15.

Janis, I. L. (1958). *Psychological stress: Psychoanalytic and behavioral studies of surgical patients.* New York: Academic Press.

Johnson, J. E. (1973). Effects of accurate expectations about sensations on the sensory and distress components of pain. *Journal of Personality and Social Psychology, 27,* 261-275.

Johnson, J. E. (1996). Coping with radiation therapy: Optimism and the effect of preparatory interventions. *Research in Nursing and Health, 19,* 3-12.

Johnson, J. E. (1999). Self-regulation theory and coping with physical illness. *Research in Nursing & Health, 22,* 435-448.

Johnson, J. E., Christman, N. J., & Stitt, C. (1985). Personal control interventions: Short- and long-term effects on surgical patients. *Research in Nursing and Health, 8,* 131-145.

Johnson, J. E., Fieler, V. K., Jones, L. S., Wlasowicz, G. S., & Mitchell, M. L. (1997). *Self-regulation theory: Applying theory to your practice.* Pittsburgh, PA: Oncology Nursing Press.

Johnson, J. E., Fuller, S. S., Endress, M. P., & Rice, V. H. (1978). Altering patients' responses to surgery: An extension and replication. *Research in Nursing and Health, 1,* 111-121.

Johnson, J. E., Kirchhoff, K. T., & Endress, M. P. (1975). Altering children's distress behavior during orthopedic cast removal. *Nursing Research, 24,* 404-410.

Johnson, J. E., & Leventhal, H. (1974). Effects of accurate expectations and behavioral instructions on reactions during a noxious medical examination. *Journal of Personality and Social Psychology, 29,* 710-718.

Johnson, J. E., Morrissey, J. F., & Leventhal, H. (1973). Psychological preparation for an endoscopic examination. *Gastrointestinal Endoscopy, 19,* 180-182.

Johnson, J. E., Nail, L. M., Lauver, D., King, K. G., & Keys, H. (1988). Reducing the negative impact of radiation therapy on functional status. *Cancer, 61,* 46-51.

Johnson, J. E., & Rice, V. H. (1974). Sensory and distress components of pain: Implications for the study of clinical pain. *Nursing Research, 23,* 203-209.

Johnson, J. E., Rice, V. H., Fuller, S. S., & Endress, M. P. (1978). Sensory information, instruction in a coping strategy, and recovery from surgery. *Research in Nursing and Health, 1,* 4-17.

Kessler, T. A. (1998). The Cognitive Appraisal of Health Scale: Development and psychometric evaluation. *Research in Nursing & Health, 21,* 73-82.

Killeen, M. (1990). The influence of stress and coping on family caregivers' perceptions of health. *International Journal of Aging and Human Development, 30,* 109-117.

Kim, H., Garvin, B. J., & Moser, D. K. (1999). Stress during mechanical ventilation: Benefit of having concrete objective information before cardiac surgery. *American Journal of Critical Care, 8,* 118-126.

Lazarus, R. S. (1966). *Psychological stress and the coping process.* New York: McGraw-Hill.

Lazarus, R. (1981). The stress and coping paradigm. In C. Eidsdorfer, D. Cohen, A. Kleinman, & P. Maxim (Eds.), *Models for clinical psychopathology* (pp. 177-214). New York: Spectrum.

Lazarus, R. (1991). *Emotion and adaptation.* New York: Oxford University Press.

Lazarus, R. (1998). *Fifty years of the research and theory of R. S. Lazarus: An analysis of historical and perennial issues.* London: Lawrence Erlbaum.

Lazarus, R., & Folkman, S. (1984). *Stress, appraisal, and coping.* New York: Springer.

Leventhal, H. (1970). Findings and theory in the study of fear communication. In L. Berkowitz (Ed.), *Advances in experimental social psychology* (Vol. 5, pp. 107-270). New York: Academic Press.

Leventhal, H., & Johnson, J. E. (1983). Laboratory and field experimentation: Development of a theory of self-regulation. In P. J. Wooldridge, M. Schmidt, J. K. Skipper, & R. C. Leonard (Eds.), *Behavioral science and nursing theory* (pp. 189-262). St. Louis, MO: C. V. Mosby.

Mandler, G., & Watson, D. (1966). Anxiety and the interruption of behavior. In C. D. Spielberger (Ed.), *Anxiety and behavior.* New York: Academic Press.

Mason, J. W. (1975). Endocrine parameters and emotion. In L. Levi (Ed.), *Emotions—Their parameters and measurement* (pp. 143-181). New York: Raven Press.

Mishel, M. H. (1981). The measurement of uncertainty in illness. *Nursing Research, 30,* 258-263.

Mishel, M. H. (1984). Perceived uncertainty and stress in medical patients. *Research in Nursing and Health, 7,* 163-171.

Monat, A., & Lazarus, R. S. (Eds.). (1977). *Stress and coping: An anthology.* New York: Columbia University Press.

Moos, R. H. (1986). *Coping with physical illness.* New York: Plenum.

Munkres, A., Oberst, M. T., & Hughes, S. H. (1992). Appraisal of illness, symptom distress, self-care burden, and mood states in patients receiving chemotherapy for initial and recurrent cancer. *Oncology Nursing Forum, 19*(8), 1201-1209.

Murphy, S. P. (1982). *Factors influencing adjustment and quality of life of hemodialysis patients: A multivariate approach.* Unpublished doctoral dissertation, University of Illinois, Chicago.

Murphy, S. P., Powers, M. J., & Jalowiec, A. (1985). Psychometric evaluation of the hemodialysis stressor scale. *Nursing Research, 34,* 368-371.

Nisbett, R., & Schachter, S. (1966). Cognitive manipulation of pain. *Journal of Experimental Social Psychology, 2,* 227-236.

Nolan, M. R., Grant, G., & Ellis, N. C. (1990). Stress is in the eye of the beholder: Reconceptualizing the measurement of caregiver burden. *Journal of Advanced Nursing, 15,* 544-555.

Norbeck, J. S., & Tilden, V. P. (1983). Life stress, social support, and emotional disequilibrium in complications of pregnancy: A prospective, multivariate study. *Journal of Health and Social Behavior, 24,* 30-46.

Northouse, L. L., Templin, T., Mood, D., & Oberst, M. T. (1998). Couples' adjustment to breast cancer and benign breast disease: A longitudinal analysis. *Psycho-Oncology, 7,* 37-48.

Oberst, M. T., Hughes, S. H., Chang, A. S., & McCubbin, M. A. (1991). Self-care burden, stress appraisal, and mood among persons receiving radiotherapy. *Cancer Nursing, 14*(2), 71-78.

Oberst, M. T., Thomas, S. E., Gass, K. A., & Ward, S. E. (1989). Caregiving demands and appraisal of stress among family caregivers. *Cancer Nursing, 12*(4), 209-215.

Pearlin, L. I., & Schooler, C. (1978). The structure of coping. *Journal of Health & Social Behavior, 19,* 2-21.

Pellino, T. A., & Oberst, M. T. (1992). Perception of control and appraisal of illness in chronic low back pain. *Orthopedic Nursing, 11,* 22-26.

Plutchik, R., Kellerman, H., & Conte, H. R. (1979). A structural theory of ego defenses and emotions. In C. E. Izard (Ed.), *Emotions in personality and psychopathology.* New York: Plenum.

Powers, M. J., & Jalowiec, A. (1987). Profile of the well-controlled, well-adjusted hypertensive patient. *Nursing Research, 36,* 106-110.

Rice, V. H. (1990). Coping: An important construct for nursing. *Search: Improved Nursing Care Through Research, 14,* 1-3.

Rice, V. H., Caldwell, M., Butler, S., & Robinson, J. (1986). Relaxation training and response to cardiac catheterization: A pilot study. *Nursing Research, 35,* 39-43.

Rice, V. H., Mullin, M. H., & Jarosz, P. (1992). Preadmission self-instruction effects on postadmission and postoperative indicators in CABG patients: Partial replication and extension. *Research in Nursing & Health, 15*(4), 253-259.

Rice, V. H., Sieggreen, M., Mullin, M., & Williams, J. (1988). Development and testing of an arteriogram information intervention for stress reduction. *Heart & Lung, 17,* 23-28.

Roman, L. A., Lindsay, J. K., Boger, R. P., DeWys, M., Beaumont, E. J., Jones, A. S., & Haas, B. (1995). Parent-to-parent support initiated in the neonatal intensive care unit. *Research in Nursing & Health, 18,* 385-394.

Roy, C., & Roberts, L. L. (1981). *Theory construction in nursing: An adaptation mode.* Englewood Cliffs, NJ: Prentice Hall.

Scott, D. W., Oberst, M. T., & Bookbinder, M. I. (1984). Stress-coping response to genitourinary carcinoma in men. *Nursing Research, 33*(6), 325-329.

Scott, D. W., Oberst, M. T., & Dropkin, M. J. (1980). A stress-coping model. *Advances in Nursing Science, 3,* 9-23.

Selye, H. (1936). A syndrome produced by diverse nocuous agents. *Nature, 138,* 32.

Sigg, E. B. (1975). The organization and functions of the central sympathetic nervous system. In L. Levi (Ed.), *Emotions—Their parameters and measurement* (pp. 93-122). New York: Raven Press.

Stetler, C. B. (1994). Refinement of the Stetler/Marram model for application of research findings into practice. *Nursing Outlook, 42,* 15-25.

Suls, J., & Fletcher, B. (1985). The relative effects of avoidant and nonavoidant coping strategies: A meta-analysis. *Health Psychology, 3,* 249-288.

Swanson, J. A. (1982). *Compliance and coping in hemodialysis patients.* Unpublished master's thesis, University of Illinois, Chicago.

University of San Francisco School of Nursing Symptom Management Faculty Group. (1994). A model for symptom management. *Image: Journal of Nursing Scholarship, 26,* 272-276.

Ward, S. E., Carlson-Dakes, K., Hughes, S. H., Kwekkeboom, K. L., & Donovan, H. S. (1998). The impact on quality of life of patient-related barriers to pain management. *Research in Nursing & Health, 21,* 405-413.

Weisman, A. D. (1979). *Coping with cancer.* New York: McGraw-Hill.

Wikoff, R. L., & Miller, P. (1989). Analysis of the Jalowiec scale with cardiac patients' spouses. *Nursing Research, 38,* 221-222.

Williams, M. A., Oberst, M. T., Bjorklund, M. C., & Hughes, S. H. (1996). Family caregiving in cases of hip fracture. *Rehabilitation Nursing, 21*(3), 124-131, 138.

Wilson, I. B., & Cleary, P. D. (1995). Linking clinical variables with health-related quality of life. *Journal of the American Medical Association, 273,* 59-65.

Wong, C. A., & Bramwell, L. (1992). Uncertainty and anxiety after mastectomy for breast cancer. *Cancer Nursing, 15*(5), 363-371.

CHAPTER 11

Stress, Coping, and Health in Children

Nancy A. Ryan-Wenger, Vicki W. Sharrer, and Christine A. Wynd

tressful situations and attempts to cope with these experiences have a direct and observable impact on psychological, behavioral, and physiological systems. Therefore, these experiences are of interest to nursing and other health care professionals. Effective coping strategies may help to prevent maladaptive stress responses. Because lifelong patterns for coping with stress are begun in childhood, it is important to understand children's stressors, coping patterns, outcomes, and the environmental and individual factors that influence the stress-coping process (Haggerty, Sherrod, Garmezy, & Rutter, 1996). For the purpose of this chapter, a *child* is generally defined as a person between the ages of 6 to 18 years, unless otherwise noted. Extant knowledge about children's stress-coping processes is derived primarily from the disciplines of nursing, psychology, and medicine. This chapter, although not all-inclusive, is a synthesis of key findings from these disciplines.

➤ THEORETICAL FRAMEWORK

There are no specific models or theories to explain the entire process of children's stress and coping; the transactional model developed for adults (Lazarus & Folkman, 1984), however, is the theory most commonly applied to research in children. This dynamic transactional stress-coping process fits well within an ecological and growth and developmental model, which is critical when studying children. In an ecological model, environmental and individual characteristics interact to influence a child's behavior, and like any systems model, a change in one system (cellular, individual, family, or community) influences change in other systems (Bahg, 1990). The concepts of growth and development are critical to any model that explains children's behavior because of the tremendous changes in cognitive, physical, social, and psychological status that occur during childhood (Berk, 1997).

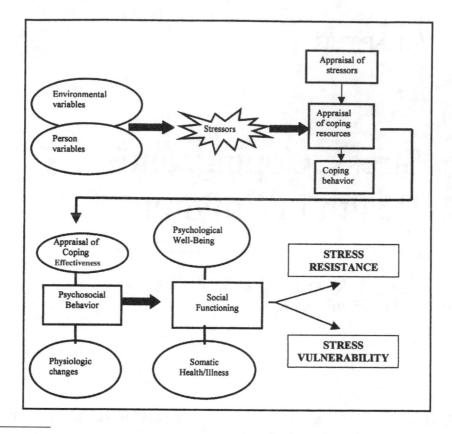

Figure 11.1. A Transactional Model of the Stress-Coping Process (adapted with permission from Lazarus, 1990)

The framework shown in Figure 11.1 is an adaptation of Lazarus's model of stress and emotion processes (Lazarus, 1990). Each child represents a unique combination of individual and environmental variables. Stressors result from person-environment interactions, which cause a child to appraise the situation, appraise the coping resources that are available to him or her, and employ a repertoire of coping behaviors. Short-term effects of the child's reaction include appraisal of the effectiveness of coping behavior, psychosocial behavior, and physiological changes. Long-term effects are manifested as psychological well-being, social functioning, and somatic health or illness. The overall effectiveness of the stress-coping process places children in a position of being relatively resistant or vulnerable to additional stress. The assumption underlying the model is that the actual stress-coping process is dynamic and interrelated—not as simplistic or linear as is reflected in the model.

Lazarus's (1990) theory has been applied to children by many researchers, but it has not specifically been tested for its adequacy with respect to children. The extent to which research and theory fit within the model and support the proposed linkages between concepts can serve as a beginning for the evaluation of the logical adequacy of the model (Walker & Avant, 1988). The key concepts in the stress-coping process model in Figure 11.1 serve as an outline for this chapter.

➤ STRESSORS

The literature reveals two major categories of stressors in children, normative and nonnormative. *Normative* refers to the common, developmental stressors of daily life (e.g., being left out of the group, parents fighting, or getting bad grades). *Nonnormative* stressors arise from unusual or traumatic experiences (e.g., serious illness of the child or parent, child abuse, or community disasters). Sources of stress are closely related to age, gender, and developmental level. In addition, growth, maturation, and expansion of environmental influences that occur with increasing age change the nature of stressful experiences (Berk, 1997). For example, "being larger than others your age" is more stressful for adolescent girls than for adolescent boys. Troubled peer relationships with same-sex friends are very stressful for school-age children, whereas the most stressful relationships for adolescents are usually with the opposite sex. In research and clinical practice, children's stressors are typically measured with various forms of checklists.

Stress in preschool, elementary, junior high, and high school children was first quantified by Coddington (1972), who developed the widely used Life Event Scales (LES) consisting of 30 to 42 stressful life events. The events were derived from the literature about adult coping behavior, the popular Holmes and Rahe (1967) Social Readjustment Rating Scale, and the author's experience with children. The amount of "life change" likely to be incurred by each stressful event was estimated by other professionals who worked with children. "Death of a parent" was assigned the highest number of "life change units." The child's total stress score was the sum of life change units for each stressor experienced in the past year. Other instruments with items derived from adults' perspective were developed, including a revision of the LES (Table 11.1).

Later, new instruments were developed that included events that children identified as stressful to them. To obtain stressors for a new instrument, children were asked to identify events that were stressful or made them "feel bad, nervous, or worried" (Lewis, Siegel, & Lewis, 1984). Children's responses were incorporated into the 20-item Feel Bad Scale (FBS). A comparison of the children's list of stressors with those identified by adults reveals very few similarities; in fact, there are only 4 items in common between the LES and the FBS (Ryan, 1988). School-age children report that their most frequently occurring stressors are feeling sick, having nothing to do, not having enough money to spend, being pressured to get good grades, and feeling left out of the group (Lewis et al., 1984). Children identified more normative, daily events related to parents, school, peers, and self, whereas adults tended to list mostly family-related, nonnormative catastrophic events. Research designed to examine children's responses to "life stress" requires instruments that tap the range of stressors that are most relevant to children.

Nurses have examined stress related to illness or hospitalization for many years; most notably is the classic work by Visintainer and Wolfer (1975). The stress of separation from parents has been reduced by more liberal visiting policies. As medical technology has advanced, however, so have the potential sources of stress to children, most notably the many invasive, frightening, and painful diagnostic tests and treatments. Children's medical fears have not changed significantly, however. When asked, children continue to identify separation from parents, needle and other "sticks," being told that something is wrong with them, and uncertainty (Broome, Hellier, Wilson, Dale, & Glanville, 1988; Hart & Bossert, 1994). Table 11.1 presents a detailed description of many instruments developed during the past 27 years to measure stressors in children from preschool age to adolescence.

Most instruments contain different types of stressors and are specifically designed for selected age groups. Despite the large number of instruments available, most were developed for and tested on largely white, middle-class children and published more than a decade ago. Sociopolitical changes have made it likely that new stressors have arisen, such as personal safety, community violence, homelessness, threat of war, AIDS, and increased availability of drugs to younger children

TABLE 11.1 Instruments for Measurement of Stressors in Children and Adolescents

Author	Instrument	Target Group	Original Source of Items	Format	Instrument Completed By	Meaning of Scores
Coddington (1972)	Life Event Record	Preschool, elementary, junior high, senior high	Author, literature (life change units determined by adults)	30-42 items; yes/no in past 12 months	Parent or adolescent	Total number of life change units = amount of social readjustment
Yamamoto (1979)	Stressful Experiences Scale	7- to 11-year-olds	Literature, classroom teachers	20 items; ranked for severity and frequency	Children	Sum of scores for each subscale = stress severity and frequency
Monaghan, Robinson, and Dodge (1979)	Children's Life Events Inventory	Children	Coddington Scales and authors (Life change units determined by adults)	40 items; check if experienced in past 12 months	Parent or child	Total number of life change units = amount of social readjustment
Yeaworth, York, Hussey, Ingle, and Goodwin (1980)	Adolescent Life Change Event Scale	Junior high, senior high	Authors (life change units determined by adolescents)	31 items; check if occurred in past 12 months	Adolescent	Sum of life change units = amount of life change
Johnson and McCutcheon (1980)	Life Events Checklist	12-17 years	Coddington scales and authors	46 items; check if occurred in past 12 months; circle if good or bad; 0-3 scale for impact of event on life	Adolescents	Sum of impact ratings for positive and negative events = positive and negative change scores
Newcomb, Huba, and Bentler (1981)	Life Events Questionnaire	7th-12th grades	Literature	39 items; rated 1-5 on a "happiness" scale; yes/no in past 12 months and before the past 12 months	Adolescents	Sum of item scores = severity score; total number of items selected = frequency score
Coddington (1984)	Life Event Scale for Children	School-age children	Adults, literature	31-47 items; yes/no in 3-month intervals (summer, fall, autumn, and spring)	Children	Total number of life change units = amount of social readjustment
	Life Event Scale for Adolescents	Adolescents		Adolescents		

TABLE 11.1 Continued

Author	Instrument	Target Group	Original Source of Items	Format	Instrument Completed By	Meaning of Scores
Beal and Schmidt (1984)	Youth Adaptation Rating Scale	Junior high, high school	Adolescents determined the items and severity ratings for each one	59 items; checked if occurred; time period not specified	Adolescents	Sum of severity ratings = degree of adaptation required
Lewis, Siegel, and Lewis (1984)	Feel Bad Scale	8- to 12-year-olds	Children	20 items; rated 1-5 for how bad it is, and how often it happens	Children	Product of total scores for severity subscale times frequency subscale = level of stress
Elwood (1987)	Stressor Inventories	4th and 7th grades	Children	Major events: 7 or 8 items; daily hassles: 16-24 items; rated on scale of 0-4 for amount of upsettingness or stressfulness	Children	Sum of scores for each event = level of stressfulness
Compas, Davis, Forsythe, and Wagner (1987)	Adolescent Perceived Events Scale—Jr. High version	Junior high	Junior high school students	142 items; yes/no during this school year; −4 to +4 on bad to good scale (desirability)	Adolescents	Total weights of positive and negative events = cognitive appraisal of stressors
Compas et al. (1987)	Adolescent Perceived Events Scale—High School version; College version	High school, college	High school and college students	200-210 items; yes/no in past 3 months; −4 to +4 on desirability, impact, and frequency	Adolescents	Sum of product of total weights for desirability times impact events = cognitive appraisal of stressors
McCubbin and Patterson (1987)	A-FILE: Adolescent-Family Inventory of Life Events and Changes	12- to 18-year-olds	Other stress scales, group of 11th graders	50 items; scored as yes/no in past 12 months and before the past 12 months	Adolescents	Sum of yes responses = amount of stressful change in family

(continued)

TABLE 11.1 Continued

Author	Instrument	Target Group	Original Source of Items	Format	Instrument Completed By	Meaning of Scores
Dise-Lewis (1988)	Life Events and Coping Inventory	12- to 15-year-olds	Adolescents	125 items; scored on scale of 1-9 for amount of stress it caused	Young adolescents	Sum of item scores = amount of stress
Broome, Hellier, Wilson, Dale, and Glanville (1988)	Child Medical Fear Scale	5- to 12-year-olds	Clinical experience of children	17 items; scale of 0-2 for level of fear	Children; parent version also available	Sum of item scores = level of medical fear
Gullone and King (1992), Burnham and Gullone (1997)	Fear Survey Schedule for Children	2nd through 12th grades	Theory, clinical experience, literature	80 items; scale of 0-2 for amount of fear perceived for each event	Children, adolescents	Sum of items scores = total level of fear
Hockenberry-Eaton, Manteuffel, and Bottomley (1997)	Childhood Cancer Stressors Inventory	7- to 13-year-olds	Literature, clinical experience	18 items; true/false for experience of each stressor; scale of 0-3 for bothersomeness of each stressor	Children	Number of stressors = frequency of stress; sum of bothersome scores = intensity of stress; sum of frequency × intensity scores = total perceived stress

(Carroll & Ryan-Wenger, 1999; Gullone & King, 1993; Neff & Dale, 1996).

➤ APPRAISAL OF STRESSORS

Lazarus and Folkman (1984) describe the individual's cognitive appraisal of person-environment interactions as irrelevant, benign-positive, or stressful. If the encounter is appraised as stressful or potentially stressful, the individual further appraises it as harm or loss, threat, or challenge. These are not necessarily mutually exclusive, which further illustrates the importance of considering the individual perspective when studying the stress-coping process. It is this appraisal that helps to determine the actual effect of the stressor on the individual. It makes little sense to ask one individual to appraise or evaluate "stress" for another.

Two studies illustrate this assertion. Yamamoto (1979) asked fourth, fifth, and sixth graders to rate 20 academic and personal stressors for level of "upsettingness." Then, he ranked the items from high to low. Seven items were similar to events on the Coddington scale; therefore, he compared the children's rankings with adult's rankings for the same items that were obtained during development of the original Coddington scale. Children ranked 2 events as much more stressful for them, 4 events were much less stressful, and 1 event was approximately the same (death of a parent) as the adults' ranking. Rende and Plomin (1991) compared parents' perception of the upsettingness of 25 life events from Coddington's scale to their first-grade children's perceptions of the same events. Parents rated 4 events as significantly higher in upsettingness than did the children. Total scores were also significantly higher for parents, suggesting that overall parents overestimated their children's level of stress.

Although most instruments measure the source of stress, and perhaps the frequency with which stressors occur, many instruments fail to measure the appraisal aspect—that is, they do not ask "how bad is it for you?" Fewer than half of the instruments listed in Table 11.1 ask children to appraise the degree of "badness," upsettingness, "desirability," or "happiness" related to each stressor listed. Lewis and others (1984) examined the relationship between badness and frequency with which stressors occurred. There was a predictable linear relationship with 10 of the 20 items on the FBS in that perceived severity increased as frequency of the stressors increased. Interestingly, children who had never experienced them ranked two items, "separation of parents" and "being pressured to try something new," highest in badness.

Children's sense of control over a stressor is part of their appraisal of the stressor. For example, being witness to parents arguing looms larger than their own arguments with a playmate. The issue of control has only recently received attention in the theoretical and research literature, but the few studies illustrate that sense of control over a stressor has an impact on well-being, coping behavior, and outcomes. In one study, children who believed that they had no control over daily stressors responded with more avoidance behaviors

than did children who perceived some control (Hardy, Power, & Jaedicke, 1993).

The primary-secondary control model was tested on a group of children with leukemia. The model assumes that many medical stressors are outside of children's control, and that children adjust their coping behavior accordingly (Wiesz, McCabe, & Dennig, 1994). Primary control coping involved attempts to alter the stressor, whereas secondary control coping included attempts to adjust oneself to the stressor or to make no attempt to cope at all (relinquished control). Children's reports of their coping strategies revealed that use of secondary control during painful medical procedures was associated with better behavioral and illness-specific adjustment.

The cognitive diathesis-stress model of depression was studied in 439 children aged 10 or 11 years (Hilsman & Garber, 1995). The stressor was receipt of unacceptable grades on a report card with resultant negative parental reactions to the grade report. The model suggests that negative thoughts and lack of control over a stressor are associated with high levels of depression. In the study, children who had negative thoughts about their low grades and felt little control over their grades experienced depressive symptoms that lasted for 5 days. Children with more positive cognitions and a sense of control reported fewer depressive symptoms and recovered more rapidly from the stress of unacceptable grades. They had more confidence in themselves and believed they could remedy the poor grades.

Few instruments are available that measure children's perceptions of control. One exception is the Student Perceptions of Control Questionnaire related to academic achievement developed by E. A. Skinner and colleagues at the University of Rochester (cited in Hilsman & Garber, 1995). It would be useful to identify children's perceptions of control over their stressors, and, where there is potential for change in perceptions, clinicians can help children find ways to regain some control and thus change maladaptive responses. Also, examination of the relationships between control, types of coping strategies used, and outcomes is greatly needed.

➤ APPRAISAL OF COPING RESOURCES

Once a stressor has been identified and appraised, individuals appraise coping resources that are available to manage the stressor. There is little research to support whether a large or small repertoire of coping strategies is best, and there is also little research on the extent to which a child uses different strategies in different situations. Lazarus and Folkman (1984) emphasize that, in adults, coping behaviors differ according to whether one is anticipating, experiencing, or managing the aftermath of a stressor. In one study, children (ages 8-12 years) were asked to list ways that they managed stressors before, during, and after the stressful event to determine the domain of coping behavior for future instrument development (Ryan, 1989). Children were not asked to reveal the specific stressor they were thinking about, but their responses suggested that they followed the instructions. In general, Ryan notes,

> Anticipation of stressors causes children to marshal coping strategies which serve to avoid the situation (isolation, avoidance), to tackle the situation (cognitive behaviors), or to seek support from others (social support). During the stressful event, behaviors related to social support are still apparent, cognitive behaviors are most prevalent, and physical exercise and emotional behaviors are also frequently identified. After the stressor, behaviors which help to forget the stressor, such as distracting behaviors and avoidant behaviors, are common. Emotional behaviors, and, for the first time, relaxation behaviors are frequently identified, which suggests that built-up tension is released through use of these strategies. (p. 115)

The Coping Resources Inventory for older adolescents and adults is the only instrument found that measures the resources currently available to manage stressors (i.e., precursors to stress), as opposed to coping strategies actually selected and implemented (Hammer, 1988). Additional research is needed to (a) develop global measures of children's coping resources, (b) examine the extent to which coping repertoires expand or contract with age and experience, (c) determine the relative effectiveness, and (d) evaluate the relative merits of a large or small repertoire of coping strategies.

➤ COPING BEHAVIOR

Coping behaviors or strategies are "constantly changing cognitive and behavioral efforts" to manage stressors (Lazarus & Folkman, 1984, p. 141). Coping strategies are inherently neutral; they can be viewed as positive or negative only in the context of the situation and outcomes. In other words, "ignore it" may be the best strategy for a stressor the child cannot change but is relatively short lived, such as being ridiculed by a group of children at summer camp. A pattern of stressful peer relationships at school, however, is not a stressor that can be ignored.

Lazarus and Launier's (1978) early work differentiated between problem-focused and emotion-focused coping strategies. Problem-focused strategies are used to manage or change the stressor, whereas emotion-focused strategies are used to manage the emotions generated by the stressor. Implementation of these definitions is difficult without knowing the intent behind the strategy—that is, coping strategies are not inherently problem focused or emotion focused. For example, "talk to someone" could be a strategy intended to obtain advice about how to handle the problem or to complain bitterly about the problem, and "think about it" could be to think about ways to handle the problem or ways to "get even" with the perpetrators. Most coping instruments include general strategies similar to these examples. Inclusion of multiple possibilities for "intent" behind each strategy would result in extremely lengthy instruments.

A nonhierarchical taxonomy of children's coping behaviors was developed from a synthesis of 16 published research studies of primarily healthy children (Ryan-Wenger, 1992). All coping strategies mentioned in the research studies were inductively sorted into categories, resulting in 15 mutually exclusive categories. The categories, their definitions, and examples are shown in Table 11.2.

A similar review of research studies that focused on coping behavior of children with acute or chronic illness showed that the same 15 categories of coping strategies were used (Ryan-Wenger, 1996). The development of instruments to measure children's coping has followed a similar pattern as that of measurement of children's stressors, beginning with items derived from adults' perspective, literature on adult coping behavior, or observation of children. Later, instruments began to include coping strategies that children say they use. Table 11.3 lists coping instruments that have been used in research or clinical practice.

Coping strategies are learned in infancy and childhood, and many continue into adulthood. Several cross-sectional studies across age groups of 8- to 12-year-olds indicate that older children use cognitive and problem-solving strategies more often than younger children in a variety of stressful situations, which reflects an increased ability to think abstractly (Altshuler & Ruble, 1989; Band & Weisz, 1988; Ryan, 1989). Compas (1988), however, found the opposite trend in use of problem-solving strategies in a study of 10- to 15-year-old children. Additional research is needed to determine situations in which problem solving is used and most appropriate for children of different ages. A longitudinal study of 8- to 11-year-olds, who were age 10 to 13 at the second data collection point, showed no difference in coping frequency scores over time, but there was a significant interaction between age and time for coping effectiveness scores (Sharrer & Ryan-Wenger, 1995). Nine-year-olds had the highest scores at Time 1, and 12-year-olds had the lowest

scores at Time 2, suggesting that as age increases, children's perceptions of their coping effectiveness decrease. Coping strategies can be taught to children, as evidenced by research and case studies that focus on teaching relaxation skills (LaMontagne, Mason, & Hepworth, 1985), self-regulation by hypnosis (Sugarman, 1996), and psychoeducational group training in coping skills (Jones & Selder, 1996).

In studies of adults and children, the availability and quality of parental support play a significant role in the types of coping strategies used to manage stressors and in both short- and long-term outcomes of the stress-coping process. One study showed that maternal support and a structured parenting style may play a role in the number of coping strategies that children use and in the use of avoidant and aggressive strategies (Hardy et al., 1993). Unexpectedly, these behaviors were more evident when mothers provided a high level of support, defined as behavior that makes the child feel comfortable, accepted, and secure (i.e., listening, comforting, and approving of the child). One explanation for this finding might be that children who feel secure and supported tend to avoid or are perhaps not as concerned about daily stressors that are perceived as being outside their control. Their use of aggressive behavior is not as easy to interpret.

Two separate critical reviews of the literature examined the coping strategies used by children with acute or chronic illness (Ryan-Wenger, 1996) and the determinants and consequences of children's coping with painful medical stressors (Rudolph, Dennig, & Weisz, 1995). Much of the data are inconsistent, suggesting that additional research is needed, particularly with regard to differentiating coping behavior from outcomes. The most commonly reported coping strategy in many studies was the use of social support, although most of the reports did not indicate from whom such support was sought (Ryan-Wenger, 1996). Other common coping strategies included stressor modification, which included taking control or direct action against the stressor; cognitive

TABLE 11.2 Taxonomy of Children's Coping Strategies

Category	Definition	Examples of Coping Strategies
Aggressive activities	Verbal or motor activities that may be hurtful to persons, animals, or objects	Aggression, motor aggression, heavy-handed persuasion
		Moderate persuasion, indirect display of anger, attacks
		Physical attacks, destroy, verbal aggression, yell, argue
Behavioral avoidance	Behavior other than isolating that is a deliberate attempt to keep oneself away from a stressor	Escape, escape from family contact, temporary escape
		Escape from social contact, avoidance, go somewhere else
		Don't do anything about it, sleep, leave the situation
		Try to get out of it, change the topic, look away
		Limit setting, inhibition of action
Behavioral distraction	Behavior other than isolating or avoidant that delays the need to deal with a stressor	Distraction, do something else, watch TV
		Strenuous activities, quiet activities, animals
		Motor distraction, play, play alone
		Group activities, music, inanimate objects
Cognitive avoidance	Deliberate cognitive attempts to avoid acknowledging the existence of a stressor	Deny that situation exists, don't think about it
		Reject it, information limiting, ignore it
		Forget about it
		Thought stopping
Cognitive distraction	Deliberate cognitive attempts to keep thoughts away from a stressor	Diversionary thinking, visual distraction
		Cognitive distraction, think about something else
		Read, fantasy, humor
Cognitive problem solving	Thoughts focused on ways to modify, prevent, or eliminate the stressor	Focus on the situation, processing information
		Analyze, learn, problem solving
		Reality-oriented working through, think, reason
		Stress recognition, decision making
Cognitive restructuring	Thoughts that alter one's perception of the characteristics of the stressor	Positive restructuring, emphasize the positive
		Think about a reward, reward-oriented cognition
		Wishful thinking, tell self it's OK, convince self
		Defensive reappraisal, hope enhancement

TABLE 11.2 Continued

Category	Definition	Examples of Coping Strategies
Emotional expression	Behavior other than aggressive motor and verbal activities that expresses feelings or emotions	Ventilate feelings, act the way you want to feel Cry, empathize
Endurance	Behavior that causes one to face the stressor and accept its consequences	Expose self to fear, peaceful acquiescence Comply/cooperate, submit, endurance Relinquish control
Information seeking	Behavior that involves obtaining information about the stressor	Information seeking, programs, media, parents Explore, investigate, touch, clarify other's feelings Questioning, vigilant behavior, orienting
Isolating activities	Behavior that serves to separate the individual from the presence of others	Solitary, time-out, go to a special place Exclusion, isolate self
Self-controlling activities	Behavior or cognitions that serve to reduce tension or control one's behavior or emotions	Behavior-regulating cognitions Emotion-regulating cognitions, emotion management Self-soothing activities, think about relaxing Self-destruction, repetitive actions/habits Self-protection, tension reducing, eating, drinking Self-focusing, relax
Spiritual support	Behavior that suggests an appeal to a higher being	Spiritual support, pray
Stressor modification	Noncognitive behavior that eliminates the stressor or modifies the characteristics of the stressor	Propose a compromise, alter the situation Conflict mitigation

SOURCE: Reprinted, with permission, from the *American Journal of Orthopsychiatry.* Copyright © 1992 by the American Orthopsychiatric Association, Inc.

and behavioral distraction; and cognitive restructuring, which involved changing one's perception of the stressor.

Recent research studies indicated that avoidant coping behaviors were associated with poor metabolic control in children with diabetes (Grey, Lipman, Cameron, & Thurber, 1997). Coping strategies used by children with chronic illnesses are similar to strategies they use to deal with non-illness-related stressors (Spirito, Stark, Gil, & Tyc, 1995), and even during repeated hospitalizations they are relatively stable (Boyd & Hunsberger, 1998). No longitudinal, prospective studies were found that had examined the mechanisms by which coping strategies are

TABLE 11.3 Instruments for Measurement of Coping Strategies and Coping Resources in Children and Adolescents

Author	Instrument	Target Group	Original Source of Items	Format	Instrument Completed By	Meaning of Scores
Mooney, Graziano, and Katz (1984)	Nighttime Fears Coping Checklist	8- to 13-year-olds	Literature, children, parents	36 items; scored yes/no	Children	Sum of items scores for five subscales = frequency and variety of coping strategies used
Wertlieb, Weigel, and Feldstein (1987)	Stress and Coping Interview	7- to 10-year-olds	Scoring method derived from theory	Semistructured interview; 10 categories of coping behavior	Interviewer and child	Child's responses sorted into 1 of 10 categories reflecting focus, function, and mode of child's coping behavior
Patterson and McCubbin (1987)	A-COPE: Adolescent Coping Orientation for Problem Experiences	12- to 18-year-olds	10th- to 12th-grade students	95 items; scale of 1-5 for frequency of use	Adolescents	Sum of item scores for 12 subscales = frequency and variety of coping strategies used
Ritchie, Caty, and Ellerton (1988)	Children's Coping Strategies Checklist	Hospitalized 2- to 6-year-olds	Scoring method derived from literature, theory	Observation of hospitalized preschoolers; 40 behaviors scored as yes/no	Observer	Total number of coping behaviors observed for each of six subscales = variety and type of coping behavior
Spirito, Stark, and Williams (1988)	KIDCOPE (Brief Coping Checklist)		Adult coping scales		Children, adolescents	Sum of item scores = total frequency and efficacy of coping strategies
	School-age version	7- to 12-year-olds		School age: 15 items; yes/no for frequency; 0-2 for efficacy		
	Adolescent version	13- to 18-year-olds		Adolescent: 10 items; scale of 0-3 for frequency and efficacy		

Author	Instrument	Population	Source	Items/Scale	Subjects	Scoring
Hammer (1988)	Coping Resources Inventory	High school	Clinical practice, literature	60 items; scale of 0-3 for extent to which items are descriptive of subject during the past 6 months	Adolescents	Sum of item scores = amount of resources; standard scores profile plots of five dimensions
Dise-Lewis (1988)	Life Events and Coping Inventory	12- to 14-year-olds	Junior high students	52 items; scale of 1-9 for likelihood that one would use each strategy	Children	Sum of items scores = amount of coping strategies that are likely to be used
Ryan-Wenger (1990)	Schoolagers' Coping Strategies Inventory	8- to 12-year-olds	Elementary school children	26 items; scale of 0-3 for frequency of use and effectiveness	Children	
Austin, Patterson, and Huberty (1991)	Coping Health Inventory for Children	8- to 12-year-olds with chronic illness	Theory, literature, parents, children	45 items; scale of 1-5 for frequency of use	Parents of children with chronic illness	Sum of item scores for five subscales = frequency and variety of coping strategies
Gil, Abrams, Phillips, and Keefe (1989)	Coping Strategies Questionnaire for Sickle Cell Disease (SCD)	Children and adolescents with chronic pain due to SCD	Adult instrument, clinical practice	42 items; scale of 0-6 for frequency of use; overall level of control over pain and overall effectiveness of each strategy	Children, adolescents	Item scores converted to composite scores on two factors: coping attempts and pain control/rational thinking

acquired, retained, or abandoned. Social learning theory (Bandura, 1977) suggests that the process involves observation of others, such as parents and peers. Therefore, research on similarities and differences between individual coping behavior and coping behavior of one's parents, siblings, peers, and significant others would reveal useful information. The cognitive processes involved in deciding which coping behaviors should be used to manage stressors are also largely unknown.

► PERSON AND ENVIRONMENTAL FACTORS

A variety of individual and environmental factors play a role in determining the stress-coping process and outcomes, and it is outside the scope of this chapter to describe them all. These factors include age, gender, socioeconomic status, parental support, health status, and personality characteristics. One factor that will be briefly reviewed is the child's coping style.

An individual's repertoire of coping strategies is probably partially determined by his or her's coping style, which is not to be confused with coping behavior. Coping style, or temperament, is a relatively stable personality characteristic that typifies one's style of managing person-environment interactions (Thomas & Chess, 1984). Coping styles are usually described in unidimensional, dichotomous terms, such as monitors versus blunters (Miller, 1989), avoidant versus vigilant (Cohen & Lazarus, 1973), or internalizers versus externalizers (Boyd & Johnson, 1981). Temperament is usually defined in terms of nine characteristic ways of responding to one's environment: activity, rhythmicity, approach or withdrawal, adaptability, threshold of responsiveness, intensity of reaction, mood, distractibility, and persistence. Difficult infants tend to have biological irregularity, withdrawal, slow adaptability, and negative reactions of high intensity (Chess, 1990). Difficult school-aged children are those with low adaptability and negative mood (Hegvik, McDevitt, & Carey, 1982).

Research that will be reviewed in the following sections tends to focus either on children's coping strategies and outcomes or on coping styles and outcomes. Little is known, however, about how coping strategies, styles, and outcomes interact. Clinicians who desire to help children acquire more effective coping strategies would probably benefit by examining the compatibility of new coping strategies with the child's inherent coping style. To advance theory about the origin and maintenance of coping strategies, and inform practice, it is essential to study the contribution of coping style to this process. There are many instruments that have been developed to measure coping styles for children of all ages, as shown in Table 11.4.

► SHORT-TERM RESPONSES IN THE STRESS-COPING PROCESS

Appraisal of Coping Effectiveness

Children are capable of evaluating the effectiveness of their coping strategies (Ryan-Wenger, 1990). Little is known, however, about many aspects of children's appraisal of coping effectiveness, including when and how often this appraisal occurs, the criteria that they use to define "effectiveness," how these differ from adults' definitions of effectiveness, or how children alter their coping behaviors based on periodic appraisal of their effectiveness. The theoretical model shown in Figure 11.1 suggests that the relative effectiveness of coping strategies influences psychological behavior, social functioning, and somatic health outcomes of stressful person-environment interactions. To date, little empirical research has adequately tested this proposition.

Psychosocial Behavior

One outcome of the stress-coping process is a change in affect and social behavior (Lazarus, 1990). Sometimes, these changes are short lived and are viewed as the normal "ups and downs" of childhood and adolescence. A review article by Grey and Hayman (1987) provides a list of instruments to measure children's anxiety, depression, and generalized affect. School stress has received the most attention in the literature as a source of psychosocial upset. Hilsman and Garber (1995) found that poor grades on a report card resulted in varying levels of depression in school-age children, but for most children such symptoms disappear after 5 days. Fear of examinations, in particular, served as a major source of stress, with responses including increased tension, disorganization, less productive schoolwork, anxiety, insecurity, uneasiness, and uncertainty (Schuller, 1994). Kleine (1994) studied mood states following a math examination in 61 ninth graders. A negative mood was clearly established in the children as a result of the testing. The children were then randomly assigned to scheduled physical education classes or to a special literature class. The mood states of the children taking the literature class remained negative, but children in the exercise classes experienced elevated moods and decreased tension. Boys' mood states improved to a greater extent than those of girls, probably because boys are more likely to identify physical activity as an effective coping strategy (Ryan, 1989).

Advances in health technology, medical management, and nursing care have dramatically increased survival rates and decreased mortality for children suffering from chronic disease and disability. At the same time, ethical questions have been raised about such medical interventions with respect to the stress of chronic illness and the impact on quality of life, especially social adaptation, growth and development, and cognitive functioning (Blakeney et al., 1998; Bloom, Wright, Morris, Campbell, & Krawiecki, 1997).

Children respond to the stress of their own illnesses in a variety of ways. Canning, Canning, and Boyce (1992) discovered that children with chronic illness reported fewer or similar depressive symptoms when compared to a group of healthy controls. It was hypothesized that ill children cope by using denial and repression, reporting lower levels of distress

and anxiety. The children were also found to be highly defensive. The researchers concluded that a repressive style of coping may be a protection against psychological distress, at least temporarily, and that denial of illness and defensiveness may protect children against severe depression.

When a parent has cancer, the gender of the ill parent and the gender of the child moderate stress responses (Compas et al., 1994). Adolescent girls responded with increased anxiety and depression when their mothers were diagnosed with cancer. Grant and Compas (1995) studied this situation further and found that teenage girls reported greater stress related to increasing family responsibilities. The hypothesis that adolescent girls may use ineffective coping strategies was not supported, and in fact adolescent girls successfully used distraction as a method of coping with their mothers' illnesses by engaging in household tasks and family responsibilities. Although more tasks and responsibilities enhanced reported stress, they also provided a mechanism for effective coping.

Physiologic Changes

In infants and children, as well as adults, experiences of stressful situations and attempts to cope with stressors have a direct and observable impact on physiological systems. Physiologically, stressful experiences activate the hypothalamic-pituitary-adrenocortical (HPA) system (Gunnar, 1998). The HPA system enhances stress resistance by increasing energy needed to cope and by modulating other body systems that are sensitive to stress including emotions. Studies of laboratory-induced stress provide useful data for studies of the physiologic impact of real-life stressors on children.

Three related laboratory studies were conducted to examine relationships among cardiovascular responsivity to laboratory-induced stress, age, ethnicity, gender, and family history of cardiovascular (CV) disease (Allen & Mathews, 1997; Malpass et al., 1997; Musante, Treiber, Davis, Levy, & Strong,

TABLE 11.4 Instruments for Measurement of Coping Styles in Children and Adolescents

Author	Instrument	Target Group	Original Source of Items	Format	Instrument Completed By	Meaning of Scores
Rose (1972)	Level of Involvement in the Coping Process	1½- to 7-year-olds, at home and hospital	Theory, literature	Observation of child's coping behaviors	Observer, child	Observations sorted into three categories: precoping, active coping, inactive coping
Murphy and Moriarty (1976)	Comprehensive Coping Inventory	3- to 5-year-olds	Theory, literature, clinical practice	999 items; scoring methods not reported	Children, parents, and team of professionals	Scores represent typical coping style
Carey and McDevitt (1978)	Infant Temperament Questionnaire	4- to 8-month-olds	Theory	95 items; scale of 1-6 for frequency of behavioral occurrence	Mother	Sum of item scores for nine subscales = child's typical temperament or coping style
McDevitt and Carey (1978)	Behavioral Style Questionnaire	3- to 7-year-olds	Theory	100 items; scale of 1-6 for frequency of behavioral occurrence	Mother	Sum of item scores for nine subscales = child's typical temperament or coping style
Zeitlan (1980, 1985a)	Coping Inventory—Observation	3- to 5-year-olds	Theory	48 items; scale of 1-5 for frequency of occurrence	Observation by parent, teacher	Sum of item scores = subscale scores on three dimensions: productive/ nonproductive, flexible/ rigid, active/passive
Boyd and Johnson (1981)	Analysis of Coping Style	Form C: 8-12 years Form Y: 13-18 years	Theory	Projective test; children's reactions to 20 drawings	Interviewer, child	Responses sorted into six categories: internalized attack, denial, and avoidance and externalized attack, denial, and avoidance
Hegvik, McDevitt, and Carey (1982)	Middle Childhood Temperament Questionnaire	8- to 12-year-olds	Theory	99 items; scale of 1-6 for frequency of behavioral occurrence	Mother	Sum of item scores for nine subscales = child's typical temperament or coping style

Author (Date)	Instrument	Age Group	Basis	Format	Respondent	Scoring/Interpretation
Fullard, McDevitt, and Carey (1984)	Toddler Temperament Scale	12- to 36-month-olds	Theory	97 items; scale of 1-6 for frequency of behavioral occurrence	Mother	Sum of item scores for nine subscales = child's typical temperament or coping style
LaMontagne (1984, 1987)	Preoperative Mode of Coping Interview	8- to 18-year-olds hospitalized, prior to surgery	Theory	Structured interview; character of responses reduced to a score from 1 to 10	Interviewer, child	Low score = avoidant; High score = active coping style
Zeitlan (1985b)	Coping Inventory: Self-Rated Form	Adolescents, adults	Theory	48 items; scale of 1-5 for frequency of occurrence	Observation by parent, teacher	Sum of item scores = three subscales: productive/nonproductive, flexible/rigid, active/passive
Peterson and Toler (1986)	Coping Strategies Interview	5- to 11-year-olds hospitalized, prior to surgery	Literature, theory, children	Structured interview; count number of info-seeking responses	Interviewer, child	Compare number of info-seeking versus avoiding responses
Meisgeier and Murphy (1987)	Murphy-Meisgeier Type Indicator for Children	2nd to 8th grade	Theory	70 items; forced choice between two responses	Children	Responses profiled into 16 type dimensions
Zeitlan, Williamson, and Szczepanski (1988)	Early Coping Inventory	4- to 36-month-olds	Theory	48 items; scale of 1-5 for frequency of occurrence	Observation by parent, teacher	Sum of item scores = subscale scores on three dimensions: productive/nonproductive, flexible/rigid, active/passive
Martin (1988)	Temperament Assessment Battery for Children	3- to 7-year-olds	Theory	48 items; scale of 1-7 for frequency of behaviors	Parent, teacher, and clinician each complete a form	Sum of item scores = subscale scores; standardized into T scores; profile plots for temperament style
Miller (1989)	Kiddie Choice Survey (Monitoring-Blunting Scale for Children)	Not stated	Theory	Structured interview; responses consistent with blunting are identified	Interviewer, child	Compare number of responses in categories of blunting versus monitoring

1995). Researchers evaluated a cross-cultural sample of 159 children (ages 8-19) and adolescents (ages 15-17) in a laboratory protocol consisting of a reaction time task, a mirror tracing task, a cold forehead challenge, and a stress interview. Results demonstrated that adolescents were more reactive than children when comparing hemodynamic responses for blood pressure (BP) and cardiac output during clinical stressors. The children showed greater increases in temperature, pulse, and respiration (TPR). Results suggested that β-adrenergic reactivity may peak in young adults after the pubertal transition, with a gradual decline during the adult years. White adolescents exhibited greater systolic BP and TPR changes than did black adolescents. Black adolescents had greater diastolic BP changes and vagal withdrawal along with greater heart rate increases during cold forehead challenge. Pubertal status affected black-white differences in vascular responding. Surprisingly, white female children had a greater diastolic BP response across tasks than did black female children. These results support the suggestion that pubertal transition is important in the development of gender differences in CV reactivity to behavioral challenges, although age, social roles, and psychological maturation may be intervening variables.

Recent research has focused on the measurement of cortisol in response to stressful stimuli. Cortisol is a key hormone produced in response to physiological and psychosocial stressors (Mason, 1968; Seyle, 1976). Salivary cortisol is a reliable and valid measure of unbound plasma cortisol and therefore of adrenocortical reactivity (Laudat et al., 1988). Cortisol increases during various physical and emotional stressors, and measurements of salivary cortisol have frequently been used to determine the effects of the stress response on the health of children. For example, Flinn and England (1997) investigated the relationships among socioeconomic conditions, family, environment, stress, and health in a rural Caribbean village. Longitudinal monitoring of cortisol in this natural environment was used to identify specific psychosocial antecedents and consequences of childhood stress. The physiological stress response was assessed by salivary cortisol levels in children age 2 months to 18 years ($N = 22,438$). Elevated cortisol levels were not always associated with traumatic or negative events. Eating meals, difficult physical work, basketball, and the return of a family member who was temporarily absent were associated with temporary moderate increases (10%-100%) in cortisol levels. High-stress events (cortisol increases from 100% to 2000%), however, were associated with family trauma, conflict, or change. Punishment, quarreling, and residence change substantially increased cortisol levels.

➤ LONG-TERM EFFECTS OF THE STRESS-COPING PROCESS

Some children develop frequent or exaggerated psychological symptoms, illnesses, social isolation, or other long-term manifestations of the internalization of stress. Some commonly used instruments to measure these long-term outcomes are listed in Table 11.5.

Psychological Well-Being and Social Functioning

Normative stressors for school-age children frequently involve peer problems and academic failures. Repetti (1996) investigated the stress of perceived academic and social failures at school and found that children reported their own behaviors as more demanding and aversive toward parents. Much of this behavior represented attempts to secure parental attention and gain reassurance after problems occurred in school. Children under stress of school failures were also more prone to behave aversively with mothers than with fathers. There is evidence that children make greater efforts to control their behavior when in the company of their fathers, and often children feel predisposed to seek their mothers in times of stress. Children may feel more comfortable turning to their mothers for caring and emotional security (Repetti, 1994).

In contrast, Campbell, Pierce, Moore, Marakovitz, and Newby (1996) investigated boys exhibiting behavior problems starting at age 4 and followed them to ages 6 and 9 ($N =$ 102). Externalizing problems included aggression toward peers, noncompliance, overactivity, and lack of impulse control. These behaviors were associated with concurrent family stress, particularly negative maternal control. As the boys grew older, they continued to report receiving negative discipline and were exposed to chronic family stress characterized by negative life events, marital dissatisfaction, and maternal depression.

Behavior during a "strange situation" (maternal separation and a strange adult female who comforts the infant if he or she becomes distressed) revealed attachment classifications for thirty-eight 19-month-old infants (Hertsgaard, Gunnarm, Erickson, & Nachmias, 1995). This study provides support that disorganized attachment behavior (Type D attachment) reflects a vulnerability to stressful stimulation. Type D attachments are expected to occur most often in infants who are at risk for poor parenting or whose lives are characterized by a high degree of familial stress (Carlson, Cicchetti, Barnett, & Braunwald, 1989). The results may be a reflection of the lack of an organized set of attachment-related coping responses. The researchers postulate that the vulnerability of this particular group of infants to stress may result in disorders related to their social and emotional development.

Steward (1998) hypothesized that for some infants who live in a chaotic or non-nurturing environment, overuse of the normal conservation-withdrawal coping mechanism (shutdown of reaction to the environment) results in decreased demand for attention, underfeeding, and a decreased growth rate.

Although the coping behavior is effective in dealing with the stressful environment, it may be related to the development of nonorganic failure to thrive (NOFTT) syndrome. Steward supports this hypothesis with research findings indicating that infants with NOFTT sleep more, are more difficult, and are less responsive to their environments than healthy infants. Prospective studies are needed, however, to determine whether these characteristics develop before, during, or after growth failure reaches a level at which the diagnosis of NOFTT is made.

Finally, posttraumatic stress syndrome and other psychosocial problems are receiving attention related to traumatic experiences, such as having cancer, severe burns, child abuse, or witnessing the ravages of war. Children who survive cancer may have difficulty with intellectual, academic, emotional, adaptive, and social functioning (Morris, Krawiecki, Wright, & Walter, 1993). Twenty-five children between the ages of 2 and 25 years were followed, and the majority showed low average to deficient levels of performance on neuropsychologic achievement and adaptive behavior measurements. Duration of cancer and medical risk scores significantly correlated with decreased functioning. Behavior problems were not often observed in these children, although several demonstrated characteristics of hyperactivity. The extent to which these changes are due to stress versus the long-term effects of chemotherapy treatment is not known.

Psychosocial adjustment in survivors of massive pediatric burn injuries was examined as part of a longitudinal study initiated in 1986 (Blakeney et al., 1998). These young burn victims were mildly diminished in academic and social competence, but the majority were adapting satisfactorily and the children appeared to have no more behavioral problems than those reported in an age-matched healthy control group. Burned children also reported positive self-esteem. Decreased activity competence, as in athletic sports, was associated only with the level of

TABLE 11.5 Instruments for Measurement of Stress Responses in Children and Adolescents

Author	Instrument	Target Group	Original Source of Items	Format	Instrument Completed By	Meaning of Scores
Horowitz, Wilner, and Alvarez (1979)	Impact of Event Scale (for posttraumatic stress disorder [PTSD])	Children, adults who have experienced a traumatic event	Theory, clinical practice	30 items; scale of 0-3 for extent to which symptoms are experienced	Children, adults	Sum of item scores = subscale scores on intrusiveness and avoidance (PTSD)
Chandler, Shermis, and Marsh (1985)	Stress Response Scale	5- to 14-year-olds	Derived from theory and *DSM-III* categories	40 behavioral items; scale of 0-5 for frequency of occurrence	Children	Sum of frequency scores = total and subscale scores = amount of stress response; profiles indicate four common response patterns
Hockenberry-Eaton, Manteuffel, and Bottomley (1997)	Children's Adjustment to Cancer Index	7- to 13-year-olds	Derived from literature and experience of primary author	30 items; scale of 1-5 for frequency of ability to do things	Children	Sum of item scores = level of adjustment to cancer
Achenbach and Edelbrock (1983)	Child Behavior Checklist: Behavior Problem Scale	2- or 3-year-olds; 4- to 16-year olds	Theory, clinical practice, literature	113 items; scale of 0-2 for extent to which item is true for the child	Parent, teacher, adolescent	Sum of item scores = subscale scores on nine dimensions; standardized scores profiled for specific behavior problem areas

Achenbach and Edelbrock (1983)	Child Behavior Checklist: Social Competence Scale	2- or 3-year-olds; 4- to 16-year-olds	Theory, clinical practice, literature	Eight sections; multiple-response choices for characteristics descriptive of the child	Parent, teacher, adolescent	Sum of item scores = subscale scores on six dimensions; standardized scores profiled for specific social competence areas
Elliott, Jay, and Woody (1987)	Observation Scale for Behavioral Distress	3- to 13-year-olds undergoing medical procedures	Literature, other observation instruments	Eight behavior categories	Observation by health care provider	Modal categories of observed behaviors most descriptive of child's response to medical procedures
Merrell and Walters (1998)	Internalizing Symptoms Scale for Children	8- to 13-year-olds	Theory, literature, clinical practice	48 items; scale of 0-3 for extent to which statement is true of the child	Child, adolescent	Sum of item scores = subscale scores; standardized and plotted on profile for Negative Affect/General Distress and Positive Affect

physical impairment. Unfortunately, it was difficult for researchers to determine if decreased psychosocial and behavioral competencies (reported in 37% of the sample) were due to the burn impairment and disfigurement or due to lower socioeconomic and educational backgrounds of families. Because of the pervasiveness and horror of the war in their country, children in Croatia, Bosnia, and Herzegovina are at great risk for post-traumatic stress disorder (PTSD). A study of 1,787 children, ages 6 to 15 years, showed high levels of PTSD reactions among the children, with girls scoring higher on both intrusion and avoidance dimensions (Dyregrov, Kuterovac, & Barath, 1996).

HPA axis disturbance was evaluated via blood samples for corticotropin (ACTH) and cortisol in 13 depressed and nonabused children, 13 normal control children, and 13 depressed and abused children (Kaufman et al., 1997). Although a blunting effect was expected, the depressed and abused children (when compared to the depressed and nonabused and normal control children) had a significantly augmented ACTH response to corticotropin-releasing hormone (CRH) challenge. All children who were in the high responder groups were found to be currently living in homes in which there was ongoing emotional maltreatment (chronic ongoing adversity), whereas all low responders were not. The abused children that showed blunted ACTH secretion post-CRH were living in relatively stable environments. Results indicate that experiences of abuse in combination with ongoing stressors and an absence of positive supports promote significant dysregulation of the HPA axis system. Although HPA activity is adaptive in the short term, prolonged stress and concomitant prolonged HPA activity leave the infant or child physiologically and psychologically vulnerable (Gunnar, 1992). Findings also suggest that it may not be the chronicity of stress exposure but rather the developmental timing of exposure that is critical in determining the long-term consequences.

Somatic Health and Illness

Numerous studies summarized by Boyce and others indicate that consistently, and across settings, a small portion (15%-20%) of the child population accounts for most of the school absentee rate, more than half of the morbidity, and half of the health services utilization of that population (Boyce, 1992; Kornguth, 1990; Weitzman, Walker, & Gortmaker, 1986). Children with chronic illnesses or disabilities account for only approximately 5%; the remainder comprises children with frequent and various physical and psychological morbidity conditions. One longitudinal study showed that the same childhood patterns of illness and health services utilization persist into adulthood (Lewis & Lewis, 1989). Some hypothesized determinants of frequent illnesses are parental anxiety regarding the child's health, constitutional vulnerability to stress (illness-prone), or internalization of stress (Boyce, 1992). Research on children with frequent illnesses, frequent absence from school due to illness, and frequent use of health services is needed to examine their relationships to coping behavior.

Drummond and Hewson-Bower (1997) investigated the association between psychosocial stress and susceptibility to upper respiratory tract infections. This relationship was demonstrated through measurement of the concentration of secretory immunoglobulin A (sIgA) and its ratio to albumin in saliva in 45 children with a history of recurrent colds and flu and in 45 healthy children. The purpose was to investigate the differences between ill and healthy children in terms of their degree of life events stress and their personality and mood profiles. Secretory IgA is regarded as a first line of defense against the invasion of antigens into the lining of the upper respiratory tract (Ahl & Reinholdt, 1991; Bienenstock, Croitoru, Ernst, & Stanisz, 1989; Borysenko, 1987). High preinfection levels of sIgA correlate well with protection against viral infection (Isaacs, Webster, & Valman, 1984; Rossen et al., 1970). Results indicated a lower sIgA:albumin ratio and greater psychological distress in children with a history of recurrent colds and flu. The findings support the view that psychosocial stress increases susceptibility to colds and flu by decreasing mucosal immunity in the upper respiratory tract. The findings also suggest a multidimensional relationship between stress and susceptibility to colds and flu. Variables that may have an impact include stressful life events, personality traits, and signs of emotional disturbance, such as anxiety and depression.

Immune changes of children experiencing the normative stressor of entering kindergarten were the focus of another study (Boyce et al., 1995). Adrenocortical and behavioral predictors of immune responses were measured by salivary cortisol level, quantitative counts of T cell subsets, and behavioral difficulty with school adjustment ($N = 39$). Findings supported previous studies (Gunnar, Mangelsdorf, Larson, & Hertsgaard, 1989; Larson, Gunnar, & Hertsgard, 1991; Lewis & Thomas, 1990) with a moderate increase in salivary cortisol in response to low-level psychologic stress. Immunologic function exhibited a modest increase in cell numbers and diminution in function, although all scores remained within the realm of normal ranges for children of this age.

A surprising finding was that children of more highly educated mothers showed greater adrenodcortical activation and larger increases in T cell subsets than those peers with mothers who were less educated. The researchers postulated that there may be greater expectation placed on children of more highly educated parents. Parent-reported behavioral difficulties and adrenocortical responses to school entry were associated with alterations in both enumeration and functional measures of immune status. The results suggest that behavioral and adrenocortical responses may be associated with different profiles of immunological effects that influence susceptibility to immune-mediated disease. Previous research suggests that individual differences in temperament, sociocultural environment, and psycho-social factors influence the coping and adaptive capacity of the child.

➤ STRESS RESISTANCE AND STRESS VULNERABILITY

Research in the area of stress and coping in children has focused as much on positive as on negative outcomes. Some research concerns a special subset of "resilient" children who have experienced many unusually severe stressors and yet function exceptionally well despite the great odds against them (Masten, Best, & Garmezy, 1990). The majority of research concerns a different and larger group of resilient or stress-resistant children who come from a variety of environments and manage stressors of varying frequency and severity without unusual physical or psychosocial problems. This type of sustained competence is a capacity that develops over time in the context of person-environment interactions (Masten & Coatsworth, 1998). Other children appear to be more vulnerable to stressful situations and environments. Stress vulnerability is defined as a "condition of unusual or exaggerated susceptibility to the environmental agents of disease or disorder, including psychosocial stressors" (Boyce, 1992, p. 4).

Many children conduct their daily lives in a socially and behaviorally competent manner at home and at school despite the presence of family stressors. Smith and Prior (1995) operationally defined this competence as "child stress resilience." Attributes of child temperament, self-esteem, ability, gender, and mother-child warmth were studied in relation to family stress involving poverty, family discord, and stressful life events. Although age, gender, ability, and self-concept were not significant for adaptation, positive temperament, lower levels of maternal stress, and a warm maternal-child relationship predicted more adaptive responses to stress. Phipps and Mulhern (1995) were interested in the stress resilience of children undergoing bone marrow transplants (BMT). Forty-one children were studied prospectively at prehospitalization and 6 and 12 months post-BMT. Social competence and self-concept were diminished after facing the stress of BMT; pre-BMT family characteristics of cohesion and expressiveness, however, significantly predicted improved child adjustment outcomes and therefore promoted child resilience. Family conflict proved to be a risk factor that adversely influenced the child's response to stress.

We argue that "ineffective coping strategies" contribute to internalization of stress. In his work with adults, Lazarus stated that the ways that people cope with stress are probably more directly related to health and illness than are the frequency and severity of stressors (Lazarus & Launier, 1978). Studies have shown that children with a history of recurrent abdominal pain or other stress-related symptoms used less effective coping strategies or had significantly lower coping effectiveness scores than children with no stress-related symptoms (Ryan-Wenger, 1990). The effectiveness (and social acceptability) of children's coping strategies may determine the extent to which children are vulnerable or resilient to current and future stressful situations. Even successful coping takes a psychological toll on children; therefore, it is important to examine the amount of coping children have to do over time (Emery & Coiro, 1997). It may be that although emotional regulation buffers against certain stressors, it also increases vulnerability to others, and successful coping in one realm may not be indicative of positive coping and overall psychological well-being (Thompson & Calkins, 1996).

It is important to identify factors that cause children to be resistant to stress. It is tempting to assume that protective factors are simply the opposite of risk factors, and that stress resistance and vulnerability are opposite poles of a single dimension. In the absence of a body of research to support either assumption, Rutter (1996) suggests that in the search for causality, stress resistance and vulnerability should be treated as separate constructs, and that exploration of causal factors include physical, psychological, social, and environmental variables.

➤ IMPLICATIONS FOR RESEARCH, THEORY DEVELOPMENT, AND PRACTICE

What is known about stress and coping in children was generated from the perspective of several disciplines, and typically new research in each discipline is informed by a synthesis of this knowledge. Because the stress-coping process influences a child's psychological, behavioral, and physiological systems simultaneously, more research should be interdisciplinary, in which the problem, design, method, and interpretation of findings are approached from multiple perspectives. More research is needed to understand children's appraisal of stressors and coping resources; children's motivations for selecting coping strategies; linkages between stressors, coping behavior, and outcomes; and interventions to decrease vulnerability or increase children's stress resistance.

Stress-coping theories developed specifically for children are overdue. Although researchers have typically applied theories that explain adult stress and coping behavior to research and practice with children, children's cognitive, physical, and social realities are dramatically different from those of adults. If one accepts that appraisal plays a significant role in the stress-coping process, then theories are needed to explain differences in appraisal as children move through stages of cognitive development. Children's stressors are not the same as adults' stressors, nor is their level of control over stressors the same. Theories should account for sources of stress such as height, weight, appearance, and agility, which are of extreme importance to children and adolescents when peer acceptance begins to take priority over family relationships or relationships with significant others. It may be helpful to begin by comprehensively analyzing and perhaps revising each proposition of an adult-level theory with respect to obvious differences between children and adults.

Nurses and other health care providers should always consider potential interactions among stress, coping, health, and illness. Include in history-taking the sources of stress and typical coping strategies from the child's and the parents' perspectives. Children can be taught new coping strategies in individual or group settings. Helping children relate specific coping strategies to desirable and undesirable outcomes may be the first step in assisting children to manage their own stress-related responses. Scholars interested in children's stress-coping processes will want more in-depth discussion than could be provided in this chapter. Additional work by the following authors with programs of research in this area should be examined: J. Austin, M. Grey, M. Hockenberry-Eaton, L. LaMontagne, N. Ryan-Wenger, and R. C. Yeaworth in nursing; B. Compas, A. Spirito, W. T. Boyce, and N. Garmezy in psychology; and C. Lewis, M. Masten, L. Peterson, and M. Rutter in medicine.

➣ REFERENCES

Achenbach, T. M., & Edelbrock, C. (1983). *Manual for the Child Behavior Checklist and Revised Child Behavior Profile.* Burlington: University of Vermont, Department of Psychiatry.

Ahl, T., & Reinholdt, J. (1991). Subclass distribution of salivary secretory immunoglobulin A antibodies to oral streptococci. *Infection and Immunity, 59,* 3619-3625.

Allen, M., & Matthews, K. (1997). Hemodynamic responses to laboratory stressors in children and adolescents: The influences of age, race and gender. *Psychophysiology, 34,* 329-339.

Altshuler, J. L., & Ruble, D. N. (1989). Developmental changes in children's awareness of strategies for coping with uncontrollable stress. *Child Development, 60,* 1347-1349.

Austin, J. K., Patterson, J. M., & Huberty, T. J. (1991). Development of the Coping Health Inventory for Children. *Journal of Pediatric Nursing, 6,* 166-174.

Bahg, C. (1990). Major systems theories throughout the world. *Behavioral Science, 35,* 79-107.

Band, E. B., & Weisz, J. R. (1988). How to feel better when it feels bad: Children's perspectives on coping with everyday stress. *Developmental Psychology, 24,* 247-253.

Bandura, A. (1977). *Social learning theory.* Englewood Cliffs, NJ: Prentice Hall.

Beal, S., & Schmidt, G. (1984). Development of a Youth Adaptation Rating Scale. *Journal of School Health, 54,* 197-200.

Berk, L. E. (1997). *Child development* (4th ed.). Boston: Allyn & Bacon.

Bienenstock, J., Croitoru, K., Ernst, P., & Stanisz, A. (1989). Nerves and neuropeptides in the regulation of mucosal immunity. In B. Askonas, B. Moss, G. Torrigiani, & S. Gorini (Eds.), *The immune response to viral infections* (pp. 19-27). New York: Plenum.

Blakeney, P., Meyer, W., Robert, R., Desai, M., Wolf, S., & Herndon, D. (1998). Long-term psychosocial adaptation of children who survive burns involving 80% or greater total body surface area. *Journal of Trauma: Injury, Infection, and Critical Care, 44,* 625-634.

Bloom, A. A., Wright, J. A., Morris, R. D., Campbell, R. M., & Krawiecki, N. S. (1997). Additive impact of in-hospital cardiac arrest on the functioning of children with heart disease. *Pediatrics, 99,* 390-398.

Borysenko, M. (1987). The immune system: An overview. *Annals of Behavioral Medicine, 7,* 3-10.

Boyce, W. T. (1992). The vulnerable child: New evidence, new approaches. *Advances in Pediatrics, 39,* 1-33.

Boyce, W. T., Adams, S., Tschann, J. M., Cohen, F., Wara, D., & Gunnar, M. R. (1995). Adrenocortical and behavioral predictors of immune responses to starting school. *Pediatric Research, 38,* 1009-1017.

Boyd, H. F., & Johnson, G. O. (1981). *Analysis of coping style: A cognitive-behavioral approach to behavior management.* Columbus, OH: Merrill.

Boyd, J. R., & Hunsberger, M. (1998). Chronically ill children coping with repeated hospitalizations: Their perceptions and suggested interventions. *Journal of Pediatric Nursing, 13,* 330-342.

Broome, M. E., Hellier, A., Wilson, T., Dale, S., & Glanville, C. (1988). Measuring children's fears of medical experiences. In C. F. Waltz & O. L. Strickland (Eds.), *Measurement of nursing outcomes: Vol. 1. Measuring client outcomes* (pp. 201-214). New York: Springer.

Burnham, J. J., & Gullone, E. (1997). The Fear Survey Schedule for Children-II: A psychometric investigation with American data. *Behavior Research and Therapy, 35,* 165-173.

Campbell, S. B., Pierce, E. W., Moore, G., Marakovitz, S., & Newby, K. (1996). Boys' externalizing problems at elementary school age: Pathways from early behavior problems, maternal control, and family stress. *Development and Psychopathology, 8,* 701-719.

Canning, E. H., Canning, R. D., & Boyce, W. T. (1992). Depressive symptoms and adaptive style in children with cancer. *Journal of the American Academy of Child and Adolescent Psychiatry, 31,* 1120-1124.

Carey, W. B., & McDevitt, S. C. (1978). Revision of the Infant Temperament Questionnaire. *Pediatrics, 61,* 735-739.

Carlson, V., Cicchetti, D., Barnett, D., & Braunwald, K. (1989). Disorganized/disoriented attachment relationships in maltreated infants. *Developmental Psychology, 25,* 525-531.

Carroll, M. K., & Ryan-Wenger, N. A. (1999). School-age children's fears, anxiety, and human figure drawings. *Journal of Pediatric Health Care, 13,* 24-31.

Chandler, L. A., Shermis, M. D., & Marsh, J. (1985). The use of the Stress Response Scale in diagnostic assessment with children. *Journal of Psychoeducational Assessment, 3,* 15-29.

Chess, S. (1990). Studies in temperament: A paradigm in psychosocial research. *Yale Journal of Biology and Medicine, 63,* 313-324.

Coddington, R. D. (1972). The significance of life events as etiologic factors in the disease of children. II. A study of a normal population. *Journal of Psychosomatic Research, 16,* 205-213.

Coddington, R. D. (1984). Measuring the stressfulness of a child's environment. In J. H. Humphrey (Ed.), *Stress in childhood* (pp. 97-126). New York: AMS Press.

Cohen, F., & Lazarus, R. S. (1973). Active coping processes, coping dispositions, and recovery from surgery. *Psychosomatic Medicine, 35,* 375-389.

Compas, B. E. (1988). Coping with stress during childhood and adolescence. *Annual Progress in Child Psychiatry and Child Development,* 211-237.

Compas, B. E., Davis, G. E., Forsythe, C. J., & Wagner, B. M. (1987). Assessment of major and daily stressful events during adolescence: The Adolescent Perceived Events Scale. *Journal of Consulting and Clinical Psychology, 55,* 534-541.

Compas, B. E., Worsham, N. S., Grant, K. E., Mireault, G., Howell, D. C., Epping, J. E., & Malcarne, V. L. (1994). When mom or dad has cancer: Markers of psychological distress in cancer patients, spouses, and children. *Health Psychology, 13,* 507-515.

Dise-Lewis, J. E. (1988). The Life Events and Coping Inventory: An assessment of stress in children. *Psychosomatic Medicine, 50,* 484-499.

Drummond, P., & Hewson-Bower, B. (1997). Increased psychosocial stress and decreased mucosal immunity in children with recurrent upper respiratory tract infections. *Journal of Psychosomatic Research, 43,* 271-278.

Dyregrov, A., Kuterovac, G., & Barath, A. (1996). Factor analysis of the Impact of Event Scale with children in war. *Scandinavian Journal of Psychology, 37,* 339-350.

Elliott, C. H., Jay, S. M., & Woody, P. (1987). An observational scale for measuring children's distress during medical procedures. *Journal of Pediatric Psychology, 12,* 543-551.

Elwood, S. W. (1987). Stressor and coping response inventories for children. *Psychological Reports, 60,* 931-947.

Emery, R. E., & Coiro, M. J. (1997). Some costs of coping: Stress and distress among children from divorced families. In D. Cicchetti & S. L. Toth (Eds.), *Developmental perspectives on trauma: Theory, research and intervention* (pp. 435-462). Rochester, NY: University of Rochester Press.

Flinn, M., & England, B. (1997). Social economics of childhood glucocorticoid stress response and health. *American Journal of Physical Anthropology, 102,* 33-53.

Fullard, W., McDevitt, S. C., & Carey, W. B. (1984). Assessing temperament in one- to three-year-old children. *Journal of Pediatric Psychology, 9,* 205-217.

Gil, K. M., Abrams, M. R., Phillips, G., & Keefe, F. J. (1989). Sickle cell disease pain: Relations of coping strategies to adjustment. *Journal of Consulting and Clinical Psychology, 57,* 725-731.

Grant, K. E., & Compas, B. E. (1995). Stress and anxious-depressed symptoms among adolescents: Searching for mechanisms of risk. *Journal of Consulting and Clinical Psychology, 63,* 1015-1021.

Grey, M., & Hayman, L. L. (1987). Assessing stress in children: Research and clinical implications. *Journal of Pediatric Nursing, 2,* 316-327.

Grey, M., Lipman, T., Cameron, E., & Thurber, F. W. (1997). Coping behaviors at diagnosis and in adjustment one year later in children with diabetes. *Nursing Research, 46,* 312-317.

Gullone, E., & King, N. J. (1992). Psychometric evaluation of a revised fear survey schedule for children and adolescents. *Journal of Child Psychology and Psychiatry, 33,* 987-998.

Gullone, E., & King, N. J. (1993). The fears of youth in the 1990s: Contemporary normative data. *Journal of Genetic Psychology, 154,* 137-153.

Gunnar, M. R. (1992). Reactivity of the hypothalamic-pituitary-adrenocortical system to stressors in normal infants and children. *Pediatrics, 90,* 491-497.

Gunnar, M. R. (1998). Quality of early care and buffering of neuroendocrine stress reactions: Potential effects on the human brain. *Preventive Medicine, 27,* 208-211.

Gunnar, M., Mangelsdorf, S., Larson, M., & Hertsgaard, L. (1989). Attachment, temperament and adrenocortical activity in infancy: A study of psychoendocrine regulation. *Developmental Psychology, 25,* 355-363.

Haggerty, R. J., Sherrod, L. R., Garmezy, N., & Rutter, M. (1996). *Stress, risk and resilience in children and adolescents: Processes, mechanisms, and interventions.* New York: Cambridge University Press.

Hammer, A. L. (1988). *Manual for the Coping Resources Inventory.* Palo Alto, CA: Consulting Psychologists Press.

Hardy, D. F., Power, T. G., & Jaedicke, S. (1993). Examining the relation of parenting to children's coping with everyday stress. *Child Development, 64*(6), 1829-1841.

Hart, D., & Bossert, E. (1994). Self-reported fears of hospitalized school-age children. *Journal of Pediatric Nursing, 9,* 83-90.

Hegvik, R. L., McDevitt, S. C., & Carey, W. B. (1982). The Middle Childhood Temperament Questionnaire. *Developmental and Behavioral Pediatrics, 3,* 197-200.

Hertsgaard, L., Gunnarm, M., Erickson, M., & Nachmias, M. (1995). Adrenocortical responses to the strange situation in infants with disorganized/disoriented attachment relationships. *Child Development, 66,* 1100-1106.

Hilsman, R., & Garber, J. (1995). A test of the cognitive diathesis-stress model of depression in children: Academic stressors, attributional style, perceived competence, and control. *Journal of Personality and Social Psychology, 69*(2), 370-380.

Hockenberry-Eaton, M., Manteuffel, B., & Bottomley, S. (1997). Development of two instruments examining stress and adjustment in children with cancer. *Journal of Pediatric Oncology Nursing, 14,* 178-185.

Holmes, T. H., & Rahe, R. H. (1967). The social readjustment rating scale. *Journal of Psychosomatic Research, 11,* 213-218.

Horowitz, M., Wilner, N., & Alvarez, W. (1979). Impact of Event Scale: A measure of subjective stress. *Psychosomatic Medicine, 41,* 209-218.

Isaacs, D., Webster, A., & Valman, H. (1984). Immunoglobulin levels and function in pre-school children with recurrent respiratory infections. *Clinical Experience in Immunology, 58,* 335-340.

Johnson, J. H., & McCutcheon, S. (1980). Assessing life stress in older children and adolescents: Preliminary findings with the Life Events Checklist. In I. G. Sarason & C. D. Spielberger (Eds.), *Stress and anxiety, Vol. 7* (pp. 111-125). Washington, DC: Hemisphere.

Jones, F. C., & Selder, F. (1996). Psychoeducational groups to promote effective coping in school-age children living in violent communities. *Issues in Mental Health Nursing, 17,* 559-571.

Kaufman, J., Birmaher, B., Perel, J., Dahl, R., Moreci, P., Nelson, B., Wells, W., & Ryan, N. (1997). The corticotropin-releasing hormone challenge in depressed abused, depressed nonabused and normal control children. *Biological Psychiatry, 42,* 669-679.

Kleine, D. (1994). Sports activity as a means of reducing school stress. *International Journal of Sports Psychology, 22,* 366-380.

Kornguth, M. L. (1990). School illnesses: Who's absent and why? *Pediatric Nursing, 16,* 95-99.

LaMontagne, L. L. (1984). Children's locus of control beliefs as predictors of preoperative coping behavior. *Nursing Research, 33,* 76-85.

LaMontagne, L. L. (1987). Children's preoperative coping: Replication and extension. *Nursing Research, 36,* 163-167.

LaMontagne, L. L., Mason, K. R., & Hepworth, J. T. (1985). Effects of relaxation on anxiety in children: Implications for coping with stress. *Nursing Research, 34,* 289-292.

Larson, M., Gunnar, M., & Hertsgaard, L. (1991). The effects of morning naps, car trips and maternal separation on adrenocortical activity in human infants. *Child Development, 62,* 362-372.

Laudat, M. H., Cerdas, S., Fournier, C., Guiban, D., Guilhaume, B., & Luton, A. P. (1988). Salivary cortisol measurement: A practical approach to assess pituitary-adrenal function. *Journal of Clinical Endocrinology and Metabolism, 66,* 343-348.

Lazarus, R. S. (1990). Theory-based stress measurement. *Psychological Inquiry, 1,* 3-13.

Lazarus, R. S., & Folkman, S. (1984). *Stress, appraisal and coping.* New York: Springer.

Lazarus, R. S., & Launier, M. R. (1978). Stress related transaction between person and environment. In L. A. Pervin & M. Lewis (Eds.), *Perspectives in interactional psychology.* New York: Plenum.

Lewis, C. E., & Lewis, M. A. (1989). Educational outcomes and illness behaviors of participants in a child-initiated care system: A 12-year follow-up study. *Pediatrics, 84,* 845-850.

Lewis, C. E., Siegel, J. M., & Lewis, M. A. (1984). Feeling bad: Exploring sources of distress among preadolescent children. *American Journal of Public Health, 74,* 117-122.

Lewis, M., & Thomas, D. (1990). Cortisol release in infants in response to inoculation. *Child Development, 61,* 50-59.

Malpass, D., Treiber, F. A., Turner, J. R., Thompson, W., Levy, M., & Strong, W. B. (1997). Relationships between children's cardiovascular stress responses and resting cardiovascular functioning 1 year later. *International Journal of Psychophysiology, 25,* 139-144.

Martin, R. P. (1988). *The Temperament Assessment Battery for Children.* Brandon, VT: Clinical Psychology Press.

Mason, J. (1968). A review of psychoendocrine research on the pituitary-adrenal-cortical system. *Psychosomatic Medicine, 30,* 576-607.

Masten, A. S., Best, K. M., & Garmezy, N. (1990). Resilience and development: Contributions from the study of children who overcome adversity. *Development and Psychopathology, 2,* 425-444.

Masten, A. S., & Coatsworth, J. D. (1998). The development of competence in favorable and unfavorable environments: Lessons from research on successful children. *American Psychologist, 53,* 205-220.

McCubbin, H. I., & Patterson, J. M. (1987). A-FILE: Adolescent Family Inventory of Life Events and Changes. In H. I. McCubbin & A. I. Thompson (Eds.), *Family assessment inventories for research and practice* (pp. 100-109). Madison: University of Wisconsin Press.

McDevitt, S. C., & Carey, W. B. (1978). The measurement of temperament in 3-7 year old children. *Journal of Child Psychology and Psychiatry, 19,* 245-253.

Meisgeier, C., & Murphy, E. (1987). *Murphy-Meisgeier Type Indicator for Children.* Palo Alto, CA: Consulting Psychologists Press.

Merrell, K. W., & Walters, A. S. (1998). *Internalizing Symptoms Scale for Children.* Austin, TX: Pro-Ed.

Miller, S. M. (1989). Cognitive informational styles in the process of coping with threat and frustration. *Advances in Behavioural Research and Therapy, 11,* 223-234.

Monaghan, J. H., Robinson, J. O., & Dodge, J. A. (1979). The Children's Life Events Inventory. *Journal of Psychosomatic Research, 23,* 63-68.

Mooney, K. C., Graziano, A. M., & Katz, J. N. (1984). A factor-analytic investigation of children's nighttime fear and coping responses. *Journal of Genetic Psychology, 111,* 205-215.

Morris, R. D., Krawiecki, N. S., Wright, J. A., & Walter, L. W. (1993). Neuropsychological, academic, and adaptive functioning in children who survive in-hospital cardiac arrest and resuscitation. *Journal of Learning Disabilities, 26,* 46-51.

Murphy, L. B., & Moriarty, A. E. (1976). *Vulnerability, coping and growt'..* New Haven, CT: Yale University Press.

Musante, L., Treiber, F. A., Davis, H., Levy, M., & Strong, W. B. (1995). Temporal stability of children's cardiovascular reactivity: Role of ethnicity, gender and family history of myocardial infraction. *International Journal of Psychophysiology, 19,* 281-286.

Neff, E. J. A., & Dale, J. C. (1996). Worries of school-age children. *Journal of the Society of Pediatric Nurses, 1,* 27-32.

Newcomb, M. D., Huba, G. J., & Bentley, P. M. (1981). A multidimensional assessment of stressful life events among adolescents: Derivation and correlates. *Journal of Health and Social Behavior, 22,* 400- 415.

Patterson, J. M., & McCubbin, H. I. (1987). A-COPE: Adolescent Coping Orientation for Problem Experiences. In H. I. McCubbin & A. I. Thompson (Eds.), *Family assessment inventories for research and practice* (pp. 226-241). Madison: University of Wisconsin Press.

Peterson, L., & Toler, S. M. (1986). An information seeking disposition in child surgery patients. *Health Psychology, 5,* 343-358.

Phipps, S., & Mulhern, R. K. (1995). Family cohesion and expressiveness promote resilience to the stress of pediatric bone marrow transplant: A preliminary report. *Developmental and Behavioral Pediatrics, 16,* 257-263.

Rende, R. D., & Plomin, R. (1991). Child and parent perceptions of the upsettingness of major life events. *Journal of Child Psychology and Psychiatry, 32,* 627-633.

Repetti, R. L. (1994). Short-term and long-term effects of processes linking perceived job stressors to father-child interaction. *Social Development, 3,* 1-15.

Repetti, R. L. (1996). The effects of perceived daily social and academic failure experiences on school-age children's subsequent interactions with parents. *Child Development, 67,* 1467-1482.

Ritchie, J. A., Caty, S., & Ellerton, M. (1988). Coping behaviors of hospitalized preschool children. *Maternal Child Nursing Journal, 17,* 153-171.

Rose, M. H. (1972). *The effects of hospitalization on coping behaviors of children.* Unpublished doctoral dissertation, University of Chicago, Chicago.

Rossen, R., Butler, W., Walkman, R., Alford, R., Hornick, R., Togo, Y., & Kasel, J. (1970). The proteins in nasal secretion. II. A longitudinal study of IgA and neutralizing antibody levels in nasal washings from men infected with influenza virus. *Journal of the American Medical Association, 211,* 1157-1161.

Rudolph, K. D., Dennig, M. D., & Weisz, J. R. (1995). Determinants and consequences of children's coping in the medical setting: Conceptualization, review and critique. *Psychological Bulletin, 118,* 328-357.

Rutter, M. (1996). Stress research: Accomplishments and tasks ahead. In R. J. Haggerty, L. R. Sherrod, N. Garmezy, & M. Rutter (Eds.), *Stress, risk and resilience in children and adolescents: Processes, mechanisms, and interventions* (pp. 354-385). New York: Cambridge University Press.

Ryan, N. M. (1988). The stress-coping process in school-age children: Gaps in the knowledge needed for health promotion. *Advances in Nursing Science, 11,* 1-12.

Ryan, N. M. (1989). Stress-coping strategies identified from school-age children's perspective. *Research in Nursing & Health, 12*(2), 111-122.

Ryan-Wenger, N. A. (1990). Development and psychometric properties of the schoolagers' coping strategies inventory. *Nursing Research, 39*(6), 346-349.

Ryan-Wenger, N. A. (1992). A taxonomy of children's coping strategies: A step toward theory development. *American Journal of Orthopsychiatry, 62,* 256-263.

Ryan-Wenger, N. A. (1996). Children, coping and the stress of illness: A synthesis of the research. *Journal of the Society of Pediatric Nurses, 1,* 126-138.

Schuller, S. (1994). Load and stress in school: Their sources and possibility of coping with them. *Studia Psychologica, 26,* 41-54.

Seyle, H. (1976). *The stress of life* (Rev. ed.). New York: McGraw-Hill.

Sharrer, V. W., & Ryan-Wenger, N. A. (1995). A longitudinal study of age and gender differences in school-age children's stressors and coping strategies. *Journal of Pediatric Health Care, 9,* 123-130.

Smith, J., & Prior, M. (1995). Temperament and stress resilience in school-age children: A within-families study. *Journal of the American Academy of Child and Adolescent Psychiatry, 34,* 168-179.

Spirito, A., Stark, L. J., Gil, K. M., & Tyc, V. L. (1995). Coping with everyday and disease-related stressors by chronically ill children and adolescents. *Journal of the American Academy of Child and Adolescent Psychiatry, 34,* 283-290.

Spirito, A., Stark, L. J., & Williams, C. (1988). Development of a Brief Coping Checklist for use with pediatric populations. *Journal of Pediatric Psychology, 13,* 555-574.

Steward, D. (1998). *Biophysical correlates of non-organic failure to thrive in infants.* Unpublished doctoral dissertation, Ohio State University, College of Nursing, Columbus.

Sugarman, L. I. (1996). Hypnosis: Teaching children self-regulation. *Pediatrics in Review, 17,* 5-11.

Thomas, A., & Chess, S. (1984). *Temperament and development.* New York: Brunner/Mazel.

Thompson, R. A., & Calkins, S. D. (1996). The double-edged sword: Emotional regulation for children at risk. *Development and Psychopathology, 8,* 163-182.

Visintainer, M. A., & Wolfer, J. A. (1975). Psychological preparation for surgical pediatric patients: The effect on children's and parents' stress response and adjustment. *Pediatrics, 56,* 187-202.

Walker, L. O., & Avant, K. C. (1988). *Strategies for theory construction in nursing.* Norwalk, CT: Appleton-Century-Crofts.

Weisz, J. R., McCabe, M. A., & Dennig, M. D. (1994). Primary and secondary control among children undergoing medical procedures: Adjustment as a function of coping style. *Journal of Consulting and Clinical Psychology, 62,* 324-332.

Weitzman, M., Walker, D. K., & Gortmaker, S. (1986). Chronic illness, psychosocial problems, and school absences: Results of a survey of one county. *Clinical Pediatrics, 25,* 137-141.

Wertlieb, D., Weigel, C., & Feldstein, M. (1987). Measuring children's coping. *American Journal of Orthopsychiatry, 57,* 548-560.

Yamamoto, K. (1979). Children's ratings of the stressfulness of experiences. *Developmental Psychology, 15,* 581-582.

Yeaworth, R. C., York, J., Hussey, M. A., Ingle, M. E., & Goodwin, T. (1980). The development of an adolescent life change event scale. *Adolescence, 57,* 91-97.

Zeitlan, S. (1980). Assessing coping behavior. *American Journal of Orthopsychiatry, 50,* 139-144.

Zeitlan, S. (1985a). *Coping Inventory: A measure of adaptive behavior (observation form).* Bensenville, IL: Scholastic Testing Service.

Zeitlan, S. (1985b). *Coping Inventory: A measure of adaptive behavior (self-rated form).* Bensenville, IL: Scholastic Testing Service.

Zeitlan, S., Williamson, G. G., & Szczepanski, M. (1988). *Early Coping Inventory: A measure of adaptive behavior.* Bensenville, IL: Scholastic Testing Service.

CHAPTER 12

Stress, Coping, and Family Health

Rosanna DeMarco, Marilyn Ford-Gilboe,
Marie-Luise Friedemann, Hamilton I. McCubbin,
and Marilyn A. McCubbin

T he ways in which people cope is the most significant mediating factor in determining conse- quences of life stress on their health (Bomar, 1996). To date, much of the stress, coping, and health research has focused on the individual as the unit of analysis. Rarely, however, does a person manage life's demands on his or her own. Individuals also belong to a family, and it is within this context that they deal with day- to-day life stressors. Of necessity, what the in- dividual does or feels can affect the whole family unit, just as the family unit is an impor- tant influence on individual behavior. Pender (1996) wrote,

Health values, attitudes, and behaviors are learned in the family context. The place of health in the family value structure and the extent to which health-promoting knowl- edge and [coping] skills are transmitted to offspring determine the degree of impact

that families have on the health potential of future generations. (p. 80)

Helping families to learn to cope successfully with the stressors that they face in their day- to-day lives is a formidable task as family practitioners examine the many perspectives and interpretations of family stress, coping, and health. In this chapter, theoretical models of family stress, coping, and health are de- tailed and critiqued. Conceptual definitions are presented, issues of measurement and logical and empirical adequacy are reviewed, and the contributions of respective research findings to nursing knowledge are evaluated.

➤ TRADITIONAL FRAMEWORKS OF FAMILY STRESS, COPING, AND HEALTH

Interest in family stress and coping originated within the social sciences. Formal theorizing can be traced to Reubin Hill's (1949, 1958) classic ABCX model of family stress. On the basis of research conducted with families who had experienced separation during war, Hill proposed three interrelated factors that were thought to precipitate family crisis. The concept of "crisis" (or "X" factor), Hill argued, was intended to mark the point at which a family unit is disrupted and disorganized in the face of both normative and nonnormative stressor-induced situations. The three critical factors that best explain the "crisis proneness" of families are the stressor and related hardships ("A" factor), the family's resources needed to manage the stressor ("B" factor), and the family's definition of the stressor ("C" factor). According to the theory, families who are crisis prone tend to experience more stressors, particularly those that pose major challenges. In addition, these families tend to have fewer coping resources available to them and are more likely to view stressors as crises in family life rather than as manageable events. Within the ABCX model, families are proposed to follow a roller-coaster course of adjustment with a trajectory of disorganization, crisis, reorganization, and recovery (Hill, 1949, 1958). Not all families, however, progress to the point of a family crisis in which the family system changes and reorganization is necessary. The ABCX components of the Hill model were introduced as explanatory or predictor variables to account for the variability in family functioning in the face of a stressor and to determine which families deteriorated to the point of experiencing a crisis and which families did not. Thus, Hill's model focuses on precrisis variables or what has been referred to in the later literature as protective factors.

On the basis of both qualitative and quantitative longitudinal investigations conducted on families faced with war-induced separations, Hill's ABCX model evolved into the double ABCX model (McCubbin & Patterson, 1983a). This evolution was based on several fundamental observations. First, in the face of conditions of chronic stress, families, operating as a system, are forced into a crisis

and called on to reorganize and change their patterns of operation. Second, the ABCX factors defined in the Hill model were not sufficient to explain the variability in postcrisis family functioning involving reorganization and recovery. Therefore, additional factors were identified. Third, the outcome of family postcrisis behavior and processes appeared to be that of adaptation. Families need to achieve a different level of functioning as a result of changes in the family system. This level of functioning, referred to as adaptation (XX factor), reflects the family's effort to balance demands placed on the family unit referred to as "pileup" (AA factor) with the family's resources and capabilities (BB factor). Family appraisal (CC factor) involves an overall assessment of the family situation, including the stressor and its hardships, changes made, the family's capability, the compatibility of family changes with member needs and development, and the coordination and synergism of these family changes with all aspects of family functioning and system needs. Coping is the family's operating arm for producing these changes, reducing tension, and achieving family harmony and balance.

With the added focus on the family processes involved in adaptation, namely, the family's postcrisis behaviors, the double ABCX model took on a subsequent transformation referred to as the Family Adjustment and Adaptation Response (FAAR) model (McCubbin & Patterson, 1983b). In this framework, family processes involved in adaptation are introduced and described. The family's movement through postcrisis recovery involves a set of processes inclusive of change, synergism, congruency, coordination, assimilation, accommodation, and coping. Interestingly, research on family protective factors and processes emerged as the FAAR model was being introduced and subjected to scrutiny and additional study. Family protective processes gained prominence as family scientists examined the patterns of functioning that served to protect families from being "crisis prone" and that also served to foster the ease of family recovery in the face of a crisis situation (McCubbin, 1987; Olson et al., 1984). The FAAR model also was being tested for its applicability to the study of families faced with childhood chronic illnesses, namely, cystic fibrosis, myelomeningocele, and cerebral palsy. Family patterns or typologies (T factor) of family functioning emerged as important predictors of family postcrisis adaptation and functioning. Most prominent among the typologies were family patterns of regenerativity, resiliency, traditionalism, and rhythmicity. With these sets of dramatic findings, depicting both protective and recovery patterns of family functioning that served to predict family adaptation, the T-Double ABCX model, which was inclusive of the FAAR elements, was given recognition and advanced for additional study and application for practice.

The development and evolution of family stress theory took another bold step with the emergence of the Resiliency Model of Family Stress, Adjustment, and Adaptation. Not only did risk, protective, and recovery factors gain prominence in the resiliency model but also the conceptual framework evolved as a result of research on families of different ethnic groups and cultures as well as emerging interest in multiple levels of family appraisal found to be relevant in understanding and explaining family adaptation (McCubbin & McCubbin, 1993; McCubbin, McCubbin, Thompson, & Thompson, 1995/1996). In the Resiliency Model of Family Stress, Adjustment, and Adaptation, the assumption that families manage stressful situations over time emphasizes the family's ability to recover from stressful events and crises by drawing on patterns of functioning, strengths, capabilities, appraisal processes, coping, resources, and problem solving to facilitate adaptation. Because of the centrality of the resiliency model in the study of family stress and coping in nursing, it is reviewed in depth later.

Using a symbolic interactionist perspective, Boss (1987) proposed that although the meaning of an event to the family is the most important factor influencing family stress, it is the least well understood. Furthermore, be-cause families do not live in a vacuum, the context of family life is critical in shaping experiences of stress. The Contextual Model of Family Stress (Boss, 1987) develops the concept of family context, situated as two concentric circles surrounding the concepts of the ABCX model. In the innermost circle, internal context relates to factors that the family can change and control and includes three dimensions: (a) structural context, including the family boundaries, roles, and rules; (b) psychological context—the family's perception (both cognitive and affective) of the stressful event; and (c) philosophical context, or the family's values and beliefs. Unlike the internal context, the family has little or no control over its external context—the broader environment in which the family is situated. This outermost circle includes the elements of culture, history, economics, development, and heredity. Boss also differentiates between family stress and crisis. Family stress is a neutral concept that simply describes pressure experienced by families that changes family equilibrium in some way. Two outcomes of stress are possible within Boss's model: crisis or coping. Crisis is a serious disturbance in the functioning of the family such that the family is immobilized. Coping refers to the family's management of the stressful event such that there are no detrimental effects on family members. Although this definition of coping is tied to effectiveness or success in management (an outcome), Boss also refers to coping as a process of managing the stressful situation, leading to confusion about the nature of this concept.

Burr, Klein, and associates (1994) developed a systems-oriented model of family stress as a means of addressing inconsistency between family theories that emphasize systems processes and the deterministic assumptions of the ABCX model and theories that have evolved from it that have guided much of the research about family stress and coping. For these theorists, stress is viewed as a process that is intrinsically linked to other family systems processes. Family stress occurs when usual rules for managing family life (i.e., rules of transformation) are not sufficient for the family to handle change or a new input to the system. As a result, normal activities and routines are disrupted, and attention is focused on the stressful situation and how the family will manage it. Using this perspective, Burr et al. studied stress processes of 50 families experiencing six different stressful events: bankruptcy, institutionalized handicapped child, troubled teenager, chronically ill child (muscular dystrophy), infertility, and displacement as a homemaker. Data were collected using in-depth interviews, observation, and questionnaires in participants' homes during a 3-month period. Study findings provided support for complexity and variation in family stress and coping processes. The following theoretical insights have been proposed from this work: (a) families exhibit many different patterns of response to stressful situations; (b) families that are quick to allocate resources for managing a stressful situation tend to cope more effectively than those that wait; (c) the emotional subsystem (communication, cohesion, bonding, and togetherness) may improve as a result of experiencing stress; (d) if families focus on changes in their emotional systems during stress, they tend to cope more effectively; (e) although specific coping strategies tend to be generally helpful or harmful, this determination is context specific; and (f) there are some general differences in men's and women's approaches to coping with stressful events (Burr et al., 1994).

In summary, this brief overview of family stress and coping theories that have evolved within social science provides a glimpse into foundational work in this area. For in-depth descriptions of these theories, the reader is directed to the original texts. Although much theorizing about family stress and coping evolved from the ABCX model, there is a clear indication that scholarship within this domain is shifting its focus to consider the impact of systems thinking, the role of family strengths and resiliency, and the role of context in family stress experience. Foundational work conducted within the social sciences has been influential in nursing's approach to family stress and coping. Although family stress and coping theories that have evolved within nursing bear some similarity to social science perspectives, they have been less bound to these theories and, therefore, provide unique ways of understanding family stress and coping.

► EVOLVING PERSPECTIVES IN NURSING

It is no accident that theories of family stress, coping, and resiliency emerged within nursing. The durability of the family system in the face of adversity has profound implications for both the short- and long-term health and well-being of family members, who may be living with disease or disability. Nurses are challenged to promote the health and development of both family members and the family as a unit. In the following sections, three theories that have advanced nursing's ability to understand, predict, and work with families under stress are examined. The theories reviewed vary in both perspective and stage of development and are presented as examples of nursing's unique contribution to understanding family stress and coping.

The Resiliency Model of Family Stress, Adjustment, and Adaptation

Origins and Evolution

One of the important developments in family stress theory is advancement of theories that explain resiliency in the family unit. Family resiliency theory, a natural extension of family stress theory, was developed to shed light on our understanding of how and why some families, when faced with the adversity of illnesses and traumatic conditions, are able to cope, endure, and survive. It also plays a vital and positive role in explaining support and in-home care to promote the well-being of family members who may be threatened or affected by the situation. For the purpose of developing and applying intervention strategies, nursing and other disciplines are cultivating the development of resiliency theories that answer the complex question of which combination of risk factors, protective factors, and recovery factors determines which families are more likely to adapt to a family crisis involving a traumatizing illness or medical condition.

The combined research and theory-building efforts of nursing and family scientists, encompassing a period of 15 years at the endowed Institute for the Study of Resiliency in Families and the Family Stress, Coping, and Health Project at the University of Wisconsin-Madison, have resulted in the Resiliency Model of Family Stress, Adjustment, and Adaptation (McCubbin & McCubbin, 1993, 1996). This framework has been used to guide research by nursing and behavioral scientists throughout the world working both individually and collectively to isolate protective and recovery factors in the family unit that may affect physical and psychological outcomes of family members affected by medical conditions. In addition, the resiliency model and derived findings have fostered the parallel research efforts directed at the development and testing of reliable and valid measures to assess risk, protective, and recovery factors to be used in family and health-related investigations. The development of family measures to study stress, coping, and resiliency has been in progress for the past 20 years (McCubbin & Thompson, 1987, 1991; McCubbin, Thompson, & McCubbin, 1996; Olson et al., 1984).

Resiliency and Family Nursing

In the context of family nursing, *family resiliency* is defined as the property of the family system that enables the family unit to respond constructively to (a) a stressor (in combination with risk factors) and, in so doing, maintain its positive functioning and ensure the well-being and development of the family unit and its members (i.e., protective), and (b) disorganization (family crisis brought about by a stressor in combination with risk factors) and, in doing so, bounce back and restore its positive functioning and ensure the well-being and development of the family unit and its members (i.e., recovery).

The concept of family resiliency has a rich history embedded in the longitudinal research on resilience in children (Werner, 1984; Werner & Smith, 1982), the study of resiliency in children at risk for adverse developmental outcomes (Garmezy, 1991a, 1991b; Rutter, 1990), investigations of children's competence as a protective factor in the face of risk situations (Garmezy, 1987; Garmezy & Masten, 1991; Luthar & Zigler, 1992), and the study of resiliency in inner-city adolescents (Luthar, 1991; Luthar, Doernberger, & Zigler, 1993).

There has been a proliferation of research on resiliency in children and youth with investigations designed to determine which aspects in the family milieu emerge as central protective factors in the development of resiliency in children (Baldwin, 1990; Conrad & Hammen, 1993; Richters & Martinez, 1993; Wyman, Cowen, Work, & Parker, 1991). In the past decade, nursing and family scientists have expanded this earlier focus to investigate and advance theories to explain variability in resiliency of the family system in the face of normative (McCubbin, 1999) and nonnormative life events and changes (McCubbin, McCubbin, Thompson, Han, & Allen, 1997).

Drawing from two decades of family stress, coping, and resiliency research to which they are sustained contributors, McCubbin and McCubbin (1993, 1996) in collaboration with their colleagues (McCubbin et al., 1995/1996, 1997) developed and tested the Resiliency Model of Family Stress, Adjustment, and Adaptation. This conceptual framework has been used to guide both family science and nursing studies throughout the world. The 36 copyrighted research instruments developed by the McCubbin and McCubbin team and tested for reliability and validity have been used to measure various dimensions of the resiliency framework, particularly risk, protective, and recovery factors.

Normative data are available for many of these measures, and some have been translated into foreign languages, including Korean, Chinese, Spanish, Hebrew, Japanese, and Russian for application in cross-cultural studies (McCubbin et al., 1996).

As described previously, the Resiliency Model of Family Stress, Adjustment, and Adaptation is rooted in Hill's (1949, 1958) ABCX model and has evolved systematically for a period of 20 years. This evolution has been fostered by both qualitative and quantitative studies of families faced with life events such as war-induced separation (McCubbin, Dahl, Hunter, & Plag, 1975), having a child member with a chronic illness (McCubbin & McCubbin, 1993), and normative transitions and changes (McCubbin, Thompson, Pirner, & McCubbin, 1988). The inductively derived conceptual model of family resiliency focuses on the role of risk, protective, and recovery factors in the prediction and explanation of family resiliency (McCubbin et al., 1997). The McCubbin and McCubbin framework seeks to explain why some families endure life's hardships and traumas with minor adjustment and appear to be buffered by protective factors. The framework is also intended to explain why families in crisis, or those who experience disorganization and a need for change due to life events, are able to bounce back, recover, and adapt through the use of recovery factors in the process of restoring, changing, and introducing new patterns of family functioning.

A more complete diagram of the family resiliency model (McCubbin & McCubbin, 1996), which has also been developed to have predictive and explanatory value in the study of families of different ethnic groups, is presented in Figure 12.1 (adjustment phase) and Figure 12.2 (adaptation phase).

Family Adjustment:
A Short-Term Response

In the face of a diagnosis and the demands of caring for a member with an illness or disability, the family's initial reaction is predictably to maintain the "status quo" with minimal changes in how the family typically operates and behaves. In this "adjustment phase" of the resiliency model, the family system draws from its existing patterns of functioning, strengths, and protective factors (e.g., accord, hardiness, time and routines, celebrations, and traditions). The interacting components in this phase of family resiliency are seen as (a) the stressor event (e.g., diagnosis, illness, and disability); (b) the family's vulnerability (risk factors and the pileup of concurrent life changes, such as marital conflict, abuse, and history of violence); (c) the family's established patterns of functioning (e.g., family time and routines and family traditions); (d) the family's resources, both internal and external to the family unit (e.g., cohesiveness and social support); (e) the family's appraisal of the stressor and its severity; and (f) the family's coping repertoire and problem-solving communication (e.g., seeking consultation, openness to medical advice, and seeking support from support groups). In the short term, the family directs its energy and does all that is possible to keep family system changes to a minimum and attempts to maintain healthy functioning in the family unit. The family seeks to maintain harmony and balance among its four basic components—namely, the family's interpersonal relationships, the family's development and member well-being (including spirituality), the family's structure and functioning, and the family's relationship with the community.

The confirmation of a diagnosis or disability or both, combined with ever-increasing demands on the family unit to modify its established patterns of functioning, to introduce new patterns, and to find harmony and balance in the family system will often move the family into a crisis situation. Family crisis is not a pejorative term. Rather, it represents a state of temporary disorganization accompanied by a demand for changes in the family's expectations, rules, and overall patterns of functioning. At this point, the family struggles to modify the old and introduce new patterns of functioning to achieve family adaptation—

Figure 1

Adjustment Phase of the Resiliency Model of Family Stress, Adjustment and Adaptation and the Relational Processes of Balance and Harmony

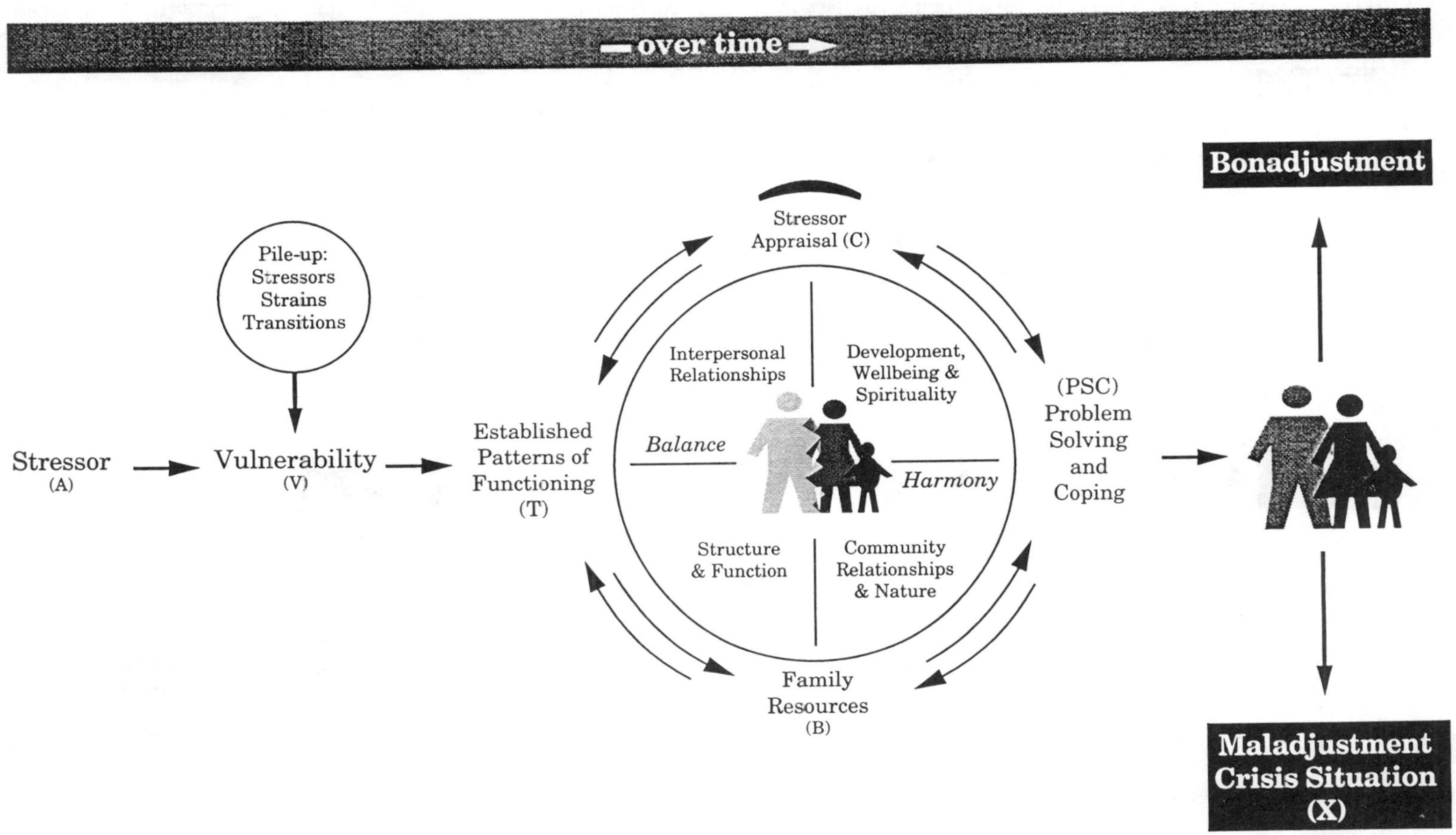

Figure 12.1. Adjustment Phase of the Resiliency Model of Family Stress, Adjustment, and Adaptation and the Relational Processes of Balance and Harmony (reproduced with permission from McCubbin & McCubbin, 1996)

Figure 2

Adaptation Phase of the Resiliency Model of Family Stress, Adjustment and Adaptation and the Relational Processes of Balance and Harmony

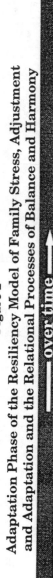

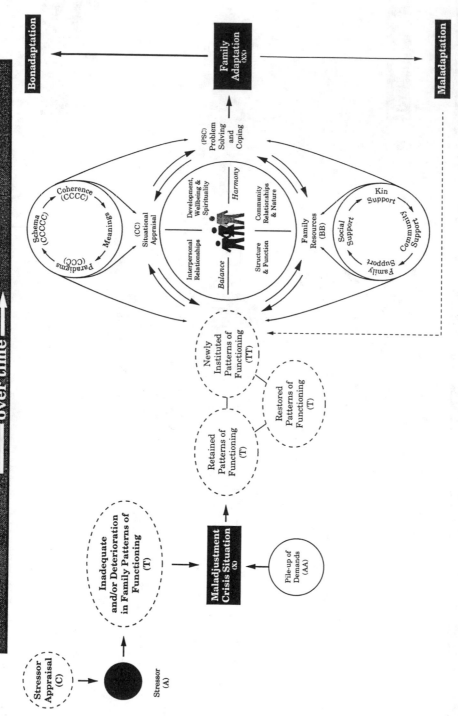

Figure 12.2. Adaptation Phase of the Resiliency Model of Family Stress, Adjustment, and Adaptation and the Relational Processes of Balance and Harmony (reproduced with permission from McCubbin & McCubbin, 1996)

the point at which harmony and congruency at the interpersonal, developmental, structural, and community levels of family functioning are achieved.

Family Adaptation: The Long-Term Response

The level and ease of family adaptation, according to McCubbin and McCubbin (1988a, 1988b, 1993, 1996), is determined by many interacting factors. These moderating and mediating factors include the pileup of family demands and risk factors extant to the family unit (e.g., prior marriage with stepchildren in the household) and its history as well as demands created by an illness situation (e.g., home care regimen and treatment plans). The family continues to develop, and normal family life cycle transitions (e.g., having an adolescent in the home), prior strains (e.g., conflict regarding religious beliefs and spending money), unresolved conflicts and issues (e.g., marital conflict), the positive and unexpected side effects of a family's efforts to cope (e.g., conflict because spouse takes on additional work to make ends meet) also come into play and influence the family's response and adaptation. The concurrent normal and abnormal life events (e.g., death in the extended family) and the ambiguity regarding what the future will hold for the family unit must all be taken into account in evaluating the family's capability for managing the diagnosis and future course of treatment for the ill member. The accumulation of life changes and hardships determines the extent to which the family's capabilities and protective resources (e.g., income, psychological and interpersonal strengths, and established patterns of family functioning that serve to creates stability and predictability) are disrupted, deteriorated, drawn down, or depleted and what remains of these patterns to be applied to helping the family to adapt to the current family crisis situation.

Family recovery factors are also important in the resiliency model. Efforts to create and adopt new and necessary patterns of functioning are important to consider in an assessment of family resiliency. For example, the family's ability to comprehend and integrate a home care medical regimen into their pattern of functioning, while maintaining or restoring family harmony and balance is an important consideration in the family's ability to achieve a satisfactory level of adaptation. The family unit may need to establish a supportive network of friends and associates to help them to cope with the situation. The medical community of physicians and nurses may be a new part of the family's network of support—a social group that did not exist or that was not previously important. Family system resources of flexibility and problem-solving communication that ensure a mutually supportive and encouraging rather than a conflictual pattern of communication may become even more important to the family unit in a crisis situation.

The resiliency model, which also draws from Aaron Antonovsky's exemplary theory building and research on "sense of coherence" (see Chapter 8 of this book) also underscores the importance of the family's appraisal processes in achieving a satisfactory level of family adaptation. Families are also called on to reconcile differences and conflicts that may emerge when the family unit, through a trial-and-error process, adopts patterns of functioning to cope that may not be congruent with the family's strongly held beliefs and values. The family's worldview, or what McCubbin and McCubbin (1996) call family schema, must also be congruent with the family's newly instituted patterns of functioning. For example, McCubbin and McCubbin note that family members may find meaning and value in raising the nation's consciousness about a disease or disability a family member may have with the hope that more research funding could lead to new and effective treatments. To champion this national cause, however, may move a family unit farther apart because some members may be "on the road" while the remaining members struggle to achieve balance and harmony on their own. This may create an incongruous situation between the family's schema of working together as a unit and a family member's efforts to make the disease or disability a national priority.

The family unit is also called on to give meaning to the health problem. Family meanings are the collective views of the family unit cultivated, developed, and adopted (actively and passively) by family members to render legitimacy and acceptability to the current situation (e.g., illness and disability). These values relate to the family's efforts to cope, to the family's adopted patterns of functioning, and to the family's hopes and beliefs for the future, given the crisis that has altered the family's original life course to a substantial degree.

Family paradigms may also change to give legitimacy and meaning to the new patterns of functioning. Families may have shaped and adopted a family paradigm for work that affirms family members' individuality to do what is necessary to promote their own professional or work careers. In the face of a family health problem, this paradigm may be cast aside and replaced by a shared commitment to have one member devote his/her full-time efforts to the care of a member who is ill or disabled with the agreement that, at some time in the future, this member may pursue his or her own career goals. Family paradigms, according to the resiliency model, serve a vital role in stabilizing and giving predictability to the family unit. They are most commonly created and adopted to guide the family's central areas of functioning—namely, the family's marital or partner communication, sexual relationship, parenting relationship, work and family relationships, financial management, in-laws and relatives relationships, and social relationships.

The resiliency model includes a family's cultural and ethnic history that may be embedded in the personal history of its members. McCubbin and McCubbin (1996) argue that culture and ethnicity play a critical role in shaping the family's response to family crises and the adoption of patterns of functioning

needed to achieve a satisfactory level of adaptation. By drawing from and conducting studies of African American, Filipino, Asian American, and Native Hawaiian families under stress, McCubbin and McCubbin isolate the importance of culture and ethnicity in the family schema (e.g., values, beliefs, and rules) and sense of coherence (e.g., trust, control, and manageability), both of which are confirmed to be important to the family process of adaptation in the face of family crises.

Instrument Development and Use

The Resiliency Model of Family Stress, Adjustment, and Adaptation emerged from and continues to be shaped by an inductive process with research informing theory. Consequently, the development of family measures to study risk, protective, and recovery factors in the process of adaptation has been continuous since the introduction of the initial versions of the theoretical framework in 1978. Throughout the years, the Family Stress, Coping, and Health Project has generated 36 reliable and valid self-report and family system-focused research instruments. In testing the evolving theory, a host of family adaptation measures have been used, including the family APGAR (Adaptation, Partnership, Growth, Affection, Resolve) (Smilkstein, 1978), FACES (Family and Cohesion Evaluation Scales I, II, IIA, III) (Olson, Portner, & Bell, 1978, 1982), Family Index of Regenerativity and Adaptation-General (McCubbin & Thompson, 1987), Family Member Well-Being Index (McCubbin & Patterson, 1982/1996), Family Distress Index (McCubbin, Thompson, Thompson, & McCubbin, 1993), and Family Attachment and Changeability Index (McCubbin, Thompson, & Elver, 1995/1996a). In addition, measures of family risk factors, family protective factors, and family recovery factors, presented in the book *Family Assessment: Resiliency, Coping and Adaptation—Inventories for Research and Practice* (McCubbin, Olson, & Larson, 1996) include the following:

1. Risk factors or pileup: the Family Inventory of Life Events and Changes (FILE; McCubbin & Patterson, 1983a), the Adolescent–Family Inventory of Life Events and Changes (AFILE; McCubbin, Patterson, Bauman, & Harris, 1981/1996), the Young Adult Family Inventory of Life Events and Strains (YAFILE; McCubbin, Patterson, & Grochowski, 1984/1996), and the Family Pressures Scale–Ethnic (McCubbin, Thompson, & Elver, 1993/1996)

2. Protective factors: the Family Hardiness Index (McCubbin, McCubbin, & Thompson, 1988), the Family Inventory of Resources for Management (McCubbin, Comeau, & Harkins, 1991), the Family Time and Routines Index (McCubbin, McCubbin, & Thompson, 1988), the Family Traditions Scale (McCubbin & Thompson, 1986a/1996), the Family Celebrations Index (McCubbin & Thompson, 1986b/1996), the Social Support Index (SSI; McCubbin, Patterson, & Glynn, 1981/1996), and the Young Adult Social Support Index (YA-SSI; McCubbin et al., 1984/1996)

3. Recovery factors: the Coping Health Inventory for Parents (McCubbin, McCubbin, Nevin, & Cauble, 1983/1996; McCubbin et al., 1983), the Family Crisis Oriented Personal Evaluation Scales (McCubbin, Olson, & Larsen, 1981/1996), the Family Coping Index (McCubbin, Thompson, & Elver, 1995/1996b), the Adolescent Coping Orientation for Problem Experiences (Patterson & McCubbin, 1983/1996), the Youth Coping Index (McCubbin, Thompson, & Elver, 1995/1996c), the Family Problem Solving Communication (McCubbin et al., 1988), the Dual-Employed Coping Scales (Skinner & McCubbin, 1981), and the Family Schema–Ethnic Inventory (McCubbin, Thompson, Elver, & Carpenter, 1992/1996)

Nursing Research

The evolution of nursing research using the resiliency model resulted from the profession's interest in exploring family change and adaptation over time. Although the theoretical framework had its origin in war-induced family traumas, the resiliency model gained currency by virtue of its relevance to the study of families coping with many health problems, including myelomeningocele (McCubbin, 1988a, 1989), handicaps (McCubbin, 1988b), cystic fibrosis (McCubbin, McCubbin, Mischler, & Svavarsdottir, in press), and cerebral palsy (McCubbin et al., 1981).

Carr (1995) affirmed the value of the resiliency model as a guide to nursing research. Many nursing studies have examined family stress and adaptation within the framework of the resiliency model. For example, the resiliency model has been used to guide research on families coping with acute health problems, such as myocardial infarction (Carr, 1995), severe trauma, and head injuries (Kosciulek, McCubbin, & McCubbin, 1993; Leske & Jiricka, 1998). The model has also been used to study family responses to chronic childhood conditions in many contexts, including those caring for infants with chronic apnea at home, children with congenital heart conditions, and children with a variety of illnesses participating in early discharge programs after rehabilitation (Svavarsdottir & McCubbin, 1996; Youngblut, Brennan, & Swegart, 1994). In addition, the model has been used to examine life changes such as retirement (Smith, 1997).

Critique of the Model and Special Considerations

Originally, Hill's ABCX model offered simplicity and a charted, linear approach to knowledge development about family stress and family crises. McCubbin, McCubbin, and associates (McCubbin & McCubbin, 1988a, 1988b, 1996; McCubbin et al., 1997) have made the case for looking beyond family crises. They have fostered a line of research designed to isolate those risk, protective, and recovery factors that provide nursing with the best possible predictors of family adaptation in the face of a range of illnesses, disabilities, and life situations. Ironically, although the complexity of the Resiliency Model of Family Adjustment and Adaptation has shed new light on critical factors that shape the outcome of family adaptation, particularly for those families of different ethnic backgrounds, the model has also been difficult to test as a whole. Although a few investigations have examined the model in a comprehensive way by defining dimensions of the model as latent variables underlying broader constructs, there is much to be learned about the direct and indirect effects of risk factors and about the moderating and mediating influences of protective and recovery factors (Lavee, McCubbin, & Patterson, 1985; McCubbin & McCubbin, 1988a, 1988b, 1996).

As noted by the developing authors, but also emphasized here, there is much to learn about families under stress, including why and under what conditions families "bounce back." The resiliency model needs to be expanded or competitive frameworks introduced or both to explain the variability in perceptions and meanings of events by the family and individual members. Furthermore, the contribution of daily hassles to the cluster of risk factors that families must deal with on a day-to-day basis needs to be examined. Studies that address the complexity of coping behaviors and repertoires and identify when they serve as protective and recovery factors in the processes of family adjustment and adaptation are also needed. Finally, the issue of potential deliberateness of family crises needs to be studied. Do some families allow themselves to enter a crisis as a planned strategy so as to change and transform themselves for their own good? Nursing has much to offer the advancement of the resiliency theory as we move toward greater understanding of family risk, protective, and recovery factors and the conditions under which they operate most effectively.

The Framework of Systemic Organization

Origins and Evolution

A second family model, the Framework of Systemic Organization, draws on principles derived from open systems theory (Von Bertalanffy, 1968) and social ecology (Bronfenbrenner, 1977). In contrast to other models discussed in this chapter, its origin is not rooted in theories of stress and coping. In fact, neither term appears in Friedemann's theoretical articles or textbook (Friedemann, 1989a, 1989b, 1995). Instead, the framework presents an explanation and visualization of general family functioning. Within the total family process, coping is seen as a series of actions undertaken to resolve incongruence or disharmony within family members, between members, and between the family and its environment. Friedemann (1995) claims that everyone affected feels incongruence; it can therefore be defined as stress. Friedemann offers the idea that coping is embedded in the family process (Anderson & Tomlinson, 1992) and suggests that coping represents the entire family process as it unfolds day after day. This implies that the process is indivisible and responds to an innate, often unconscious, need of the systems (family and individuals) to gain congruence. Coping is not linear or circular but rather three-dimensional in its complexity; it is not a response to a stimulus but rather a series of strategies of the entire family system and its members to respond to changes from within or from the environment.

The development of the Framework of Systemic Organization started with the discovery of four distinct dimensions of family functioning as a result of a factor analysis done for the purpose of testing an instrument to measure family functioning (Friedemann, 1991a). Family maintenance and coherence address the stability of the system or homeostasis, whereas family change and individuation refer to family growth or morphogenesis. These four dimensions are easily detected in family therapy literature. Homeostasis is discussed as the outcome of two groups of behaviors. The first, described by Bowen (1976), represents system maintenance, or collective behavior patterns such as decision making, enforcing rules, caring for the sick, or screening information. These behaviors are grounded in a set of values and beliefs that are

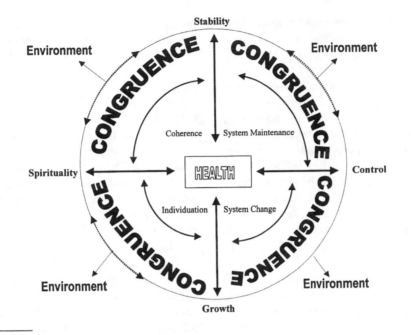

Figure 12.3. Framework of Systemic Organization

learned and taught to each new generation. The second group of behaviors, coherence, is played out at the interpersonal level and refers to sharing time, space, emotional energy, and material goods (Kantor & Lehr, 1975).

Growth or morphogenesis is also easily divided into two groups of behaviors—those that are enacted at the family system level and those enacted at the individual level. At the individual level, family members engage in individuation as they develop interests, commit themselves to goals outside the family, and connect with other people. At the system level, the family then adjusts to the diversity of its members through system change. It accepts information from outside and integrates it by making the necessary organizational changes (Kantor & Lehr, 1975).

In addition to stability and growth, Friedemann complements the model with two other systemic targets, control and spirituality. These she conceptualized inductively by examining her own family and nursing practice and deductively based them on the work of Kantor and Lehr (1975). From this perspective, the family is seen as a system composed

of individuals and interpersonal units, all having unique qualities of their own. The interactions of family members occur as sequences of acts and purposeful repetitive patterns. The notion that family strategic patterns are relatively stable and basic to a larger overall family life process is central to the framework of systemic organization (Friedemann, 1989a, 1991a). This life process is represented graphically in Figure 12.3.

The Model

According to Friedemann (1995), coping with any type of change is intimately fused with the life processes of the family and its individuals. All systems seek *congruence,* a state in which all interacting systems and subsystems function harmoniously in that their rhythms and spatial patterns are attuned to each other. Because change is ongoing and occurring at a rapid pace, a state of congruence is utopian. Nevertheless, systems strive to at least approach congruence to the extent of feeling its effect as peace of mind, calmness, and well-being. Friedemann claims that a major motivator for change is the need to control anxiety that results from incongruence. Anxiety can become evident as physical and mental distress in any form. Consequently, individuals and families strive to find a desired level of stability and growth, control, and spirituality to ward off anxiety and reach a sense of congruence that is defined as *health*. The emphasis individuals and families place on each of the targets differs among families and defines the family's style of functioning. Health, therefore, is the subjective experience of congruence. It increases as families reach an approximation of their desired balance between stability and growth, control, and spirituality.

Coping with change, therefore, pertains to four distinct processes. The first process is maintaining stability through the continuation of values, traditions, and daily routines. Growth, the second process, occurs through adaptation and readjustment of the system's operation to changes from within and outside. Growth implies a change of attitudes and values (second-order change) and not simply a readjustment of roles and minor behaviors to keep the family functioning (first-order change) (Watzlawick, Weakland, & Fisch, 1974). The third process is control, a reaction to change that attempts to eliminate or minimize threats to stability, with homeostasis being the goal. Examples are disciplining children, screening information, or seeking medical care. Finally spirituality is defined as changing one's own system (individual or family) to find meaning and congruence. As a result, the family accepts the change and incorporates it into its overall life process. Spirituality implies connecting with and becoming a part of other systems, be it other individuals, organizations, nature, or a higher being, and thereby finding a new identity and meaning (Friedemann, 1995).

In the family, these processes of coping can be observed as behaviors that pertain to the process dimensions in the inner circle of the model (Figure 12.3). System maintenance involves organizational strategies and includes concepts such as power structure and problem negotiation patterns (Haley, 1976); family structure and generational boundaries (Minuchin, 1974); coalitions, rules, and roles (Haley, 1976; Lewis, Beavers, Gossett, & Phillips, 1976); and family organization and control (Moos & Moos, 1984). Coherence entails behaviors used to establish and maintain emotional bonds. Related concepts are closeness and empathy (Lewis et al., 1976), cohesion (Moos & Moos, 1984; Olson et al., 1984), and enmeshment (Minuchin, 1974). System change behaviors are necessary to adjust to change from within and the environment. Concepts such as morphogenesis (Buckley, 1967), adaptability (Olson et al., 1984), and family growth and flexibility (Kantor and Lehr, 1975; Lewis et al., 1976) address these processes. Individuation consists of behaviors that individuals employ to follow their interests and search for meaning. On the family level, individuation relates to the family's accommodation to members' differences in values, opinions, lifestyles, and schedules. Individuation is implied in concepts such as self-differentiation (Bowen, 1976), self-disclosure, and expressiveness (Lewis et al., 1976).

The Nursing Process

The task of categorizing behaviors according to these process dimensions may be formidable because the same behavior could be categorized in more than one process dimension, depending on the reason why it is undertaken. For example, a family walk in the woods could be system maintenance if done for the sake of physical exercise, coherence if its purpose is to find togetherness, individuation if a family member seeks a connection to nature in his or her search for meaning, or system change if the walk is to provide a new identity and reorganization of priorities for the family. Consequently, nurses need the family's interpretation of their own behaviors to reach conclusions. Nursing within the Framework of Systemic Organization is therefore a client-driven, holistic, and in-depth approach to individuals and families. Nurses assess with the family its life process before the change (illness, crisis, etc.), its life process after the change, and the optimal life process they would like to achieve considering the situation.

Friedemann (1995) explains that for a family to be healthy, all members need to express a reasonable level of satisfaction with the family or well-being. To achieve well-being, each person's developmental needs have to be honored by the family. Although developmental needs differ with age, all refer to growth and change. Friedemann claims that every crisis in a family occurs when growth is inhibited, and thus every crisis is a developmental crisis.

Be it for the sake of crisis resolution or simply to enhance the life process, the goal of nursing is not the family's health but the facilitation of the process the family chooses to achieve its health (congruence) and allow each person to grow and develop freely. The entire process is coping and occurs within the dimensions of the life process described previously. The challenge for the nurse is to make an assessment that represents the family's reality, not the nurse's.

Friedemann (1995) promotes open discussion in which the nurse reveals her or his theoretical thinking by explaining the major concepts of the model in simple terms and then encourages the family to explore how everyday strategies and specific coping attempts may fit into the four process dimensions. An agreement about necessary changes is reached jointly. Strategies to enhance the family process that lead to a balance of targets that the family considers optimal are developed by examining the family's successes in using strategies in the past. The nurse then assists the family in using familiar strategies or in the creation of new ones. Interventions such as teaching, practicing interactions, or procuring new resources are used if the family discovers a need for new strategies. Friedemann has specified a step-by-step approach in an intervention model for substance abusing families (Friedemann, 1989b, 1992). This model also has been applied in other areas of nursing

(Friedemann, 1995; Friedemann, Jozefowicz, Schrader, Collins, & Strandberg, 1989).

The Framework of Systemic Organization is appropriate for families of various cultures, structures, and/or economic situations. Whereas the general life process depicted in Figure 12.3 is generally applicable to all families, vast differences are found in the specific strategies used and in the emphasis placed on certain targets among various types of families. Within the Framework of Systemic Organization, culture is defined as two processes occurring simultaneously—namely, culture maintenance and culture transformation. These processes are inherent in the pursuit of stability versus growth or the maintenance of cultural tradition versus adaptation of life patterns to a changed environment. Consequently, culture is lived within the family life process. To assess cultural patterns, the nurse simply follows the dimensions of the life process and examines how certain strategies are used to pursue family targets (Friedemann, 1991b, 1995). Because many of these may be unfamiliar to the nurse, the unbiased use of the model has the potential for promoting cultural awareness.

The use of the framework reduces the comparison of client families along preset norms that may not be valid for all. Instead of using norms, the nurse can let the family judge its own level of health or effectiveness. He/she may disagree with the family's self-assessment based on signs of congruence or stress within the system. In such cases, the nurse is encouraged to point out inconsistencies and suggest reevaluation of the situation. Ultimately, however, it is the family who makes the decision to change and to make change happen.

Instrument Development and Use

To use the major concepts of the Framework of Systemic Organization as a theoretical basis for research, they need to be operationalized and measured. Key concepts are family health and congruence. Friedemann (1995) states that health can only be estimated and that the sole expert of health is the family. According to the framework, there is evidence of health if (a) the family pursues strategies pertaining to all four process dimensions, (b) the family is reasonably satisfied with family functioning, (c) the anxiety level of family members is low, and (d) there is congruence between the family's pursuits and environmental expectations.

The Assessment of Strategies in Families-Effectiveness (ASF-E) instrument is available for initial screening of family health. The ASF-E (Friedemann, 1991a; Friedemann & Smith, 1997) represents a subjective assessment of family effectiveness in all four dimensions. Respondents mark statements of family functioning ranked according to levels of effectiveness that are most like their family. The latest version has 20 items and subscores for the targets of stability, growth, spirituality, and individuation (Friedemann 1998). The ASF-E has been examined for content, construct, and concurrent validity (Friedemann, 1991a, 1998). Internal consistency of the ASF-F is satisfactory, with Cronbach's alpha coefficients ranging from .69 to .78 for the subscales and .82 for the total scale. Furthermore, respondents' scores on the ASF-E have been found to converge with their descriptions of family process dimensions specified in the framework (Friedemann & Smith, 1997). The ASF-E has also been translated into three foreign languages and tested in four countries with families experiencing different life and health situations. The four targets of the framework were clearly defined through exploratory factor analysis in all studies. This provides substantial evidence of the instrument's cultural applicability. Because the evaluation of family effectiveness is subjective, a high score also implies satisfaction.

In addition to its use in research, the ASF-E has shown merit as a clinical tool. It provides a basis for general discussion, the selection of a focal dimension (scored lower than the others), and the determination of needed changes. The tool may also be used to facilitate discussion about differences in perceptions among various family members and

to seek a clarification of a desired life process that satisfies all members. Having defined such an ideal, the nurse can then work with the family in determining what coping strategies to use to arrive at their goal.

The family APGAR (Smilkstein, 1978) has also been used successfully as a complementary measure of satisfaction. A variety of existing standardized anxiety measures and measures of negative emotions, such as anger or depression, are recommended to explore the existence of personal and interpersonal conflicts that may or may not be family based.

Within the Framework of Systemic Organization, the family process is also seen as the major determining factor of outcomes such as quality of parenting, caregiving, or adjustment to difficult situations. A tool to measure the family process at this level needs to delineate strategies without judging their effectiveness. Such a tool (ASF-F [Function]) is under development by Friedemann and others but needs refinement. Challenges faced in development of the ASF-F include the need to ensure cross-cultural relevance of the items and difficulty related to categorizing each activity with a specific process dimension.

Research Testing the Framework of Systemic Organization

Throughout her book, Friedemann (1995) cites hundreds of studies that provide support for theoretical tenets of the Framework of Systemic Organization. In addition, many studies have been undertaken specifically to test propositions deduced from the theory. There are three issues of concern to researchers working with this and other systemic frameworks. First, systemic models defy linear causality, which is the basis of empirical research. Second, the framework uses a reciprocal interaction worldview (Fawcett, 1995). Therefore, the family process is constantly evolving. This implies that there is no objective truth of the kind that empirical research seeks to discover. Finally, the framework of systemic organization stresses the importance of understanding diversity, whereas most statistical methods that are based on central tendency neglect the exploration of differences from the norm.

Unfortunately, there is no research method that circumvents these issues. Friedemann (1995) advocates between-methods triangulation to group data generated by more than one method, thereby converging partial truths. While using innovative approaches, including qualitative methodology guided by the framework, close attention to the sampling procedures, sequencing of the methods, and interpretation of the data is imperative (Floyd, 1993). A few examples of such research exist. Pierce (1998) conducted an ethnographic study of African American families to examine their experience of caring and the meaning they found in the process. The Framework was used as a template along which emerging themes and behaviors of caregivers were grouped. The experience of caring involved eight caring actions pertaining to the four process dimensions (physical work, sacrifice, taught and shared actions, structure of caring, communication, accommodation, mutuality, and learning). Meaning was described by the way the caregivers pursued and balanced the four targets to find congruence. The meaning of caring encompassed 13 expressions (emotional burden, evasion of conflicts, motivations concerned with love and duty, approval of the care recipient, philosophical introspection, self-development, fairness, filial ethereal value, self-contemplation, Christian piety, living in the moment and hoping for the future, and purpose). The findings supported the notion of culture in that patterns were maintained and transformed within the domains of caring actions, family functions, and expressions of caring of these caregivers.

Similarly, Friedemann's study of family involvement in nursing homes showed that family functioning measured with the ASF-E and certain items of the Family Environment Scale (Moos & Moos, 1984) were the strongest predictor of families' expectations to be involved (Friedemann, Montgomery, Rice, & Farrell, 1999). A qualitative inquiry associated with the same study complemented these results by showing that families tried to maintain their family style even in the nursing home and desired involvement that was congruent with the emphasis they placed on the four family process dimensions. Whereas coherence was important to most and maintained through visiting, direct care was related to an emphasis on system maintenance. Activities of learning and patient advocacy were related to families' emphasis on growth and connecting with their environment (Friedemann, Montgomery, Maiberger, & Smith, 1997).

Smith and Friedemann (1999) showed that the framework is well suited to the development of family process models at the midrange level in a study involving families with members who suffered from chronic pain. Both the ASF-E and in-depth interviews were used to assess family functioning and the role that pain plays in the family and in regulating interactive patterns (Friedemann & Smith, 1997). The interviews were minimally structured, and the Framework of Systemic Organization was used mainly for interpretation of the results. Dominant themes pointed to the struggle of the family in finding congruence—a struggle that was played out by the individual with pain and on the family level. The informants with pain reported a great need to belong and to be heard. In their family life, this need remained unmet resulting in distress, loneliness, and confusion. This emotional climate set the stage for ensuing family strategies. Several processes were evident. A cycle of obligations was evident as the individuals with pain sacrificed themselves for others, thereby gaining charismatic power and the ability to bind others through obligation to serve and reciprocate. A second dynamic was extreme closeness at the expense of individuation of the family members and the third was family isolation from the environment. From these phenomena, it was evident that healing as defined by the respondents meant approaching congruence by breaking the cycle of obligation and freeing the individual from the emotional bondage. In support of the framework, families that reported healing engaged in individuation and allowing each other to grow. They shifted the emphasis from the target of control to spirituality and found a new sense of health and happiness. The pain was no longer the dominant force in the family even if it still existed.

DeMarco (1997) extended the framework by applying it to staff teams in acute care hospital units. Without prior theorizing, focus groups were used to explore the nature of staff nurses' interactional behaviors. Results were used to create items that were organized according to the four process dimensions of the Framework of Systemic Organization and then tested conventionally (DeMarco & Friedemann, 1995). This approach resulted in a valid and reliable instrument. In her dissertation, DeMarco (1997) refined the instrument and tested a model that she explicated using the Framework of Systemic Organization in which relationships between family function and workgroup function and between family intimacy and work relationships were hypothesized. Significant positive correlations were found between relational patterns in the family and at work. Silencing the self in the family was related to keeping silent at work and being compliant with expected feminine roles which subsequently led to inner hostility. These emotions were conceptualized as negative coherence or lack of individuation. Nurses who found personal meaning in their work and incorporated new knowledge experienced personal growth and demonstrated positive individual coherence or individuation at the workplace. DeMarco's findings clearly speak to the process of seeking congruence or failing to do so.

Critique and Summary

The approach to nursing practice within the Framework of Systemic Organization leads away from a narrow focus on the causes of distress and methods to deal with the stressors to a direct intervention with the system influenced by the stressors in the context of the entire situation. Likewise, research uses multiple methods to interpret process as it unfolds. The approach to practice and research needs to be family process-specific and, therefore, sensitive to the families' subjective stress appraisal. Research and practice methods must accommodate vast differences in reactions related to cultural, developmental, and economic factors that can be assessed only through open-ended, in-depth interviewing.

Unfortunately, linear approaches to nursing care that are preferred by nurses for the sake of simplicity and ease of application are not congruent with this framework. Thus, any situation that appears to be easy may become immensely complex when multiple confounding factors are added. Nevertheless, Friedemann's (1995) book provides assessment and intervention examples so that nurses can learn to shift their thinking from cause-and-effect decision making to a more complex systems approach.

Research studies with the framework have the potential of revealing novel types of information, but the danger of getting lost in a complex maze of mutually interacting forces exists. Designs need to maintain a fine balance of simplicity and depth to be useful and interpretable. Few guidelines currently exist for the convergence of various research methods, and the results derived from such methods and carefully planned designs are greatly needed. Research with the Framework of Systemic Organization is still in the experimental stage, and its quality needs to be carefully monitored. Nevertheless, this framework tends to appeal to independent thinkers who dare to take their research efforts beyond existing parameters and experiment with new approaches in the search for new solutions.

The Developmental Health Model

Origins and Evolution

Another family theory, the Developmental Health Model (DHM), is a theoretical extension and refinement of the McGill Model of Nursing, a curriculum model first developed by Moyra Allen and faculty at the

McGill University School of Nursing in the 1970s. Initially developed from grounded theory analysis of nurse-family interactions while working together on health matters, the McGill model emphasizes a particular style or approach to working with families, called situation-responsive nursing (SRN) (Allen, 1983, 1994; Gottlieb & Rowat, 1987), that has been applied and evaluated in a variety of clinical settings since its inception (Ezer, McDonald, & Gros, 1991; Feeley & Gerez-Lirette, 1992). A collection of papers reviewing the development and application of the McGill model was recently published in book form (Gottlieb & Ezer, 1997). The need to further develop concepts and test hypotheses derived from the model, however, was proposed as a logical next step in theory development (Gottlieb & Rowat, 1987).

At the Nursing Theory Congress in 1986, Allen presented early theoretical work, which grounded SRN within an evolving system of concepts that she called the Developmental Health Model. Since 1989, Ford-Gilboe and colleagues at the University of Western Ontario have been extending Allen's work by more formally describing theory concepts and their relationships and by testing hypotheses derived from the DHM. An explanation of key theoretical concepts and their relationships based on a model developed by Ford-Gilboe (1998) follows (Figure 12.4).

The aim of the DHM is the development of knowledge about the nature of healthy development in individuals and families and the role of the nurse in facilitating this process (Allen, 1994). An early health-promotion model, the McGill model, was originally developed as a means of fully articulating a complementary role for nursing that was distinct from that of medicine (Allen, 1977). Many theoretical influences can be identified. Families are viewed from a systems perspective in which the interaction and influence of individual members, the family unit, and the broader environment on each other are considered (Allen, 1983, 1994). Consistent with the World Health Organization's (1978) view of health promotion, the DHM emphasizes

process and adopts a strengths perspective that focuses on how families develop capabilities needed for healthy living within the context of everyday life events and the social conditions within which they live. Social learning theory (Bandura, 1977) provides a frame of reference for understanding how families cope with and learn from life events and how this learning is transferred from one situation to another (Allen, 1994). Ford-Gilboe (1998) contends that the DHM is an "empowerment model" because its emphasis on strengths, process, and shared power between the nurse and family fosters reflection and self-awareness while building the skills needed to effectively manage life events and work toward health goals that are important to the family. Thus, this approach may be particularly well suited to families who have been disenfranchised in some way (e.g., those living in poverty, single-parent families, and survivors of abuse).

Key Concepts and Their Relationships

In the DHM, health is a multidimensional construct composed of many concepts and processes (Gottlieb & Rowat, 1987). At least four characteristics contribute to a family's overall pattern of health: health work, health potential, competence in health behavior, and health status (Ford-Gilboe, 1998). Furthermore, health is viewed as a characteristic of the family—a way of living—that is learned and shaped within the context of family life. When viewed in this way, it becomes possible for families to learn how to be healthy as they experience and deal with life events. These situations offer opportunities for families to develop health. Illness is one such situation, as are other expected and unexpected life events, such as the birth of a baby, managing a period of unemployment, or adapting to life as a single-parent family. Thus, health and illness are separate concepts in the model (Allen, 1983, 1994).

Two of the most important attributes of health are coping and development (Allen,

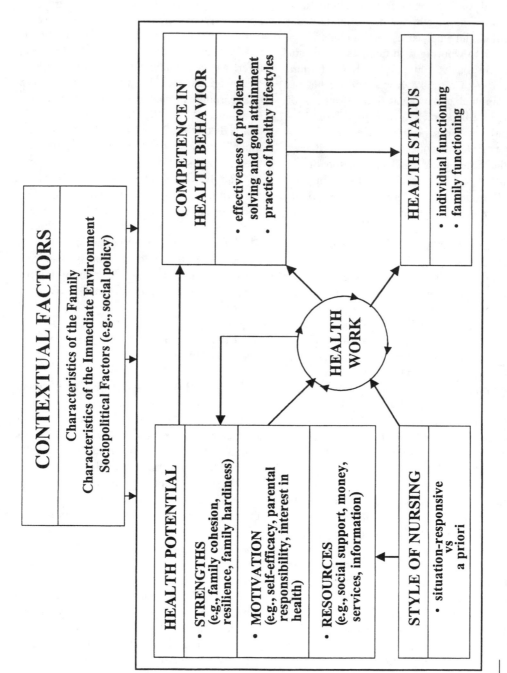

Figure 12.4. Relationship of Key Concepts in the Developmental Health Model (DHM) (reproduced from Ford-Gilboe, 1998)

1983, 1994; Gottlieb & Rowat, 1987). Coping is viewed as a function of problem-solving—a process of attempting to deal with or solve challenging health situations—whereas development relates to the growth-seeking behavior seen in the family's ability to mobilize strengths and resources to achieve health goals (Warner, 1981).

Health Work. Health work, the central concept in the theory, reflects the process through which families develop or learn problem-solving and growth-seeking skills over time. Health work is a universal process that reflects essential human qualities—the desire to learn from and cope with life experiences and to develop one's potential. Although families engage in health work on their own, the nurse may share this activity when assistance has been sought to support the family's efforts for managing a particular situation.

As participation in health work increases, families become more active in experimenting with new ways of coping and developing and make conscious choices to seek healthier ways of living. Thus, health work may be represented on a fluid continuum from lower degrees to higher degrees with many variations evident between these two extremes. In general, lower degrees of health work are associated with lack of interest in or conscious thought about health matters, a preference for established health routines over new ideas regardless of their effectiveness, a focus on weaknesses or barriers to achieving goals, and a tendency to base health decisions primarily on expert opinion or default (doing nothing). Families who demonstrate lower degrees of health work engage in limited or inconsistent problem solving when faced with a challenging health situation.

In contrast, higher degrees of health work are reflected by interest and active involvement in health matters, a focus on family strengths and abilities, and experimenting with alternative approaches for promoting health in collaboration with experts as needed (Ford-Gilboe, 1997a, 1998). Thus, these families use a proactive, problem-solving approach to manage health situations that includes a constellation of behaviors, such as observing the situation and gathering information, examining and analyzing the situation, generating new and existing alternatives for managing the situation, selecting options by weighing the pros and cons and fit with the family's lifestyle, trying out and evaluating the plan, and modifying the approach as necessary.

Health work is both situation specific and general. Because health work develops over time, families learn to deal with particular situations using both new and established ways of coping and developing. As these behaviors are learned in one situation, they become integrated into the family's ways of living and may be translated into new situations that occur. Thus, when the health work of a family is examined across different situations, a general pattern or style emerges.

Furthermore, the degree to which a family engages in health work is influenced by at least three factors: the health potential of the family and its members, the broader context of family life, and, when present, the way in which the nurse works with the family (i.e., the style of nursing).

Health Potential. Health potential refers to the strengths, motivation, and resources of the family and its members (Allen, 1983, 1994; Ford-Gilboe, 1994). Family strengths are the internal capabilities of the family and its members that are exhibited as a unique family functioning style (Ford-Gilboe, 1998). Qualities of family members, such as personality dispositions, are also important sources of family strength. All families, even those faced with what seem to be insurmountable challenges, possess strengths (Dunst, Trivette, & Deal, 1994). Motivation refers to the family's overall interest in health matters as reflected by the priority given to health issues, the family's desire to change health behavior based on current needs, and family members' beliefs about their ability to influence health (Allen, 1994). The motivational aspect of health potential is closely tied to family values. Resources are external sources of assistance in health matters and may include access to information, economic sufficiency, and social support from extended family, friends, and the community as well as needed time, energy, and support services (Allen, 1994; Ford-Gilboe, 1998).

Because higher degrees of health work require active involvement and a view of health situations as family rather than individual issues, participating in this process over time also enhances the health potential of the family and its members by (a) building new strengths, (b) cultivating motivation through the experience of success, and (c) developing resources of information and support.

Broader Context of Family Life. The broader social context in which the family is embedded may affect the extent and pattern of health work. The nature of this influence is thought to be situation-dependent. Consistent with an ecological systems perspective (Bronfenbrenner, 1977), at least three levels of the environment can be considered when describing the context of family life: (a) characteristics of the family (e.g., cultural background, stage of the family life cycle, and family history), (b) characteristics of the immediate environment (e.g., stressors or chronic demands imposed by a particular situation, safety of the neighborhood, and availability of needed services), and (c) broader sociopolitical forces that affect family life (e.g., changes in social programs or policies and cultural biases or stereotypes that work to disenfranchise certain groups).

Style of Nursing. The role of nursing in the DHM is to assist the family to develop healthy ways of living by structuring experiences that assist the family to actively engage in the process of health work. The method of nursing that accompanies this goal, called situation-responsive nursing (SRN), is presented as an alternative to a more traditional, a priori approach to practice. Key characteristics of SRN include a view of the family as client, an orientation to the health aspects of

situations (i.e., how a family copes with situations), a belief in the need to work with families over time, development of a collaborative relationship between nurse and client, use of an exploratory approach that focuses on the family members' perceptions of their situation as information is collected, and a focus on family potential as opposed to deficits (Allen, 1994; Gottlieb, 1982; Gottlieb & Rowat, 1987). This approach contrasts with a more traditional method of nursing that is characterized by an individual focus, the nurse as expert, use of an a priori assessment framework, episodic care in which interventions are delivered to the client during a brief period of time, and a focus on deficits as opposed to strengths (Allen, 1994).

Allen further emphasizes the importance of identifying and building on the health potential of the family by structuring opportunities for learning new health behaviors that capitalize on existing family strengths, motivation, and resources. Thus, the nurse indirectly fosters health work by assisting the family to build its health potential. Once developed, these capabilities can be drawn on to facilitate health work. Using a SRN approach is, therefore, theoretically more effective in assisting families to build health potential and to engage in health work than the use of more traditional practice approaches. Over time, improvements in both health potential and health work will translate into better health outcomes (i.e., competence in health behavior and improved health status) for these families (Ford-Gilboe, 1998).

Nursing process within the Developmental Health Model builds on the principles of collaboration, negotiation, and inquiry. Assessment is guided by five broad questions that focus on describing the health situations with which the family is dealing and providing some structure for exploration and dialogue. The goal of assessment is to arrive at an understanding of how family members view the situation for which help has been sought, their goals for managing the situation, and their current ways of coping, including their use of resources. As the nurse works with a family over time, the assessment is broadened to focus on understanding how the broader context of family life (e.g., general functioning, past experience, cultural background, and social placement) affects the family's ability to manage the situation at hand (Laforêt-Fleisser & Ford-Gilboe, 1996). As the family's goals become clearer, the nurse and family negotiate a plan for working toward those goals that draws on the unique strengths and resources of both the family and the nurse. The health work plan differs from a nursing care plan in that it reflects the combined perspective of the nurse and family and specifies how each will contribute to the achievement of the family's goals. The family's major task is to become actively involved in learning to cope with the health situation. The nurse's major role is to structure learning experiences that are directed toward meeting the family's objectives while enhancing its participation in health work and fostering health potential (Ford-Gilboe, 1998). Many specific strategies may be used by the nurse to facilitate this process (Gottlieb, 1997; Gottlieb & Feeley, 1996). Strategies are tailored to complement the family's style of functioning and its health potential and are introduced based on the family's readiness to move forward with new activities (Allen, 1994; Gottlieb & Rowat, 1987). Evaluative processes are integrated with activities and based on feedback related to the family's response to the plan and progress made toward identified goals.

Outcomes of Health Work: Competence in Health Behavior and Health Status. As families engage in health work over time, they develop the skills used as part of the health work process (i.e., problem solving and goal attainment), and, as their interest in health and awareness of health issues increases, they begin to adopt healthier lifestyle practices (e.g., improved exercise, nutrition, and stress management). Therefore, competence in health behavior implies that families are effective in managing health situations and achieving health goals and in making and sus-

taining lifestyle changes that are important to them.

The health potential of the family contributes to the development of competence. Families who have a well-developed reservoir of capabilities at their disposal are more likely to view themselves as competent and to ensure that their actions are consistent with their self-perceptions. Over time, increased competence in health behavior may ultimately result in improvements in health status. Health status refers to the functioning of the family and its members, as indicated by concepts such as quality of life, satisfaction with family life, or ability to engage in activities of daily living (Ford-Gilboe, 1998).

Instrument Development and Use

The Health Options Scale (HOS; Ford-Gilboe, 1997b), a 21-item summated rating scale, was developed as a measure of Health Work. This instrument is currently being used as part of a program of research testing the DHM. Participants indicate the extent to which their families engage in behaviors consistent with health work using a 4-point Likert-type scale from "strongly disagree" (1) to "strongly agree" (4). Higher scores reflect higher degrees of health work. Items representing both extremes of the health work continuum are included, necessitating reverse scoring for some. Items are arranged in three subscales: (a) Attending, which reflects active involvement in health matters (8 items); (b) Goal Attainment, which reflects identification and pursuit of health goals (6 items); and, (c) Experimenting, the extent to which the family uses a problem-solving approach to resolve health problems (7 items).

Confirmatory factor analysis was used to assess the dimensional structure of the HOS using data from a community sample of 325 parents. The proposed three-factor solution supported the data (GFI = .89) and accounted for 98% of item variance. Internal consistency of total and subscale HOS scores has been acceptable ($\alpha > .70$). Concurrent validity has been established through moderate correlations with several established measures of theoretically related concepts, including the Problem-Solving Inventory, a measure of problem-solving style (Heppner, 1988), and the Health-Promoting Lifestyle Profile II (Walker, 1997), a measure of individual healthy lifestyle practices (Ford-Gilboe, 1997b). The HOS has been used in many different family contexts with similar results (Table 12.1).

The reliability and validity of the HOS with children (ages 10-17 years) are currently being examined using data collected from 200 children in school and community settings. A clinical version of the HOS has been developed and is currently being tested by undergraduate nursing students working with families in the community.

There is a good fit between many existing instruments and the theoretical definitions of health potential, competence in health behavior, and health status proposed in the Development Health Model. The following are examples of instruments that have been used to measure these constructs:

1. Health potential

   Strengths: Resilience Scale (Wagnild & Young, 1993), Family Hardiness Index (McCubbin et al., 1988), and Cohesion Scale of the FACES III (Olson et al., 1985)

   Motivation: General Self-Efficacy Scale (Scherer et al., 1982)

   Resources: Personal Resources Questionnaire (PRQ85)(Weinert, 1987), Financial Strain Index (Avison, 1997), and Family Social Support Index (Fink, 1993)

2. Competence in health behavior: Health Promoting Lifestyle Profile (HPLP) (Walker, Sechrist, & Pender, 1987) and HPLP II (Walker, 1997)

3. Health status: Family APGAR (Smilkstein, 1978) and the General Scale of the Family Assessment Device (FAD) (Epstein, Baldwin, & Bishop, 1983), both measures of family functioning; and Quality of Life Index, a measure of individual quality of life (Ferrans & Powers, 1985, 1992)

Research Testing the Developmental Health Model

The positive impact of situation-responsive nursing (SRN) has been documented using a variety of approaches. Both process and outcomes of SRN have been examined in ambulatory care units and community nursing centers (called health workshops) in which the model was initially demonstrated and evaluated (Allen, Frasure-Smith, & Gottlieb, 1980; Frasure-Smith, 1997; Frasure-Smith, Allen, & Gottlieb, 1997). Across these studies, nurses who adopted a situation-responsive approach to practice were found to focus more on helping clients cope with challenging life situations and less on treatment of illness. Furthermore, clients reported that these nurses were more helpful than those who employed more traditional approaches. The clinical usefulness of SRN in a variety of clinical settings has also been described (Carnavale, 1997; Feeley & Gerez-Lirette, 1992; Grossman, 1997; Meister, 1997; Tyler, 1997). Pless et al. (1994) compared the effects of a 1-year health-promoting intervention based on the principles of SRN to usual care on psychosocial adjustment of 332 chronically ill children recruited from hospital speciality clinics. Analysis of covariance was used to test the hypothesis that the intervention would be effective in either reducing or preventing maladjustment, with baseline scores on several child outcome measures used as covariates. As hypothesized, after 1 year, children in the intervention group were less dependent, less anxious, and less depressed than those in the control group.

Concept development and formal testing of the DHM continue. At the University of Western Ontario, Canada, the DHM is well integrated into the undergraduate curriculum, and lessons learned from using the model in practice provide vital information necessary for theory refinement. Much of the theory-testing and refinement work is being conducted by faculty and graduate students as part of the Family Health Promotion Research Program within the school of nursing. Formal deductive testing of propositions from the DHM is in the early stages. Several studies have been undertaken or are in progress that test aspects of the model with varying populations, including single-parent families with school-aged children (Ford-Gilboe, 1994, 1997a, 1997b; Ford-Gilboe, Berman, Laschinger, & Laforêt-Fleisser, 1999); and those with chronic health problems (Chambers, 1999); families with preschool children (Monteith, 1997); families with an adult member with chronic inflammatory bowel disease (Moore-Hepburn, 1997); and Latin American Mennonite families (Burrill, 1998). A summary of these studies is presented in Table 12.1. In all of these studies, cross-sectional, correlational survey designs were used to examine specific relationships between concepts in the DHM. Data were enhanced by the use of in-depth qualitative interviews in three studies. In one study, simultaneous testing of many theoretical relationships was undertaken using path analysis (Ford-Gilboe et al., 1999).

Although the number of studies testing propositions derived from the DHM is limited, findings from these studies provide consistent support for the theory propositions. A positive relationship between health potential and health work has been found in the five studies in which this relationship was examined. Many individual and family strengths have been used to operationalize health potential, such as resilience, optimism, family hardiness, family cohesion, and social support. Furthermore, seven measures of health potential were found to significantly predict 22% of the variance in health work in a sample of 138 families with preadolescent children (67 single-parent families and 68 two-parent families) (Ford-Gilboe, 1997a, 1997b). Support for the relationship between health work and competence in health behavior has been provided through positive relationships found between health work and health-promoting lifestyle practices (four studies) as well as between health work and both problem-solving effectiveness and goal-attainment effectiveness (one study). The positive influence of health potential on competence in health behavior has been supported through relationships found between mothers' resilience and healthy lifestyle (Monteith, 1997) and between many health potential variables and healthy lifestyle, problem-solving effectiveness, and goal-attainment effectiveness (Ford-Gilboe et al., 1999). In two separate studies, positive relationships were found between health work and health status measured using quality of life and family functioning. Finally, relationships in a causal model that included the concepts of health potential, health work, competence in health behavior, and health status were tested in a sample of 236 single-parent families using structural equation modeling (Ford-Gilboe et al., 1999). The model was found to fit the data (GFI = .987; adjusted GFI = .934), and all specified paths were moderate and significant ($r = .45$ to .55, $p < .05$). Health potential, health work, and competence in health behavior were found to predict 30% of the variance in family functioning.

The consistency of these results with samples of families who differ in terms of family form, stage of the lifecycle, and socioeconomic status suggests that the model is applicable to a wide range of family units. With the exception of Burrill's (1998) study, samples have been predominantly English speaking, with the majority of participants identifying most closely with Canadian culture and reporting British or European ancestry. Although cultural variations in the model are expected, little research has been conducted in this area. Findings from Burrill's (1998) study of Latin American Mennonite families suggest that the goal attainment aspect of health work may be less culturally relevant for this group than for families who have been integrated into the dominant culture. The issue of applicability of the theory to families in other countries, who experience different cultural and social realities, needs to be studied. Despite these limitations, the DHM has proven utility as a guide for clinical practice. As theory development continues, the Development Health Model is emerging as a potentially im-

TABLE 12.1 Research Testing the Developmental Health Model

Reference	Purpose	Sample	Design	Results	Support for Theory
Ford-Gilboe (1994, 1997)	To examine the extent to which selected strengths, motivations, and resources predict health work for all families and by family type	Community sample of 138 families with preadolescent children (10-14 years old); 68 single-parent families; 70 two-parent families Wide variation in annual income (range $10,000-$250,000/year; $\bar{x}$ = $46,651); 46% of mothers had some college education; 90% Caucasian	Predictive survey; mailed questionnaire of standardized measures completed by mother and index child (10-14 years old) in each family plus in-depth semistructured interviews with subsample of families (n = 16)	Indicators of health potential predicted 22% of variance in health work for the total sample (27% for single-parent families and 25% for two-parent families). Family cohesion and pride, mother's sex role orientation, network support, and community support were all related to health work (r = .20-.44). Qualitative findings were consistent with quantitative findings.	There was a relationship between health potential and health work.
Monteith (1997)	To examine relationships among family hardiness, family health work, and mother's health-promoting lifestyle practices	Community sample of 67 families with preschool children recruited from day care centers in a rural setting 96% married; 81% employed; 62% had some college education; predominantly middle class ($\bar{x}$ annual income = $66,570, SD = $23,670); all Caucasian	Descriptive correlational; mailed survey completed by mother	A weak but significant relationship was found between resilience and health work (r = .21). Moderate relationships were found between health work and healthy lifestyle (r = .52) and resilience and healthy lifestyle (r = .42). Resilience and health work predicted 37% of variance in mothers' healthy lifestyle.	There were relationships between health potential and health work, health potential and competence, and health work and competence.
Moore-Hepburn (1997)	To examine relationships among family hardiness, health work, and quality of life of persons living with inflammatory bowel disease (IBD)	61 families with an adult member living with IBD; convenience sample drawn from specialty clinics	Descriptive correlational; mailed survey completed by member with IBD	Moderate positive relationships were found between family hardiness and both health work (r = .51) and quality of life (r = .63).	There were relationships between health potential and health work and health work and health status.

Study	Purpose	Sample	Design/Method	Findings
		57% female; 67% married; 54% completed some college; wide variation in income (range \$15,000-\$110,000/year; $\bar{x}$ = \$62,539, SD = \$28,852)		A weak but significant relationship was found between health work and quality of life (r = .24).
Burrill (1998)	To describe health conceptions, health work, and health-promoting lifestyle practices of families from a minority culture To examine the relationship between health work and health-promoting lifestyle practices	Community sample of 36 Latin American Mennonite families contacted through a church-sponsored help center 81% married; 86% unemployed; limited education (range 4-12 years; $\bar{x}$ = 6.7, SD = 1.89); predominately low income (range \$7,000-\$54,000/year; $\bar{x}$ = \$29,981, SD = \$11,886); 60% received social assistance; English primary language for approximately half of sample	Descriptive correlational; standardized measures administered using interview format and open-ended questions; mothers reported for their families	There was a moderate relationship found between health work and mother's healthy lifestyle practices (r = .40). Mothers reported a range of activities consistent with varying levels of health work. There was difficulty in translating the term "goal" into Low German; mothers described needs and how they were attempting to meet needs, however. Cultural relevance of health work needs additional study.
Ford-Gilboe, Berman, Laschinger, and Laforêt-Fleisser (1999)	To test a causal model specifying the impact of health potential on health work and, subsequently, health outcomes	Community sample of 238 single-parent families with school-age children (5-14 years) 65% separated or divorced; 54% completed some college; 67% employed; average annual income approximately one half of average Canadian family income ($\bar{x}$ = \$24,799, SD = 14.97); 91% Caucasian	Predictive survey; mailed questionnaire of standardized measures completed by mothers and in-depth semistructured interviews conducted with a subsample of families (n = 13)	There was a good fit between the model and data (χ^2 = 5.90, p = .05; GFI = .987, AGFI = .934). All paths were significant and moderate. Health potential, health work, and competence in health behavior predicted 30% of variance in family functioning. There was overall support for the major component of the theory as a whole and for relationships between health potential and health work, health potential and competence, health work and competence, and competence and health status.

portant perspective in better understanding the role of family competencies and strengths in fostering family coping and development and the collaborative, health-promoting role of the nurse in facilitating this process.

Discovering Family Stress, Coping, and Health Experiences Through Qualitative Research and Atheoretical Approaches

The Need for Qualitative Inquiries

Questions about how families experience and cope with stressful events as well as the expected and unexpected outcomes of coping over time could be addressed using qualitative methods. Qualitative research has the potential to increase understanding of family behaviors, motivations, and experiences within a context of multiple environments of influence. Qualitative research encompasses an array of methodological approaches that are bound together by common purposes and characteristics. Because qualitative methods are used to describe experiences from the perspectives of the family and its members within the context of their lives, they are ideally suited to discovery and exploration of family processes and relationships (Deatrick, Faux, & Moore, 1993; Morse & Field, 1995).

The principal critique of intervention research through integrated reports or meta-analysis is that the outcome measures are gathered from a single-family member as "reporter" of family functioning (Gillis & Davis, 1993, p. 265; Feetham, 1990; Feetham, Perkins, & Caroll, 1993). There is further need to address effective types of interventions for different types of families and clinical problems and, most important, which outcomes can be influenced the most by specific or combined interventions. Despite these specific critiques related to methodological concerns, the most important issue is the need for a connection between stressor specificity and the intervention choice. Ogden-Burke, Kauffmann, Costello, Wiskin, and Harrison (1998)

state that when nurses can identify stressors with specificity, they can focus on interventions that can make a difference for families and individual members.

According to Ogden-Burke and colleagues (1998), the current theoretical approaches supporting family stress and coping relationships and predictions lack a basic sense of connection with each other. This, in turn, suggests the need for inductive, qualitative research to expose the nature, patterns, beliefs, values, and experiences of stress and coping to build knowledge in the practice area. There is a real need to move away from heavy reliance on theoretically based structured questionnaires that are lengthy and often inflexible. Stressors do not occur in a standardized order, nor do families experience stressors in the same way. Thus, interventions can only be inductively discovered based on exploration of current and unique stress and coping variables of families and individual family members.

To understand what is known inductively about families with a child with a chronic condition, qualitative studies were reviewed and then compared to a stress and coping theoretical framework (Ogden-Burke et al., 1998). The findings supplied family researchers with not only a formidable review of many qualitative studies but also a synthesis of qualitative findings that strengthens transferability of the data in relationship to extant theoretical frameworks.

Qualitative Research Involving Families With a Child With a Chronic Condition

Qualitative studies that have explored how families cope with children with attention deficit hyperactivity disorder (ADHD) and insulin-dependent diabetes mellitus (IDDM) provide good examples of how specific interventions can be created and implemented to enhance adaptation and to help build or validate theory (Kendall, 1998; Smith, 1998). Kendall found through a grounded theory approach that parents could outlast the disruption they experienced in themselves and in their families by a process called reinvesting (i.e., relinquishing the "good ending"). Findings also suggested a developmental trajectory of how parents adjust over time as a helpful way for clinicians to plan and negotiate interventions. Smith interviewed 14 siblings of children with IDDM using an existential-phenomenological approach. Findings indicated that the siblings were dramatically affected by an aura of a "protective shield" that was imposed on their life and development. One of the key findings was the need to address interventions and outcomes that are specific for different family members, specifically other brothers and sisters.

These are two examples of how the open process dimension of rich, thick data derived from the family participants supplies researchers with specific, tangible experiences. The nature of the actual engagement of researchers with families can also become a therapeutic connection with families and specific family members who have not been able to tell their stories to others because their stories did not fit a questionnaire schedule or their responses became diluted in the controversial issues regarding scoring of "family" data (Loveland-Cherry, Horan, Burman, Youngblut, & Rodgers, 1993).

Other qualitative studies have enlightened understanding of family experiences of stress and coping, such as (a) families and children who were technology-dependent at home (Allen, Simone, & Wingenbach, 1994; Petr & Barney, 1993; Young, Creighton, & Suave, 1988), (b) families with children who are developmentally disabled or have behavior problems (Snowdon, Cameron, & Dunham, 1994; Deatrick, Knafl, & Guyer, 1993; Petr & Barney, 1993; Strauss & Munton, 1985), and (c) families with children experiencing life-threatening illnesses and uncertainty in the context of chronic illnesses, such as rheumatoid arthritis, Crohn's disease, lupus, and scleroderma (Barnes, Bandak, & Beardslee, 1990; Charmaz, 1990; Cohen,

1993; Gallo & Knafl, 1998; Graves & Hayes, 1996; Knafl, Breitmayer, Gallo, & Zoeller, 1996).

Through survey research, Hentinen and Kyngas (1998) were able to identify and describe adaptation of parents with children who had chronic conditions. Although many family stress and coping theories have emphasized the need for health care staff to support and give parents information about strategic resources in dealing with crises, the findings of this study indicate that emotional and instrumental support are much more important to parents.

Essentially, the previously mentioned studies create a map that allows researchers to understand that parents (a) often feel incapable; (b) need help dealing with equipment vendors; (c) need help with insurance companies, government funding, and travel; (d) have to deal with others offering help but are not really being available; (e) have to deal with the child's fears and developmental changes superimposed on illness; and (f) have to cope with other people's attitudes regarding care for a child at home (Ogden-Burke et al., 1998).

Other Qualitative Research in Family Stress and Coping

There is a body of qualitative research that explores caregiver and patient experiences as they relate to chronic mental illnesses (schizophrenia), cognitive changes (Alzheimer's disease), and the coping patterns and needs of caregivers described through the "burden" they experience (Brown, 1993). Caregiver burden has been studied extensively for clients who suffer from dementia or Alzheimer's disease (Chou, 1997; Grassel, 1998; Gwyther, 1998; Kane, 1997; Vrabec, 1997). Caregiver burden has been explained as an objective burden (disruption of family life) and a subjective burden (e.g., caregiver response to the situation) (Vrabec, 1997). It is known that objective burden is reflected by disruptions in finances, roles, and neighbor relations, whereas subjective burden refers to the experience of embarrassment and being trapped, resentful, and overloaded. From an economic perspective, family caregiving is largely uncompensated in the United States beyond claiming an exemption on taxes (Morton-Robinson, 1997). Costs of family caregiving are difficult to track. Expenditures for goods, insurance copayments, prescriptions, and indirect increases in utility bills are difficult to analyze because of the shared nature of payment in many cases between the caregivers and clients (Fisher, 1998; Knox, 1998; Sanchez, 1998). The value of time and the valuing of women caregivers also reflect indirect cost to peoples lives both personally and professionally (Ward, 1990).

It is unclear whether the experience that caregivers have in relation to Alzheimer's disease and dementia is similar to or different from that of caregivers of clients with other chronic illnesses. The following is the key question: How do caregivers experience the responsibility of caregiving at this point in time in health care delivery? The experiences of caregiving with chronically ill populations are not anecdotal in nature but provide evidence of strong personal voices that can direct health policy research and family-based interventions.

Research Priorities

A three-round Delphi study of families and children in families revealed a need for qualitative research designs and methods to explore stress and coping (Broome, Woodring, & O'Connor-Von, 1996). The highest levels of consensus for researchable topics on children with acute illnesses and chronic conditions included (a) factors that influence health-seeking behaviors and habits in children, (b) factors that influence the abilities of families to balance the demands of chronic illnesses and the psychological effects of trauma on children, families, and health care providers, (c) service needs for families with children living with HIV/AIDS, (d) effects of family decision making and child competence

on treatment outcomes, and (e) influences of family values on use of primary care health services. Although these research priorities address the child-family interface specifically, they also have applicability to other relationships within aging families (e.g., filial responsibility with parents) and adult-adult relationships in general.

Although each of the research priorities is presented as the "effect" or "influence" of a factor on a behavior or health outcome, each can be viewed as a potential research question about patterns, experiences, values, and attitudes that are shaped through facets of family life. Finally, although it is an assumption of this part of the chapter that research priorities are universal questions for all people, differences in race, ethnicity, class, and gender are formidable reasons to continue to enhance transferability of findings with and through different populations of peoples and families using qualitative family stress and coping research.

➣ FUTURE IMPLICATIONS

This chapter has guided the reader through the development of theory and research with families and has discussed current approaches to practicing nursing and designing nursing research. Certain trends have become visible with the passage of time.

Historically, the perspectives of stress and coping theory and research differed significantly from the systemic perspective of family systems and family therapy theory and research. Family stress, first perceived as one or more stress-inducing events (Holmes and Rahe, 1967), later became a mutually reinforced pileup of changes (McCubbin, 1987/ 1996) that affected family functioning or family health (Pearlin, 1991). Even with the introduction of the concepts of appraisal and style of coping (Sorensen, 1993), the process of coping was considered to be linear and to occur along a timeline. A shift to more systemic thinking occurred with the new understanding that families seek to maintain functioning that fits with their own definition of "normalcy" (Loveland-Cherry, 1996). Nevertheless, linear notions have not disappeared entirely. The search to identify influencing factors or moderators in the linear progression toward health or maladaptation continues.

In nursing, scholars have adopted certain common views about the family that depart from the linear perspective. Family health is conceptualized as a complex process and coping as overall problem solving. Interventions are viewed as family driven, with the goal of empowering families to use their own resources to become healthy. This has resulted in a shift in the role of the nurse from the expert who diagnoses problems to a partner who can work with the family to mutually explore family strengths. Finally, the importance of viewing the family in a broader context of culture and community life has been reinforced.

Thus, newer trends in nursing include the notion that the overall family process signifies coping (Anderson & Thomlinson, 1992; Friedemann, 1995). Research is seemingly several steps behind such theory development, however. Even self-proclaimed systemic researchers rely on linear models that explore coping as an independent or dependent variable or as a mediator because traditional research has few solutions for the exploration of systemic, mutually reinforcing processes. Qualitative methods have gained importance in family nursing research because they lead to a broader understanding of people's experience, motivation, and the meaning ascribed to certain situations.

It can be anticipated that the previously mentioned trends will continue into the future. Nursing at the family system level will provide many benefits to patients discharged from hospitals and rehabilitation centers, family caregivers, parents with young children, families of the mentally ill, and others. Nevertheless, such care will remain a luxury rather than the norm within the United States' money-driven health care system. Some nurse practitioners will practice family nursing un-

officially and will seek creative ways to be reimbursed. Some nursing schools may be inclined to push family nursing theory into the background of their advanced nursing curricula, however, and scientific and medically oriented course requirements will prevail. This stands in stark contrast to an urgent need for effective family interventions as patients are discharged with more serious health problems and families are expected to provide more of their care.

Family stress theory will need to be further developed in a systematic way so that it will slowly converge with other types of systemic family theory. Researchers from various disciplines need to work together and add their individual perspectives to complex family research projects conducted in the context of different health and illness situations, such as drug abuse prevention, oncology care, diabetes maintenance, cardiovascular disease prevention, and the parenting of chronically ill children. Family researchers will need to focus on family processes while they work with other experts who are knowledgeable about various health problems and developmental issues. Together, they will find creative solutions for symptom maintenance, disease prevention, health promotion, or rehabilitation. These interdisciplinary teams also need to include researchers skilled in a variety of research methods. Projects that combine methods, such as those undertaken by Friedemann and her team (1997), need to be undertaken more frequently. Most important, such projects will have to be longitudinal to explore the ongoing evolution of the family process as situations change. Such research will not only focus on commonalties and average performance but also will describe variations in family processes based on age, culture, or socioeconomic status. In fact, studies addressing distinctions between such groups in terms of perceptions, motivation for self-care, caregiving processes, or parenting approaches will become the center of attention. Much creativity will be required to render justice to the complexity and variety of family interactions and the pursuit of family health.

➤ REFERENCES

Allen, M. (1977). Comparative theories of the expanded role in nursing and implications for nursing practice: A working paper. *Nursing Papers, 9*(2), 38-45.

Allen, M. (1983). Primary care nursing: Research in action. In L. Hockey (Ed.), *Recent advances in nursing: Primary care nursing* (pp. 32-77). Edinburgh, UK: Churchill-Livingstone.

Allen, M. (1994). *A developmental health model— Nursing as continuous inquiry.* Unpublished manuscript.

Allen, M., Frasure-Smith, N., & Gottlieb, L. (1980). *Models of nursing practice in a changing health care system: A comparative study in three ambulatory care settings. Part I: Research report; Part II: Appendices.* Montreal: McGill University, School of Nursing.

Allen, N. L., Simone, J. A., & Wigenbach, G. F. (1994). Families with a ventilator-assisted child: Transitional issues. *Journal of Perinatology, 14,* 48-55.

Anderson, K., & Tomlinson, P. (1992). The family health system as an emerging paradigmatic view for nursing. *Image, 23,* 57-63.

Avison, W. (1997). Roles and resources: The effects of family structure and employment on women's psychological distress. *Research in Community and Mental Health, 8,* 233-256.

Bandura, A. (1977). Self-efficacy: Toward a unifying theory of behavioral change. *Psychological Review, 84*(2), 191-215.

Barnes, C. M., Bandak, A. G., & Beardslee, C. I. (1990). Content analysis of 186 descriptive case studies of hospitalized children. *Maternal Child Nursing Journal, 19*(4), 281-296.

Bomar, P. (1996). *Nurses and family health promotion: Concepts, assessment, and interventions* (2nd ed.). Philadelphia: Saunders.

Boss, P. (1987). *Family stress management.* Newbury Park, CA: Sage.

Bowen, M. (1976). Theory in the practice of psychotherapy. In P. J. Guerin (Ed.), *Family therapy: Theory and practice* (pp. 42-90). New York: Gardner.

Bronfenbrenner, U. (1977). Toward an experimental ecology of human development. *American Psychologist, 32*(7), 513-531.

Broome, M. E., Woodring, B., & O'Connor-Von, S. (1996). Research priorities for the nursing of children and their families: A Delphi study. *Journal of Pediatric Nursing, 11*(5), 281-287.

Brown, M. A. (1993). Caregiver stress in families of person with HIV/AIDS. In S. L. Feetham, S. B. Meister, J. M. Bell, & C. L. Gillis (Eds.), *The nursing of families* (pp. 211-223). Newbury Park, CA: Sage.

Buckley, W. (1967). *Sociology and modern systems theory.* Englewood Cliffs, NJ: Prentice Hall.

Burr, W., Klein, S., & Associates. (1994). *Reexamining family stress: New theory and research.* Thousand Oaks, CA: Sage.

Burrill, E. (1998). *Health conception, health work and health-promoting lifestyle practices in Latin American Mennonite families.* Unpublished master's thesis, University of Western Ontario, London, Ontario, Canada.

Carnavale, F. (1997). The McGill Model of Nursing in the intensive care setting. In L. Gottlieb & H. Ezer (Eds.), *A perspective on health, family, learning and collaborative nursing: A collection of writings on the McGill Model of Nursing* (pp. 323-326). Montreal: McGill University, School of Nursing.

Carr, M. A. (1995). *Effect of a family crisis intervention program on family need satisfaction, family functioning, and patient stress following an acute myocardial infarction.* Unpublished doctoral dissertation, Catholic University of America, Washington, DC.

Chambers, A. (1999). *Mother's resilience, social support and health work in single-parent families with a chronically ill child.* Master's research project proposal, University of Western Ontario, London, Ontario, Canada.

Charmaz, K. (1990). Discovering chronic illness: Using grounded theory. *Society, Science, & Medicine, 30*(11), 1161-1172.

Chou, K. R. (1997). A psychometric assessment of caregiver burden: A cross-cultural study. *Journal of Pediatric Nursing, 12*(6), 352-362.

Cohen, M. H. (1993). The unknown and the unknowable—Managing sustained uncertainty. *Western Journal of Nursing Research, 15,* 77-96.

Conrad, M., & Hammen, C. (1993). Protective and risk factors in high and low risk children: A comparison of children with unipolar, bipolar, medically ill, and normal mothers. *Development and Psychopathology, 5,* 593-607.

Deatrick, J. A., Faux, S. A., & Moore, C. M. (1993). The contribution of qualitative research to the study of families' experiences with childhood illness. In S. L. Feetham, S. B. Meister, J. M. Bell, & C. L. Gillis (Eds.), *The nursing of families* (pp. 61-69). Newbury Park, CA: Sage.

Deatrick, J. A., Knafl, K. A., & Guyer, K. (1993). The meaning of caregiving behaviors: Inductive approaches to family theory development. In S. L. Feetham, S. B. Meister, J. M. Bell, & C. L. Gilliss (Eds.), *The nursing of families: Theory, research, education, practice* (pp. 38-45). Newbury Park, CA: Sage.

DeMarco, R. (1997). *The relationship between family life and workplace behaviors: Exploring the gendered perceptions of staff nurses in acute care.* Doctoral dissertation, Wayne State University. [*Dissertation Abstracts International, 58*(3B), 9725823]

DeMarco, R., & Friedemann, M. L. (1995). *The Staff Nurse Workplace Behaviors Scale (SMWBS): Using qualitative to quantitative research paradigms in instrument development.* Unpublished manuscript, Northeastern University, Boston.

Dunst, C., Trivette, C., & Deal, A. (1994). *Supporting and strengthening families.* Cambridge, MA: Brookline.

Epstein, N., Baldwin, L., & Bishop, D. (1983). The McMaster Family Assessment Device. *Journal of Marital and Family Therapy, 9*(2), 171-180.

Ezer, H., McDonald, J., & Gros, C. (1991). Follow-up of generic master's graduates: Viability of a model of nursing practice. *Canadian Journal of Nursing Research, 23*(3), 9-20.

Fawcett, J. (1995). *Analysis and evaluation of conceptual models of nursing* (3rd ed). Philadelphia: Davis.

Feeley, N., & Gerez-Lirette, T. (1992). Development of professional practice based upon the McGill Model of Nursing in an ambulatory care setting. *Journal of Advanced Nursing, 17,* 801-808.

Feetham, S. (1990). Conceptual and methodological issues in research of families. In J. Bell, W. Watson, & L. Wright (Eds.), *The cutting edge of family nursing* (pp. 35-49). Calgary, Alberta: Family Nursing Unit Publications.

Feetham, S., Perkins, M., & Carroll, R. (1993). Exploratory analysis: A technique for the analysis of dydactic data in research of families. In S. Feetham, S. Meister, J. Bell, & C. Gilliss (Eds.), *The nursing of families: Theory, research, education, practice* (pp. 99-107). Newbury Park, CA: Sage.

Ferrans, C., & Powers, M. (1985). Quality of Life Index: Development and psychometric properties. *Advances in Nursing Science, 8,* 15-24.

Ferrans, C., & Powers, M. (1992). Psychometric assessment of the Quality of Life Index. *Research in Nursing and Health, 15,* 29-38.

Fisher, I. (1998, June 7). Families providing complex medical care, tubes and all. *New York Times,* pp. 1, 30.

Floyd, J. (1993). The use of across-method triangulation in the study of sleep concerns in healthy older adults. *Advances in Nursing Science, 16*(2), 125-141.

Ford-Gilboe, M. (1994). Family strengths, motivation and resources as predictors of health promotion behavior in single-parent and two-parent families. (Doctoral dissertation, Wayne State University, 1994). *Dissertation Abstracts International, 56*(2), 741B.

Ford-Gilboe, M. (1997a). Family strengths, motivation and resources as predictors of health promotion behavior in single-parent and two-parent families. *Research in Nursing and Health, 20,* 205-217.

Ford-Gilboe, M. (1997b, April). *Development of an instrument to measure family health promotion behaviour: The Health Options Scale.* Paper presented at the Midwest Nursing Research Society Conference, Minneapolis, MN.

Ford-Gilboe, M. (1998). *An overview of the Developmental Health Model.* London, Ontario, Canada: University of Western Ontario, School of Nursing.

Ford-Gilboe, M., Berman, H., Laschinger, H., & Laforêt-Fleisser, Y. (1999, June). *Testing a causal model of family health promotion in single-parent families led by mothers.* Paper presented at the International Nursing Research Conference, Edmonton, Canada.

Frasure-Smith, N. (1997). The workshop: A comparative study of patient's perceptions of nursing in four ambulatory care settings. In L. Gottlieb & H. Ezer (Eds.), *A perspective on health, family, learning and collaborative nursing: A collection of writings on the McGill Model of Nursing* (pp. 113-129). Montreal: McGill University, School of Nursing.

Frasure-Smith, N., Allen, M., & Gottlieb, L. (1997). Models of nursing practice in a changing health care system: Overview of a comparative study in three ambulatory care settings. In L. Gottlieb & H. Ezer (Eds.), *A perspective on health, family, learning and collaborative nursing: A collection of writings on the McGill Model of Nursing* (pp. 31-74). Montreal: McGill University, School of Nursing.

Friedemann, M. L. (1989a). Closing the gap between grand theory and mental health practice with families. Part 1: The framework of systemic organization for nursing of families and family members. *Archives of Psychiatric Nursing, 3,* 1019.

Friedemann, M. L. (1989b). Closing the gap between grand theory and mental health practice with families. Part 2: The Control-Congruence Model for mental health nursing of families. *Archives of Psychiatric Nursing, 3,* 20-28.

Friedemann, M. L. (1991a). An instrument to evaluate effectiveness in family functioning. *Western Journal of Nursing Research, 13,* 220-235.

Friedemann, M. L. (1991b). Exploring culture and family caring patterns with the framework of systemic organization. In P. L. Chinn (Ed.), *Anthology on caring.* New York: National League for Nursing Press.

Friedemann, M. L. (1992). *Enhancing families with the congruence model: A counseling/education approach.* Miami: Florida International University. (Available from the author)

Friedemann, M. L. (1995). *The framework of systemic organization: A conceptual approach to families and nursing.* Thousand Oaks, CA: Sage.

Friedemann, M. L. (1998). *1998 testing of the ASF-E.* Unpublished manuscript, Florida International University, College of Health Sciences, Miami.

Friedemann, M. L., Jozefowicz, F., Schrader, J., Collins, A., & Strandberg, P. (1989). Advanced family nursing with the Control-Congruence Model. *Clinical Nurse Specialist, 3*(4), 164-170.

Friedemann, M. L., Montgomery, R. J., Maiberger, B., & Smith, A. (1997). Family involvement in the nursing home: Family-oriented practices and staff-family relationships. *Research in Nursing & Health, 20,* 527-537.

Friedemann, M. L., Montgomery, R. J., Rice, C., & Farrell, L. (1999). Family involvement in the nursing home. *Western Journal of Nursing Research, 21,* 549-567.

Friedemann, M. L., & Smith, A. A. (1997). A triangulation approach to testing a family instrument. *Western Journal of Nursing Research, 19,* 364-378.

Gallo, A. M., & Knafl, K. A. (1998). Parents reports of "tricks of the trade" for managing childhood chronic illness. *Journal of the Society Pediatric Nursing, 3*(3), 93-100.

Garmezy, N. (1987). Stress, competence and development: Continuities in the study of schizophrenic adults, children vulnerable to psychopathology, and the search for stress resistant children. *American Journal of Orthopsychiatry, 57*(2), 159-174.

Garmezy, N. (1991a). Resilience in children's adaptation to negative life events and stressed environments. *Pediatric Annals, 20*(9), 462-466.

Garmezy, N. (1991b). Resiliency and vulnerability to adverse developmental outcomes associated with poverty. *American Behavioral Scientist, 34*(4), 416-430.

Garmezy, N., & Masten, A. (1991). The protective role of competence indicators in children at risk. In E. M. Cummings, A. L. Greene, & K. H. Karrakei (Eds.), *Perspectives on stress and coping* (pp. 151-174). Hillsdale, NJ: Lawrence Erlbaum.

Gillis, C. L., & Davis, L. L. (1993). Does family intervention make a difference? An integrative review and meta-analysis. In S. L. Feetham, S. G. Meister, J. M. Bell, & C. L. Gillis (Eds.), *The nursing of families: Theory, research, education and practice* (pp. 259-265). Newbury Park, CA: Sage.

Gottlieb, L. (1982). *Styles of nursing as practised at the workshop: A health resource.* Montreal: McGill University.

Gottlieb, L. (1997). Health promoters: Two contrasting styles in community nursing. In L. Gottlieb & H. Ezer (Eds.), *A perspective on health, family, learning and collaborative nursing: A collection of writings on the McGill Model of Nursing* (pp. 87-100). Montreal: McGill University, School of Nursing.

Gottlieb, L., & Ezer, H. (Eds.). (1997). *A perspective on health, family, learning and collaborative nursing: A collection of writings on the McGill Model of Nursing.* Montreal: McGill University, School of Nursing.

Gottlieb, L., & Feeley, N. (1996). The McGill model of nursing and children with a chronic condition: Who benefits and why? *Canadian Journal of Nursing Research, 28*(3), 29-48.

Gottlieb, L., & Rowat, K. (1987). The McGill Model of Nursing: A practice-derived model. *Advances in Nursing Science, 9*(4), 51-61.

Grassel, E. (1998). Home care of demented and nondemented patients. Health and burden of caregivers. *Gerontologic Geriatrics, 3,* 57-62.

Graves, C., & Hayes, V. E. (1996). Do nurses and parents of children with chronic conditions agree on parental needs? *Journal of Pediatric Nursing, 11*(5), 288-299.

Grossman, M. (1997). Creating a structure to support the McGill model. In L. Gottlieb & H. Ezer (Eds.), *A perspective on health, family, learning and collaborative nursing: A collection of writings on the McGill Model of Nursing* (pp. 317-322). Montreal: McGill University, School of Nursing.

Gwyther, L. P. (1998). Social issues of the Alzheimer's patient and family. *American Journal of Medicine, 104*(4A), 17S-21S.

Haley, J. (1976). *Problem solving therapy.* San Francisco: Jossey-Bass.

Hentinen, M., & Kyngas, H. (1998). Factors associated with the adaptation of parents with a chronically ill child. *Journal of Clinical Nursing, 7,* 316-324.

Heppner, P. (1988). *The problem solving inventory.* Palo Alto, CA: Consulting Psychologists Press.

Hill, R. (1949). *Families under stress.* New York: Harper & Row.

Hill, R. (1958). Generic features of families under stress. *Social Casework, 49,* 139-150.

Holmes, T. H., & Rahe, R. H. (1967). The social readjustment scale. *Journal of Psychometric Research, 11,* 213-218.

Kane, R. L. (1997). Which outcomes matter in Alzheimer disease and who should define them? *Alzheimer Disease Associated Disorders, 11*(6), 12-17.

Kantor, D., & Lehr, W. (1975). *Inside the family.* San Francisco: Jossey-Bass.

Kendall, J. (1998). Outlasting disruption: The process of reinvestment in families with ADHD children. *Qualitative Health Research, 8*(6), 839-857.

Knafl, K., Breitmayer, B., Gallo, A., & Zoeller, L. (1996). Family response to childhood chronic illness: Description of management styles. *Journal of Pediatric Nursing, 11*(5), 315-326.

Knox, R. A. (1998, July 20). The toll caring takes. *Boston Globe,* pp. C1, C3.

Kosciulek, J., McCubbin, M., & McCubbin, H. (1993). A theoretical framework for family adaptation to head injury. *Journal of Rehabilitation, 59*(3), 40-45.

Laforêt-Fleisser, Y., & Ford-Gilboe, M. (1996). Learning to nurse families using the developmental health model: Educational strategies for undergraduate students. *Journal of Family Nursing, 2*(4), 383-398.

Lavee, Y., McCubbin, H. I., & Patterson, J. (1985). The double ABCX model of family stress and adaptation: An empirical test by analysis of structural equations with latent variables. *Journal of Marriage and the Family, 47*(4), 811-825.

Leske, J. S., & Jiricka, M. K. (1998). Impact of family demands and family well-being and adaptation after critical injury. *American Journal of Critical Care, 7*(5), 383-392.

Lewis, J. M., Beavers, W. R., Gossett, J. T., & Phillips, V. A. (1976). *No single thread: Psychological health in family systems.* New York: Brunner/Mazel.

Loveland-Cherry, C. J. (1996). Family health promotion and health protection. In *Nurses and family health promotion* (pp. 22-35). Philadelphia: Saunders.

Loveland-Cherry, C. J., Horan, M., Burman, M., Youngblut, J., & Rodgers, W. (1993). Scoring family data: An application with families with preterm infants. In S. L. Feetham, S. B. Meister, J. M. Bell, & C. L. Gillis (Eds.), *The nursing of families* (pp. 90-98). Newbury Park, CA: Sage.

Luthar, S. S. (1991). Vulnerability and resilience: A study of high risk adolescents. *Child Development, 62,* 600-616.

Luthar, S. S., Doernberger, C. H., & Zigler, E. (1993). Resilience is not a unidimensional construct: Insights from a prospective study of inner-city adolescents. *Development and Psychopathology, 4,* 287-299.

Luthar, S. S., & Zigler, E. (1992). Intelligence and social competence among high-risk adolescents. *Development and Psychopathology, 4,* 287-299.

McCubbin, H., Dahl, B., Hunter, E., & Plag, A. (1975). Residuals of war: Families of prisoner of war and servicemen missing in action. *Journal of Social Issues, 31*(4), 161-182.

McCubbin, H., Nevin, R., Larsen, A., Comeau, J., Patterson, J., Cauble, A., & Striker, K. (1981). *Families coping with cerebral palsy.* St. Paul: University of Minnesota, Family Social Science.

McCubbin, H., & Thompson, A. (Eds.). (1987). *Family assessment inventories for research and practice (FAIRP).* Madison: University of Wisconsin System.

McCubbin, H., Thompson, A., Pirner, P., & McCubbin, M. (1988). *Family types and strengths: A life cycle and ecological perspective.* Edina, MN: Burgess.

McCubbin, H., Thompson, E., Thompson, A., & McCubbin, M. (1993). Family schema, paradigms, and paradigm shift: Components and processes of appraisal in family adaptation to crises. In A. Thrunbull, J. Patterson, S. Behr, D. Murphy, J. Margquis, & M. Blue-Banning (Eds.), *Cognitive coping, families and disability* (pp. 239-255). Baltimore: Brooks.

McCubbin, H. I. (1996). Family Index of Regenerativity and Adaptation-General (FIRA-G). In H. I. McCubbin, A. I. Thompson, & M. A. McCubbin (Eds.), *Family assessment: Resiliency, coping and adaptation—Inventories for research and practice* (pp. 713-722). Madison: University of Wisconsin System. (Original work published 1987)

McCubbin, H. I., Comeau, J. K., & Harkins, J. A. (1991). Family Inventory of Resources for Management (FIRM). In H. I. McCubbin & A. I. Thompson (Eds.), *Family assessment inventories for research and practice* (pp. 198-199). Madison, WI: Family Stress and Coping Health Project.

McCubbin, H. I., & McCubbin, M. A. (1988a). Family systems assessment. In E. Karoly (Ed.), *Handbook of child health assessment: Biopsychosocial perspectives* (pp. 227-261). New York: John Wiley.

McCubbin, H. I., & McCubbin, M. A. (1988b). Typologies of resilient families: Emerging roles of social class and ethnicity. *Family Relations, 37,* 245-254.

McCubbin, H. I., McCubbin, M. A., Nevin, R., & Cauble, A. (1996). Coping Health Inventory for Parents (CHIP). In H. I. McCubbin, A. I. Thompson, & M. A. McCubbin (Eds.), *Family assessment: Resiliency, coping and adaptation—Inventories for research and practice* (pp. 407-454). Madison: University of Wisconsin System. (Original work published 1983)

McCubbin, H. I., McCubbin, M. A., Patterson, J., Cauble, A. E., Wilson, L., & Warwick, W. (1983). CHIP—Coping Health Inventory for Parents: An assessment of parental coping patterns in the care of the chronically ill child. *Journal of Marriage and the Family, 45,* 359-370.

McCubbin, H. I., McCubbin, M. A., Thompson, A. I., Han, S., & Allen, C. (1997, Fall). Families under stress: What makes them resilient. *Journal of Family and Consumer Sciences,* 3-15.

McCubbin, H. I., McCubbin, M. A., Thompson, A. I., & Thompson, E. A. (1995). Resiliency in ethnic families: A conceptual model for predicting family adjustment and adaptation. In H. I. McCubbin, E. A. Thompson, A. I. Thompson, & J. Fromer (Eds.), *Resiliency in ethnic minority families: Native and immigrant American families, Volume 1* (pp. 3-48). Madison: University of Wisconsin System.

McCubbin, H. I., Olson, D., & Larsen, A. (1996). Family Crisis Oriented Personal Evaluation Scales (F-COPES). In H. I. McCubbin, A. I. Thompson, & M. A. McCubbin (Eds.), *Family assessment: Resiliency, coping and adaptation—Inventories for research and practice* (pp. 455-508). Madison: University of Wisconsin System. (Original work published 1981)

McCubbin, H. I., & Patterson, J. (1983a). The family stress process: The double ABCX model of adjustment and adaptation. In H. I. McCubbin, M. Sussman, & J. Patterson (Eds.), *Social stress and the family: Advances in developments in family stress theory and research* (pp. 7-37). New York: Haworth.

McCubbin, H. I., & Patterson, J. (1983b). The family stress process: The double ABCX model of adjustment and adaptation. *Marriage and Family Review, 6*(1/2), 7-27.

McCubbin, H. I., & Patterson, J. (1996). Family Member Well-Being (FMWB). In H. I. McCubbin, A. I. Thompson, & M. A. McCubbin (Eds.), *Family assessment: Resiliency, coping and adaptation—Inventories for research and practice* (pp. 753-782). Madison: University of Wisconsin System. (Original work published 1982)

McCubbin, H. I., Patterson, J., Bauman, E., & Harris, L. (1996). Adolescent Family Inventory of Life Events and Changes (A-FILE). In H. I. McCubbin, A. I. Thompson, & M. A. McCubbin (Eds.), *Family assessment: Resiliency, coping and adaptation—Inventories for research and practice* (pp. 179-212). Madison: University of Wisconsin System. (Original work published 1981)

McCubbin, H. I., Patterson, J., & Glynn, T. (1996). Social Support Index (SSI). In H. I. McCubbin, A. I. Thompson, & M. A. McCubbin (Eds.), *Family assessment: Resiliency, coping and adaptation—Inventories for research and practice* (pp. 357-390). Madison: University of Wisconsin System. (Original work published 1981)

McCubbin, H. I., Patterson, J., & Grochowski, J. (1996). Young Adult Family Inventory of Life Events and Strains (YA-FILES). In H. I. McCubbin, A. I. Thompson, & M. A. McCubbin (Eds.), *Family assessment: Resiliency, coping and adaptation—Inventories for research and practice* (pp. 213-226). Madison: University of Wisconsin System. (Original work published 1984)

McCubbin, H. I., & Thompson, A. (Eds.). (1991). *Family assessment inventories for research and practice (FAIRP)*. Madison: University of Wisconsin System.

McCubbin, H. I., & Thompson, A. (1996a). Family Traditions Scale (FTS). In H. I. McCubbin, A. I. Thompson, & M. A. McCubbin (Eds.), *Family assessment: Resiliency, coping and adaptation—Inventories for research and practice* (pp. 341-348). Madison: University of Wisconsin System. (Original work published 1986)

McCubbin, H. I., & Thompson, A. (1996b). Family Celebrations Index (FCELEBI). In H. I. McCubbin, A. I. Thompson, & M. A. McCubbin (Eds.), *Family assessment: Resiliency, coping and adaptation—Inventories for research and practice* (pp. 349-356). Madison: University of Wisconsin System. (Original work published 1986)

McCubbin, H. I., Thompson, A., & Elver, K. (1996). Family Pressures Scale-Ethnic (FPRES-E). In H. I. McCubbin, A. I. Thompson, & M. A. McCubbin (Eds.), *Family assessment: Resiliency, coping and adaptation—Inventories for research and practice* (pp. 227-236). Madison: University of Wisconsin System. (Original work published 1993)

McCubbin, H. I., Thompson, A., & Elver, K. (1996a). Family Attachment and Changeability Index (FACI). In H. I. McCubbin, A. I. Thompson, & M. A. McCubbin (Eds.), *Family assessment: Resiliency,* *coping and adaptation—Inventories for research and practice* (pp. 725-752). Madison: University of Wisconsin System. (Original work published 1995)

McCubbin, H. I., Thompson, A., & Elver, K. (1996b). Family Coping Index (FAMCI). In H. I. McCubbin, A. I. Thompson, & M. A. McCubbin (Eds.), *Family assessment: Resiliency, coping and adaptation—Inventories for research and practice* (pp. 509-536). Madison: University of Wisconsin System. (Original work published 1995)

McCubbin, H. I., Thompson, A., & Elver, K. (1996c). Youth Coping Index (YCI). In H. I. McCubbin, A. I. Thompson, & M. A. McCubbin (Eds.), *Family assessment: Resiliency, coping and adaptation—Inventories for research and practice* (pp. 585-612). Madison: University of Wisconsin System. (Original work published 1995)

McCubbin, H. I., Thompson, A., Elver, K., & Carpenter, K. (1996). Family Schema-Ethnic (FSCH-E). In H. I. McCubbin, A. I. Thompson, & M. A. McCubbin (Eds.), *Family assessment: Resiliency, coping and adaptation—Inventories for research and practice* (pp. 639-686). Madison: University of Wisconsin System. (Original work published 1992)

McCubbin, H. I., Thompson, A. I., & McCubbin, M. A. (Eds.). (1996). *Family assessment: Resiliency, coping and adaptation—Inventories for research and practice*. Madison: University of Wisconsin System.

McCubbin, M. A. (1988a). Family stress, resources, and family types: Chronic illness in children. *Family Relations, 37,* 203-210.

McCubbin, M. A. (1988b). Family stress and family strengths: A comparison of single and two parent families with handicapped children. *Research in Nursing and Health, 12,* 101-110.

McCubbin, M. A. (1989). Theoretical orientations to family stress and coping. In C. R. Figley (Ed.), *Treating stress in families* (pp. 3-43). New York: Brunner/Mazel.

McCubbin, M. A. (1999). Normative family transitions and health outcomes. In A. Hinshaw, S. Feetham, & J. Shauer (Eds.), *Handbook of clinical nursing research* (pp. 201-230). Newbury Park, CA: Sage.

McCubbin, M. A., & McCubbin, H. I. (1993). Families coping with illness: The Resiliency Model of Family Stress, Adjustment and Adaptation. In C. B. Danielson, B. Hamel-Bissell, & P. Winstead-Fry (Eds.), *Families, health, and illness: Perspectives on coping and intervention* (pp. 21-63). St. Louis, MO: C. V. Mosby.

McCubbin, M. A., & McCubbin, H. I. (1996). Resiliency and families: A conceptual model of family adjustment and adaptation in response to stress and crises. In H. I. McCubbin, A. I. Thompson, & M. A. McCubbin (Eds.), *Family assessment: Resiliency, coping and adaptation—Inventories for research and practice* (pp. 1-64). Madison: University of Wisconsin System.

McCubbin, M. A., McCubbin, H. I., Mischler, E., & Svavarsdottir, E. (in press). Family relationships in cystic fibrosis. In B. Lask, M. Bluebond-Langer, & D. Angst (Eds.), *Psychosocial aspects of cystic fibrosis.* London: Chapman & Hall.

McCubbin, M. A., McCubbin, H. I., & Thompson, A. I. (1996). Family Problem Solving Communication Index (FPSC). In H. I. McCubbin, A. I. Thompson, & M. A. McCubbin (Eds.), *Family assessment: Resiliency, coping, and adaptation—Inventories for research and practice* (pp. xx-xxi). Madison: University of Wisconsin System. (Original work published 1988)

Meister, C. (1997). The fit of the McGill Model of Nursing to the practice of psychiatric nursing. In L. Gottlieb & H. Ezer (Eds.), *A perspective on health, family, learning and collaborative nursing: A collection of writings on the McGill Model of Nursing* (pp. 327-332). Montreal: McGill University, School of Nursing.

Minuchin, S. (1974). *Families and family therapy.* Cambridge, MA: Harvard University Press.

Monteith, B. (1997). *The relationships among mother's resilience, family health work and mother's health promoting lifestyle practices in families with preschool children.* Unpublished master's thesis, University of Western Ontario, London, Ontario, Canada.

Moore-Hepburn, J. (1997). *The relationships between hardiness, health work and quality of life in families experiencing chronic inflammatory bowel disease.* Unpublished master's research project, University of Western Ontario, London, Ontario, Canada.

Moos, R. H., & Moos, B. S. (1984). *Family Environment Scale: Manual* (2nd ed.). Palo Alto, CA: Consulting Psychologists Press.

Morse, J., & Field, P. A. (1995). *Qualitative research methods for health professionals.* Thousand Oaks, CA: Sage.

Morton-Robinson, K. (1997). Family caregiving: Who provides the care, and at what cost? *Nursing Economics, 15*(5), 243-247.

Ogden Burke, S., Kauffmann, E., Costello, E., Wiskin, N., & Harrison, M. B. (1998). Stressors in families with a child with a chronic condition: An analysis of qualitative studies and a framework. *Canadian Journal of Nursing Research, 30,* 71-95.

Olson, D. H., McCubbin, H. I., Barnes, H. L., Larsen, A. S., Muxen, M. J., & Wilson, M. A. (1984). *Families: What makes them work.* Beverly Hills, CA: Sage.

Olson, D. H., Portner, J., & Bell, R. (1978). *Family adaptability and cohesion evaluation scales.* St. Paul: University of Minnesota, Family Social Science.

Olson, D. H., Portner, J., & Bell, R. (1982). *FACES II: Family Adaptability and Cohesion Evaluation Scales.* St. Paul: University of Minnesota, Family Social Science.

Patterson, J., & McCubbin, H. (1996). Adolescent Coping Orientation for Problem Experiences (A-COPE). In H. I. McCubbin, A. I. Thompson, & M. A. McCubbin (Eds.), *Family assessment: Resiliency, coping and adaptation—Inventories for research and practice* (pp. 537-584). Madison: University of Wisconsin System. (Original work published 1983)

Pearlin, L. I. (1991). Life strains and psychological distress among adults. In A. Monat & R. S. Lazarus (Eds.), *Stress and coping: An anthology* (3rd ed., pp. 319-336). New York: Columbia University Press.

Pender, N. (1996). *Health promotion in nursing practice* (3rd ed.). Stamford, CT: Appleton & Lange.

Petr, C. G., & Barney, D. D. (1993). Reasonable efforts for children with disabilities: The parents' perspective. *Social Work, 38*(3), 247-254.

Pierce, L. L. (1998). *The experience and meaning of caring for urban family caregivers of persons with stroke.* Unpublished doctoral dissertation, Wayne State University, Detroit, MI.

Pless, I., Feeley, N., Gottlieb, L., Rowat, K., Dougherty, G., & Willard, B. (1994). A randomized trial of a nursing intervention to promote the adjustment of children with chronic physical disorders. *Pediatrics, 94,* 70-75.

Richters, J. E., & Martinez, P. E. (1993). Violent communities, family choices, and children's chances: An algorithm for improving the odds. *Development and Psychopathology, 5,* 609-627.

Rutter, M. (1990). Psychsocial resilience and protective mechanisms. In J. Rolf, A. Masten, D. Cicchetti, K. Nuechterlein, & S. Weintrab (Eds.), *Risk and protective factors in the development of psychopathology* (pp. 181-214). Cambridge, UK: Cambridge University Press.

Sanchez, M. C. (1998, July 4). Cuts threaten community lifelines. *Boston Globe,* pp. B1, B6.

Scherer, M., Maddux, J., Mercandante, B., Prentice-Dunn, S., Jacobs, B., & Rogers, R. (1982). The Self-Efficacy Scale: Construction and validation. *Psychological Reports, 51,* 663-671.

Skinner, D., & McCubbin, H. (1981). *Dual-Employed Coping Scales (DECS).* St. Paul: University of Minnesota.

Smilkstein, G. (1978). The family APGAR: A proposal for a family function test and its use by physicians. *Journal of Family Practice, 6,* 1231-1239.

Smith, A. A., & Friedemann, M. L. (1999). Perceived family dynamics of persons with chronic pain. *Journal of Advanced Nursing, 30,* 543-551.

Smith, M. E. (1998). Protective shield: A thematic analysis of the experience of having an adult sibling with insulin-dependent diabetes mellitus. *Issues in Mental Health Nursing, 19*(4), 317-335.

Smith, S. D. (1997). The retirement transition and the later life family unit. *Public Health Nursing, 14*(4), 207-216.

Snowdon, A. W., Cameron, S., & Dunham, K. (1994). Relationships between stress, coping resources and satisfaction with family functioning in families of children with disabilities. *Canadian Journal of Nursing Research, 26*(3), 63-76.

Sorensen, E. S. (1993). *Children's stress and coping: A family perspective.* New York: Guilford.

Strauss, S. S., & Munton, M. (1985). Common concerns of parents with disabled children. *Pediatric Nursing, 11,* 371-375.

Svavarsdottir, E., & McCubbin, M. A. (1996). Parenthood transition for parents of an infant diagnosed with a congenital heart condition. *Journal of Pediatric Nursing, 11*(4), 207-216.

Tyler, L. (1997). The McGill Model of Nursing in a hospital ambulatory setting. In L. Gottlieb & H. Ezer (Eds.), *A perspective on health, family, learning and collaborative nursing: A collection of writings on the McGill Model of Nursing* (pp. 333-342). Montreal: McGill University, School of Nursing.

Von Bertalanffy, L. (1968). *General systems theory.* New York: Brazeller.

Vrabec, N. J. (1997). Literature review of social support and caregiver burden, 1980 to 1995. *Image, 29*(4), 383-388.

Wagnild, G., & Young, H (1993). Development and psychometric evaluation of the Resilience Scale. *Journal of Nursing Measurement, 1,* 165-178.

Walker, S. (1997). *Revised Health Promoting Lifestyle Profile II.* Unpublished data.

Walker, S., Sechrist, K., & Pender, N. (1987). The Health-Promoting Lifestyle Profile: Development and psychometric characteristics. *Nursing Research, 36*(2), 76-81.

Ward, D. (1990). Gender, time, and money in caregiving. *Scholarly Inquiry for Nursing Practice: An International Journal, 4*(3), 223-239.

Warner, M. (1981). Health and nursing: Evolving one concept by involving the other. *Nursing Papers, 13,* 10-17.

Watzlawick, P., Weakland, C. E., & Fisch, R. (1974). *Change: Principles of problem formation and problem resolution.* New York: Norton.

Werner, E. (1984). Resilient children. *Young Children, 10,* 68-72.

Werner, E. E., & Smith, R. S. (1982). *Vulnerable but invincible: Longitudinal study of resilient children and youth.* New York: Adams, Bannister, Cox.

World Health Organization. (1978). *Alma Ata Declaration.* Copenhagen: Author.

Wyman, P. A., Cowen, E. L., Work, W. C., & Parker, G. R. (1991). Developmental and family milieu correlates of resilience in urban children who have experienced major life stress. *American Journal of Community Psychology, 19*(3), 405-426.

Young, L. Y., Creighton, D. E., & Suave, R. S. (1988, May/June). The needs of families of infants discharged home with continuous oxygen therapy. *Journal of Obstetric, Gynecologic, and Neonatal Nursing,* 187-193.

Youngblut, J. M., Brennan, P. F., & Swegart, L. A. (1994). Families with medically fragile children: An exploratory study. *Pediatric Nursing, 20*(5), 463-468.

PART V

Stress, Coping,
and Health:
Mediating Factors

CHAPTER 13

Attitudes, Beliefs, Values, and Culture as Mediators of Stress

Judith A. Cohen and Lorraine M. Welch

 ttitudes, beliefs, values, and culture are antecedent factors for understanding patient resources and behaviors and are among those variables that are very important for coping with threats to health. The models of health behaviors selected for this chapter are not all inclusive but were derived from many assumptions about the inherent value that each theory contributes to understanding the ways in which nursing can assist clients in their quest for health. The theories of health behavior provide a range of ideas about what is useful to clients as they live in a stressful health care environment that places more responsibility on them to care for themselves. One assumption is that people will act to reduce a threat to their health to protect their well-being. This assumption leads to a presentation of the expectancy-value models of health behavior. Another assumption is that interpersonal processes mediate stress and influence the adoption of new health behaviors. A reciprocal interpersonal process, the foun-

dation of nursing, recognizes the clients' competency and mastery in acquiring new health behaviors. A presentation of the models that emphasize the interpersonal process broadens the idea of mediating stress from managing threats (inherent in the expectancy-value models) to validating unique human health potential. A third assumption is that cultures have unique care values, beliefs, and practices that define health. The models of health behaviors that emphasize culture incorporate the meaning of health and illness experience to preserve health behaviors or direct change to new behaviors that are culturally congruent. A fourth assumption is that people value growth in a direction that is health promoting. A model that has as its focus health promotion rather than health protection is based on the belief that health is more than the absence of disease. Such a model serves the client who is health promoting even without a defined threat to health. All the models presented have unique emphases but have in common the incorporation of attitudes, beliefs, values, and culture as variables that are relevant to the mediation of stress and health. These factors will be explicated.

Conceptualizations of attitudes lend themselves to numerous definitions depending on theoretical origins of the term (Doganis & Theodorakis, 1995). Learning theorists conclude that an attitude is a learned implicit anticipatory response gained from experience (Doob, 1947). Cognitive theory treats attitude as a filter through which we perceive reality (Chein, 1948). Behaviorists have formulated that attitudes are the outcome of behavior (Bem, 1972). This three-dimensional structure of attitudes means that individuals can have similar attitudes on one level, such as the cognitive domain (convictions, ideas, or knowledge about an object, person, or concept), but differ on the affective domain (expresses an appreciation, wish, or feelings of the individual toward an object or person; Doganis & Theodorakis, 1995). When there is agreement between the cognitive and affective elements, there is a stronger relationship between attitudes and behavior.

Fishbein and Ajzen (1975) believe that attitudes are formed as the corresponding beliefs are developed. In this way, they connect belief formation to attitudes. Beliefs are classified by Fishbein and Ajzen as descriptive or inferential. Doganis and Theodorakis (1995) note,

> Descriptive beliefs are primarily formed by direct observation and direct experience, and are shaped by interaction with other individuals. Additionally, the beliefs are formed by the effect of external sources such as newspapers, books, journals, radio, television, friends, and so forth. (p. 29)

Inferential beliefs, however, are secondary interpretations of descriptive beliefs gained through repetition, judgment, or attempts to understand new information. All beliefs are not equally important in the formation of attitudes. Therefore, attitudes are seen as the product of beliefs about the consequences of a particular behavior and the evaluation of these consequences.

Values are standards that people use to assess themselves and others. Value orientations are a means to understanding variations among cultures. The common value orientations involve the person's relationship to nature, understandings of human nature, ways of relating to others, orientation to time, and orientation to activity (being vs. doing; Lantz, 1996). Each value orientation will affect health-related behaviors often in ways that the person may not be fully aware of. Various models are derived from the hypothesis that behavior depends on two central notions: the value placed by an individual on a particular goal and the individual's estimate of the likelihood that a given action will achieve that goal (Abraham & Sheeran, 1994). When these positions are conceptualized in terms of health-related behaviors, value is viewed as the desire to avoid illness and belief is viewed as a specific health notion that will prevent illness.

Culture is a universal experience and is a multifaceted concept referring to the total of acquired beliefs, values, traditions, artifacts, knowledge, language, and patterns that allow individuals to interact effectively with their unique environments (Lantz, 1996; Leininger, 1988). Beliefs that are strongly related to one's culture are important aspects in the formation of one's intention to do a health-related behavior. Cultural influences on health behavior are conceptualized as personal normative beliefs (feelings of personal responsibility for carrying out the health-related behavior) and role beliefs (one's perception of a how a person such as oneself should behave; Godin et al., 1996).

Understanding and predicting behavior is the central goal of theories that explain why individuals engage in and adhere to specific health recommendations. Developing models that have increasing reliability to predict behavior forms the core of research efforts that frame a variety of specific behaviors. Researchers are seeking to identify the factors and relationships among these factors that are the most potent predictors of health behaviors, whether that behavior is related to exercise adherence, smoking cessation, safe sex, reduction of cardiac risk through low-fat diets, breast self-examination, or bulimia prevention.

➤ MODELS OF HEALTH BEHAVIOR

Four models from psychology that consider attitudes, beliefs, and values that mediate stress, coping, and health are the Health Belief Model (HBM) (Becker, 1974; Rosenstock, 1966, 1974), the theories of reasoned action and planned behavior (Ajzen, 1985; Ajzen & Fishbein, 1980), and the theory of interpersonal behavior (Triandis, 1977, 1980). These theories are based on the assumption that a threat to health calls forth a behavioral response (threats arouse coping strategies) and are grouped as such as expectancy-value models. Expectancy-value models provide a framework for understanding the relationship between a person's attitudes and his or her underlying beliefs. Specifically, expectancy-value models imply that it is expected that a change in health behavior will produce an outcome that is of value to the individual.

Models/theories were developed in nursing that also addressed the factors of attitudes, belief, values, and culture. These will be explicated as well. They are Cox's Interaction Model of Client Health Behavior (Cox, 1982), Pender's (1996) Health Promotion Model, and Leininger's (1991) theory of cultural care diversity and universality. Each of these theories or models reflects the philosophy and values of the nursing discipline, which is committed to a humanistic, holistic worldview and an emphasis on wellness and health promotion rather than the traditional disease model.

The Health Belief Model

The Health Belief Model (HBM) (Figure 13.1) is derived from Lewin, Dembo, Festinger, and Sears's (1944) level of aspiration theory, which attempted to explain and predict health behaviors by focusing on attitudes and beliefs of individuals. The HBM was originally proposed in the 1950s by social scientists for the United States Public Health Service to explain a person's lack of engagement in preventive health behaviors (e.g., free immunizations). These preventive health behaviors were generally time-specific actions and had public health as the area of concern.

The HBM proposed by Rosenstock (1966, 1974) and Becker (1974) hypothesizes that health-related action depends on the simultaneous occurrence of the following factors:

1. Sufficient motivation (or health concern) exists to make health issues salient or relevant.
2. There is a belief that one is susceptible (vulnerability) to a serious health problem or to the sequelae of that illness or condition (perceived threat). Perceived threat is identified by two key variables, perceived susceptibility and perceived severity.
3. There is a belief that following a particular health recommendation is beneficial (perceived benefit) in reducing the perceived threat at a subjectively acceptable cost. Cost refers to perceived barriers that must be overcome to follow the health recommendation.

The model proposes that clients are more likely to engage in health behaviors if they have high perceived threat, high benefits from engaging in the related preventive action, and low cost. Although the relational structure has not been well specified, the elements are usually considered as additive (Kirsch & Joseph, 1989).

The HBM was modified over time to address prevention both from secondary and tertiary perspectives. Problems involved in changing lifelong habits of eating, drinking, exercising, and smoking are obviously more difficult to alter. Preventive behaviors that predict or explain change over time required modification of the HBM. It became evident that the HBM, as originally proposed, did not consider two subsequent developments in so-

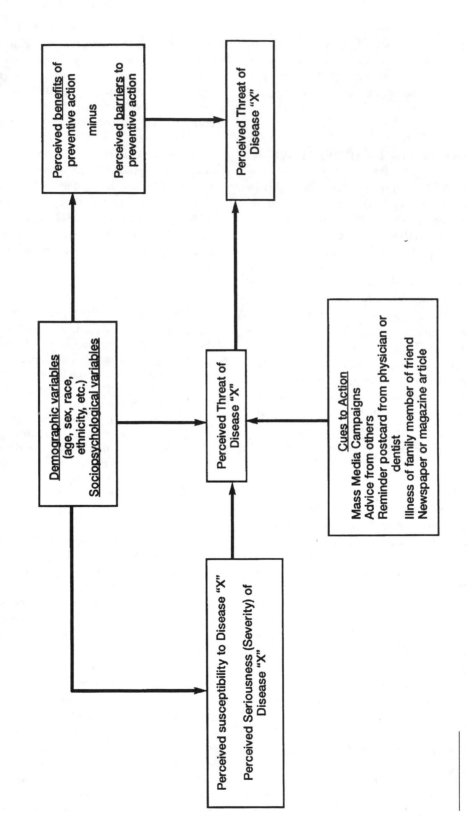

Figure 13.1. Health Belief Model (reproduced with permission from Janz & Becker, 1984)

cial cognitive theory that have contributed to explanations of health-related behavior. Rosenstock, Strecher, and Becker (1988) describe the first as the emphasis on the several sources of information for acquiring expectations and the second as the introduction of the self-efficacy concept (Bandura, 1977). The delineation of reinforcement and role modeling as sources of expectations provides important avenues for altering expectations (Rosenstock et al., 1988).

The concept of self-efficacy stipulates that the person must be able to produce the behavior that will yield the outcome. For example, if a woman wants to perform breast self-exam for health reasons, she must believe that it will benefit her health and that she is capable of doing the exam (efficacy expectation). The concept of self-efficacy contributes to the HBM because it limits the cost (barrier) dimension (Rosenstock et al., 1988).

The HBM has consistently been the focus of theory development and research attention. Janz and Becker (1984) presented a critical review of 29 HBM-related investigations dated from 1974 to 1984. They grouped studies under three headings: preventive health behaviors (PHB), sick role behaviors (SRB), and clinic visits. In the post-1974 studies, the HBM dimension "barriers" was identified as the most powerful predictor for both PHB and SRB. The reviews identified "susceptibility" as more important in PHB than in SRB. Finally, they noted that "perceived severity" was a less powerful predictor, with the exception of the SRB studies. They combined the pre- and post-1974 findings to conclude, "Overall, these investigations provide very substantial empirical evidence supporting HBM dimensions as important contributors to the explanation and prediction of individuals' health-related behaviors" (Janz & Becker, 1984, p. 41).

Recently, there has been interest in using the HBM to predict HIV-related risk behaviors (Bakker, Buunk, Bram, Siero, & van Den Eijnden, 1997; Falck, Siegal, Wang, & Carlson, 1995; Steers, Elliot, Nemiro, Ditman, & Oskamp, 1996). The HBM has

been useful as a theoretical framework to examine health care utilization in sickle cell disease patients (Reese & Smith, 1997), identify perceived barriers for completing a living will (VandeCreek & Frankowski, 1996), study the use of mammography and breast self-exam (Savage & Clarke, 1996), examine risk factors related to youth alcohol initiation (Werch, Carlson, Pappas, Dunn, & Williams, 1997), analyze social identity and health promotion (Storer, Cychosz, & Anderson, 1997), study skin cancer protective behaviors (Carmel, Shani, & Rosenberg, 1996), and assess maternal attitudes toward physicians' role in child health promotion (Cheng et al., 1996). Population subjects have been diverse in terms of age, including children (Palermo & Drotar, 1996) and older women (Thomas, Fox, Leake, & Roetzheim, 1996), race (Brown & Segal, 1996; Brunswick & Banaszak-Holl, 1996; Champion & Scott, 1997), and ethnicity (Thorpe, Ford, Fajans, & Wirawan, 1997).

Research guided by the HBM has not yielded consistent support for the model. Lauver (1992) noted that the model's variable perceived severity has been consistently associated with illness behavior but less well associated with prevention behavior. She also noted that tests of HBM variables with breast self-examination performance have revealed inconsistent relationships. Lack of similar measurement of the HBM variables may account for some of the differences in findings.

Theory of Reasoned Action

The theory of reasoned action (TRA) (Figure 13.2), a model designed by Ajzen and Fishbein (1980), is based on the assumption that behavior is under volitional control. It is also assumed in the theory that people act on the basis of the information that is available to them. According to the theory, the best predictor of behavior is the intention to perform a specific behavior. As noted by Reinecke, Schmidt, and Ajzen (1997), "Intentions are assumed to capture the motivational factors that influence a behavior; they are indications of how hard people are willing to try, of how much of an effort they are planning to exert in order to perform the behavior" (p. 744). The TRA contends that intention is related to two constructs, expectations and beliefs, about the consequences of performing a specific behavior and about the social expectations regarding the behavior. Attitude toward enacting the behavior is the sum of the products of specific beliefs about the outcome, or consequences of performing the behavior (expectancy), and the corresponding evaluation of that outcome (value). The relative weight of an individual's attitude toward performing the behavior and the individual's perceived social normative expectations regarding performing the behavior determines intention. The theory recognizes that not all intentions are behavioral intentions and that not all intentions are good predictors of behavior (Fishbein & Middlestadt, 1990). For example, the theory distinguishes behavioral intention from intentions to reach a goal (Fishbein et al., 1992). Fishbein et al. tested the theory of reasoned action in terms of its applicability to predicting and understanding intimate (affective) behaviors as they examined the relationship between attitudinal and normative factors (subjective norm) and intention in HIV risk behaviors of gay men. They demonstrated that attitudes were the more important determinant of intentions to engage in intimate sexual behavior. In cities in which different normative influences were measured, strong subjective norms were also correlated with behavioral intention factors. Environmental or economic factors may also influence health behaviors. The model does not address the influence of social norms and peer influences on peoples' decisions regarding their health behaviors. Behavioral categories represented by studies using TRA included cigarette smoking (Hanson, 1997; Van Oss Marin, Marin, Perez-Stable, Otero-Sabogal, & Sabogal, 1990), condom use (Fisher, Fisher, & Rye, 1995; Gold, 1993; Jemmott & Jemmott, 1991), clinical and screening behaviors (Michels, Taplin, Carter, & Kulger, 1995), exercise (Blue, 1995;

Courneya & McAuley, 1995; Godin, 1994), and oral hygiene behaviors (Tedesco, Keffer, & Fleck-Kandath, 1991). Fisher et al., Michels et al., and Courneya and McAuley found that the theory performs well with respect to explaining intention. The efficiency for prediction of behavior varied across health-related behavior categories. The research demonstrated that perceived behavioral control (i.e., self-efficacy) was as important as attitude across health-related behavior categories.

Theory of Planned Behavior

The theory of planned behavior (TPB) is an extension of TRA, which is limited by the assumption that behavior is under complete volitional control. TRA is also challenged by developments in social cognitive theory, particularly the work on self-efficacy (Bandura, 1977). Ajzen (1985) expanded TRA (Figure 13.2) by adding the concept of self-efficacy, which he identified as the construct perceived behavioral control. TPB has been shown to yield greater explanatory power than the original TRA for goal-directed behaviors (Ajzen & Madden, 1986). New lines for research and practice have emerged that explore the added value of prediction and explanation with the construct perceived behavioral control (Reinecke et al., 1997).

Godin and Kok (1996) completed a 1985 to 1995 review of the social and behavioral sciences literature and the clinical medicine literature that applied the theory of planned behavior. They scrutinized the literature in terms of the strength of the association between each of the theoretical constructs with intention and behavior and the explained variation in intention and behavior. Their review attempted to describe the importance of perceived behavioral control to explain a significant portion of variance in intention and the contribution of other theoretical constructs to explain intention and predict behavior. Finally, they sought to explain the influence of how perceived behavioral control was

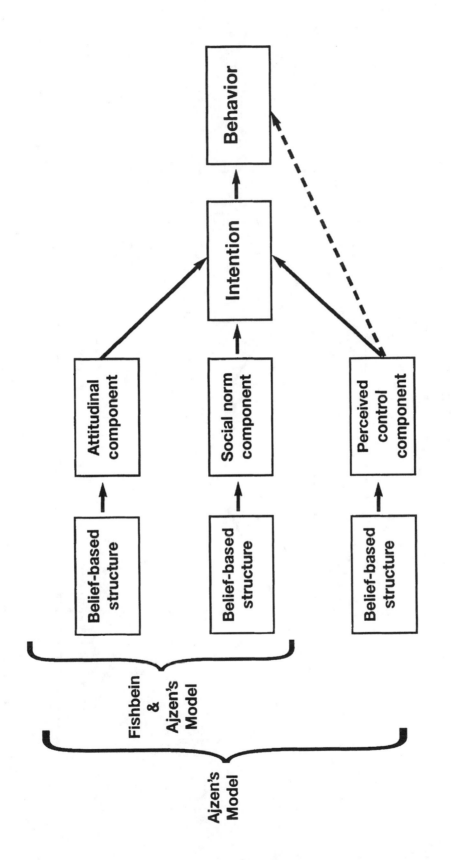

Figure 13.2. Schematic Representation of Fishbein and Ajzen's Theory of Reasoned Action and Ajzen's Theory of Planned Behavior (reprinted with permission from *Journal of Applied Social Psychology*, Vol. 26, No. 17, pp. 1556-1586. © V. H. Winston & Son, Inc., 360 South Ocean Boulevard, Palm Beach, FL 33480. All rights reserved.)

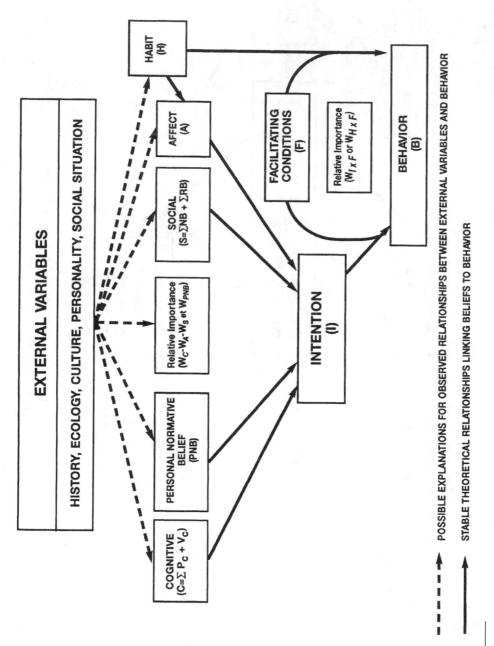

EXTERNAL VARIABLES

HISTORY, ECOLOGY, CULTURE, PERSONALITY, SOCIAL SITUATION

HABIT
(H)

AFFECT
(A)

SOCIAL
$(S=\Sigma NB + \Sigma RB)$

Relative Importance
$(W_C \cdot W_A \cdot W_S \text{ et } W_{PNB})$

PERSONAL NORMATIVE
BELIEF
(PNB)

COGNITIVE
$(C=\Sigma P_C + V_C)$

FACILITATING
CONDITIONS
(F)

Relative Importance
$(W_{I \times F} \text{ or } W_{H \times F})$

INTENTION
(I)

BEHAVIOR
(B)

----→ POSSIBLE EXPLANATIONS FOR OBSERVED RELATIONSHIPS BETWEEN EXTERNAL VARIABLES AND BEHAVIOR

——→ STABLE THEORETICAL RELATIONSHIPS LINKING BELIEFS TO BEHAVIOR

Figure 13.3. Schematic Representation of Triandis's Theory of Interpersonal Behavior (reprinted with permission from *Journal of Applied Social Psychology*, Vol. 26, No. 17, pp. 1556-1586. © V. H. Winston & Son, Inc., 360 South Ocean Boulevard, Palm Beach, FL 33480. All rights reserved)

assessed on the relationships between the variables. They examined 58 behavioral applications to verify the efficiency of the theory of planned behavior to explain intention or predict behavior. These applications were classified into the following categories: addictive (cigarette, alcohol, drugs, and eating disorders), automobile, clinical and screening (cancer screening and health check), eating, exercising, HIV/AIDS, and oral hygiene. Godin and Kok determined that "the overall average correlations between intention and attitude, subjective norm and perceived behavioral control were .46, .34, and .46, respectively" (p. 92). The average explained variance in intention was 40.9%, varying from 32.0% (eating behavior) to 46.8% (oral hygiene). Intention is thereby retained as the most important variable. Godin and Kok concluded that health-related behaviors remain largely within one's personal motivation except where perceived behavioral control plays a more important role than intention, as in the categories addictive and clinical and screening.

Triandis's Theory of Interpersonal Behavior

The theory of interpersonal behavior (Triandis, 1977, 1980) (Figure 13.3), like HBM, TRA, and TPB, focuses on intention to do a specific behavior. Triandis (1980) explains intention using four constructs: cognition (personal and subjective analysis of performing a certain behavior), affect (feelings associated with thoughts of performing the behavior), social factors (includes normative beliefs and beliefs about specific social roles), and personal normative beliefs (a moral norm, the obligation to do or not to do a behavior). Social factors as a predictor variable are important because they include the individual's internalization of the referent group's culture and interpersonal agreements that have been made with others regarding the behavior. The cognitive factor is conceptually similar to the attitudinal concept in TRA and TPB in that

there is a personal and subjective analysis of the outcomes of performing a health behavior. The affective factor, the results of feelings generated from previous experiences related to the behavior, is one of the distinctive elements used to explain intention. Triandis also includes other normative influences in addition to the normative belief or motivation to comply to explain intention, such as personal normative beliefs and role beliefs. Finally, Triandis predicts specific behavior based on a wider range of factors in addition to intention, such as motivation, facilitating conditions, and past behavior or habit. Facilitating conditions may be responsible for one not performing the behavior even when intention is high, habits are well entrenched, and the situation is relevant to one's values. Triandis's model may be more helpful in explaining health behaviors than the HBM or the TRA because it is more comprehensive.

As noted by Godin et al. (1996), Triandis's theory has gained much attention following its initial applications in the 1970s. Some authors (Godin & Kok, 1996; Parker, Manstead, & Stradling, 1995) suggest that Ajzen's theory of planned behavior incorporates some of Triandis's theoretical construct (particularly role beliefs and moral norms). Applications include intentions to seek care for a breast cancer symptom (Lauver & Chang, 1991), using condoms (Boyd & Wandersman, 1991), getting a mammogram (Baumann, Brown, Fontana, & Cameron, 1993), and driving behavior (Parker et al., 1995). The cross-cultural validity of the Triandis model has been tested with Mexican and American women to understand fertility-related intentions (Davidson, Jaccard, Triandis, Morales, & Diaz-Guerrero, 1976); with Anglo, migrant, and aboriginal high school students in New South Wales to predict intention to complete high school (McInerney, 1991); and with three Canadian ethnocultural communities to predict and explain intention for condom use for each instance of sexual intercourse with a new partner (Godin et al., 1996). Facione (1993) suggested that the

Triandis model "offers exceptional promise to nurse researchers whose goal is to achieve cultural sensitivity in their research investigations" (p. 49).

Cox's Interaction Model of Client Health Behavior

Cox (1982) identified the need for a client-focused model of health behavior that would

(a) recognize the client's individuality and uniqueness in the attainment of positive health behaviors, (b) address the elements that constitute client-professional interaction and their role in determining health behavior, and (c) guide the development of nursing interventions that would be specifically tailored to the individual client and the expressed health care need. (p. 42)

A central construct in explaining health behavior within her model is intrinsic motivation. Its definition is similar to that of the HBM (Rosenstock et al., 1988) and cognition evaluation theory (Deci & Ryan, 1985). Cox, however, wanted to address the limitations of existing models originating within the psychological and sociological paradigms. The psychology paradigm emphasizes the effect of cognition on behavior, with little attention given to the roles of the affective and social influences. The sociological paradigm emphasizes the social and environmental influences on health and illness, with little attention given to important individual client variables and cognitive processes that impact decision making and behavior. Most models are based on the disease model, which does not reflect the wellness and health-promotion concerns that currently exist. The disease model depicts clients as passive non-participants because of their limited knowledge of disease, making them dependent on the greater knowledge of health care professionals. These models also assume a philosophy that excluded personal freedom and choice in the exercise of health behaviors. A final factor that the model was designed to address is the lack of explicit examination of the role of the client-provider interaction in effecting client behavior and health outcomes.

The Interaction Model of Client Health Behavior (IMCHB) is depicted in Figure 13.4. It is organized around three major elements: client singularity, client professional interaction, and health outcomes. Client singularity recognizes the uniqueness and holism of the client when explaining actions directed toward risk reduction and health promotion. Each client brings differing variables of demographic characteristics, social influences, previous health care experience, and environmental resources (e.g., personal financial resources and access to health care). Although not explicitly stated, cultural influences can be inferred in this element. There is a time ordering of the variables so that the background variables are antecedent to subsequent variables and elements. Therefore, culture would form the context for attitudes, beliefs, and values, which are inherently found within intrinsic motivation, cognitive appraisal, and affective response.

Intrinsic motivation in the model "recognizes choice, desire, and the need for competency and self-determinism as causal factors in behavior" (Cox, 1982, p. 49). The experience of feeling competent and self-determining provides intrinsic rewards and reinforces the motivation to continue with health-seeking behavior. This feeling of mastery and competence is similar to the concept of self-efficacy within Bandura's social cognitive theory and the HBM.

Cognitive appraisal is operationalized as perceived health status (Carter & Kulbok, 1995), and these perceptions reflect beliefs about self-concept, culture, the ability to function in society, and values and commitments. Subsuming affective response within cognitive appraisal, as was done in earlier models, led to interventions that did not address the problem. Therefore, Cox supports affective responses to health concerns as a totally sepa-

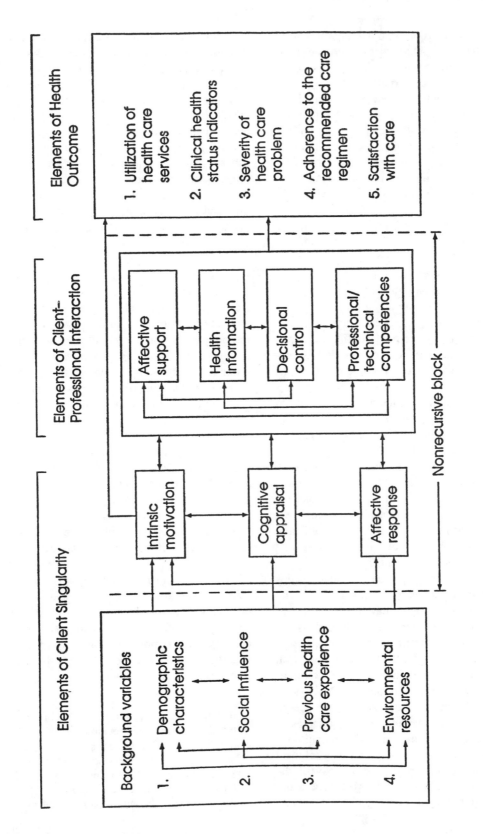

Figure 13.4. Interaction Model of Client Health Behavior (from Pender, *Health Promotion in Nursing Practice*, 1996, Appleton & Lange. Reproduced with permission from The McGraw-Hill Companies)

rate construct from cognitive appraisal. She emphasizes the interplay between the background variables and the relationships among beliefs, motivation, and affect.

The elements of client-professional interaction are affective support, health information, decisional control, and professional and technical competencies. These components define the interaction and the strength of the components within the interaction and vary according to the client's singularity and the expressed health care need (Cox, 1982). These elements recognize that although knowledge is necessary for positive health behaviors, it is not sufficient to change behavior. It is the client's relationship with the provider, the amount of choice and perceived decisional control that exist, the amount of social support, and aspects of client singularity and nurse singularity (competency of the nurse) that will influence how information is processed and used (Cox, 1986). Therefore, the model depicts the elements of client-professional interaction together with intrinsic motivation, cognitive appraisal, and affective response as nonrecursive or reciprocal in nature (Carter & Kulbok, 1995).

Health outcomes include (a) use of health care services, (b) clinical health status indicators, (c) severity of health care problem, (d) adherence to the recommended care regimen, and (e) satisfaction with care. Positive health outcomes or health behavior are those that maintain or promote health.

Studies have explored the relationships among the variables of client singularity and health outcomes. Some have explored the interplay between demographic characteristics, social influence, intrinsic motivation, cognitive appraisal, and affective response with health outcomes (adherence to a recommended regimen) (Farrand & Cox, 1993; Locke & Vincent, 1995). Others have focused on the relationships between the variables of client singularity and other client health outcomes, such as use of health services, clinical health status indicators, and severity of the health care problem (Cox, Miller, & Mull, 1987; Troumbley & Lenz, 1992).

Only two published studies have examined the relationships between the variables of client singularity and the elements of client-professional interaction. Cox, Sullivan, and Roghmann (1984) explored how demographic characteristics, social influence, previous health care experience, environmental resources, cognitive appraisal, and affective responses related to affective support and health information within the client-professional interaction. A multivariate approach to analysis provided these researchers with a fuller explanation for nonuse of amniocentesis in older women. They also showed that the IMCHB was successful in identifying approaches that support informed client decision making about a specific health risk. Brown (1992) examined demographic characteristics, intrinsic motivation, cognitive appraisal, and affective response to all four aspects of the client-professional interaction. Brown interpreted the findings of her study as empirical evidence supporting "tailoring of the client-nurse interaction to the client's individuality as a central concept in Cox's interaction model of client health behavior" (p. 39).

Only one published study was found that had tested the IMCHB exploring relationships among all three elements of the model. Cox and Roghmann (1984) examined how the use of health care services was explained by the client singularity variables (demographic characteristics of patients, social influence, previous health care experience, environmental resources, intrinsic motivation, cognitive appraisal, and affective response) and aspects of client-professional interaction (decisional control and professional and technical competencies). In a sample of women ($N = 203$) older than age 34, she found that for the decision to request amniocentesis,

first, both the individuality of the client and the client-professional relationship/interaction are significant determinants of health decisions and subsequent health behavior. Second, not only do these elements directly influence behavior, but in addition, they appear to have reciprocity with one another;

and professional response likewise influences client singularity. (p. 283)

Samples have been diverse with respect to age and have included children (Cox, Cowell, Marion, & Miller, 1990; Farrand & Cox, 1993); adolescents (Locke & Vincent, 1995); adults, including prenatal clients and members of the military (Brown, 1992; Cox, 1985; Cox & Roghmann, 1984; Cox et al., 1984; Cox & Wachs, 1985; Troumbley & Lenz, 1992); and elders (Cox, 1986; Cox et al., 1987). No studies were found that tested the IMCHB in other countries. Studies (Cox, 1986; Cox et al., 1984) have reflected incorporation of clients by race (black) but not by cultural background.

Designs of the studies have been qualitative (phenomenology; Brown, 1992) and quantitative. Statistical analyses have included stepwise regression (Cox et al., 1987; Cox & Wachs, 1985; Farrand & Cox, 1993; Troumbley & Lenz, 1992), multiple regression (Cox & Roghmann, 1984; Locke & Vincent, 1995), hierarchical regression (Cox, 1986; Troumbley & Lenz, 1992), factor analysis (Cox, 1985; Cox et al., 1987), discriminant analysis (Cox & Roghmann, 1984), and structural modeling or LISREL (Cox & Roghmann, 1985; Cox et al., 1984; Locke & Vincent, 1995). Twenty-four studies testing the IMCHB have been evaluated (Carter & Kulbok, 1995). The model has been used to explain the decision of at-risk prenatal clients requesting amniocentesis (Cox & Roghmann, 1984; Cox et al., 1984), with more than half of the variance being explained by the model. Many studies have explored the relationships between the numerous variables within the element of client singularity. Some (Cox, 1985; Cox & Wachs, 1985) explored the relationships between demographic characteristics and intrinsic motivation. Cox (1986) focused on describing the interplay between the demographic characteristics of community-based elders and intrinsic motivation, cognitive appraisal, and affective response to identify those at risk for decreased health and well-being.

Pender's Health Promotion Model

Similar to Cox, Pender developed her model during the early 1980s when attention was turning to promoting high-level wellness and personal health. Pender also noted there was little attention in the literature paid to what motivates people to seek their health potential. She found the concept of perceived threat in earlier models (i.e., the health belief model) to be of limited usefulness in motivating people who were healthy.

Pender's Health Promotion Model (HPM) depicts "the multidimensional nature of persons interacting with their environment as they pursue health" (Pender, 1996, p. 53). The influence of Bandura and social cognitive theory is readily evident in the model, with self-efficacy being a central construct. Cognition, affect, actions, and environmental events are proposed as operating interactively to determine behavior (Pender, Walker, Sechrist, & Frank-Stromborg, 1990). Fishbein's theory of reasoned action asserts that beliefs, attitudes, and sociocultural norms impact health behavior, and this is also important to the development of this model. Pender integrated many of the constructs from earlier theories into a nursing paradigm that emphasizes humanism and holism.

The 1987 version of the HPM is shown in Figure 13.5 (Pender, 1987). Pender identified seven cognitive and perceptual factors in individuals that are amenable to change. The importance of health reflects the value one places on health. Perceived control of health is the belief that health is self-determined (similar to the concept of internal locus of control), influenced by others (similar to the concept of external locus of control), or the result of chance. Perceived self-efficacy is the belief that one has competence and mastery to carry out specific health behaviors. Definition of health reflects the meaning of health to the individual. Perceived health is the self-evaluation of current status as a subjective state. Perceived benefits are the personal desirability of outcomes, and perceived barriers reflect unde-

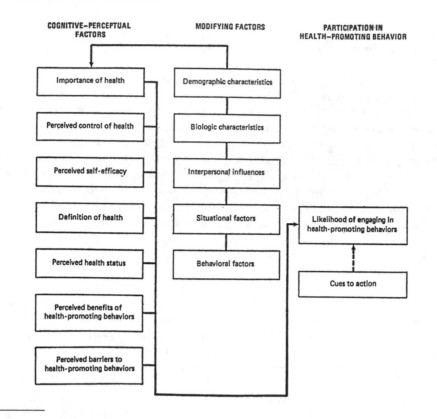

Figure 13.5. Health Promotion Model (from Pender, *Health Promotion in Nursing Practice,* 1996, Appleton & Lange. Reproduced with permission from the McGraw-Hill Companies)

sirable blocks to health-promoting behavior (Pender et al., 1990).

The cognitive and perceptual factors interact with other modifying factors less amenable to change to determine health behavior. Pender (1987) asserted that "the modifying factors exert their influence through the cognitive/perceptual mechanisms that directly affect behavior" (p. 68). The modifying factors, therefore, are not considered to have a direct effect on health behavior. Examples of demographic characteristics include age, gender, marital status, income, education, and cultural background; biologic characteristics are body weight and composition. Interpersonal influences include expectations of significant others and the norms of the social group. Situational factors are defined as access to health-promoting options within the environment, and behavioral factors include prior ex-

perience with health actions. Cues to action are specified as external or internal triggers for health-related behavior (Pender et al., 1990).

Pender's (1996) revised model is shown in Figure 13.6. On the basis of analyses of studies using the HPM, the concepts of importance of health and perceived control of health were deleted due to their inability to explain specific health behavior and cues to action. This was believed to be related to difficulty in identification and measurement. Definition of health, perceived health status, and demographic and biologic characteristics were combined into personal factors to increase flexibility in selecting and measuring particular variables that may be relevant to a particular behavior or population. Personal factors may have a direct influence on both behavior-specific cognitions and affect as well as

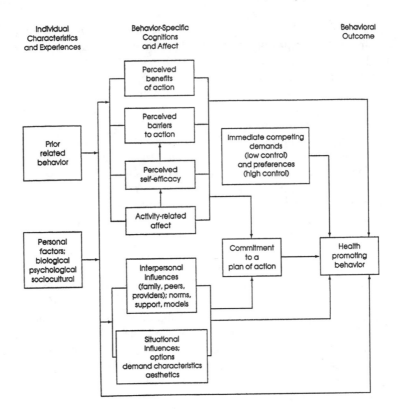

Figure 13.6. Revised Health Promotion Model (from Pender, *Health Promotion in Nursing Practice,* 1996, Appleton & Lange. Reproduced with permission from the McGraw-Hill Companies)

health-promoting behavior. The concept of behavioral factors of the earlier model has been renamed as prior related behavior. Prior related behavior has both direct and indirect effects on health-promoting behavior. The direct effect results from habit formation and engaging in the behavior with little thought. The indirect effect results from its positive impact on self-efficacy, perceived benefits of action, perceived barriers to action, and activity-related affect.

Pender (1996) considers behavior-specific cognitions and affect to be "of major motivational significance" (p. 68) and amenable to modification through nursing intervention. A new variable within this category in the revised model is "activity-related affect." This concept is defined as subjective feelings associated with a particular behavior that directly influences the performance of the behavior or

indirectly influences it by impacting self-efficacy.

"Commitment to a plan of action" is a second new variable in the revised model and is similar to the concept of intention in Fishbein's theory of reasoned action (Pender, 1996, p. 72). Pender defined this concept as "commitment to carry out a specific action irrespective of competing preferences and the identification of strategies for accomplishing and reinforcing the behavior" (p. 72).

"Immediate competing demands and preferences" is the third new variable to be incorporated into the revised model. These refer to alternatives to planned behavior that occur just prior to the intended activity. Competing demands are conflicts over which the person has low control because of work or family responsibilities. Competing preferences are alternative behaviors with high personal control and that generally reinforce behavior. Pender defined "health-promoting behavior" as the outcome of the HPM (p. 73). It is directed toward achieving positive health outcomes and results in a positive health experience throughout one's life.

Pender (1996) identified research studies focused on predicting health-promoting lifestyles and specific behaviors, such as exercise and use of hearing protection. These studies reflected the 1987 version of the model. The health-promoting lifestyles studies were of blue-collar workers (Weitzel, 1989), white-collar workers (Pender et al., 1990), community-dwelling elders (Walker, Kerr, Pender, & Sechrist, 1990), cardiac rehabilitation patients (Pender et al., 1990), ambulatory cancer patients (Frank-Stromborg, Pender, & Walker, 1990), and participants in the National Survey of Personal Health Practices and Consequences (Johnson, Ratner, Bottorff, & Hayduk, 1993). Five to seven variables were selected to be tested as predictors in each of these studies, with demographic characteristics, perceived control of health, and perceived health status being common to all studies. Participants in these studies were adults or elders. Weitzel (1989) included in her sample individuals of differing racial or ethnic backgrounds, including European American, Hispanic, and African American participants. She examined the prediction of health-promoting lifestyle. The scores of the Health Promoting Lifestyle Profile were regressed on four of the seven cognitive-perceptual factors (importance of health, perceived control of health, perceived self-efficacy, and perceived health status) and the modifying factors. The cognitive-perceptual factors were more predictive than the demographic factors in explaining health-promoting behaviors (Pender, 1996; Weitzel, 1989).

Statistical methods used in these studies were multiple regression (Frank-Stromborg et al., 1990; Pender et al., 1990; Weitzel, 1989), hierarchic regression (Sechrist, 1990; Walker et al., 1990), and causal path modeling using LISREL for structural equation analysis

(Frank-Stromborg et al., 1990; Johnson et al., 1993; Pender et al., 1990; Sechrist, 1990; Walker et al., 1990). From 20% to 38% of variance was explained by the variables within the model. Pender (1995) used the outcomes of the causal path modeling using LISREL to revise her model. She determined that the "demographic characteristics of age and gender have significant direct paths as well as significant indirect paths to health-promoting lifestyles. The direct paths from the modifying factors to health-promoting health behavior were not consistent with the HPM" (p. 56).

Six published studies focused on explaining and predicting specific behaviors—five on exercise (Frank-Stromborg et al., 1990; Garcia et al., 1995; Pender, 1990; Sechrist, 1990; Walker et al., 1990) and one on hearing protection (Lusk, Ronis, Kerr, & Atwood, 1994). Almost all the variables were tested from the model (except cues to action) as predictors for the specific behaviors. The sample in the first study included preadolescents and adolescents (Garcia et al., 1995). The rest used adults and elders. Study participants were all from a European American background except those for one study (Garcia et al., 1995), in which participants also came from African American and other racial backgrounds. Pender (1996) cited an unpublished study (Kerr, 1994) that tested the cross-cultural applicability of the HPM among Mexican American workers.

Statistical analyses in these studies were regression (Garcia et al., 1995), hierarchic multiple regression (Frank-Stromborg et al., 1990; Pender, 1990), structural equation analysis using LISREL (Frank-Stromborg et al., 1990; Lusk et al., 1994; Pender, 1990; Sechrist, 1990; Walker et al., 1990), and path analysis (Garcia et al., 1995). The variance explained in these published studies ranged from 19% to 55%. When exploratory causal modeling was used, in which modifying factors were allowed to directly affect the target behaviors, the explained variance increased from a range of 25% to 36% to a range of 51%

to 55%. The higher percentage reflected the greater explanatory power of the modifying factors when allowed to directly affect the specific behavior (hearing protection).

Pender (1996) concluded that "behavior-specific variables of perceived self-efficacy, benefits, and barriers were empirically supported as predictors of health behaviors in the majority of studies in which they were included. Self-efficacy and barriers received the largest support, with benefits receiving moderate support" (p. 65). On the basis of her analysis of the studies using her 1987 model, Pender (1996) decided that some health-specific variables needed "to be reevaluated as to their centrality in predicting health-promoting and protecting behaviors" (p. 65). The revised HPM reflected this decision. No published works were found using the revised model.

Leininger's Theory of Cultural Care: Diversity and Universality

A third theory or model, which incorporates attitudes, beliefs, values, and culture, is Leininger's theory of cultural care: diversity and universality (TCCDU). Care is the central construct of this theory, which is supported by concepts of health and environmental contexts. Leininger (1988) defines culture as the "learned, shared, and transmitted values, beliefs, norms, and life practices of a particular group that guides thinking, decisions, and actions in patterned ways" (p. 156). Cultural care, then, is the understanding of known values, beliefs, and patterned expressions that "assist, support, or enable another individual or group to maintain well-being, improve a human condition or lifeway, or face death and disabilities" (p. 156). The concepts of diversity and universality refer to both the variability and the common meanings of patterns and values that people culturally derive for health and well-being.

Unlike Cox's and Pender's models that reflected the influence of social cognitive theory, Leininger's TCCDU clearly reflects her anthropological grounding with new formulations made within the nursing perspective. Leininger developed the Sunrise Model to depict the essential elements of TCCDU as shown in Figure 13.7. The historical, cultural, and social contexts of human beings are represented in the top half of the circle. These factors influence care expressions and patterns and practices of holistic health and well-being through language, ethnohistory, and environmental contexts. These factors also influence folk, professional, and nursing systems, with nursing mediating between the folk and professional systems.

Leininger (1988) identified the following dominant modes to guide nursing decisions and actions to provide culturally congruent care or care that fits with the clients' cultural beliefs, values, and lifeways: cultural care preservation or maintenance, cultural care accommodation, and cultural care repatterning or restructuring. Cultural care preservation or maintenance is defined as those professional actions or decisions that support the preservation of relevant care values so that people can maintain their well-being. Cultural care accommodation or negotiation is defined as those professional actions and decisions that assist clients to adapt to or to negotiate for a satisfying health outcome. Cultural care repatterning or restructuring refers to those professional actions and decisions that help clients change their lifeways for new or different patterns that are culturally meaningful, satisfying, and support healthy life patterns.

Leininger's Sunrise Model is much more explicit about the role that culture plays in health than the previous models. She (1988) asserted,

> Cultures have folk and professional care values, beliefs, and practices that influence cultural care practices in Western and non-Western cultures. Knowledge of meanings and practices derived from worldviews, social structure factors, cultural values, environmental context, and language uses are essential to guide nursing decisions and ac-

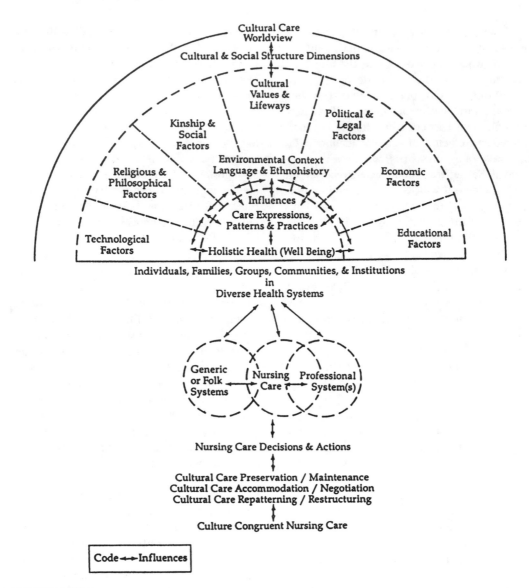

Figure 13.7. Leininger's Sunrise Model to Depict Theory of Cultural Care Diversity and Universality (Leininger, M. M. [Ed.], *Culture Care Diversity & Universality: A Theory of Nursing,* 1991: National League for Nursing Press and Jones & Bartlett Publishers, Sudbury, MA. *www.jbpub.com.* Reprinted with permission)

tions in providing culturally congruent care. (p. 155)

Leininger's theory of cultural care diversity and universality has been tested widely throughout the world in more than 14 major cultures and 100 subcultures. In more than 20 years of research studies based on her theory, more than 140 care constructs have been developed, and more continue to be developed (Leininger, 1991). These care constructs include stress alleviation, trust, comfort, succorance, attention, presence, engrossment, and empathy (Leininger, 1988). Research studies have predominantly used qualitative methods, such as phenomenology and ethnonursing. The latter method was developed by Leininger to fit the theory. She used the anthropological methodology, ethnography, and adapted it to focus on the viewpoints, beliefs, practices, health patterns, and nursing care phenomena of a particular culture. The use of this method allows for the "discovery of people's emic (local or insider's) views of the meanings, symbols, patterns, and expressions of cultural care and nursing from a holistic perspective" (Leininger, 1988, p. 153). The focus on the emic perspective to gain and test new knowledge in lived human contexts is counter to the notions of testing theory through preconceived (etic) views of the researcher.

➤ PHASE OF THEORY DEVELOPMENT OF THE NURSING MODELS

Walker and Avant (1988) identified four phases of theory development: description, explanation, prediction, and control. In addition, they identified three basic approaches to theory construction: analysis, synthesis, and derivation. They blended these with the three elements of theory (concepts, statements, and theory) to identify nine strategies or approaches in theory development. Each of the three nursing theories will be examined according to the phase of, and strategies used in, the theory development.

Cox's Interaction Model of Client Health Behavior

Cox (1982) proposed the IMCHB as a "theoretical prescription for nursing" (p. 41) that would equate to the final phase of theory development, control. This phase of theory development assumes that desired outcomes can be identified and prescribes specific health outcomes and the process to achieve these outcomes. A prescriptive theory re-

quires concepts and relationships between all concepts to be well identified and tested. To date, this has not been achieved within the IMCHB. As Carter and Kulbok (1995) point out in their evaluation of the first decade of research using the IMCHB,

> Testing to this point has emphasized the elements of client singularity and health outcomes with less focus on the interaction elements. More testing of the model is necessary—with possible model modifications—before the IMCHB can meet the criteria of a theory. (p. 65)

Cox has defined and explained concepts of client singularity, client-professional interaction, and health outcomes. The large number of studies focusing on the element of client singularity suggests that "researchers are already using the IMCHB as a multiphasic model for the descriptive portion of their research" (Carter & Kulbok, 1995, p. 69) to better design interventions that address the uniqueness of clients.

Concept derivation is evident in Cox's (1982) selection of intrinsic motivation as the central construct of her model. Deci and Ryan's (1985) notion of intrinsic motivation was transposed and reconceptualized in the model to mean self-determinism in health judgment and behavior, perceived competency in health, and responsiveness to internal and external cues. Perceived competency as a part of intrinsic motivation is also similar to Bandura's (1977) and the health belief model's (Becker, 1974) concept of self-efficacy.

The concept of health outcomes needs further clarification and refinement before the model can predict and prescribe specific health outcomes. For example, health outcomes has been operationalized to include five behaviors: use of health care services, clinical health status indicators, severity of health care problem, adherence to the recommended care regimen, and satisfaction with care. In reality, only two of these represent behavioral constructs—use of health care services and adherence to the recommended care regimen.

Most research studies have lent support for the proposed linkages or relationships among the concepts, with the explanatory power of these relationships being quite strong, generally approximately 40% to 60%. Cox (1982) theorized that there is a reciprocal relationship between the elements of client singularity (intrinsic motivation, cognitive appraisal, and affective response) and those of the elements of client-professional interaction. Only two studies explore these two elements (Brown, 1992; Cox et al., 1984), and only one study (Cox & Roghmann, 1984) examined the relationships among concepts in all three elements. Carter and Kulbok (1995) encouraged the addition of a feedback loop within the model in which relationships between health outcomes and client singularity could be asserted and examined. Cox noted the complexity of model and that it must be complex to address the complexity of health behavior. It is clear that there is a need for much more empirical support and testing of the model before it can be viewed as predictive and prescriptive.

Pender's Health Promotion Model

The HPM is also an extensive model proposed as a framework to describe, explain, and predict health-promoting behaviors. It is structurally very similar to the HBM (Rosenstock, 1974). It seems that theory derivation strategies were initially used by Pender, whereby a whole structure was moved from one field and modified to fit another— nursing. The HBM did not prove helpful in describing, explaining, and predicting health-promoting behaviors because of its reliance on threat or fear as the primary motivating force. Pender inductively derived her model using theory synthesis strategies from existing research on health-promoting behavior that had greater relevance to nursing. The model clearly reflects a major emphasis on self-reflection and self-regulation as well as percep-

tions of self-efficacy consistent with the research of social cognitive theory (Bandura, 1986).

Pender described many concepts, which define the construct cognitive-operational definitions. The vagueness of some theoretical definitions has been addressed in the revised model. She also defined the construct modifying factors through several concepts.

Pender stipulated the relationships that exist between the cognitive-perceptual factors and health-promoting behaviors. As primary motivational factors, they exert a direct effect on health-promoting behaviors. The modifying factors exert an indirect influence on health-promoting behaviors, only through the cognitive-perceptual factors. No direct effects are hypothesized by Pender to exist between the modifying factors and health-promoting behaviors, but statistical analyses using regression have allowed modifying factors, such as gender, age, and marital status, to show direct relationships with health-promoting behaviors (Johnson et al., 1993). The relational inconsistencies using more sophisticated statistical analyses such as structural equation modeling (LISREL) have been identified (Johnson et al., 1993) as has direction for future modification and extension of the existing theory. Pender has used structural equation modeling in recent studies to clearly specify causal paths, clearer relationships among existing concepts, and the need for additional concept development within the model. This ongoing theory analysis has led to the development of a newer version of the model that incorporates three new concepts and defines additional relationships among the concepts.

Leininger's Theory of Cultural Care: Diversity and Universality

Leininger's TCCDU reflects mainly the use of concept synthesis, concept derivation, and theory synthesis strategies (Cohen, 1991). Development of her taxonomy of caring constructs demonstrates the use of concept synthesis. Through the study of 100 cultures and subcultures using the ethnonursing method or other qualitative approaches, library data, and direct observations, she combined clusters of phenomena that seemed to relate closely and identified more than 135 major care constructs.

Concept derivation is evident in Leininger's transformation of the anthropological concept and methodology of ethnography into a new concept and methodology that is more applicable to nursing—that is, ethnonursing. Her construction of the Sunrise Model to depict the essential elements of the TCCDU reflects another example of concept derivation. She uses the concepts (anthropological social structure and worldview) of a social anthropologist to emphasize the importance of understanding caring from both an individual and a group cultural viewpoint (Cohen, 1991).

Finally, Leininger used theory synthesis strategies in the development of the TCCDU. She used ethnonursing methods to obtain the emic or indigenous viewpoint of the people about care. She pictorially represented the symmetrical interrelationships between the model's concepts (technological factors, religious and philosophical factors, kinship and social factors, cultural values and beliefs, political and legal factors, educational factors, and economic factors) and their influence within language and environment contexts on care expressions, patterns, practice, and wellbeing. She depicted how care and health patterns relate to nursing care principles and interventions. The nursing system can act as a bridge between the folk and personal health systems through three types of nursing care actions: cultural care preservation, cultural care accommodation, and cultural care repatterning (Cohen, 1991).

Theory generation may occur at multiple levels, studying individuals, groups, families, and communities or cultures. This model uses both inductive strategies at the micro level based on empirical data and deductive strategies at the macro level while studying multiple cultures worldwide. The model also incorporates two phases of generating research knowledge: discovering substantive knowledge (Phase 1) and applying the knowledge to practice situations (Phase 2). It was during Phase 2 that Leininger classified many of her constructs into a taxonomy to help nurses conceptualize, order, and study types of caring phenomena (Cohen, 1991). The significance of the model is that it is the "only known model in nursing to combine both theory and method and to distinguish different levels of abstraction and methodological approaches" (Leininger, 1985, p. 44).

➤ INSTRUMENTS TO ASSESS ATTITUDES, BELIEFS, VALUES, AND CULTURE

Many instruments or tools have been developed and/or tested with the respective models. In the theories from social psychology (the HBM, the theory of interpersonal behavior, the theory of planned behavior, and the theory of reasoned action), the authors of each theory have provided specifications for measuring each variable.

The Health Belief Model

The HBM has the advantage of specifying a set of six key predictors of health behaviors that appear amenable to measurement and seem to mediate relationships between preventive behavior and nonmodifiable variables, such as demographic characteristics and prior sexual experience (Abraham & Sheeran, 1994). Russell (1991) tested an instrument based on the HBM that assessed injury prevention health beliefs in which all six scales showed internal consistency and test-retest reliability. The instrument may be useful to nurse researchers and nurse clinicians developing nursing interventions to prevent injuries in young children.

Bernstein and Keith (1991) reexamined Eisen, Zellman, and McAlister's Health Belief Model Questionnaire (a 22-item scale to measure four HBM constructs). Bernstein and Keith's reevaluation contradicted the authors' findings that the scales were deficient because the criteria used were not appropriate for categorical item responses. They also suggested that factor analysis would be more appropriate than the exploratory methods that were employed by Eisen et al.

Theories of Reasoned Action and Planned Behavior

Ajzen and Fishbein (1980) established instrument development guidelines. The approach to the instrument development process is grounded in the qualitative findings of in-depth interviews with members of the target population. Data derived from the population of interest ensure inclusion of salient beliefs, which are beliefs that serve as determinants of one's attitude at any given moment (Fishbein & Ajzen, 1975). Questionnaires are then developed to measure from the identified salient beliefs normative beliefs for TRA and salient beliefs, normative beliefs, and perceived control beliefs for TPB.

Young, Lierman, Powell-Cope, Kasprzyk, and Benoliel (1991) examined the relationships between components of a changed theory of reasoned action. They changed TRA by adding two components of the Triandis model, personal normative belief and facilitating conditions. The instrument used to measure breast self-exam (BSE) behavior was developed from the guidelines established by Ajzen and Fishbein (1980). Content and face validity were established for the instrument that measured behavior, behavior intention, affect, attitude, and social norm as well as the two components of the Triandis model. Where multiple items were used to measure a model component, internal consistency reliability was evaluated. The Cronbach's alpha coefficients were .82 (affect scale), .70 (attitude scale), and .89 (social norm scale). Young et al. (1991) found that "despite the iterative process of instrument development, a number of threats to reliability remain as a theory is ap-

plied to the empirical world" (p. 142). Among the concerns of these authors are the reliability of attitude scores when a specific belief is not endorsed by a participant; questions that require a contextual response, such as the circumstances regarding the performance of BSE; and the appearance of seemingly redundant questions that create frustration for a respondent. It was also noted that the study of an expected health behavior might introduce a bias that is not measured by the structure of the items. For example, avoidance of highly valued health behaviors such as BSE may not be reflected in the items, or the sample population may not be willing to admit to such actions.

Godin et al. (1996) did cross-cultural testing of the TRA and the TPB using the specific guidelines for instrument development by Ajzen and Fishbein (1980) for TRA and the method described by Ajzen (1991) for TPB. They constructed questionnaires to measure attitude (with a semantic differential scale), subjective norm (with three questions, each on a 5-point scale), and perceived behavior control (a variable specific to TRA) with three questions for which the answers were ranked on a 5-point scale. The Cronbach's alpha coefficients for the attitude measure were .79, .81, and .84 for the Latin American, English-speaking Caribbean, and South Asian communities, respectively (Godin et al., 1996). For the subjective norm measures, the Cronbach's alpha coefficients were .69, .79, and .87 for the three samples, respectively, and for perceived behavior control they were .79, .63, and .83, respectively.

Interaction Model of Client Health Behavior

The Health Self-Determinism Index (HSDI; Cox, 1985) attempted to capture the multidimensionality of motivational components of health behavior. The HSDI is based on Deci and Ryan's (1985) cognitive evaluation theory of intrinsic motivation. It has 20 items, 5 each for four subscales: self-determined health judgments, self-determined health behaviors, perceived sense of competency in health matters, and responsiveness to internal and external cues. Half of the items are worded such that "strongly agree" responses indicate a strong sense of self-determinism and competency regarding health behavior. The other half of the items are worded more extrinsically so that "strongly agree" responses reflect little or no self-determinism in health judgments and behavior, decreased feelings of competency about their health, and a greater responsiveness to extrinsic motivation.

The initial psychometric properties of the instrument were determined in a sample of 202 adults randomly selected from the general population (Cox, 1985). An alpha coefficient of .82 was obtained for the full 20-item scale, and the scale was reduced to 16 items after item-total correlations for four items were determined to be lower than the .30 criterion for acceptability (Nunnally, 1978). There was an associated increase in the alpha coefficient to .84 with the 16-item instrument that is higher than the .70 reliability standard for newer scales. Using .30 as the minimum acceptable loading factor score, Cox (1985) reported the average significant loadings for the four factors as .49 for self-determinism in health judgment, .52 for self-determinism in health behavior, .61 for perceived competency in health matters, and .45 for internal and external cue responsiveness. The data supported the multidimensionality of the construct of motivation.

The Health Self-Determinism Index for Children (HSDI-C; Cox et al., 1990) is an adaptation of the adult version that allows examination of the dimensions of a child's motivation for health behavior and the relative strength on an intrinsic-extrinsic continuum within each of the dimensions. Scoring was done on a 1 to 4, intrinsic-extrinsic ordinal scale. Factor analysis yielded four separate but related scales: behavior and goal setting, competency, internal-external cue responsiveness, and health judgment. The average loadings on the factors was .59 for behavior and goal setting, .48 for competency, .55

for internal-external cue responsiveness, and .51 for health judgment. These values provide strong support for the hypothesized scales. In two administrations of the HSDI-C, the alphas were .90 and .92, .84 and .88, .84 and .88, and .63 and .77 for the four respective subscales. Although Cox et al. recognized the need for continued application and testing of the tool, they concluded that it would allow for the exploration of "the link between psychosocio-environmental antecedents and correlated of intrinsic motivation" (p. 245).

The Health Promotion Model

The Health-Promoting Lifestyle Profile (HPLP) was developed by Pender (1982) to measure positive health behaviors. She developed the precursor to the HPLP that she called the Lifestyle and Health Habits Assessment (LHHA). The LHHA was a 100-item checklist arranged in 10 categories that reflected positive health behaviors from the literature. To evaluate the LHHA, she pilot-tested the instrument for clarity and response variance and to estimate reliability (Walker, Sechrist, & Pender, 1987). Four nursing faculty members who were familiar with the concept of health-promoting lifestyle established content validity. As a result of these steps in instrument development, Pender began empirical validation of the HPLP 107-item tool using the approach advocated by Nunnally (1978). Pender identified six dimensions of health-promoting lifestyle as the final structure of the 48-item HPLP: self-actualization, health responsibility, exercise, nutrition, interpersonal support, and stress management. The total instrument had a high internal consistency (alpha coefficient .92), with the reliability of the six subscales ranging from .70 to .90 (Walker et al., 1987).

Walker et al. (1990) developed a Spanish-language version of the HPLP to "facilitate the identification of some commonalties in wellness-oriented health behaviors across cultures and economic groups" (p. 272). Walker (as cited in Kulbok, Baldwin, Cox, & Duffy,

1997) has also psychometrically evaluated the newly revised Health-Promoting Lifestyle Profile II (HPLP II). The HPLP II is used to measure health-promoting behavior; as noted by Kulbok et al. (1997), however, several items measure perceptions, knowledge, and actions and are not solely behavioral indicators.

➤ IMPLICATIONS OF THE MODELS OF HEALTH BEHAVIOR FOR NURSING

Theory Development

The implications of the models of health behavior for nursing are considered as the theories develop from a linear to a process orientation, evolve a distinct language, embrace cultural perspectives, and demonstrate empirical adequacy. Four theories from social cognitive theory and three theories from nursing seek to explain, predict, and influence behavior. Most models have evolved over time in terms of the context and purpose for which they are used. The purpose of the social cognitive theories was to explain the failure of people to engage in prevention or early detection of asymptomatic illness. Later, the models were used to explain responses to illness and compliance with prescribed medical therapies. Recently, the use of the models has shifted to modifying lifelong behaviors. Some of the models build on social learning theory but add the context of wellness (the HPM), interpersonal variables (theory of interpersonal behavior and the IMCHB), and culture (TCCDU, the theory of interpersonal behavior, and the HBM). Many of the theories discussed previously have added the concept of self-efficacy (HBM and TRA) or identified self-efficacy (HPM) as a distinct dimension to explain and predict health behavior. The models advance nursing science in that they provide worthwhile theoretical constructs for research, education, and practice. The use of the previously discussed models of health behav-

ior by nursing contributes to the testing and evolution of an understanding of our ability to explain, predict, and influence behavior.

All the theories described previously, with the exception of the TCCDU, are frameworks that have their origins in social cognitive theory and expectancy-value theory. HBM and IMCHB seek to explain health promotion behavior but go beyond the frameworks found in other disciplines by viewing the person holistically and as an active partner in the health promotion process. The Triandis and Cox models have the greatest complexity, with multiple variables and reciprocity among variables. Cox's IMCHB, in particular, loses aesthetic appeal that is found with simpler and more parsimonious models. Cox (1986) acknowledges that her model

> could be reduced substantially to conform to the statistical ideal using factor analysis, structural equation modeling, and the development of instrumental variables . . . [but] such an approach would miss the interplay and polarities of the variables . . . the statistical ideal would sacrifice the advancement of nursing knowledge. (p. 56)

Linearity

A concept of importance to theory development is that of internal cognitive processing of experience over time. The awareness that changes in lifelong behaviors require adaptations over time emphasizes a process perspective. Understanding behavioral change as incremental adaptations implies a shift from linear to process modeling. As noted by Facione (1993), there is a linearity common to models that predate later insights on the recursive nature of cognitive processing. One response to this problem is to combine models such as the Triandis model with Ajzen and Fishbein's theory of reasoned action. As in the case of Cox's IMCHB, the model accounts for cognitive processing through the interplay between the client singularity and that of the nurse.

Interactional Process

One of the most significant contributions that the IMCHB makes to nursing theory that explains health promotion behaviors is its emphasis on interactional processes—the processes by which clients and health professionals come together to determine a health decision or action (Cox, 1982). This interactional process orientation highlights the centrality of the concept of singularity for both the client and the health professional. It is our singularity that defines us both as individuals and as health professionals, and it is the interplay between the client's singularity and the nurse's singularity that strongly impacts coping and health behavior. Whereas Cox emphasizes the interactional process between the client and the health care professional, Pender highlights the importance of the interpersonal influences, situational influences, and immediate competing demands and preferences when describing the context for health promotion decisions and behaviors. Pender recognizes the uniqueness of individuals in variables such as individual characteristics and experiences (prior related behavior, personal, biological, and psychological and sociocultural factors).

Triandis's model of interpersonal behavior, however, considers interaction from a cultural and interpersonal perspective in its definition of social factor. Social factor, a predictor variable, is described as the individual's internalization of the referent group's subjective culture and specific interpersonal agreements that the individual has made with others regarding the performance of certain behaviors (Facione, 1993). The Triandis model therefore directs the health care provider to examine interpersonal and cultural relevance from a within-group perspective.

Culture

The understanding of diverse cultural groups as it relates to the provision of nursing and health care is critical to the outcomes of the efforts of providers. Transcultural nursing is a synthesis of concepts from anthropology, sociology, biology, and nursing that provides a rich interdisciplinary perspective. This perspective improves "the quality of care given by learning to focus on the ways in which illness and health are expressions of a particular culture and how culture influences patients' expectations of nursing care" (Herberg, 1995, p. 5). Understanding health from a cultural context extends thinking from the largely social behavioral perspectives of the HBM, TRA, TPB, and the HPM.

The Triandis model offers exceptional promise to nurse researchers whose goal is to achieve cultural sensitivity in their research investigations (Facione, 1993). Facione believes that instruments that include culturally relevant items within the six components of the model could capture diverse explanations for health behaviors. The cross-cultural validity of the Triandis model has been documented empirically (Davidson et al., 1976; Godin et al., 1996; McInerney, 1991).

Leininger's TCCDU generates theory that demonstrates a macroperspective of families, communities, and cultures. The understanding of the uniqueness and singularity of clients and their worldviews, whether they be individuals or larger groups, is achieved by gaining the emic perspective—the ways of knowing and meanings of care within their cultural and social structure, environmental context, language, and ethnohistory. Tripp-Reimer (1984) has also advocated the role of the nurse as mediator between the biomedical (etic) model and the patient (emic) model. The explicit focus on how values, attitudes, beliefs, and practices are embedded within a culture is the hallmark and strength of the TCCDU. Culturally congruent care can be designed and delivered only in context with an understanding of these values, attitudes, beliefs, and practices.

The impact of culture or ethnicity is built into the IMCHB (background variables) and HPM (individual characteristics and experiences) but often is not explicitly studied with respect to how culture influences values, attitudes, beliefs, and practices. When samples are described in research testing these two models, terms such as race are often used interchangeably with culture. Both cross-cultural and intracultural testing is required so that a range of subculture characteristics, such as race, geographic region, and social class, are considered. In so doing, the values, beliefs, and attitudes of individuals within the larger group are actually represented. Although the IMCHB, HPM, and TCCDU differ with respect to emphasis, they all stress "not only the structure and outcomes of nursing interventions but also the process by which interventions are developed and implemented" (Cox, 1986, p. 56). They refocus attention away from illness models to models that recognize the multidimensional nature of health.

Language

Models based in social cognitive theory use similar concepts, although the language varies between models. Weinstein (1993) offers a review of four competing models of health-protective behavior, two of which are the HBM and the TRA. His review highlights similarities, such as the assumption that anticipation of negative health outcomes and the desire to avoid such outcomes creates motivation for self-protection. The HBM includes the variable as "perceived severity," whereas the TRA uses the language "negative evaluation." Beliefs about the likelihood of negative health outcomes are described as "perceived vulnerability" in the HBM and as "expectancy" in the TRA. These differing terms have the same underlying meanings. Both theories assume that expected benefits in risk reduction must be weighed against the costs or barriers of acting to predict changes in behavior. In the HBM, various costs are represented by a single variable, whereas the TRA considers a much wider range of consequences of continuing current behavior. Some of the consequences can be seen as costs, some as health outcomes, and others as nonhealth outcomes (Weinstein, 1993).

The nursing models also recognize the interrelationships of cognitive appraisal, affective response, and motivation in health behavior. For example, cognitive appraisal in the IMCHB has been operationalized as perceived health status, but cognitive appraisal may well include more than perceived health status (Carter & Kulbok, 1995). Perceived health status is found in Pender's original HPM, but it has been reconceptualized as a personal factor that can directly or indirectly affect health behavior in her revised model. Affective response in the IMCHB means emotional arousal associated with the health concern, but the activity-related affect in the revised model of the HPM is emotional arousal regarding a specific behavior and not the outcome of the behavior. Intrinsic motivation in the IMCHB includes concepts of self-determinism and competency. Perceived self-efficacy in the HPM seems to equate to the concept of self-competence. Concept clarification would help to differentiate similar although not identical concepts across the models. Concept clarification would be particularly useful with the construct "elements of health outcome" in the IMCHB. In addition to health outcomes (health status indicators), the identified elements also reflect health behaviors (use of health care resources and adherence to the recommended care regimen) and perceptions (severity of health care problems and satisfaction with care regimen; Carter & Kulbok, 1995). Concept clarification would also facilitate the cumulative construction of knowledge based on a universal understanding of the concepts.

Empirical Adequacy

There is an impressive body of health promotion literature that operationalizes and examines the usefulness of these theories. Each health promotion behavior has engendered many researchers who have generated an expanding awareness of the use of these models. Researchers in the social sciences and in nursing are building a body of knowledge that transitions health care from an illness focus to one that values prevention of illness and promotion of a higher level of wellness for a longer life span.

Considerable empirical work, however, is needed largely due to problems in model testing and the previously mentioned problems of concept clarification. Young et al. (1991) documented reliability issues of instruments used to measure attitudes and beliefs in TPB. Reinecke et al. (1997) noted in their study of condom use that it is important to target intervention at a specific behavior of interest, such as birth control versus AIDS prevention. Their study suggests that models are applicable to context and specific health behavior. Weinstein (1993) questions the adequacy of experimental manipulations in that experimental treatments are often quite brief. Ethical considerations may also limit the differences between experimental and control conditions.

Of the three nursing models, Leininger's TCCDU has the greatest amount of empirical support. It has been used in more than 100 cultures primarily through qualitative research methodology, and more than 135 caring constructs have been identified. More than 20 studies have tested the IMCHB during the past decade (Carter & Kulbok, 1995). More than half of these studies explored the direct linkages between background variables and health outcomes, even though no direct linkages between these two concepts exist in the model. Only one study (Cox & Roghmann, 1984) has examined the relationship between all three elements of the IMCHB model. Most studies have confirmed proposed linkages within the IMCHB model, but because of its comprehensiveness and complexity the model has never been tested in its entirety. Study subjects samples have included a diverse age range but limited racial backgrounds. There has been limited testing with diverse cultures.

Previous studies used regression analysis to explore relationships among the variables, but future relationships between variables can be more clearly delineated with more advanced statistical techniques, such as struc-

tured equation modeling or LISREL. With this technique, complex models can be evaluated, exploring both the direct and the indirect effects of several variables on one or more outcome variables. In addition, structured equation modeling assesses the overall fit of the empirical data to the hypothesized model (Musil, Jones, & Warner, 1998). Weinstein (1993) also noted that there is a need to test models in their entirety, examining whether the hypothesized relationships hold.

The value of advanced statistical analysis was demonstrated in the HPM. The model has not been tested in its entirety, although 5 to 12 variables of the original model have been tested in earlier research. Through the use of statistical techniques, Pender revised her model to better reflect the empirical data. Three new variables were added, although the overall number of variables or determinants of behavior decreased from 13 to 10. Direct and indirect relationships and paths were clearly identified in the revised model.

Pender (1996) notes that the revised model needs to be tested empirically:

> Relationships among the variables should be tested in predictive studies. Where there is already evidence supporting the predictive validity of constructs in the HPM, such as perceived barriers to action, perceived benefits of actions, perceived self-efficacy, interpersonal influences, and situational influences, health promotion intervention studies should be designed incorporating these variables. The extent to which the revised HPM is useful in explaining, predicting, and altering health-promoting behaviors will be determined through further empirical studies. (p. 73)

The static qualities of the research studies, which undergird these models, present important implications for future research. Prior research has examined a moment in time to explore and explain the influences on clients' health decisions. The models do not reflect the dynamic nature of the multitude of variables that can influence health decisions and outcomes. Future research studies should examine how the variables change over time. Additions of a feedback loop from health outcomes to the variables that reflect client singularity or uniqueness (depending on the individual model) would introduce a temporal dimension to the models (Carter & Kulbok, 1995). Weinstein (1993) notes that health behaviors may be explained as several distinct steps taken at varied stages. Weinstein concludes,

> Stage theories thus require specification of the different stage (how they are defined; how they can be assessed; how people at one stage differ from those at another) and specification of the rules that govern transitions from one stage to another. (p. 331)

➤ IMPLICATIONS FOR NURSING PRACTICE

The previously discussed nursing models provide important contributions to nursing practice by focusing on the process by which and context in which clients make decisions about health and their health care. They have confronted the challenge of redefining health promotion by moving away from the traditional disease-oriented worldviews and the emphasis on secondary and tertiary prevention that has been prevalent in our society (Kulbok, Baldwin, Cox, & Duffy, 1997). They have sought to understand the determinants of health-related behaviors to ultimately achieve not only protection from illness but also high-level wellness.

These models have particular relevance for helping clients cope in that they focus on perceptions or cognitive appraisal, meanings, attitudes, emotional response, and values within a sociocultural context and group norms. They recognize the multidimensionality of coping and health and seek to emphasize the reciprocal relationship between the client and nurse that maximizes high-level wellness and health outcomes.

These models provide frameworks by which nurses can recognize and honor the uniqueness of their clients and understand how this individuality impacts clients' health decisions and care. They demonstrate a shift from the outmoded philosophical assumptions of earlier health behavior models that excluded personal freedom and choice to ones that no longer recognize compliance as a reasonable goal. The models recognize the client's role as an active, informed participant and partner and the nurse's uniqueness and competencies in the role of partner in health and wellness. Perhaps the most significant contribution of these frameworks in today's tumultuous health care environment is the explicit recognition of the importance of the interaction process between the client and the nurse in achieving wellness. The use of these frameworks can help redefine and demonstrate nursing's value to the health and wellness of people.

➤ REFERENCES

Abraham, C., & Sheeran, P. (1994). Modeling and modifying young heterosexuals' HIV-preventive behavior: A review of theories, findings and educational implications. *Patient Education and Counseling, 23,* 173-186.

Ajzen, I. (1985). From intentions to action: A theory of planned behavior. In J. Kuhl & J. Beckmann (Eds.), *Action-control: From cognition to behavior* (pp. 11-39). Heidelberg, Germany: Springer-Verlag.

Ajzen, I. (1991). The theory of planned behavior. *Organizational Behavior and Human Decision Processes, 50,* 179-211.

Ajzen, I., & Fishbein, M. (1980). A theory of reasoned action. In I. Ajzen & M. Fishbein (Eds.), *Understanding attitudes and predicting social behavior* (pp. 1-17). Englewood Cliffs, NJ: Prentice Hall.

Ajzen, I., & Madden, T. (1986). Prediction of goal-directed behavior: Attitudes, intentions and perceived behavioral control. *Journal of Experimental Social Psychology, 22,* 453-474.

Bakker, A. B., Buunk, B. P., Bram, P., Siero, F. W., & van Den Eijnden, R. J. J. M. (1997). Application of a modified health belief model to HIV preventive behavioral intentions among gay and bisexual men. *Psychology & Health, 12*(4), 481-492.

Bandura, A. (1977). Self-efficacy: Toward a unifying theory of behavior change. *Psychological Review, 84,* 191-215.

Bandura, A. (1986). *Social foundations of thought and action: A social cognitive theory.* Englewood, NJ: Prentice Hall.

Baumann, L., Brown, R., Fontana, S., & Cameron, L. (1993). Testing a model of mammography intention. *Journal of Applied Social Psychology, 23,* 1733-1756.

Becker, M. (Ed.). (1974). *The health belief model and personal health behavior.* Thorofare, NJ: Charles B. Slack.

Becker, M. H. (1988). AIDS and behavior change. *Public Health Reviews, 16*(1/2), 1-11.

Bem, D. J. (1972). Self-perception theory. In L. Berkowitz (Ed.), *Advances in experimental social psychology* (pp. 1-62). New York: Academic Press.

Bernstein, I. H., & Keith, J. B. (1991). Reexamination of Eisen, Zellman and McAlister's Health Belief Model Questionnaire. *Health Education Quarterly, 18*(2), 202-220.

Blue, C. L. (1995). The predictive capacity of the theory of reasoned action and the theory of planned behavior in exercise research: An integrated literature review. *Research in Nursing & Health, 18,* 105-121.

Boyd, B., & Wandersman, A. (1991). Predicting undergraduate condom use with the Fishbein and Ajzen and the Triandis attitude-behavior models: Implications for public health interventions. *Journal of Applied Social Psychology, 21,* 1818-1830.

Brown, C. M., & Segal, R. (1996). The effects of health and treatment perceptions on the use of prescribed medication and home remedies among African American and white hypertensives. *Social Science & Medicine, 43*(6), 903-917.

Brown, S. (1992). Tailoring nursing care to the individual client: Empirical challenge of a theoretical concept. *Research in Nursing and Health, 15,* 39-46.

Brunswick, A. F., & Banaszak-Holl, J. (1996). HIV risk behavior and the health belief model: An empirical test in an African-American community sample. *Journal of Community Psychology, 24,* 44-65.

Carmel, S., Shani, E., & Rosenberg, L. (1996). Skin cancer protection behaviors among the elderly: Explaining their responses to a health education program using the health belief model. *Educational Gerontology, 22*(7), 651-668.

Carter, K. F., & Kulbok, P. A. (1995). Evaluation of the interaction model of client health behavior through the first decade of research. *Advances in Nursing Science, 18,* 62-73.

Champion, V. L., & Scott, C. R. (1997). Reliability and validity of breast cancer screening belief scales in African American women. *Nursing Research, 46*(6), 331-337.

Chein, I. (1948). Behavior therapy and the behavior attitudes: Some critical comments. *Psychological Review, 55,* 175-188.

Cheng, T. L., Savageau, J. A., Bigelow, C., Charney, E., Kumar, S., & Dewitt, T. G. (1996). Assessing mother's attitudes about the physician's role in child health promotion. *American Journal of Public Health, 86*(12), 1809-1812.

Cohen, J. A. (1991). Two portraits of caring: A comparison of the artists, Leininger and Watson. *Journal of Advanced Nursing, 16,* 899-909.

Courneya, K. S., & McAuley, E. (1995). Cognitive mediators of the social influence-exercise adherence relationship: A test of the theory of planned behavior. *Journal of Behavioral Medicine, 18*(5), 499-515.

Cox, C. L. (1982). An interaction model of client health behavior. *Advances in Nursing Science, 5,* 41-56.

Cox, C. L. (1985). The Health Self-Determinism Index. *Nursing Research, 34,* 177-183.

Cox, C. L. (1986). The interaction model of client health behavior: Application to the study of community-based elders. *Advances in Nursing Science, 9,* 40-57.

Cox, C. L., Cowell, J., Marion, L., & Miller, E. (1990). The Health Self-Determinism Index for children. *Research in Nursing and Health, 13,* 237-246.

Cox, C. L., Miller, E. H., & Mull, C. S. (1987). Motivation in health behavior: Measurement, antecedents and correlates. *Advances in Nursing Science, 9*(4), 1-15.

Cox, C. L., & Roghmann, K. (1984). Empirical test of the interaction model of client health behavior. *Research in Nursing and Health, 7,* 275-285.

Cox, C. L., Sullivan, J., & Roghmann, K. (1984). A conceptual explanation of risk-reduction behavior: Use of prenatal diagnoses. *Nursing Research, 33,* 168-173.

Cox, C. L., & Wachs, J. (1985). Motivation: Vehicle for public health nursing interventions? *Public Health Nursing, 2,* 202-212.

Davidson, A. R., Jaccard, J. J., Triandis, H. C., Morales, M. L., & Diaz-Guerrero, R. (1976). Cross-cultural model testing toward a solution of the etic-emic dilemma. *International Journal of Psychology, 11,* 1-13.

Deci, E. L., & Ryan, R. M. (1985). *Intrinsic motivation and self-determinism in human behavior.* New York: Plenum.

Doganis, G., & Theodorakis, Y. (1995). The influence of attitude on exercise participation. In S. J. H. Biddle (Ed.), *European perspectives on exercise and sport psychology* (pp. 26-49). Champaign, IL: Human Kinetics.

Doob, L. W. (1947). The behavior of attitudes. *Psychological Review, 54,* 135-156.

Facione, N. C. (1993). The Triandis model for the study of health and illness behavior: A social behavior theory with sensitivity to diversity. *Advances in Nursing Science, 15*(3), 49-58.

Falck, R. S., Siegal, H. A., Wang, J., & Carlson, R. G. (1995). Usefulness of the health belief model in predicting HIV needle risk practices among injection drug users. *AIDS Education & Prevention, 7*(6), 523-533.

Farrand, L., & Cox, C. L. (1993). Determinants of positive health behavior in middle childhood. *Nursing Research, 42*(4), 208-213.

Fishbein, M., & Ajzen, I. (1975). *Beliefs, attitude, intention and behavior.* Don Mills, Ontario, Canada: Addison-Wesley.

Fishbein, M., Chan, D. K.-S., O'Reilly, K., Schnell, D., Wood, R., Beeker, C., & Cohn, D. (1992). Attitudinal and normative factors as determinants of gay men's intentions to perform AIDS-related sexual behaviors: A multisite analysis. *Journal of Applied Social Psychology, 22*(13), 999-1011.

Fishbein, M., & Middlestadt, S. E. (1990). Using the theory of reasoned action as a framework for understanding and changing AIDS-related behaviors. In V. M. Hays, G. Albee, & S. Schneider (Eds.), *Psychological approaches to primary prevention of acquired immunodeficiency syndrome* (pp. 93-110). Newbury Park, CA: Sage.

Fisher, W. A., Fisher, J. D., & Rye, B. J. (1995). Understanding and promoting AIDS-prevention behavior: Insights from the theory of reasoned action. *Health Psychology, 14*(3), 255-264.

Frank-Stromborg, M., Pender, N. J., & Walker, S. N. (1990). Determinants of health-promoting lifestyles in ambulatory cancer patients. *Social Science Medicine, 31,* 1159-1168.

Garcia, A., Norton-Broda, M. A., Frenn, M., Coviak, C., Pender, N. J., & Ronis, D. L. (1995). Gender and developmental differences in exercise beliefs among youth and prediction of their exercise behavior. *Journal of School Health, 65*(6), 213-219.

Godin, G. (1994). Theories of reasoned action and planned behavior: Usefulness for exercise promotion. *Medicine and Science in Sports and Exercise, 26*(11), 1391-1394.

Godin, G., Adrien, A., Willms, D., Maticka-Tyndale, E., Manson-Singer, S., & Cappon, P. (1996). Crosscultural testing of three social cognitive theories: An application to condom use. *Journal of Applied Social Psychology, 26*(17), 1556-1586.

Godin, G., & Kok, G. (1996). The theory of planned behavior: A review of its applications to health-related behaviors. *American Journal of Health Promotion, 11*(2), 87-98.

Gold, R. S. (1993). On the need to mind the gap: On-line versus off-line cognitions underlying sexual risk-taking. In D. J. Terry, C. Gallos, & M. McCamish (Eds.), *International series in experimental social psychology* (pp. 227-252). Elmsford, NY: Pergamon.

Hanson, M. J. S. (1997). The theory of planned behavior applied to cigarette smoking in African-American, Puerto Rican and non-Hispanic white teenage females. *Nursing Research, 46*(3), 155-162.

Herberg, P. (1995). Theoretical foundations of transcultural nursing. In M. M. Andrews & J. S. Boyle (Eds.), *Transcultural concepts in nursing care* (pp. 3-47). Philadelphia: J. B. Lippincott.

Janz, N., & Becker, M. (1984). The health belief model: A decade later. *Health Education Quarterly, 11,* 1-47.

Jemmott, L. S., & Jemmott, J. B., III. (1991). Applying the theory of reasoned action to AIDS risk behavior: Condom use among black women. *Nursing Research, 40*(4), 228-234.

Johnson, J., Ratner, P., Bottorff, J., & Hayduk, L. (1993). An exploration of Pender's Health Promotion Model using LISREL. *Nursing Research, 42*(3), 132-138.

Kerr, M. J. (1994). Factors related to Mexican-American worker's use of hearing protection. *Dissertation Abstracts International, 55,* 083. (University Microfilms No. 9501083)

Kirsch, J. P., & Joseph, J. G. (1989). The health belief model: Some implications for behavior change, with reference to homosexual males. In V. M. Mays, G. W. Albee, & S. F. Schneider (Eds.), *Primary prevention of AIDS* (pp. 111-125). Newbury Park, CA: Sage.

Kulbok, P. A., Baldwin, J. H., Cox, C. L., & Duffy, R. (1997). Advancing discourse on health promotion: Beyond mainstream thinking. *Advances in Nursing Science, 20,* 12-20.

Lantz, J. J. (1996). Family culture and ethnicity. In P. J. Bomar (Ed.), *Nursing and family health promotion* (pp. 60-69). Philadelphia: W. B. Saunders.

Lauver, D. (1992). A theory of care-seeking behavior. *IMAGE: Journal of Nursing Scholarship, 24*(4), 281-287.

Lauver, D., & Chang, A. (1991). Testing theoretical explanations of intentions to seek care for a breast cancer symptom. *Journal of Applied Social Psychology, 21*(17), 440-458.

Leininger, M. M. (1985). Ethnography and ethnonursing: Models and modes of qualitative data analysis. In M. Leininger (Ed.), *Qualitative research methods in nursing* (pp. 33-71). Orlando, FL: Grune & Stratton.

Leininger, M. M. (1988). Leininger's theory of nursing: Culture care diversity and universality. *Nursing Science Quarterly, 1*(4), 152-160.

Leininger, M. M. (1991). *Cultural care diversity and universality: A theory of nursing.* New York: National League for Nursing.

Lewin, K., Dembo, T., Festinger, L., & Sears, P. (1944). Level of aspirations. In J. Hunt (Ed.), *Personality and the behavior disorders* (pp. 333-378). New York: Ronald Press.

Locke, S., & Vincent, M. (1995). Sexual decision making among rural adolescent females. *Health Values, 19,* 47-58.

Lusk, S. L., Ronis, D., Kerr, M. J., & Atwood, J. R. (1994). Test of the health promotion model as a causal model of worker's use of hearing protection. *Nursing Research, 43*(3), 151-157.

McInerney, D. M. (1991). The Behavioral Intention Questionnaire: An examination of face and etic validity in an educational setting. *Journal of Cross-Cultural Psychology, 22,* 293-306.

Michels, T. C., Taplin, S. M., Carter, W. B., & Kugler, J. P. (1995). Barriers to screening: The theory of reasoned action applied to mammography use in a military beneficiary population. *Military Medicine, 160,* 431-437.

Musil, C., Jones, S. L., & Warner, C. D. (1998). Structural equation modeling and its relationship to multiple regression and factor analysis. *Research in Nursing & Health, 21,* 271-281.

Nunnally, J. C. (1978). *Psychometric theory* (2nd ed.). New York: McGraw-Hill.

Palermo, T. M., & Drotar, D. (1996). Prediction of children's postoperative pain: The role of presurgical expectations and anticipatory emotions. *Journal of Pediatric Psychology, 21*(5), 683-698.

Parker, D., Manstead, A. S. R., & Stradling, S. G. (1995). Extending the theory of planned behavior: The role of personal norm. *British Journal of Social Psychology, 34,* 127-137.

Pender, N. J. (1982). *Health promotion in nursing practice.* Norwalk, CT: Appleton-Century-Crofts.

Pender, N. J. (1987). *Health promotion in nursing practice* (2nd ed.). Norwalk, CT: Appleton & Lange.

Pender, N. J. (1990). Expressing health through lifestyle patterns. *Nursing Science Quarterly, 3*(3), 115-122.

Pender, N. J. (1996). *Health promotion in nursing practice* (3rd ed.). Stamford, CT: Appleton & Lange.

Pender, N. J., Walker, S. N., Sechrist, K. R., & Frank-Stromborg, M. (1990). Predicting health-promoting lifestyles in the workplace. *Nursing Research, 39*(6), 326-332.

Reese, F. L., & Smith, W. R. (1997). Psychosocial determinants of health care utilization in sickle cell disease patients. *Annals of Behavioral Medicine, 19*(2), 171-178.

Reinecke, J., Schmidt, P., & Ajzen, I. (1997). Birth control versus AIDS prevention: A hierarchical model of condom use among young people. *Journal of Applied Psychology, 27*(9), 743-759.

Rosenstock, I. M. (1966). Why people use health services. *Milbank Memorial Fund Quarterly, 44,* 94-124.

Rosenstock, I. M. (1974). Historical origins of the health belief model. *Health Education Monographs, 2*(4), 328-335.

Rosenstock, I. M., Strecher, V. J., & Becker, M. H. (1988). Social learning theory and the health belief model. *Health Education Quarterly, 15*(2), 175-183.

Russell, K. M. (1991). Development of an instrument to assess maternal childhood injury health beliefs and social influence. *Issues in Comprehensive Pediatric Nursing, 14*(3), 163-177.

Savage, S. A., & Clarke, V. A. (1996). Factors associated with screening mammography and breast self-examination intentions. *Health Education Research, 11*(4), 409-421.

Steers, W. N., Elliot, E., Nemiro, J., Ditman, D., & Oskamp, S. (1996). The influences of knowledge of HIV/AIDS and self-esteem on the sexual practices of college students. *Journal of Social Psychology, 136,* 99-110.

Storer, J. H., Cychosz, C. M., & Anderson, D. F. (1997). Wellness behaviors, social identities and health promotion. *American Journal of Health Behavior, 21*(4), 260-268.

Tedesco, L. A., Keffer, M. A., & Fleck-Kandath, C. (1991). Self-efficacy, reasoned action, and oral health behavior reports: A social cognitive approach to compliance. *Journal of Behavioral Medicine, 14*(4), 341-355.

Thomas, L. R., Fox, S. A., Leake, B. G., & Roetzheim, R. G. (1996). The effects of health beliefs on screening mammography utilization among a diverse sample of older women. *Women & Health, 24*(3), 77-94.

Thorpe, L., Ford, K., Fajans, P., & Wirawan, D. N. (1997). Correlates of condom use among female prostitutes and tourist clients in Bali, Indonesia. *AIDS Care, 9*(2), 181-197.

Triandis, H. C. (1977). *Interpersonal behavior.* Monterey, CA: Brooks/Cole.

Triandis, H. C. (1980). Value, attitudes and interpersonal behavior. In M. M. Page (Ed.), *Nebraska Symposium on Motivation: Beliefs, attitudes and values* (Vol. 1, pp. 195-259). Lincoln: University of Nebraska Press.

Tripp-Reimer, T. (1984). Reconceptualizing the construct of health: Integrating emic and etic perspectives. *Research in Nursing and Health, 7,* 101-109.

Troumbley, P. F., & Lenz, E. R. (1992). Application of Cox's interaction model of client health behavior in a weight control program for military personnel: A preintervention baseline. *Advances in Nursing Science, 14*(4), 65-78.

VandeCreek, L., & Frankowski, D. (1996). Barriers that predict resistance to completing a living will. *Death Studies, 20,* 73-82.

Van Oss Marin, B., Marin, G., Perez-Stable, E. J., Otero-Sabogal, R., & Sabogal, F. (1990). Cultural differences in attitudes toward smoking: Developing messages using the theory of reasoned action. *Journal of Applied Social Psychology, 20*(6), 478-493.

Walker, L., & Avant, K. (1988). *Strategies for theory construction in nursing* (2nd ed.). Norwalk, CT: Appleton & Lange.

Walker, S. N., Kerr, M. J., Pender, N. J., & Sechrist, K. R. (1990). A Spanish language version of the health-promoting lifestyle profile. *Nursing Research, 39*(5), 268-273.

Walker, S. N., Sechrist, K. R., & Pender, N. J. (1987). The Health Promoting Lifestyle Profile: Development and psychometric characteristics. *Nursing Research, 36*(2), 76-81.

Weinstein, N. D. (1993). Testing four competing theories of health-protective behavior. *Health Psychology, 12*(4), 324-333.

Weitzel, M. H. (1989). A test of the Health Promotion Model with blue-collar workers. *Nursing Research, 38*(2), 99-104.

Werch, C., Carlson, J. M., Pappas, D. M., Dunn, M., & Williams, T. (1997). Risk factors related to urban youth stage of alcohol initiation. *American Journal of Health Behavior, 21*(5), 377-387.

Young, H. M., Lierman, L., Powell-Cope, G., Kasprzyk, D., & Benoliel, J. Q. (1991). Operationalizing the theory of planned behavior. *Research in Nursing and Health, 14,* 137-144.

CHAPTER 14

Social Support

The Promise and the Reality

Patricia W. Underwood

The belief in the potential of social support to decrease stress and enhance coping has been widely supported in both the professional and lay literature during the past three decades. No other coping resource has received such widespread attention. In fact, two reviews of stress and coping research in nursing literature from 1980 to 1990 (Artinian, 1993b) and from 1991 to 1995 (Ruiz-Bueno & Underwood, in press) found that social support was the most frequently mentioned coping resource included in 81% and 66%, respectively, of the studies reviewed. The second percentage reflects a doubling of the actual number of studies that focused on social support as a variable during the time period from 1991 to 1995.

The prevalence of both lay and professional support groups for all manner of health and social challenges attests to an inherent belief in the positive difference this factor can make. Often, however, research findings appear equivocal. Explanations frequently center on lack of consistent conceptualization,

use of different measurement tools, often without sufficient psychometric strength, and lack of clarity about the theoretical underpinnings and the role that social support plays (Artinian, 1993b; Ruiz-Bueno & Underwood, in press; Stewart & Tilden, 1995).

This chapter includes a discussion of the historical development of the conceptualization of social support and an examination of different models explaining the effect of the construct. Major tools to measure social support are compared, and research in nursing and related disciplines is reviewed. A model of the effect of social support components within the stress and coping framework is proposed.

➤ HISTORICAL DEVELOPMENT

The attention to the role of social integration in health and well-being began as early as 1897 with Durkheim's (1938, 1897/1951) study linking suicide rates to decreased social

367

ties. As a result of increasing industrialization and urbanization in the 1920s, attention was drawn to the negative effects of disruption of social networks and the loss of social integration (McKenzie, 1926; Park & Burgess, 1926; Thomas & Znaniecki, 1920). The concept of social support began to receive major attention in the 1970s, principally through the work of Antonovsky (1974, 1979), Cassel (1974, 1976; Kaplan, Cassel, & Gore, 1977), Caplan (1974), Weiss (1974), and Cobb (1976) as they began to examine factors that could ameliorate the effects of negative life events.

In the 1980s, many researchers turned their attention to the conceptualization of social support and examination of the aspects that made a difference in coping with stress. Kahn and Antonucci (1980) were particularly interested in the role of social networks, whereas House (1981) examined the role of social support in coping with work stress and the saliency of various forms of support. Wortman (1984) was also interested in the components of social support that made a difference, particularly in coping with stressors such as cancer. In this regard, she built on earlier work focusing on the role of support groups for cancer patients (Dunkel-Schetter & Wortman, 1982). An inherent belief in the efficacy of support groups rather than a strong research base spurred their proliferation by both professionals and the public throughout the 1980s—a trend that has continued. Some researchers have examined the role of support groups more systematically for naturally occurring events such as bereavement (Stroebe, Stroebe, Abakoumkin & Schut, 1996) and unnatural events such as rape (Coates & Winston, 1983).

Although nursing scientists were also interested in the potential of social support to promote postoperative recovery (Eisler, Wolfer, & Diers, 1972) and coping with birth complications (Nuckolls, Cassel, & Caplan, 1972), it was not until the 1980s that programs of research began, most notably with Brandt and Weinert (Brandt & Weinert, 1981; Weinert, 1984, 1987, 1988; Weinert & Brandt,

1987), Norbeck (Norbeck & Anderson, 1989; Norbeck, Lindsey, & Carrieri, 1981, 1983), and Tilden (1983, 1984; Tilden & Gaylen, 1987), leading to the development of instruments to measure social support. In the 1990s, Artinian (1991, 1992, 1993a), Graydon (Lee, Graydon, & Ross, 1991; Small & Graydon, 1993), and Stewart (Hirth & Stewart, 1994; Stewart, Hart, & Mann, 1995; Stewart, Ritchie, McGrath, Thompson, & Bruce, 1994) evidenced sustained research in the area of social support. The majority of researchers, however, incorporated social support as a critical variable in isolated studies examining health outcomes (Coffman, Levitt, & Deets, 1990; Ferketich & Mercer, 1990; McNett, 1987; Yarcheski & Mahon, 1989).

Jalowiec (1993) included social support as a component of her studies that focused on the development of an instrument to assess coping. She suggested that the type of support used might affect the outcomes. Other researchers began to examine the type of support needed in different situations and how needs might change during the course of an illness. Nyamathi (1987), for example, found that emotional support was needed in dealing with the diagnosis of a chronic illness, whereas more tangible help was important as the illness progressed.

➤ CONCEPTUALIZATION AND MODEL DEVELOPMENT

Critical to any discussion of the phenomenon of social support are the issues of conceptualization of the construct and consideration of the possible ways in which positive influence is exerted. Conceptualizations of social support have variously focused on the sources of support, the nature of what was provided or available, and whether it functioned in a unidirectional or reciprocal manner. Conceptualizations have also varied according to whether social support is viewed as an objective quantity or more as a function of individual perception. Functional elements have included the perceived availability of support, what is received (perceived or observed), how much is provided, satisfaction with specific forms of support, or all these.

Theoretical considerations have focused on mechanisms of influence, whether through the direct effect on an outcome or via moderating or mediating influences on other variables. These propositions have not always been clearly identified nor consistently or appropriately evaluated from a statistical standpoint. The reciprocal nature of support and the cost incurred to obtain support are recent considerations in the social support literature.

Social support has been the primary focus in some studies but often is examined as one factor within a larger framework examining stress and coping. Within this context, it is frequently identified as a resource for coping. If clinicians are to fully exploit the potential benefit of social support as either a buffer from stress or a resource for coping with threatening or challenging phenomena, they must understand what social support is and how it works. As has been amply demonstrated, simply increasing the number of studies that include social support is insufficient to provide the strong base needed for research-derived clinical interventions. Conceptual clarity is at the heart of the issue, and systematic testing of explicated components and their influence on other variables within a stress and coping framework is essential. Both the form and the source of social support should be included in any conceptualization.

Forms of Support

Lack of consistency and clarity of conceptualizations has been the single greatest problem in advancing the development of social support as a coping resource. Numerous conceptualizations have been advanced throughout the years, although most include components that reflect both physical and emotional assistance. A notable exception was that of Weiss (1974), who specified six dimensions: attachment, social integration, nurturance, reassurance of worth, and reliable alliance with kin. This conceptualization focused exclusively on emotional aspects of important relationships. Early on, Gottlieb (1978) added elements of physical intervention to the conceptualization of social support. His inductively derived categorization of the forms of support included emotionally sustaining behaviors, problem-solving behaviors, indirect personal influence, and environmental action.

Kahn (1979) and Kahn and Antonucci (1980) delineated three forms of social support: aid (direct assistance—things, money, and information), affect (expression of caring, respect, and love), and affirmation (acknowledgment of the appropriateness or rightness of acts or statements). Norbeck (1981, 1984) built on these dimensions in her research. House (1981) divided the dimension of aid into two components: instrumental or direct help and informational support. Affect and affirmation were labeled emotional and appraisal support, but they were conceptually the same. Wortman (1984) and Underwood (1986) added the form of listening.

Barrera (1981) built on the work of Gottlieb and proposed a conceptualization that incorporated six elements with notable similarities to those of House (1981): material aid, physical assistance, intimate interaction, guidance, feedback, and social participation.

Although the preponderance of conceptualizations have evolved deductively, inductive approaches have gained recent recognition. Gottlieb used qualitative methods to better understand support from the experiences of both cancer patients who were undergoing radiotherapy and their families (Hinds & Moyer, 1997). Three forms of social support were identified: being there (physically, emotionally, and spiritually), giving help, and giving information and advice. These findings helped confirm deductively derived conceptualizations.

Lugton (1997) also used qualitative approaches to examine the meaning of social support to women treated for breast cancer. The women needed support to make the diagnosis appear less threatening and to assist in maintaining or changing their identities. Humor, defining abnormality, companionship, and peer comparison were forms of support designed to decrease perception of threat. Six forms of support were important to maintaining or changing identity: emotional support, companionship, practical help, opportunity for confiding, experiential support, and sexual identity support. Previously proposed elements of emotional, affirmational, and informational support and direct help were reflected in this conceptualization.

Within these conceptualizations of social support, forms were not tied to sources. Diamond (1979) stressed the importance of differentiating forms and sources of support to increase the consistency of findings across studies. Delineation of forms of support and their differentiation from sources are also important to answering the question of whether social support is a unidimensional or multidimensional resource. The more specific question, however, is whether certain forms of support are more important for coping in specific situations (Cobb, 1976). Blended conceptualizations such as that of Wandersman, Wandersman, and Kahn (1980), who described support as including group support, marital emotional support, network instrumental support, and marital instrumental support, make it more difficult to test the saliency of specific forms of support in specific situations.

Funch and Mettlin (1982) found forms of support to be differentially effective. In their study, only financial support was related to recovery among breast cancer patients. Other researchers have not found one form of support to be more effective than another (Brown, 1986; Meister, 1982; Underwood, 1986). Mitchell and Trickett (1980) suggested that the specific question is "What types of social support are most useful for which individuals in terms of what particular issues and under what environmental conditions?" Carefully and systematically planned research is needed to answer this question.

Sources of Support

Conceptualizations of social support have varied with respect to their specification of sources of support. Differentiations have been made on the basis of individual, aggregate, or network providers; support from individuals with similar experiences; and lay versus professional sources of support. Definitions of social support have ranged from the availability of a confidant (Lowenthal & Haven, 1968) to network comprehensiveness (Berkman & Syme, 1979).

Qualitative and quantitative studies, however, have found no evidence that the size of the network is related to satisfaction with social support or to enhanced outcomes (Elmore, 1984; Lambert, Lambert, Klipple, & Mewshaw, 1989; Powers, 1988).

There is evidence that differences in the benefit of social support are perceived on the basis of category of provider (Carveth & Gottlieb, 1979; Dunkel-Schetter, 1981; Lederman, 1984; Lederman, Lederman, Work, & McCann, 1979; Peck & Boland, 1977; Underwood, 1986). Sources of support, however, may be viewed differentially with respect to the forms of support they are able to provide. Support from family and friends may be valued, but they may not be the best resources for information needed to facilitate effective coping in a given situation. Therefore, professional sources may at times play a more prominent role. The degree to which professional support is valued, sought out, and used may also be a function of culture. For example, middle-class Euro/Caucasian American childbearing women frequently turn to professional and semiprofessional sources of support in dealing with the challenges of childbearing (Underwood, 1986), whereas Latinos may prefer family and lay sources of support. Vaux and Harrison (1985) noted that social support varied across subgroups of the population. To date, the sociocultural and socioeconomic influences on preferred sources of support have received insufficient attention.

Some conceptualizations of sources of social support have reflected a strong focus on the quality of relationships between providers and recipients (Brown & Harris, 1978; Qureshi & Walker, 1989; Weiss, 1975). The quality of social ties (Berkman & Syme, 1979; Shoenbach, Kaplan, Fredman, & Kleinbaum, 1986) has been studied as well. Such a focus is often directed toward the examination of social networks. Networks have been described as convoys across the life span or as existing within the context of a specific situation that is identified or perceived to be stressful. Conceptualizations of social support that incorporate the dimension of network more frequently reflect their structural as opposed to functional properties.

Valence, Cost, and Reciprocity

Historically, social support has been viewed as having a positive valence; however, social support is not a fixed commodity. It is a dynamic process that may change with circumstances. The form that social support takes and by whom it is provided may be perceived as more or less helpful in different situations (Norwood, 1996). Hinds and Moyer (1997) strongly concur that "how actions are perceived determines whether or not they are felt to be supportive" (p. 375). This conclusion was reached through the qualitative study of cancer patients undergoing radiotherapy treatments. The researchers found that even acts not intended to be supportive could be perceived as such. Conceptualizing social support as perceived satisfaction with what is given by whom provides for the recommended differentiation of forms and sources but also gives appropriate weight to individual variations in need for support, expectations of receiving it, and the relative costs of obtaining it.

Social support has generally been conceptualized as positive and cost free. Stewart and Tilden (1995) systematically explored the cost to the recipient of obtaining support and suggested the regular consideration of this element within conceptualizations of social support. Without consideration of the demands on the recipient of support, those with close-knit networks may be viewed as the automatic recipients of more support. In such networks, the positive effects of support may be ameliorated by the cost of obtaining it (Gottlieb, 1981; Norwood, 1996). Researchers and clinicians should be cautioned not to assume that support from professionals is cost free. Any social or professional relationship is open to conflict and negative interaction. Stewart and Tilden support this contention.

The importance of a reciprocal element in the conceptualization of social support is another consideration. It addresses the question of whether outcomes are enhanced when persons are able to give and receive support. It implies a burden of guilt and obligation when support is received but not returned. Thus, the cost of obtaining support may be increased. Riegel and Gocka (1995) conducted a longitudinal study of myocardial infarction patients and found that reciprocity in providing support was an important issue—but only for women. As their ability to give support decreased, stress in their supportive relationships increased. The possibility that reciprocity is a gender-specific issue warrants further investigation.

Future Conceptualizations

Greater consistency in conceptualization of social support across studies is a challenge that must be met. Research has supported the attempt to delineate forms and sources of support within any conceptualization. Although specific choices in concept labels may vary, emotional, informational, instrumental, and affirmational support appear to be common threads. Both subjective and objective elements seem desirable. Thus, conceptualizations might focus on perceptions about the support received, its availability, and a more objective assessment of network properties. Consideration of social support in terms of its cost also seems justified.

Barrera (1986) made an interesting proposal in an attempt to organize disparate elements within the definition of social support. It was suggested that social support be divided into the following categories:

1. Social embeddedness: referring to the structural elements of social support and the connections that individuals have within their social environment
2. Enacted support and perceived availability: actions that are performed to provide help to another and the perception that assistance is available
3. Satisfaction with social support: perceived adequacy of supportive ties

Enacted support seems to reflect two dimensions, whereas satisfaction as described appears to relate to social embeddedness. An alternative format might contain two categories:

1. Social currency would focus on the support network, including structural elements, quality of social ties, and perceived availability of general support.
2. Perceived enacted support would reflect satisfaction with what was provided by whom and the cost of obtaining support in a specific situation perceived as threatening or challenging. Net satisfaction with enacted support would factor in cost.

The elements of social currency and perceived enacted support might be modified by personal resources, cultural expectations, and the need for reciprocity.

Mechanisms of Effect

The ability to examine the models or mechanisms whereby social support exerts a positive influence on health is predicated on both clarity of conceptualization of social support and clarity in explication of the models. It is generally accepted that social support works through main, mediating, and moderating mechanisms. Inconsistencies in the application of the terms mediating and moderating or buffering as well as inappropriate selection of statistical tests of these relationships have increased confusion regarding the efficacy of social support. It also must be considered that a particular aspect of social support may be more relevant to one model versus another.

Main Effects

Models that hypothesize and test the main effect of social support propose that there is a direct relationship between social support and outcome variables such as well-being. The main effects of social support have been supported in many studies. For example, Hatchett, Friend, Symister, and Wadhua (1997) studied 42 end-stage renal disease patients. The Inventory of Socially Supportive Behaviors (Barrera, Sandler, & Ramsey, 1981) was used to measure the exchange of four forms of social support (emotional, instrumental, appraisal, and informational). They found that increased perceived social support from family correlated with decreased hopelessness ($r = -.25$, $p < .05$). Increased perceived support from the medical staff was correlated with increases in optimism ($r = .27$, $p < .05$). In a study of 31 mothers who delivered premature infants (Younger, Kendell, & Pickler, 1997), ratings of the helpfulness of others in providing emotional, informational, tangible, and general support (Account of Social Resources Inventory) were positively correlated with mastery ($r = .35$, $p < .05$) and negatively correlated with depression ($r = .35$, $p < .05$). Frey (1989) found significant main effects for perceived availability of social support (Norbeck Social Support Questionnaire 84) and family health among parents of diabetic children. Similar effects were not found for children's health. Chang and Krantz (1996) set out to test the mediating effect of

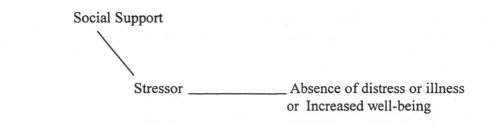

Figure 14.1. Moderating or Buffering Effect of Social Support

social support on adjustment among adult children of alcoholics. Instead, they found a main effect for social support that supported findings of Billings and Moss (1986).

Moderating or Buffering Effects

Moderating effects are at times the most misunderstood of the effects models. Antonovsky (1979) suggested that resources such as social support can increase a person's resistance to stress. A moderating effect is achieved (Figure 14.1) when a "third variable affects the zero-order correlation between two other variables" (Hurley-Wilson, 1993, p. 137). Moderators are antecedent conditions that interact with a stressor to affect the outcome. The moderating effect is best tested through an analysis of variance (ANOVA). In this model, social support is thought to protect the individual from the potentially harmful effects of exposure to a stressor. It is unclear whether it works through influencing the individual's appraisal of a potential stressor. It might be fruitful to study whether having a strong support network would act as a moderator by producing a healthier environment, by decreasing events appraised as threatening or harmful, or both. Pearlin (1989) supported the idea that social support forms a shield that insulates the individual from stress exposure. Chan and Ward (1993) suggested that social support acts to reduce the risk of illness by reducing harmful stress appraisal.

The moderating or buffering effect has been supported by several researchers (Allo-way & Bebbington, 1987; Cassel, 1976; Cobb, 1976; Cohen, 1988; Cohen & Willis, 1985; Dean & Lin, 1977; Kaplan et al., 1977). Using the Norbeck Social Support Questionnaire (NSSQ) as the measure of social support, Kang, Coe, Karaszewski, and McCarthy (1998) found that social support buffered stress among 133 well-managed middle-class asthmatic teens. Other researchers have not found support for the moderating or buffering hypothesis (Gluhoski, Fishman, & Perry, 1997) or have found varied support (Preston, 1995). For example, a study of the effect of social support in buffering the distress of bereavement among 598 gay men found that ANOVA supported only main rather than buffering effects of social support (Gluhoski et al., 1997).

Some researchers have found moderating or buffering effects in the context of studying other models. For example, Preston (1995) found that social support measured as the number of confidants had a buffering effect on health for married, elderly men. No such protective effect was found for women, however.

Sansom and Farnill (1997) did not test the buffering hypothesis but found direct, inverse relationships between network dimensions such as social integration and perceived everyday stress among recently divorced persons.

Mediating Effects

A third role for social support is that of mediator of the relationship between stress

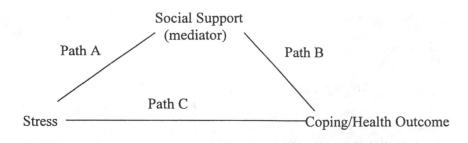

Figure 14.2. The Mediating Effect of Social Support

and health or coping outcomes (Figure 14.2). Baron and Kenny (1986) noted that the mediator effect occurs when

> variations in levels of the independent variable significantly account for variations in the presumed mediator (Path A), variations in the mediator significantly account for variations in the dependent variable (Path B), and when Paths A and B are controlled, a previously significant relationship between the independent and dependent variables is no longer significant (Path C). (p. 1178)

Multiple regression is the appropriate statistical test for this model. Eckenrode and Gore (1990) expanded on the discussion of these models in the context of their examination of work and family stress.

Several other examples of mediating effects were found. O'Brien, Wineman, and Nealon (1995) evaluated variables that mediated the relationship between the objective and subjective burden of caring for someone with multiple sclerosis and caregiver health and life satisfaction. Social support and family coping were evaluated as mediators of this relationship. The Social Network List and Support System Scale (Fiore, Becker, & Coopel, 1983; Hirsch, 1979) was used as the measure of social support. Although social support related to family coping ($r = .30$, $p < .05$), it did not mediate the relationship between burden and coping or life satisfaction. Social support did explain 7% unique variance in family satisfaction. The authors suggested that the failure to support the hypothesized relationships may have been a function of the social support measure used. This study was problematic in that the terms "mediator" and "moderator" were used interchangeably.

Oxman and Hull (1997) examined the ability of social support to mediate the relationships between activities of daily living and depression before and after heart surgery. Three measures of social support were used: the Social Network Questionnaire (SNQ; Seeman & Berkman, 1988), the Inventory of Socially Supportive Behaviors (ISSB; Barrera & Ainsley, 1983), and the Multidimensional Scale of Perceived Social Support (MSPSS; Zimet, Dahlem, Zimet, & Farley, 1988). The importance of the perceived adequacy of social support (MSPSS) was supported. The number of close network members seen (SNQ) had mediating and direct effects on activities of daily living and depression 6 months after surgery.

Runtz and Schallow (1997) used structural equation modeling to examine the role of social support in mediating the relationship between maltreatment as a child and adult adjustment. Social support was measured by the Provisions of Social Relations Scale (PSR; Turner, Frankel, & Levin, 1983). This 15-item instrument measures perceived support from family and friends. The role of social support as a mediator was confirmed. Social support explained 55% of the variance in adjustment. It is of concern that in their conclusions the authors stated that these findings supported the contentions of others that social support acts as a buffer of stress.

Future Testing of Effects

Although clarity and consistency in the conceptualization of social support are a necessary first step in building evidence of its role within the stress and coping framework, a clear understanding of the nature of effects is an immediate second step. Conceptual and statistical models must be congruent, and labels for the nature of these models must be consistently applied. Only in this way will the role of social support in relation to stress and health outcomes be explicated. Clarity in conceptualization of social support and consistency in operationalization of the concept will help determine the specific aspects of social support that produce main, moderating, or mediating effects or all three.

➤ MEASURES OF SOCIAL SUPPORT

The variations in the conceptualization of social support are reflected in the operationalization of this construct. Artinian (1993b) found that more than 30 different instruments were used to measure social support in nursing research published between 1980 and 1990. Ducharme, Stevens, and Rowat (1994) suggest that four elements of measurement should be specified: the components being measured, whether the measures are objective, the unit of measurement, and validity and reliability. A frequent criticism is that many of the instruments have not been subjected to rigorous psychometric testing (Stewart, 1989). Notable exceptions are Norbeck's SSQ (Norbeck et al., 1981, 1983), Brandt and Weinert's (1981; Wienert & Brandt, 1987) Personal Relationships Questionnaire (PRQ), and Tilden's (Tilden & Gaylen, 1987; Tilden, Nelson, & May, 1990b) Interpersonal Relationships Inventory (IPR). These instruments are compared in Table 14.1. In addition to these more widely tested instruments, four other instruments are described here because of their varied conceptualizations of social support: Barrera and Ainsley's (1983) ISSB, Norwood's (1996)

Social Support Apgar (SSA), Seeman and Berkman's (1983) SNQ, and Zimet et al.'s (1988) Multidimensional Scale of Perceived Social Support (MSPSS).

Norbeck Social Support Questionnaire (NSSQ)

This instrument was based on attachment theory. The NSSQ (Norbeck et al., 1981, 1983) provides subjects with an opportunity to list members of their support network (up to 24) and to categorize them on the basis of their relationship to the individual (e.g., "spouse," "health care provider," and "friend"). It also provides an opportunity to indicate recent loses (number lost from the network and level of support lost in the past year). Sources of support are further rated on a 5-point scale in relation to the amount (none to a great deal) of aid, affect, or affirmational support provided. Two measures are obtained for each of the forms of support. Total scores reflect functional support and network properties. Internal consistency have been reported as .89 (Norbeck & Anderson, 1989) and .78 to .84 (Frey, 1989). Test-retest reliability ranged from .85 to .92 for the subscales (Norbeck & Anderson, 1989).

Personal Relationships Questionnaire (PRQ)

The PRQ85 was built on Weiss's (1974) conceptualization of social relations (Weinert & Brandt, 1987) and has two parts. Part 1 measures support needs for the past 6 months, including who was contacted for the support and how satisfied the individual was with the support they received. Satisfaction is rated on a 6-point scale from very satisfied to very dissatisfied. Part 2 assesses five dimensions of social support—intimacy, social integration, nurturance, worth, and assistance—rated on a 7-point scale from strongly disagree to strongly agree. Items vary according to whether they measure support needs,

(text continued on page 379)

TABLE 14.1 Comparison of More Consistently Tested Measures of Social Support in Nursing Research

Measure and Author	Variables Measured	Description	Reliability	Validity	Populations Studied
Norbeck Social Support Questionnaire (NSSQ; Norbeck, Lindsey, & Carrieri, 1981, 1983)	Network properties Functional support	Listing of support network and relationship; number lost from network in past year; rating of sources on aid, affect, and affirmation	Internal consistency = .69-.97 (Norbeck et al., 1983), .89 (Kang, Coe, Karaszewski, & McCarthy, 1998; Norbeck & Anderson, 1989), .78-.84 (Frey, 1989) Test-retest = .85-.92 (Norbeck & Anderson, 1989)	Content validity via experts Construct validity	Diabetic children and parents (Frey, 1989) Families of disabled preschoolers (Failla & Jones, 1991) Families of children with disabilities (Snowdon, Cameron, & Dunham, 1994) Asthmathic teens (Kang et al., 1998) Families (Norbeck, 1981) American women (Norbeck, DeJoseph, & Smith, 1996) Widows (Robinson, 1995) Prospective heart transplant patients (Hirth & Stewart, 1994)
Personal Relationships Questionnaire 85 (PRQ85; Weinert & Brandt, 1987)	Support needs Dimensions of social support	Part 1: Who was contacted for support and rating of satisfaction Part 2: Five dimensions (intimacy, social integration, nurturance, worth, and assistance)	Internal consistency .87-.91 (Gibson, Cheavens, & Warren, 1998; Graydon & Ross, 1995; Weinert & Tilden, 1990)	Part 2 factor analysis revealed three factors: intimacy/assistance, integration/affirmation, and reciprocity Convergent validity	Chronic obstructive pulmonary disease patients (Graydon & Ross, 1995; Lee, Graydon, & Ross, 1991) Diabetics (White, Richter, & Fry, 1992) Multiple chemical sensitivity (Gibson et al., 1998)

Measure	Construct	Description	Reliability	Validity	Populations studied
Interpersonal Relationships Inventory (Tilden, 1991)	Costs and benefits of social support	39 items; three subscales (social support, reciprocity, and conflict)	Internal consistency = .83–.92 (Tilden et al., 1990b) Test-retest = .81–.91 (Tilden et al., 1990b)	Construct validity supported through factor analysis (Tilden et al., 1990b; Tilden, Hirsch, & Nelson, 1994)	Family caregivers (Hansell et al., 1998; Hughes & Caliandro, 1996; Vrabec, 1995) Males on hemodialysis (Cormier-Daigle & Stewart, 1997) Cancer patients (Douglass, 1997) Infertile couples (Jirka, Schuett, & Foxall, 1996)
Inventory of Socially Supportive Behaviors (Barrera, Sandler, & Ramsey, 1981)	Support received	40 items; three subscales (emotional support, guidance, and tangible support); 5-point rating of frequency during the preceding month	Internal consistency = .67–.94 Test-retest = .62–.88 (Barrera & Ainsley, 1983; Barrera et al., 1981; Friedman, 1997; Grossman & Rowat, 1995; Oxman, Freeman, Manheimer, & Stukel, 1994)	Concurrent validity (Barrera et al., 1981)	End-stage renal disease patients (Barrera et al., 1981; Hatchet, Friend, Symister, & Wadhua, 1997) Adolescents (Grossman & Rowat, 1995) Women and elderly with heart failure (Friedman, 1993, 1997; Friedman & King, 1994) Open-heart surgery patients (Oxman & Hull, 1997)
Multidimensional Scale of Perceived Social Support (Zimet, Dahlem, Zimet, & Farley, 1988)	Perceived adequacy of social support	12 items rated on 7-point agreement regarding adequacy of support from a significant other, family, and friends	High internal consistency and test-retest reliability (Blumenthal, Barefoot, Burg, & Williams, 1987)	Content validity (Blumenthal et al., 1987; Zimet et al., 1988)	Angiography patients (Blumenthal et al., 1987) Open-heart surgery patients (Oxman et al., 1994; Oxman & Hull, 1997) Cancer patients (Hann et al., 1995)
Social Network Questionnaire (Seeman & Berkman, 1983)	Number of close network members seen regularly	Number of children, relatives, and friends seen at least one time per month			Open-heart surgery patients (Oxman & Hull, 1997) Elderly (Seeman & Berkman, 1983)

(continued)

TABLE 14.1 Continued

Measure and Author	Variables Measured	Description	Reliability	Validity	Populations Studied
Social Support Apgar (Norwood, 1996)	Perceived satisfaction with social support	25 items; five forms (adaptation, partnership, growth, affection, and commitment); five sources (partner, parents, friends, and other acquaintances)	Internal consistency = .88–.93 (Norwood, 1996)	Content validity with experts related to NSSQ and PRQ dimensions (Norwood, 1996) Factor analysis separated on source (Norwood, 1996)	Pregnant women (Norwood, 1996)

perceived availability of support, received support, and ability to provide support. Internal consistency have ranged from .87 to .91 (Gibson, Cheavens, & Warren, 1998; Weinert & Tilden, 1990). A factor analysis of Part 2 revealed three factors: intimacy/assistance, integration/affirmation, and reciprocity (Weinert & Tilden, 1990).

Interpersonal Relationships Inventory (IPR)

Social exchange theory (Cook, 1987) and equity theory (Messick & Cook, 1983) served as the basis for the IPR (Tilden et al., 1990b). This instrument is unique in acknowledging both the costs and the benefits of social support. The IPR consists of 39 items measured on a 5-point scale. For items measuring perceived states, the response options range from "strongly agree" to "strongly disagree." Enacted behaviors are measured with respect to frequency from never to very often. The following subscales are scored separately: social support, reciprocity, and conflict (Tilden et al., 1990b). The internal consistency and construct validity of the scales have been widely supported through quantitative (Tilden, Hirsch, & Nelson, 1994) and qualitative research (Tilden, Nelson, & May, 1990a).

Additional Instruments

Inventory of Socially Supportive Behaviors (ISSB)

The ISSB is a 40-item measure of support received during the preceding month in relation to three subscales: emotional support, guidance, and tangible support. The frequency with which each item has been received in the recent past is rated on a 5-point scale from "not at all" to "about every day." Concurrent validity was supported through correlations with the Arizona Support Interview Schedule and the Moos' Family Environment Scale (Barrera et al., 1981). Internal

consistency and test-retest reliability have been supported (Barrera, 1981; Barrera & Ainsley, 1983; Oxman et al., 1994).

Social Support Apgar (SSA)

The SSA (Norwood, 1996) is a 25-item instrument developed to be an easy to use tool to assess perceived satisfaction with five forms of support (adaptation, partnership, growth, affection, and commitment) from five sources (partner, parents, other family members, friends, and other acquaintances). Each item is rated on a 3-point scale from "hardly ever" to "almost always." Content validity was established, and items were linked to dimensions of social support assessed by the NSSQ and the PRQ. Factor analysis separated items on the basis of source rather than form of support, adding to the evidence supporting the unidimensionality of social support as it related to forms. Cronbach's alpha ratings ranged from .88 to .93 across three studies by Norwood (1996). A study of pregnancy outcome variables (birth weight, weeks of gestation, and number of prenatal visits) according to level of support among a sample of 220 postpartum patients revealed no differences (Norwood, 1996). The majority of women in this study were white, nonmarried, and had just delivered their second baby. In another study of 52 white, low-income, unmarried maternity patients with less than a high school education, Norwood (1996) did find that women with higher support had lower levels of perceived life stress, supporting a buffering hypothesis. As this instrument is tested further, its sensitivity might be evaluated. A 5-point rating might increase the ability to discriminate among subjects.

Multidimensional Scale of Perceived Social Support (MSPSS)

Twelve items of perceived adequacy of social support from significant others, family, and friends are rated on a 7-point scale from "very strongly disagree" to "very strongly agree" in the MSPSS (Zimet et al.,

1988). Reliability and validity have been supported in studies of patients with angiography (Blumenthal, Barefoot, Burg, & Williams, 1987), open-heart surgery (Oxman et al., 1994), and metastatic carcinoma (Hann, Oxman, Ahles, Furstenburg, & Stukel, 1995). Alpha ratings were .93 and .94.

Summary

Significant challenges remain in the measurement of social support. First, theoretical underpinnings need to be explicated. These are clear for the NSSQ, PRQ85, and IPR Inventory but are less so for other instruments. Second, the conceptualization of social support must be specified, even if the researchers choose to measure only a component of social support rather than attempting to capture the full dimensions of the construct. Such clarification is necessary if the process by which social support positively affects outcomes is to be revealed.

The instruments have varied in their inclusion of network components and evaluation of support received. It may be useful to distinguish between reference to network meaning a general support convoy that goes along with the person and sources of support when dealing with a specific situation. Although increasing evidence supports the importance of perceptions of social support received, it may be useful to systematically explore the relevance of network quality as a buffer of stress.

Researchers should be encouraged to use well-established instruments—or components of them—to build evidence. If new instruments are developed, their rationale should be made clear. For example, the Social Support Apgar was developed to provide a quickly administered screening tool. More is not necessarily better with regard to the number of social support instruments. The challenge is to find those measures that match accepted conceptualizations and then to use these tools more consistently to build the science.

➤ RESEARCH IN NURSING AND RELATED DISCIPLINES

Social support continues to be the most widely researched coping resource both in nursing and in related disciplines. Overall, positive influences on health outcomes and protective functioning with respect to stress have been observed but with some inconsistency due to variations in conceptualization, measurement, and effects modeling. It is not the intent here to offer a complete synthesis of social support research but rather to note a few promising trends and examples.

The bulk of the researchers studying social support used descriptive or correlational designs. Few researchers attempted to manipulate social support. Researchers in social support studies also tended to examine concepts in a cross-sectional dimension. It is encouraging to note, however, that sample sizes are increasing. This is particularly critical to increasing the power of research to detect the effects of subtle differences in social support.

Roberts et al.'s (1995) study is an example of the manipulation of social support as an intervention. A randomized clinical trial compared the effectiveness of phone-call support, support through face-to-face problem-solving counseling, and routine care for 293 adults who were not well adjusted to a chronic illness. The interventions were delivered by masters' prepared nurses and measurements taken at 6 and 12 months. Main effects for social support on life satisfaction were found for both intervention groups. The phone-call group experienced the greatest improvement. Interactive effects with demographic characteristics were also found. Problem-solving counseling was most effective for those who lived alone and frequently used avoidance as opposed to problem-solving coping.

Social support researchers have tended to focus on patients or population groups coping with identified problems. The assessment of modifiers and mediators of burnout among nurses is one area in which there is considerable research focused on professionals as they carry out their roles. Duquette, Kerouac, Sandhu, and Beaudet (1994) conducted a thorough review of the literature in relation to burnout among nurses. They located eight studies that focused on the influence of social support (Constable & Russell, 1986; Dick, 1986; Duxbury, Armstrong, Drew, & Henly, 1984; Haley, 1986; Hare, Pratt, & Andrews, 1988; Mallett, 1988; Mickschl, 1984; Paredes, 1982). It was found that these studies used a consistent measure of burnout, the Maslach Burnout Index developed by Maslach and Jackson (1981). The same was not true for social support. Again, different tools were used. All studies consistently found a negative relationship between social support and burnout.

Ihlenfeld (1996) examined the support that staff nurses ($n = 24$), nursing faculty ($n = 107$), and home health nurses ($n = 128$) received from their administrators within the previous month. Both home health nurses and staff nurses wanted more support. Faculty members reported receiving little support from their deans or chairpersons but did not state that they wanted more support. In all the studies, statistically significant negative relationships were found between social support and burnout. The consistency of this finding suggests that it may be very cost-effective for nursing administrators to give conscious attention to provision of support to decrease burnout among staff.

➤ SOCIAL SUPPORT IN SPECIAL POPULATIONS

The trend for social support researchers to focus on white, middle-class, adult samples was noted in reviews of nursing research (Artinian, 1993b; Ruiz-Bueno & Underwood, in press). These samples almost exclusively are selected by convenience. It is encouraging to note an increasing interest in examining the contributions of age, gender, and ethnicity to the process of social support.

Children

There have been fewer studies specifically focused on children apart from family contexts than those with adult populations. Grossman and Rowat (1995) examined how social support mediated the relationship between stress from divorce and well-being among 244 adolescents. The ISSB (Barrera, 1981) was used as the measure of social support. When family status (married vs. divorced) was controlled, the perceived quality of the parental relationship contributed significantly to an explanation of the variance in anxiety, life satisfaction, and a sense of future. Frey (1989) studied diabetic children within a family focus. Contrary to her findings for adults, there was no main effect for social support in relation to the health of these children.

Children are a population that needs to be studied in relation to social support. The challenge is to develop appropriate measures of support that are sensitive to developmental level.

Support Needs of Families

Social support as it relates to families has been studied less frequently than at the individual level. Three studies describe support needs of the family (Baillie, Norbeck, & Barnes, 1988; Lindsey-Davis, 1990; Norbeck, 1991). In a study of organ donors (Pelletier, 1993), family members expressed differential needs for social support. Subjects sought emotional support from within their family units, whereas nurses were identified as the primary resource for informational support. Fink (1995) found that family social support in addition to hardiness and socioeconomic status explained 65% of the variance in well-being for family members who were caring for elderly parents. The study of support issues within the family is particularly critical because people draw on family members when facing harm, loss, or challenge. When the support that family members, individually and collectively, are able to give is depleted, other resources need to be made available.

Gender-Focused Studies

There is increasing evidence that social support operates differentially within the context of gender. Two studies examined the continuity of support over time for spouses whose mates experienced coronary bypass surgery (Artinian, 1992) or chemotherapy (Dodd, Dibble, & Thomas, 1993). Researchers consistently reported a decrease in support over time for men, whereas support for women was maintained.

Riegel and Gocka (1995) examined social support needs of subjects 1 month following myocardial infarction. No differences were found in support needed. Women, however, received significantly more emotional support than men. Gibson et al. (1998) and Turner (1994) confirmed the higher levels of support received by women. Allen and Stoltenberg (1995) found that college freshmen women were more supported and better satisfied with that support than were their male counterparts. Similarly, Potts (1997) reported that among 151 members of a retirement village, women had higher levels of confidant relationships than men. In contrast, Gulick (1992) found higher perceived social support in men than in women with multiple sclerosis.

In a study of patients 1 or 2 years after experiencing a myocardial infarction (Conn, Taylor, & Abel, 1991), researchers reported a negative correlation between age and social support for men ($n = 117$, $r = -.31$) but not for women ($n = 80$, $r = -.08$). Preston (1995) studied 900 persons aged 65 or older and found a positive correlation between the number of confidants and health for married men. Married women had the poorest health regardless of social support. McColl and Frieland (1994) and Willey and Silliman (1990) found gender unrelated to social support. Although these findings were not uniformly consistent, women did seem to receive more support than

did men, and gender did seem to have some differential relationship with selected variables.

In two studies, samples were limited to women. In the first study, the researchers found a relationship between form of support and outcome (Friedman, 1997). Older women with heart failure were studied to examine the relationship between support source loss, perceived enacted support, and psychological well-being. Emotional and tangible support sources were found to be stable over time for the 57 subjects. Emotional support and loss of tangible support measured by the ISSB were related to positive affect ($r = .36$ and $-.34$, respectively; $p < .01$). Stability of social relationships was also found by Kendler (1997) in a 5-year longitudinal study of female twins. In this study, social support was operationalized as relative problems, friend problems, relative support, confidants, friend support, and social integration. Kendler suggested that social support has a genetic component and that it is not just an environmental issue. Thus, women seem to have more support than men, and this support is relatively stable.

A study of 30 young men with testicular cancer used the Importance of Social Support instrument to examine social support in relation to mood (Davidson, Degner, & Morgan, 1995). No relationship was found between these two variables. The men in this study reported that they were well supported. These findings suggested that support needs to be evaluated within the context of the individuals' requirements and their perceptions of whether it does or does not meet their needs.

Cultural Implications

Few investigators have examined social support within ethnically diverse or minority targeted populations. A study by Norbeck, DeJoseph, and Smith (1996) is an exception: It examined the effect of a culturally relevant intervention on the birth weight of infants born to low-income African American women ($N = 319$). Focus groups suggested the potential efficacy of provision of support by nurses following a standard protocol in the subjects' homes. An experimental design was used to test a main effect for social support. Subjects identified as higher risk due to inadequate support (lacking support from mothers or male partners) were randomly placed in experimental and control groups. The intervention consisted of four face-to-face sessions, in which the nurses also tried to help subjects mobilize additional support from their networks. The intervention group also received follow-up phone calls in the 2-week interval between sessions. The rate of low birth weight was significantly less ($p = .045$) in the experimental group (9.1% compared to 22.4% for the control group). The effectiveness of social support in this study was consistent with the findings of Edwards et al. (1994) and Heins, Nance, and Levey-Mickens (1988) but inconsistent with those of several other studies (Bryce, Stanley, & Garner, 1991; Oakley, Rajan, & Grant, 1990; Rothberg & Lits, 1991; Spencer, Thomas, & Morris, 1989; Villar, Farnot, Barros, Victoria, & Langer, 1992). An explanation may lie in the attempt to maximize the cultural relevance of the intervention.

Linn, Poku, Cain, Holzapfel, and Crawford (1995) studied an adult African American population ($N = 255$) infected with HIV. A correlational design was used to examine the relationship between HIV symptoms and depression and anxiety. It was hypothesized that higher levels of social support would be related to lower anxiety and depression. Unfortunately, social support was measured by asking subjects if there was anyone they could talk to or count on for understanding and support and then counting the available number of confidants. Picot (1995) also focused on an African American population. A positive but weak correlation ($r = .29$, $p < .01$) was found between social support and confrontive coping in African American women who were caring for relatives with Alzheimer's disease.

Nursing research in Korea (Choi, 1994) was reviewed in relation to social support, and 11 studies were found. These studies tended to use univariate analysis techniques and different measures of social support in addition to small sample sizes, thus making it difficult to generalize across studies. Two studies examined the supportive interventions provided by nurses. M. J. Kim (1985) found that sodium excretion was lower in experimental versus control groups of hospitalized patients ($N = 66$) following a nursing intervention, although anxiety scores were not significantly different. J. A. Kim (1990), however, found that military patients ($N = 150$) with lower back pain experienced increased satisfaction, an increase in positive mood, and a decrease in depression following supportive nursing care. Choi suggests that in studying social support in Korean families, attention needs to be paid to variations in philosophy among family members and the differential effects that conflicts regarding philosophical outlook may have on the appraisal of support provided. This advice appears to be well founded. Regardless of the extent of research within a culture, it appears wise to check with members of that culture to determine the meaning and value that they as individuals ascribe to social support.

➤ FUTURE DIRECTIONS FOR THEORY DEVELOPMENT

Although the sheer amount of research on social support has continued to increase, conceptualizations have varied widely, inconsistent measures have been used, research designs and statistical models have occasionally lacked conceptual consistency, and support interventions have not been investigated extensively. Nevertheless, studies of social support continue to yield findings sufficient to validate the belief that mobilization or proffering of support will produce positive gains in coping and health. More collaborative approaches to the systematic investigation of social support are needed. A model of social support designed by this author is suggested to guide this research (Figure 14.3).

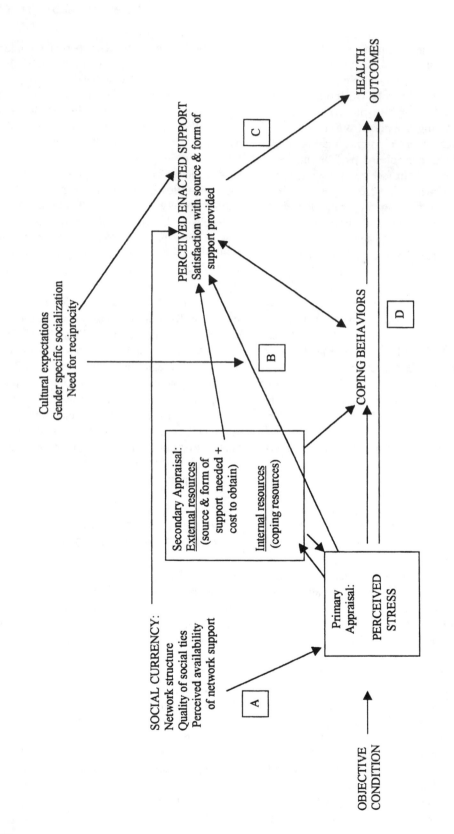

Figure 14.3. Proposed Model for the Examination of the Influence of Social Support: Path A, Buffering or Moderating Effect; Paths B and C, Mediating Effect; Path D, the Direct Effect of Appraisal on Outcome

SOURCE: Copyright held by Patricia W. Underwood.

The proposed model draws from the work of Lazarus (Lazarus, 1990; Lazarus & Folkman, 1984), House (1981), Benner and Wrubel (1989), and Lyon (1990). Objective conditions refer to those events, phenomena, or potential stressors that may produce stress if they are viewed as threatening or exceeding an individual's resources to deal with them. The key is how these conditions are perceived by the individual. The initial evaluation of the potential stressor is labeled "primary appraisal" by Lazarus. It might be helpful to attempt to categorize situations that are perceived as stressful to determine whether certain forms of support are more relevant to coping in specific situations. The individual's perceptions may be modified by both individual and situational factors. It is at this point that network variables may play a role. The ongoing presence of at least one confidant may help the individual to perceive the potential stressor as less threatening. Although "network" is a commonly misunderstood term, there may be some advantage to retaining it as a reference to structural components and labeling the broader concept "social currency" to connote a resource that may be spent. This may be especially appropriate if the definition includes perceived availability of network support and some measure of the quality of social ties. Social currency may play a greater role in the moderation or buffering of social support (Figure 14.3, Path A) than in affecting the health outcome.

The primary appraisal of an event as a threat or a challenge can trigger secondary appraisal—an assessment of the resources available to address the threat or challenge. Perception of available support may include an assessment of the form of support needed, who is available to provide it, and the cost of obtaining it. These situational variables might in turn be influenced by personal factors, such as personality, preferred coping style, personal resources, cultural expectations, need for reciprocity, and gender-specific socialization. (See Figure 14.3, Path B.)

A third component that is critical to measure is perceived satisfaction with social support (perceived enacted support). (See Figure 14.3, Path C.) Theoretically, to make this judgment people would consider their needs, what they received to address those needs, and what it cost them to get the needed help. In this model, perceived satisfaction with social support would mediate the relationship between perceived stress and health outcome (Figure 14.3, Path D). Current measures of social support would need slight modification and reassembly to capture the new conceptualization of social support. Path analysis might be used in addition to ANOVA and multiple regression techniques to test these relationships.

➢ **SUMMARY**

Social support continues to hold promise as a resource to protect against stress or to facilitate coping. To critically manipulate it in clinical situations and expect predictable outcomes, we must clearly understand how it works. Such understanding will evolve from our shared conceptualizations and the application of consistent and congruent measures within the context of research designs that maintain the integrity of the conceptualization. It is imperative that propositions such as those proposed in the suggested model of social support be systematically tested with diverse populations in varied and potentially stress-producing situations. In this way, we can identify those effects that will make the promise of social support a reality.

➢ **REFERENCES**

Allen, S., & Stoltenberg, C. (1995). Psychological separation of older adolescents and young adults from their parents: An investigation of gender differences. *Journal of Counseling and Development, 73,* 542-546.

Alloway, R., & Bebbington, P. (1987). The buffer theory of social support: A review of the literature. *Psychological Medicine, 17,* 91.

Antonovsky, A. (1974). Conceptual and methodological problems in the study of resistance resources and stressful life events. In B. Dohrenwend & B. Dohrenwend (Eds.), *Stressful life events: Their nature and effects* (pp. 245-258). New York: John Wiley.

Antonovsky, A. (1979). *Health, stress and coping.* San Francisco: Jossey-Bass.

Artinian, N. T. (1991). Stress experience of spouses of patients having coronary artery bypass during hospitalization and 6 weeks after discharge. *Heart & Lung: Journal of Critical Care, 20,* 52-59.

Artinian, N. T. (1992). Spouse adaptation to mate's CABG surgery: 1-Year follow-up. *American Journal of Critical Care, 1,* 36-42.

Artinian, N. T. (1993a). Spouses' perceptions of readiness for discharge after cardiac surgery. *Applied Nursing Research, 6,* 80-88.

Artinian, N. T. (1993b). Resources: Factors that mediate the stress-health-outcome relationship. In J. S. Barnfather & B. L. Lyon (Eds.), *Stress and coping: State of the science and implications for nursing theory, research and practice.* Indianapolis, IN: Sigma Theta Tau International.

Baillie, V., Norbeck, J., & Barnes, L. (1988). Stress, social support and psychological distress of family caregivers of the elderly. *Nursing Research, 37,* 217-222.

Baron, R. M., & Kenny, D. A. (1986). The moderator-mediator variable distinction in social psychological research: Conceptual, strategic, and statistical considerations. *Journal of Personality and Social Psychology, 51,* 1173-1182.

Barrera, M. (1981). Social support in the adjustment of pregnant adolescents: Assessment issues. In B. Gottlieb (Ed.), *Social networks and social support* (pp. 69-96). Beverly Hills, CA: Sage.

Barrera, M. (1986). *Distinctions between social support concepts, measures, and models. American Journal of Community Psychology, 14,* 413-445.

Barrera, M., & Ainsley, S. (1983). The structure of social support: A conceptual and empirical analysis. *Journal of Community Psychology, 11,* 133-143.

Barrera, M., Sandler, I., & Ramsey, T. (1981). Preliminary development of a scale of social support: Studies on college students. *American Journal of Community Psychology, 9,* 435-447.

Benner, P., & Wrubel, J. (1989). *The primacy of caring: Stress and coping in health and illness.* Reading, MA: Addison-Wesley.

Berkman, L., & Syme, L. (1979). Social networks, host resistance, and mortality: A nine year follow-up study of Alameda County residents. *American Journal of Epidemiology, 109,* 186-204.

Billings, A., & Moss, R. (1986). Children of parents with unipolar depression: A controlled 1-year follow-up. *Journal of Abnormal Child Psychology, 14,* 149-166.

Blumenthal, J., Barefoot, J., Burg, M., & Williams, R. B., Jr. (1987). Psychological correlates of hostility among patients undergoing coronary angiography. *British Journal of Medical Psychology, 60,* 349-355.

Brandt, P., & Weinert, C. (1981). The PRQ-A social support measure. *Nursing Research, 30,* 277-280.

Brown, G., & Harris, T. (1978). *Social origins of depression.* New York: Free Press.

Brown, M. A. (1986). Social support during pregnancy: A unidirectional or multidirectional construct? *Nursing Research, 35,* 4-9.

Bryce, R., Stanley, F., & Garner, J. (1991). Randomized controlled trial of antenatal social support to prevent preterm birth. *British Journal of Obstetrics and Gynecology, 98,* 1001-1008.

Caplan, G. (1974). *Support systems and community mental health.* New York: Behavioral Publications.

Carveth, W., & Gottlieb, B. (1979). The measurement of social support and its relation to stress. *Canadian Journal of Behavioral Science, 11,* 179-387.

Cassel, J. (1974). Psychosocial processes and stress: Theoretical foundations. *International Journal of Health Services, 3,* 471-482.

Cassel, J. (1976). The contribution of the social environment to host resistance. *American Journal of Epidemiology, 104,* 107-123.

Chan, T., & Ward, S. (1993). A tool to reduce stress and cardiovascular disease. *AAOHN Journal, 41,* 499-503.

Chang, J., & Krantz, M. (1996). Personal and environmental factors in relation to adjustment of offspring of alcoholics. *Substance Use & Misuse, 31,* 1401-1412.

Choi, E. C. (1994). Nursing research in Korea. *Annual Review of Nursing Research, 12,* 215-229.

Coates, D., & Winston, T. (1983). Counteracting the deviance of depression: Peer support groups for victims. *Journal of Social Issues, 39,* 169-194.

Cobb, S. (1976). Social support as a moderator of life stress. *Psychosomatic Medicine, 38,* 300-314.

Coffman, S., Levitt, M., & Deets, C. (1990). Personal and professional support for mothers of NICU and healthy newborns. *Journal of Obstetric, Gynecologic, and Neonatal Nursing, 20,* 406-415.

Cohen, S. (1988). Psychosocial models of the role of social support in the etiology of physical disease. *Health Psychology, 7,* 269-297.

Cohen, S., & Willis, T. (1985). Stress, social support and the buffering hypothesis. *Psychological Bulletin, 98,* 310-357.

Conn, V. S., Taylor, S. G., & Abel, P. B. (1991). Myocardial infarction survivors: Age and gender differences in physical health, psychosocial state and regimen adherence. *Journal of Advanced Nursing, 16,* 1026-1034.

Constable, J. F., & Russell, D. W. (1986). The effect of social support and the work environment upon burnout among nurses. *Journal of Human Stress, 12,* 20-26.

Cook, K. S. (1987). *Social exchange theory.* Newbury Park, CA: Sage.

Cormier-Daigle, M., & Sewart, M. (1997). Support and coping of male hemodialysis-dependent patients. *International Journal of Nursing Studies, 34,* 420-430.

Davidson, J., Degner, L., & Morgan, T. (1995). Information and decision-making preferences of men with prostate cancer. *Oncology Nurse Forum, 22,* 1401-1408.

Dean, A., & Lin, N. (1977). The stress-buffering role of social support. *Journal of Nervous and Mental Diseases, 165,* 403.

Diamond, M. (1979). Social support and adaptation to chronic illness: The case of maintenance hemodialysis. *Research in Nursing & Health, 2,* 101-108.

Dick, M. (1986). Burnout in nurse faculty: Relationships with management style, collegial support, and work load in collegiate programs. *Journal of Professional Nursing, 2,* 252-260.

Dodd, M. J., Dibble, S. L., & Thomas, M. L. (1993). Predictors of concerns and coping strategies of cancer chemotherapy outpatients. *Applied Nursing Research, 6,* 2-7.

Douglas, L. (1997). Reciprocal support in the context of cancer: Perspectives of the patient and spouse. *Oncology Nursing Forum, 24,* 1529-1536.

Ducharme, F., Stevens, B., & Rowat, K. (1994). Social support: Conceptual and methodological issues for research in mental health nursing. *Issues in Mental Health Nursing, 15,* 373-392.

Dunkel-Schetter, C. (1981). *Social support and coping with cancer.* Unpublished doctoral dissertation, University of Michigan, Ann Arbor.

Dunkel-Schetter, C., & Wortman, C. (1982). The role of social support in adaptation and recovery from physical illness. In S. Cohen & S. Syme (Eds.), *Social support and health* (pp. 281-302). Orlando, FL: Academic Press.

Duquette, A., Kerouac, S., Sandhu, B., & Beaudet, L. (1994). Factors related to nursing burnout: A review of empirical knowledge. *Issues in Mental Health Nursing, 15,* 337-358.

Durkheim, E. (1938). *The rules of sociological method.* New York: Free Press.

Durkheim, E. (1951). *Suicide: A study in sociology.* New York: Free Press. (Original work published 1897)

Duxbury, M., Armstrong, G., Drew, D., & Henly, S. (1984). Head nurse leadership style with staff burnout and job satisfaction in neonatal intensive care units. *Nursing Research, 33,* 97-101.

Eckenrode, J., & Gore, S. (1990). *Stress between work and family.* New York: Plenum.

Edwards, C., Cole, O., Oyemade, U., Knight, E., Johnson, A., Westney, O., Laryen, H., West, W., Jones, S., & Westney, L. (1994). Maternal stress and pregnancy outcomes in a prenatal clinic population. *Journal of Nutrition, 124,* 10065-10215.

Eisler, J., Wolfer, J., & Diers, D. (1972). Relationship between need for social approval and postoperative recovery and welfare. *Nursing Research, 21,* 520-525.

Elmore, S. (1984). The moderating effect of social support upon depression. *Communicating Nursing Research, 17,* 17-22.

Failla, S., & Jones, L. C. (1991). Families of children with developmental disabilities: An examination of family hardiness. *Research in Nursing & Health, 14,* 41-50.

Ferketich, S., & Mercer, R. (1990). Effects of antepartal stress on health status during early motherhood. *Scholarly Inquiry in Nursing Practice: International Journal, 4,* 127-149.

Fink, S. (1995). The influence of family demands on the strains and well-being of caregiving families. *Nursing Research, 44,* 139-146.

Fiore, J., Becker, J., & Coopel, D. (1983). Social network interactions: A buffer or a stress. *American Journal of Community Psychology, 11,* 423-439.

Frey, M. (1989). Social support and health: A theoretical formulation derived from King's conceptual framework. *Nursing Science Quarterly, 2,* 138-148.

Friedman, M. (1993). Social support sources and psychological well-being in older women with heart disease. *Research in Nursing and Health, 16,* 405-413.

Friedman, M. (1997). Social support sources among older women with heart failure: Continuity versus loss over time. *Research in Nursing & Health, 20,* 319-327.

Friedman, M., & King, K. (1994). The relationship of emotional and tangible support to psychological well-being among older women with heart failure. *Research in Nursing & Health, 17,* 433-440.

Funch, D., & Mettlin, C. (1982). The role of support in relation to recovery from breast surgery. *Social Science and Medicine, 36,* 352-362.

Gibson, P., Cheavens, J., & Warren, M. (1998). Social support in persons with self-reported sensitivity to chemicals. *Research in Nursing & Health, 21,* 103-115.

Gluhoski, V., Fishman, B., & Perry, S. (1997). Moderators of bereavement distress in a gay male sample. *Personality and Individual Differences, 23,* 761-767.

Gottlieb, B. (1978). The development and application of a classification scheme of informal helping behaviors. *Canadian Journal of Behavioral Sciences, 10,* 105-115.

Gottlieb, B. (1981). *Social networks and social support.* Beverly Hills, CA: Sage.

Graydon, J., & Ross, E. (1995). Influence of symptoms, lung function, mood, and social support on level of functioning of patients with COPD. *Research in Nursing & Health, 18,* 52.

Grossman, M., & Rowat, K. (1995). Parental relationships, coping strategies, received support, and well-being in adolescents of separated or divorced and married parents. *Research in Nursing & Health, 18,* 249-261.

Gulick, E. E. (1992). Model for predicting work performance among persons with multiple sclerosis. *Nursing Research, 41,* 266-272.

Haley, D. J. (1986). *The relationship among social support, alienation, religiosity, length of service and the burnout experienced by nurses' aides and licensed practical nurses employed in skilled care nursing homes.* Unpublished doctoral dissertation, Loyola University of Chicago, Chicago.

Hann, D., Oxman, T., Ahles, T., Furstenburg, C., & Stukel, T. (1995). Social support adequacy and depression in older patients with metastatic cancer. *Psycho-Oncology, 4,* 213-221.

Hansell, P., Hughes, C., Caliandro, G., Russo, P., Budin, W., Hartman, B., & Hernandez, O. (1998). The effect of a social support boosting intervention on stress, coping, and social support in caregivers of children with HIV/AIDS. *Nursing Research, 47*(2), 79-86.

Hare, J., Pratt, C. C., & Andrews, D. (1988). Predictors of burnout in professional and paraprofessional nurses working in hospitals and nursing homes. *International Journal of Nursing Studies, 25,* 105-115.

Hatchett, L., Friend, R., Symister, P., & Wadhua, N. (1997). Interpersonal expectations, social support, and adjustment to chronic illness. *Journal of Personality and Social Psychology, 73,* 560-573.

Heins, H., Nance, N., & Levey-Mickens, G. (1988). The resource mom—A program of social support for pregnant teens. *Journal of the South Carolina Medical Association, 84,* 361-363.

Hinds, C., & Moyer, A. (1997). Support as experienced by patients with cancer during radiotherapy treatments. *Journal of Advanced Nursing, 26,* 371-379.

Hirsch, B. J. (1979). Psychological dimensions of social networks: A multimethod analysis. *American Journal of Community Psychology, 7,* 263-277.

Hirth, A., & Stewart, M. (1994). Hope and social support as coping resources for adults waiting for cardiac transplantation. *Canadian Journal of Nursing Research, 26*(3), 30-47.

House, J. (1981). *Work stress and social support.* Englewood Cliffs, NJ: Prentice Hall.

Hughes, C., & Caliandro, G. (1996). Effects of social support, stress, and level of illness on caregiving of children with AIDS. *Journal of Pediatric Nursing: Nursing Care of Children and Families, 11,* 347-358.

Hurley-Wilson, B. (1993). Perception, appraisal and meaning as mediators of the stress-health linkage. In J. S. Barnfather & B. L. Lyon (Eds.), *Stress and coping: State of the science and implications for nursing theory, research and practice* (pp. 129-149). Indianapolis, IN: Sigma Theta Tau International.

Ihlenfeld, J. (1996). Nurses' perceptions of administrative social support. *Issues in Mental Health Nursing, 17,* 469-477.

Jalowiec, A. (1993). Coping with illness: Synthesis and critique of the nursing coping literature from 1980-1990. In J. Barnfather & B. Lyon (Eds.), *Stress and coping: State of the science and implications for nursing theory, research and practice* (pp. 65-83). Indianapolis, IN: Sigma Theta Tau International.

Jirka, J., Schuett, S., & Foxall, M. (1996). Loneliness and social support in infertile couples. *Journal of Obstetric, Gynecologic, and Neonatal Nursing, 25,* 55-60.

Kahn, R. (1979). Aging and social support. In M. Riley (Ed.), *Aging from birth to death.* Washington, DC: American Association for the Advancement of Science.

Kahn, R., & Antonucci, T. (1980). Convoys over the life course: Attachment, roles and social support. In P. B. Baltes & O. Brim (Eds.), *Life-span development and behavior* (Vol. 3, pp. 253-286). New York: Academic Press.

Kang, D., Coe, C., Karaszewski, J., & McCarthy, D. (1998). Relationship of social support to stress responses and immune function in healthy and asthmatic adolescents. *Research in Nursing & Health, 21,* 117-128.

Kaplan, B., Cassel, J., & Gore, S. (1977). Social support and health. *Medical Care, 15*(5 Suppl.), 47-58.

Kendler, K. (1997). Social support: A genetic-epidemiologic analysis. *American Journal of Psychiatry, 154,* 1398-1404.

Kim, J. A. (1990). *The effect of supportive nursing care in depression, mood and satisfaction in military patients with low back pain.* Unpublished doctoral dissertation, The Graduate School of Yonsei University, Seoul, South Korea.

Kim, M. J. (1985). *An experimental study of the effects of supportive nursing care on stress relief for hospitalized patients.* Unpublished doctoral dissertation, The Graduate School of Yonsei University, Seoul, South Korea.

Lambert, V., Lambert, C., Klipple, G., & Mewshaw, E. (1989). Social support, hardiness and psychological well-being in women with arthritis. *Image: The Journal of Nursing Science, 21,* 128-131.

Lazarus, R. (1990). Theory-based stress measurement. *Psychological Inquiry, 1,* 3-13.

Lazarus, R. S., & Folkman, S. (1984). *Stress, appraisal, and coping.* New York: Springer.

Lederman, R. (1984). Anxiety and conflict in pregnancy: Relationship to maternal health status. In H. Werley & J. Fitzpatrick (Eds.), *Annual review of nursing research, Volume 2* (pp. 27-62). New York: Springer.

Lederman, R., Lederman, E., Work, B., & McCann, D. (1979). Relationship of maternal anxiety, plasma catecholamines and plasma cortisol to progress in labor. *American Journal of Obstetrics and Gynecology, 132,* 495-500.

Lee, R. N. F., Graydon, J. E., & Ross, E. (1991). Effects of psychological well-being, physical status, and social support on oxygen-dependent COPD patients' level of functioning. *Research in Nursing & Health, 14,* 323-328.

Lindsey-Davis, L. (1990). Illness uncertainty, social support and stress in recovering individuals and family caregivers. *Applied Nursing Research, 3,* 69-71.

Linn, J., Poku, K., Cain, V., Holzapfel, K., & Crawford, D. (1995). Psychosocial outcomes of HIV illness in male and female African American clients. *Social Work in Health Care, 21*(3), 43-60.

Lowenthal, M., & Haven, C. (1968). Interaction and adaptation: Intimacy as a critical variable. *American Sociological Review, 33,* 20-30.

Lugton, J. (1997). The nature of social support as experienced by women treated for breast cancer. *Journal of Advanced Nursing, 25,* 1184-1191.

Lyon, B. (1990). Getting back on track: Nursing's autonomous scope of practice. In N. Chaska (Ed.), *The nursing profession: Turning points.* St. Louis, MO: C. V. Mosby.

Mallett, K. (1988). *The relationship between burnout, death anxiety and social support in hospice and critical care nurses.* Doctoral dissertation, University of Toledo, Toledo, OH.

Maslach, C., & Jackson, S. (1981). *Maslach burnout inventory research edition.* Palo Alto, CA: Consulting Psychologists Press.

McColl, M., & Frieland, J. (1994). Social support, aging, and disability. *Topics in Geriatric Rehabilitation, 9*(3), 54-71.

McKenzie, R. (1926). The ecological approach to the study of the human community. In R. Park & C. Burgess (Eds.), *The city.* Chicago: University of Chicago Press.

McNett, S. (1987). Social support, threat and coping responses and effectiveness in the functionally disabled. *Nursing Research, 36,* 98-103.

Meister, S. (1982). *Perceived social support, subnetworks and well-being at life change.* Doctoral dissertation, University of Michigan, Ann Arbor.

Messick, D., & Cook, M. (1983). *Equity theory.* New York: Praeger.

Mickschl, D. (1984). *A study of critical care nurses: The relationship among needs fulfillment discrepancy, attitudes and feelings of burnout, and unit leadership style.* Unpublished doctoral dissertation, Gonzaga University, Spokane, WA.

Mitchell, R., & Trickett, E. (1980). Social networks as mediators of social support: An analysis of the effects and determinants of social networks. *Community Mental Health Journal, 16,* 27-44.

Norbeck, J. (1981). Social support: A model for clinical research and application. *Advances in Nursing Science, 3*(4), 43-59.

Norbeck, J. (1984). The Norbeck Social Support Questionnaire. *Birth Defects: Original Article Series, 20*(5), 45-55.

Norbeck, J. (1991). Social support needs of family caregivers of psychiatric patients from three age groups. *Nursing Research, 40,* 208-213.

Norbeck, J., & Anderson, N. (1989). Psychosocial predictors of pregnancy outcomes in low-income black, Hispanic and white women. *Nursing Research, 38,* 204-209.

Norbeck, J., DeJoseph, J., & Smith, R. (1996). A randomized trial of an empirically derived social support intervention to prevent low birth weight among African American women. *Social Science & Medicine, 43,* 947-954.

Norbeck, J., Lindsey, A., & Carrieri, V. (1981). The development of an instrument to measure social support. *Nursing Research, 30,* 264-269.

Norbeck, J., Lindsey, A., & Carrieri, V. (1983). Further development of the Norbeck Social Support Questionnaire: Normative data and validity testing. *Nursing Research, 32,* 4-9.

Norwood, S. (1996). The Social Support Apgar: Instrument development and testing. *Research in Nursing & Health, 19,* 143-152.

Nuckolls, K., Cassel, J., & Kaplan, B. (1972). Psychosocial assets, life crisis and the prognosis of pregnancy. *American Journal of Epidemiology, 95,* 431-441.

Nyamathi, A. (1987). The coping responses of female spouses of patients with myocardial infarction. *Heart and Lung, 16,* 86-92.

Oakley, A., Rajan, L., & Grant, A. (1990). Social support and pregnancy outcome. *British Journal of Obstetrics and Gynecology, 97,* 155-162.

O'Brien, R., Wineman, N., & Nealon, N. (1995). Correlates of the caregiving process in multiple sclerosis. *Scholarly Inquiry for Nursing Practice, 9,* 323-342.

Oxman, T., Freeman, D., Manheimer, E., & Stukel, T. (1994). Social support and depression after cardiac surgery in elderly patients. *American Journal of Geriatric Psychiatry, 2,* 309-323.

Oxman, T., & Hull, J. (1997). Social support, depression, and activities of daily living in older heart surgery patients. *Journal of Gerontology, 52B,* 1-14.

Paredes, F. (1982). *The relationship of psychological resources and social support, occupational stress and burnout in hospital nurses.* Unpublished doctoral dissertation, University of Houston, Houston, TX.

Park, R., & Burgess, E. (Eds.). (1926). *The city.* Chicago: University of Chicago Press.

Pearlin, L. (1989). The sociological study of stress. *Journal of Health and Social Behavior, 30,* 241-256.

Peck, A., & Boland, J. (1977). Emotional reactions to radiation treatment. *Cancer, 40,* 180-184.

Pelletier, M. L. (1993). The needs of family members of organ and tissue donors. *Heart & Lung, 22,* 151-157.

Picot, S. (1995). Rewards, costs, and coping of African American caregivers. *Nursing Research, 44,* 147-152.

Potts, M. (1997). Social support and depression among older adults living alone: The importance of friends within and outside of a retirement community. *Social Work, 42,* 348-362.

Powers, B. (1988). Social networks, social support, and elderly institutionalized people. *Advances in Nursing Science, 10*(2), 40-58.

Preston, D. (1995). Marital status, gender roles, stress and health in the elderly. *Health Care for Women International, 16,* 149-165.

Qureshi, H., & Walker, A. (1989). *The caring relationship: Elderly people and their families.* New York: Macmillan.

Riegel, B. J., & Gocka, I. (1995). Gender differences in adjustment to acute myocardial infarction. *Heart & Lung, 24,* 457-466.

Roberts, J., Browne, G., Streiner, D., Gafni, A., Pallister, R., Hoxby, H., Drummond-Young, M., LeGris, J., & Meichenbaun, D. (1995). Problem-solving counseling or phone-call support for outpatients with chronic illness: Effective for whom? *Canadian Journal of Nursing Research, 27,* 111-137.

Robinson, J. (1995). Grief responses, coping processes, and social support of widows: Research with Roy's model. *Nursing Science Quarterly, 8*(4), 158-164.

Rothberg, A., & Lits, B. (1991). Psychosocial support for maternal stress during pregnancy: Effect on birth weight. *American Journal of Obstetrics and Gynecology, 165,* 403-407.

Ruiz-Bueno, J., & Underwood, P. (in press). *Resources as moderators/mediators of the stress-health outcome linkage.* Chicago: Midwest Nursing Research Society.

Runtz, M., & Schallow, J. (1997). Social support and coping strategies as mediators of adult adjustment following childhood maltreatment. *Child Abuse and Neglect, 21,* 211-226.

Sansom, D., & Farnill, D. (1997). Stress following marriage breakdown: Does social support play a role. *Journal of Divorce & Remarriage, 26*(3/4), 39-49.

Seeman, T., & Berkman, L. (1988). Structural characteristics of social networks and their relationship with social support in the elderly: Who provides support. *Social Science and Medicine, 26,* 737-749.

Shoenbach, V., Kaplan, B., Fredman, L., & Kleinbaum, D. (1986). Social ties and mortality in Evans County, Georgia. *American Journal of Epidemiology, 123,* 577-591.

Small, S., & Graydon, J. (1993). Uncertainty in hospitalized patients with chronic obstructive pulmonary disease. *International Journal of Nursing Studies, 30,* 239-246.

Snowdon, A., Cameron, S., & Dunham, K. (1994). Relationships between stress, coping resources and satisfaction with family functioning in families of children with disabilities. *Canadian Journal of Nursing Research, 26*(3), 63-76.

Spencer, B., Thomas, H., & Morris, J. (1989). A randomized controlled trial of the provision of a social support service during pregnancy: The South Manchester Family Worker Project. *British Journal of Obstetrics and Gynecology, 96,* 281-288.

Stewart, M. (1989). Social support instruments created by nurse investigators. *Nursing Research, 38,* 268-275.

Stewart, M., Hart, G., & Mann, K. (1995). Living with haemophilia and HIV/AIDS: Support and coping. *Journal of Advanced Nursing, 22,* 1101-1111.

Stewart, M., Ritchie, J., McGrath, P., Thompson, D., & Bruce, B. (1994). Mothers of children with chronic conditions: Supportive and stressful interactions with partners and professionals regarding caregiving burdens. *Canadian Journal of Nursing Research, 26*(4), 61-81.

Stewart, M., & Tilden, V. (1995). The contributions of nursing science to social support. *International Journal of Nursing Studies, 32,* 535-544.

Stroebe, W., Stroebe, M., Abakoumkin, G., & Schut, H. (1996). The role of loneliness and social support in adjustment to loss: A test of attachment versus stress theory. *Journal of Personality and Social Psychology, 70,* 1241-1249.

Thomas, W., & Znaniecki, F. (1920). *The Polish peasant in Europe and America.* New York: Knopf.

Tilden, V. P. (1983). The relation of selected psychosocial variables to emotional disequilibrium during pregnancy. *Research in Nursing & Health, 6,* 167-174.

Tilden, V. P. (1984). The relation of selected psychosocial variables to single status of adult women during pregnancy. *Nursing Research, 33,* 102-107.

Tilden, V. P. (1991). *The Interpersonal Relationship Inventory (IPRI): Instrument development summary.* Portland: Oregon Health Science University, School of Nursing.

Tilden, V. P., & Gaylen, R. D. (1987). Cost and conflict: The darker side of social support. *Western Journal of Nursing Research, 9,* 9-18.

Tilden, V. P., Hirsch, A., & Nelson, C. (1994). The Interpersonal Relationship Inventory: Continued psychometric evaluation. *Journal of Nursing Measurement, 2,* 63-78.

Tilden, V. P., Nelson, C., & May, B. (1990a). Use of qualitative methods to enhance content validity. *Nursing Research, 39,* 172-175.

Tilden, V. P., Nelson, C., & May, B. (1990b). The IPR inventory: Development and psychometric characteristics. *Nursing Research, 39,* 337-343.

Turner, H. (1994). Gender and social support: Taking the bad with the good? *Sex Roles, 30,* 521-540.

Turner, R., Frankel, B., & Levin, D. (1983). Social support: Conceptualization, measurement, and implications for mental health. *Research in Community and Mental Health, 3,* 67-111.

Underwood, P. W. (1986). *Psychosocial variables: Their prediction of birth complications and relationship to perception of childbirth.* Ann Arbor, MI: University Microfilms, International.

Vaux, A., & Harrison, D. (1985). Support network characteristics associated with support satisfaction and perceived support. *American Journal of Community Psychology, 13,* 245-267.

Villar, J., Farnot, U., Barros, F., Victoria, C., & Langer, A. (1992). A randomized clinical trial of psychosocial support during high-risk pregnancies. *New England Journal of Medicine, 327,* 1266-1271.

Vrabec, N. (1995). *Burden in rural versus urban family caregivers.* Unpublished doctoral dissertation, University of Wisconsin-Milwaukee.

Wandersman, L., Wandersman, A., & Kahn, S. (1980). Social support in the transition to parenthood. *Journal of Community Psychology, 8,* 332-342.

Weinert, C. (1984). Evaluation of the PRQ: A social support measure. In K. Barnard, P. Brandt, & B. Raff (Eds.), *Social support and families of vulnerable infants* (Birth Defects, Original Article Series No. 20, pp. 59-97). White Plains, NY: March of Dimes Defects Foundation.

Weinert, C. (1987). A social support measure: PRQ85. *Nursing Research, 36,* 273-277.

Weinert, C. (1988). Measuring social support: Revision and further development of the Personal Resource Questionnaire. In C. Waltz & O. Strictland (Eds.), *Measurement of nursing outcomes* (Vol. 1, pp. 309-327). New York: Springer.

Weinert, C., & Brandt, P. (1987). Measuring social support with the Personal Resources Questionnaire. *Western Journal of Nursing Research, 9,* 589-602.

Weinert, C., & Tilden, V. P. (1990). Measures of social support: Assessment of validity. *Nursing Research, 39,* 212-216.

Weiss, R. (1974). The provisions of social relationships. In Z. Rubin (Ed.), *Doing unto others.* Englewood Cliffs, NJ: Prentice Hall.

Weiss, R. (1975). *Marital separation.* New York: Basic Books.

White, N., Richter, J., & Fry, C. (1992). Coping, social support, and adaptation to chronic illness. *Western Journal of Nursing Research, 14,* 211-224.

Willey, C., & Silliman, R. (1990). The impact of disease on the social support experiences of cancer patients. *Journal of Psychosocial Oncology, 8,* 79-95.

Wortman, C. (1984). Social support and cancer: Conceptual and methodological issues. *Cancer, 53,* 2339-2360.

Yarcheski, A., & Mahon, N. (1989). A causal model of positive health practices: The relationship between approach and replication. *Nursing Research, 38,* 88-93.

Younger, J., Kendell, M., & Pickler, R. (1997). Mastery of stress in mothers of preterm infants. *Journal of the Society of Pediatric Nurses, 2,* 29-35.

Zimet, G., Dahlem, W., Zimet, S., & Farley, G. (1988). The Multidimensional Scale of Perceived Social Support. *Journal of Personality Assessment, 52,* 30-41.

CHAPTER 15

Type A Behavior Pattern and Cardiovascular Health

Erika Friedmann and Sue Ann Thomas

ursing is identified by the phenomena selected for study and the purposes for studying them (Lindsey, 1982). Theoretical models guide the use of variables and the design of the research and the interpretation of the findings. The biopsychosocial model (Engle, 1977, 1980) describes the multifaceted contributors to health. According to the biopsychosocial model, environmental, psychological, social, behavioral, physiological, and spiritual factors combine to contribute to the health of the individual at a given time (Audy, 1971). In the biopsychosocial model, the mind and the body are inexorably united. Factors that affect any aspect of the components can affect the status of all other aspects. Simply stated, behaviors, feelings, thoughts, and biology are interdependent, and challenges in any area can either enhance or detract from physical health.

Thomas and colleagues developed a holistic cardiovascular model based on the biopsychosocial model (Thomas & DeKeyser, 1996; Thomas & Liehr, 1995; Thomas, Liehr, DeKeyser, & Friedmann, 1993). The theory includes the combination of social, psychological, behavioral, and physiological factors interacting within the individual to determine cardiovascular health. A schematic diagram of the model is shown in Figure 15.1. Within all four realms, chronic states and acute changes affect survival. In this model, the combination of psychological, social, behavioral, and physiological factors either promotes health by moderating or promotes disease by enhancing pathological processes. Type A behavior has been identified as a behavioral risk factor for coronary heart disease. From the perspective of the biopsychosocial model, Type A behavior is conceptualized as a behavioral factor promoting the pathogenic process leading to coronary heart disease (CHD). As such, it is relevant to both the theory and the practice of nursing.

Several different psychological models of Type A behavior attempt to explain how cognition and perception influence the behavior and physiological responses characteristic of Type A behavior. These include Friedman and Rosenman's (1974) original conceptualiza-

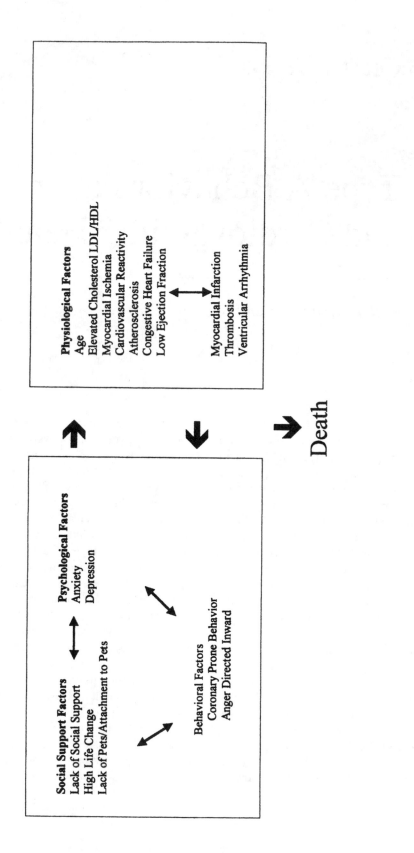

Figure 15.1. Schematic Model of the Relationship Between Behavioral, Social, Psychological, and Physiological Factors as Determinants of Cardiovascular Health

tion of Type A behavior as a style of reacting to challenging situations, Glass's (1977) model relating to uncontrollability, Scherwitz and Canick's (1988) theory based on self-involvement, and Price's (1982) complex construction of personal and social reality. These models treat Type A behavior as a stable personality trait. No matter which model is used to understand the physiological and behavioral responses of Type A individuals, the models provide ample opportunity for nurses, psychologists, or other health professionals to intervene and help individuals learn to modify their expression of this trait.

➤ HISTORY OF TYPE A BEHAVIOR

The belief that a pattern of aggressive or hostile behavior is associated with coronary heart disease can be traced back several centuries. As early as 1897 Osler suggested that a lifestyle including a "treadmill of practice" (1910, p. 698) and the difficulty inducing a man of this type to lessen "the race, an' rack, an' strain" (1910, p. 974) caused angina pectoris. Osler described the typical angina patient as "robust, vigorous in mind and body, the keen and ambitious man, the indicator of whose engine is always set at full speed ahead" (Osler, 1910, p. 839).

The scientific study of the relationship of hostile, aggressive behavior and coronary heart disease (CDH) was initiated by Friedman and Rosenman in the 1950s (Friedman & Rosenman, 1959; Rosenman & Friedman, 1961). They termed this behavior Type A or coronary-prone behavior. Type A behavior is an action-emotion complex that requires an environmental challenge to trigger the expression of the behavior (Friedman, 1969). Individuals who exhibit Type A behavior, or Type A's, were described as being engaged in a "chronic struggle to obtain an unlimited number of poorly defined things . . . in the shortest time possible," even in the face of obstacles or hindrances (Jenkins, Zyzanski, & Rosenman, 1979, p. 3). Paradoxically, they appear to be well organized, self-confident, and self-

controlled (Rosenman, 1983). The behavior pattern was characterized by competitiveness, time urgency, and aggression.

Friedman and Rosenman designed a mildly challenging interview, the Structure Interview (SI), to elicit this behavior. In the SI, the Type A behavior pattern is determined both from the content of the subjects' answers to interview questions and from the manner in which they respond. The Type A individual expresses hostility, hyperaggressiveness, competitiveness, impatience, and a sense of time urgency in answers during the interview (Rosenman, 1983). Visual clues to Type A behavior are hurried and loud speech, muscle tension, and hostile facial patterns. Individuals who generally do not exhibit most of these behaviors are called Type B's. Type B's have a less aggressive and more even-paced type of behavior that does not lead to the inappropriate hostility and competitiveness often exhibited by Type A's (Rosenman, 1983).

In 1975, the Western Collaborative Study Group (WCSG) provided the first large-scale prospective epidemiological research to demonstrate the relationship between Type A behavior and CHD incidence. In the WCGS, a sample of 3,154 essentially healthy men aged 39 to 59 who were employed were assessed with the SI for Type A behavior (Rosenman et al., 1964). Rosenman and colleagues found that during an 8½-year period the Type A men were twice as likely to experience a myocardial infarction (MI) compared to the Type B men (Rosenman et al., 1975). This was true even after controlling for the influences of other risk factors. The researchers suggested that Type A behavior was an independent risk factor of approximately the same predictive power as that of the traditional risk factors of cigarette smoking, hypertension, and elevated cholesterol.

The Review Panel on Coronary Heart Disease of the National Heart Lung and Blood Institute (1981) recognized the Type A behavior pattern as a risk factor independent of and equal in magnitude to the standard risk factors for CHD, such as smoking, high blood pressure, and hyperlipidemia. After 1981, there were an increasing number of reports on the relationship of Type A behavior and CHD and on the effects of psychological treatment of Type A behavior and CHD outcomes. The research produced conflicting results.

➣ TOOLS FOR MEASURING TYPE A BEHAVIOR

Structured Interview (Friedman & Rosenman, 1974) and the Jenkins Activity Survey (JAS; Jenkins et al., 1979) are the most frequently used measures of Type A. Other tools used less often include the Framingham Type A Scale (FAS) (Haynes, Levine, Scotch, Feinleib, & Kannel, 1978), the Bortner Scale (BS) (Bortner, 1969), and a modification of the SI called the Videotaped Structure Interview (VSI) (Thoresen, Friedman, Gill, & Ulmer, 1982). The Matthews Youth Test for Health (MYTH) (Matthews & Angulo, 1980) is a tool specifically designed to assess coronary-prone behavior in children. The origins and psychometric properties of these tools are included in Table 15.1. SI and VSI assess behavioral responses of individuals to a series of oral questions given in a specific manner during an in-person interview as a means of identifying Type A behavior. The remaining three tools used with adults (JAS, FAS, and BS) rely on individual personal evaluation of adults' attitudes, activities, and behavioral tendencies using a questionnaire. The MYTH relies on teachers' assessments of students' behaviors in their classrooms and playgrounds (Matthews & Angulo, 1980).

The self-report measures—the JAS, FAS, and BS—assess individuals' self-perceptions about their attitudes, activities, and responses, whereas the observational tools—the SI, VSI, and MYTH—assess a set of behaviors exhibited either during interviews or in everyday life. The JAS (Jenkins, Zyzanski, & Rosenman, 1971) and the BS (Bortner, 1969) were developed using questions designed to address components of the SI. For both of

these scales, a factor analysis approach was used to identify and confirm items correlated with the SI assessment of Type A behavior. The JAS concentrates on attitudes, whereas the BS emphasizes behaviors. Questions comprising the FAS were chosen to form 1 of 20 scales "to assess behavioral dimensions not measured by any one item alone" ((Haynes et al., 1978a, p. 365). These questions were selected as those most closely related to the concepts included in the SI from a group of 300 psychosocial questions.

The criterion-related validity of each of the five measures used with adults has been established through documentation of the relationship of Type A behavior to incidence of CHD (Table 15.1). Assessment of the characteristics by behavioral observation of children has been used to establish concurrent validity for teachers' classification of behavior type using the MYTH (Meininger, Stashinko, & Hayman, 1991).

The development and use of the tools to measure Type A behavior in adults have been limited primarily to samples of white, middle-class men. None of the scales has been validated through prospective association with coronary heart disease among blacks. Cross-sectional data, using the FAS to assess Type A behavior, indicate that Type A behavior is equally common among blacks and whites (Sprafka, Folsom, Burke, Hahn, & Pirie, 1990).

Although the SI, JAS, BS, and FAS have been found to be significantly related to heart disease, assessments of Type A behavior with these tools are not very consistent (Byrne, Rosenman, Schiller, & Chesney, 1985). Several authors report low agreement between Type A classification using the SI and other methods. For example, in a study of cardiac patients, SI and JAS categorization as Type A was in agreement in only 55% of 101 cases (Thomas & Friedmann, 1990). Furthermore, patterns of intercorrelations between the self-report measures of Type A behavior indicate diversity among the measures rather than homogeneity (Byrne et al., 1985). Thus, it appears that these scales are measuring different aspects of one or more common underlying constructs that put individuals at increased risk for the development of clinical CHD.

The SI has been determined to be the best Type A behavior assessment tool for prospective prediction of CHD (Booth-Kewley & Friedman, 1987; Matthews, 1988; Scherwitz, Berton, & Leventhal, 1977). As noted previously, assessment of an individual's behavior pattern with the SI was designed to rely largely on the speech characteristics of the subject. The construct and concurrent validity of this approach have been confirmed (Scherwitz et al., 1977; Schucker & Jacobs, 1977). In fact, in one study of 60 undergraduate students, 52% of the variance in Type A classification using the SI was explained by speech characteristics. In contrast, in this same sample, the interview content explained 53% of variation in Type A classification using the JAS, and speech characteristics did not contribute significantly to the explanation of variation in Type A with the JAS (Scherwitz et al., 1977). These findings suggest that speech characteristics distinctive of SI-determined Type A behavior might be related to the mechanism for the increased risk of CHD exhibited by SI-classified Type A individuals.

Summary

Five tools have been validated to assess Type A behavior by their association with increased CHD mortality or morbidity. The SI and the VSI require in-person 10- to 15-minute interviews by trained assessors. The JAS, BS, and FAS are paper-and-pencil questionnaires completed by the respondents. The JAS, BS, and FAS are easier and more economical to use than the SI.

Although each of the five scales is associated with cardiac mortality, classification of Type A behavior with these scales has not been consistent. The SI and its derivative, the VSI, use actual behaviors to classify Type A behavior, whereas the JAS, BS, and FAS rely

on individuals' self-perceptions of their attitudes and behaviors. Self-assessments are notoriously poor among Type A individuals and have questionable reliability (Byrne et al., 1985). The behavioral classification afforded by the SI most closely matches Friedman and Rosenman's original conceptualization of Type A behavior.

➤ ASSOCIATION OF TYPE A BEHAVIOR WITH CHD: PROSPECTIVE STUDIES

Research addressing the association of Type A behavior with CHD peaked during the 1980s after the Review Panel on Coronary Heart Disease of the National Heart Lung and Blood Institute recognized it as a risk factor for CHD. The conflicting evidence on the relationship of Type A behavior and CHD in epidemiological studies, however, led to questioning of the clinical utility. Three large prospective studies found confirming results: the Framingham Heart Study (Eaker, Abbot, & Kannel, 1989; Haynes & Feinleib, 1982), Belgium study (DeBacker, Kornitzer, & Kittel, 1983), and the French-Belgian Collaborative Group Study (1982). The Honolulu Study (Cohen & Reed, 1985) and reports from the Multiple Risk Factor Intervention Trial (MRFIT) study (Dembroski, MacDougall, Costa, & Grandits, 1989; Shekelle, Gale, Ostfeld, & Paul, 1983) did not support the relationship between Type A behavior and CHD. The Honolulu Study has been criticized for using an inadequate, unvalidated, unique list of questions as a tool to measure Type A behavior. MRFIT study participants were healthy, but the study was limited to individuals identified as having a high risk of developing CHD rather than using a large heterogeneous population not selected for disease-related characteristics, as was used in studies finding an association between Type A behavior and CHD. The difference in the type of populations included in the MRFIT study and the WCGS provides some explana-

TABLE 15.1 Selected Measures of Type A Behavior

Measure and Author	Variables Measured	Brief Description	Reliability	Validity	Populations Studied
Bortner (Bortner, 1969)	Type A behavior	This is a 14-item self-rated scale. Each item asks subjects to indicate their position between two statements of extreme behaviors.	Test-retest .71 over 34 weeks (Johnston & Shaper, 1983)	Type A predicted coronary heart disease and myocardial infarctions of sudden death in multivariate analysis (French-Belgian Collaborative Group, 1982)	Men ($N = 3,202$) from three European cities
Framingham Type A Scale (Haynes, Levine, Scotch, Feinleib, & Kannel, 1978)	Type A behavior	Ten items are selected by experts from a 300-item psychosocial attribute to assess individual's competitive drive, sense of time urgency, and perception of job pressures. Different questions were used for women not employed outside the home than for other women and men.	Internal reliability: men, .71; women, .70	Prevalence of coronary heart disease associated with Type A behavior in women, women not employed outside the home, and men (Haynes, Levine, Scotch, Feinleib, & Kannel, 1978b) Relative annual incidence rates A to B 1.4-2.9 depending on subgroup (Matthews, 1982)	Members of the Framingham Heart Study from 1965 to 1967, 44-64 years old ($N = 1,822$)
Jenkins Activity Survey (Jenkins, Zyzanski, & Rosenman, 1979)	Type A behavior Speed and impatience Job involvement Hard driving and competitive	This is a 52-item self-report scale. Subscales include different numbers of items: 21, 21, 24, and 24, respectively. Each item asks subjects to choose one of three or four responses to situations that best describes their behavior.	Internal consistency of scales .73-.85 Test-retest .60-.70 across 1-4 years (Jenkins, 1978)	Type A's twice as likely to exhibit clinical coronary heart disease (Rosenman et al., 1975) Type A predicted total coronary heart disease (DeBacker, Kornitzer, Kittel, et al., 1983)	Participants (middle-class men 44-64 years old) in the Western Collaborative Group Study ($N = 644$) Men 40-55 years old ($N = 1,958$) free of heart disease at beginning and followed for 5 years (DeBacker et al., 1983)

Instrument	Construct	Description	Reliability	Validity	Sample
Matthews Youth Test for Health (Matthews & Angulo, 1980)	Type A behavior	This is a 17-item teacher rating scale with three subscales: Type A, Competitiveness, and Impatience-aggression.	Internal consistency of scales .88–.90 Test-retest reliability from .73 to .86 over 3 months	Children classified as Type A acted and played in manner consistent with that behavior type	School-age children (N = 485) in Grades kindergarten, 2, 4, 6
Structured Interview (Friedman & Rosenman, 1974)	Type A behavior Categorical measure with four levels: A1 (fully developed Type A), A2 (incompletely developed Type A), X (equal representation of Types A and B), and B (not Type A)	Behavioral assessment of style of reacting to challenging situations is presented in a 25-question structured interview.	80% test-retest over 12 to 20 months; interrater reliability 75% to 90% (Rosenman, 1978)	Relative annual coronary incidence rates A to B 2.2 (Matthews, 1982)	Participants (middle-class men 44-64 years old) in the Western Collaborative Group Study (N = 3,154)
Videotaped Structured Interview (Thoresen, Friedman, Gill, & Ulmer, 1982)	Type A behavior Same categories as Structured Interview	Behavioral assessment of style of reacting to challenging situations is presented in a 25-question structured interview, similar to but administered in a less challenging manner than the Structured Interview. Specific behaviors are scored and summed.	Interrater reliability .79 among eight raters (Powell, Friedman, Thoresen, Gill, & Ulmer, 1984)		Myocardial infarction patients younger than 65 years old (N = 884)

tion for the conflicting results (Rosenman, 1993). Ragland and Brand (1988) performed a 22-year follow-up study of WCGS mortality from CHD and found that it was not related to Type A behavior, although deaths were predicted from traditional risk factors. These results suggest that Type A behavior may be useful in predicting CHD in middle-aged men, but not as well as older men.

➤ THEORETICAL MECHANISM FOR THE RELATIONSHIP BETWEEN TYPE A BEHAVIOR AND CORONARY HEART DISEASE (CHD)

It is generally assumed that the relationship between psychosocial factors, including Type A behavior, and CHD is mediated by chronic physiological arousal, repeated and excessive cardiovascular responses to stressors, or both (Contrada & Krantz, 1988; Friedman & Rosenman, 1974; Thomas & Friedmann, 1990, 1994). Type A behavior has been conceptualized as acting to increase the likelihood of developing atheroscerotic plaque and/or to triggering the acute processes that lead to myocardial infarction and sudden cardiac death (Williams, Suarez, Kuhn, Zimmerman, & Schanberg, 1991), such as plaque rupture and thrombosis (Muller, Abela, Nesto, & Tofler, 1994).

Evidence for the relationship of Type A behavior to atherosclerosis is presented here. It has been suggested that unfavorable lipid profiles and increased cardiovascular and neuroendocrine responses (Buselli & Stuart, 1999; Contrada & Krantz, 1988) are mechanisms that mediate the relationship between Type A behavior and CHD. Increased platelet and leukocyte adhesion, vascular smooth muscle cell migration, and increased lipid deposition can result from endothelial injury secondary to stress (Engler & Engler, 1995). Furthermore, elevation in cholesterol ester content of arterial walls consistent with increased catecholamines may be another

mechanism for increased promotion of atherosclerotic changes in Type A individuals (Suarez, Williams, Kuhn, Zimmerman, & Schanberg, 1991). Type A men exhibited chronic elevation of plasma neurohormones in the laboratory that generalized to more naturalistic settings, as indicated by 24-hour urinary excretion rate responses (Williams et al., 1991).

Angiographic studies directly address the end point of the long-term process of plaque development. The results of studies that include angiography, however, must be interpreted cautiously because this is usually conducted when coronary artery disease is already suspected; therefore, the sample is biased and may not be representative of the entire population (Johnston, 1993).

The association of Type A behavior with severity of angiographically documented coronary artery disease appears to depend on the method used to assess Type A behavior. In a 1988 review of 16 studies of the relationship between angiographically documented coronary artery disease and Type A behavior (Haynes & Matthews, 1988), 66% of the studies including Type A behavior classification with the SI demonstrated a relationship between Type A behavior and angiographic findings. In contrast, the majority of the studies including classification of Type A behavior with the JAS did not demonstrate a relationship between Type A behavior and angiographic findings. Three studies using the Bortner Scale did not find a relationship between severity of coronary artery disease and Type A behavior (Matthews & Haynes, 1986).

The atherosclerotic process involved in the development of CHD is expected to be accelerated in Type A individuals. Chronic sympathetic nervous system arousal among Type A individuals is related to physiological changes, including lower high-density lipoproteins and higher low-density lipoproteins and triglycerides, which are also related to the development of atherosclerosis. There appears to be an association between SI-assessed Type A behavior and the severity of atherosclerosis.

> ## TYPE A BEHAVIOR, SPEECH STYLE, AND CARDIOVASCULAR REACTIVITY

Studies of stress responses address the more acute process that could cause immediate cardiovascular effects. Exaggerated cardiovascular and epinephrine responses of Type A individuals are indicative of enhanced sympathetic nervous system arousal that could potentially damage the cardiovascular system (Contrada & Krantz, 1988). The finding that CHD patients are more reactive to some stressors than are comparable healthy adults (Corse, Manuck, Cantwell, Giordani, & Matthews, 1982) provides additional evidence for the importance of the extreme reactivity to stressors in the development of CHD (Thomas & Friedmann, 1990).

For individuals classified as Type A using both the SI and the JAS, high total serum cholesterol is associated with larger catecholamine and cortisol responses to a stressor, whereas for Type B individuals serum cholesterol is negatively associated with these responses (Suarez et al., 1991). In healthy Type A men, plasma norepinephrine during stress was correlated negatively with high-density lipoprotein and positively with triglycerides and low-density lipoprotein (Fredrikson & Blumenthal, 1992). These findings relate directly to the opportunistic development of plaque discussed previously.

As noted earlier, the extreme responses to stressors are one component of the hypothesized physiological mechanism for the increased CHD morbidity and mortality exhibited among Type A individuals. Many studies have addressed cardiovascular reactivity among Type A individuals. The association of Type A behavior with physiological reactivity appears to depend on the method used to assess Type A behavior and on the nature of the stressor. In one of the few studies of CHD patients using both the SI and JAS to identify Type A behavior, Corse et al. (1982) found that increased cardiovascular response was associated with SI categories but not with the JAS-classified Type A behavior. It appears that SI-classified Type A behavior is associated with increased cardiovascular responses to moderate stressors, whereas JAS-classified Type A behavior is not. Less stressful tasks such as reading aloud were not differentially stressful for Type A and Type B cardiac patients, however, independent of whether the JAS or SI method of assessment was used (Thomas & Friedmann, 1990). Similarly, Type As and Bs respond in parallel to physical challenges such as cold pressor tests (Contrada & Krantz, 1988). The level of the challenge and emotional arousal induced by demands during the study are also important contributors to differences in physiological reactivity of Type A and B individuals. Type As are extremely reactive when harassed while performing, in situations requiring active effort to successfully complete tasks, or when presented with emotionally challenging situations (Contrada & Krantz, 1988).

Type A behavior identified with the SI is dependent largely on the characteristics of the speech behavior during the structured interview (Scherwitz et al., 1977). Therefore, the dynamics of the characteristic speech pattern are implicated as important contributors to the excessive cardiovascular reactivity and the increased risk of CHD exhibited by Type A individuals. Studies investigating the impact of speech stylistics on cardiovascular status have examined the blood pressure during the structured interview used to diagnose Type A behavior and have also examined the relationship between specific speech stylistics characteristic of Type A behavior, such as rapid speech, and cardiovascular reactivity during the SI. In the first type of research, in nonpatient subjects, blood pressure during the structured interview was higher among SI-classified Type A individuals than Type B individuals (Blumenthal, Lake, & Williams, 1985; Matthews, 1986). In research addressing the second theme, Type A persons had more frequent periods of quick, explosive speech during the SI than did Type Bs (Sparacino, Hansell, & Smyth, 1979). Blood pressures were also higher during intervals with higher frequencies of this type of speech. Minute-to-minute blood pressures during the SI were positively correlated with loud, explosive, and rapid speech (Anderson et al., 1986). When rate of speech did not differ, as in the mildly stressful reading task, cardiovascular reactivity did not differ between Type A and Type B cardiac patients (Thomas & Friedmann, 1990). Thus, although rapid speech is more typical of Type A than Type B individuals, the exaggerated cardiovascular response generally associated with Type A behavior was actually associated with rate of speech rather than the Type A behavior pattern in general.

These results were supported by the following studies. Two groups of researchers examined rate of speech and cardiovascular responses. They demonstrated that slowing the rate of speech in an experimental situation leads to decreased cardiovascular reactivity in apparently healthy young adults (Friedmann, Thomas, Kulick-Ciuffo, Lynch, & Suginohara, 1982; Siegman, Anderson, & Berger, 1990) and in cardiac patients (Thomas & Friedmann, 1994). These findings were consistent for both men and women (Siegman et al., 1990; Thomas & Friedmann, 1994) and for SI- and JAS-classified Type A and Type B individuals (Thomas & Friedmann, 1994). This suggested that modifying the behavior (namely, rapid speech) could lead to reduced cardiovascular reactivity among Type As.

Type As are also hypothesized to experience enhanced stress responses that would increase the likelihood of acute events such as plaque rupture, thrombosis, MI, and sudden cardiac death. SI-assessed Type As are more reactive than Type Bs to moderately severe stressors; JAS-assessed Type As are not. The rapid, explosive type of speech characteristic of Type A behavior causes greater blood pressure increases than slower speech. Lowering the rate of speech of Type A individuals reduces their cardiovascular responses.

▷ COMPONENTS OF TYPE A BEHAVIOR AND CHD

In a response to some of the conflicting data and in an effort to refine and redefine Type A behavior, researchers attempted to identify the toxic components of Type A behavior. Hostility and speech stylistics were identified as the most dangerous components of Type A behavior. Dembroski and colleagues (Dembroski et al., 1989; Dembroski, MacDougall, Williams, Hanley, & Blumenthal, 1985) developed a rating scheme to obtain the components scores from tapes of SIs and applied these to existing data sets from studies of Type A behavior and coronary artery disease. They proposed that the most dangerous components of Type A behavior were speech style and hostility. From these efforts, hostility emerged as the leading candidate for the toxic core of Type A behavior.

The potential effects of hostility on CHD morbidity and mortality were addressed in studies of (a) atherosclerosis and mortality among CHD patients and (b) the incidence or mortality or both from CHD among large groups of healthy adults. In these studies, the Cook-Medley Ho Scale (Cook & Medley, 1954), a 54-item scale from the Minnesota Multiphasic Personality Inventory (MMPI), was used to assess hostility. Subjects high in hostility on this scale are often labeled HiHo.

Studies addressing the relationship of hostility to morbidity among patients with documented CHD showed consistently that hostility was positively related to morbidity. In a series of reports, Williams and colleagues related high hostility to the severity of coronary artery disease (Dembroski, MacDougall, Williams, Hanley, & Blumenthal, 1985; MacDougall, Dembroski, Dimsdale, & Hackett, 1985; Williams et al., 1980). High hostility scores in the MRFIT study also were related to subsequent reinfarction (Dembroski et al., 1989).

The results of studies examining hostility in populations that had completed the MMPI for other purposes and were contacted later to obtain information about CHD status are less consistent. Some studies show a relationship between hostility and CHD mortality and morbidity, whereas others do not. In a 25-year follow-up study of 225 physicians, hostility was associated with a five times greater incidence of angina and MI (Barefoot, Dahlstrom, & Williams, 1983). In a similar 25-year follow-up study of 478 physicians, no relationship was found between hostility and any aspect of CHD (McCranie, Watkins, Brandsma, & Sisson, 1985). Shekelle et al. (1983) related high hostility to MI and CHD mortality among a large group of employed men (N = 1,876) at 10- and 25-year follow-ups. There was a linear relationship between hostility and survival in a relatively small group of men (Barefoot, Dodge, Peterson, Dahlstrom, & Williams, 1989). To date, these studies have included only men. In contrast, hostility was not found to be related to CHD incidence mortality, morbidity, or total mortality in a 33-year follow-up study of undergraduate students (Hearn, Murray, & Luepker, 1989) or in a 30-year follow-up study of 280 men who started the study as adults (Leon, Finn, Murray, & Bailey, 1988). McCranie et al. (1985) found no relationship in terms of mortality in a 25 year follow-up study with physicians. Possible reasons for the inconsistent results were discussed extensively by Hearn et al. (1989). Their most convincing argument was that differences in the age at which hostility was assessed influenced the outcome of the prospective studies. Some contradictions remain, however, even after each of the factors are considered.

Hostility was identified as one of the potentially dangerous components of the Type A behavior pattern. A clear and consistent relationship between hostility and both the severity of atherosclerosis and the recurrence of MI was found among patients with existing CHD. Population studies (Barefoot et al.,

1983) suggest that hostility may play an important role in the development of CHD among healthy individuals, but the results of the studies were not conclusive. Matthews (1988) and Kawachi et al. (1998) argue that the failure of some studies to find a relationship between hostility and development of CHD does not justify abandoning the concept.

> ## INTERVENTIONS TO REDUCE TYPE A BEHAVIOR AND RISK OF CORONARY HEART DISEASE (CHD)

Although several studies (Frank, Heller, Kornfeld, Sporn, & Weiss, 1978; Rosenman et al., 1975; Williams et al., 1980) have linked Type A behavior, as measured with the SI, to the incidence of and mortality from CHD, questions about the feasibility of altering Type A behavior and whether such alterations would be associated with reductions in risk of CHD arose. Many studies have been designed to change the behavior of individuals who display Type A behavior (Gill et al., 1985) or patients who have documented CHD (Friedman et al., 1986; Powell, Friedman, Thoresen, Gill, & Ulmer, 1984). Nunes, Frank, and Kornfeld (1987) reviewed the literature on controlled studies of the psychological treatment of Type A behavior using a meta-analysis in which the data from a group of studies were statistically synthesized. They identified 10 studies with 17 different treatment groups that reported measures of Type A behavior. On the basis of their initial review, 5 of the 10 studies suffered from serious methodological problems ranging from subject self-selection into treatment group (Friedman et al., 1986; Powell et al., 1984) to the lack of a formal control group (Roskies et al., 1979). The generalizability of the treatments studied is limited due to the small numbers of participants, samples composed of predominantly male, middle-class volunteers, and the lack of long-term follow-up assessments (Nunes et al., 1987). Furthermore, only 2 of the studies, the Recurrent Coronary Prevention Project (Friedman et al., 1986; Powell et al., 1984) and Gill et al.'s (1985) study, used the SI with raters blind to the subjects' treatment status to assess Type A behavior after the intervention.

The meta-analysis (Nunes et al., 1987) showed a significant probability across studies for reduction in 3-year combined CHD mortality and myocardial infarction incidence. This finding was based mainly on two studies that provided comprehensive treatment of Type A behavior.

The most comprehensive treatment of Type A behavior in an intervention trial was in the Recurrent Coronary Prevention Project (RCCP). In the RCPP, standard cardiac counseling was compared to a comprehensive program of education about Type A behavior, relaxation training, cognitive therapy, behavior modification, and emotional support (Friedman et al., 1986; Powell et al., 1984). All participants in the RCCP had a documented MI 6 months before entry into the study. In this study, 270 patients elected to participate in the control group and received cardiac counseling. They attended an average of 25 counseling sessions during a period of 4.5 years. The control treatment consisted of cardiac-related advice and information concerning diet, exercise, drugs, possible surgical regimens, and cardiovascular pathophysiology. The treatment group consisted of 582 men. They attended an average of 38 counseling sessions. The treatment group received the same amount of cardiac counseling as the control group but also received Type A behavior counseling. The Type A behavior counseling consisted of progressive muscle relaxation, behavior alteration techniques, changes in certain beliefs, restrictions of various environmental situations, and cognitive affective learning. One hundred sixty-one (59.6%) of the control group and 335 (56.6%) of the treatment group participants remained in the study for 4.5 years.

Both groups experienced significant reductions in Type A behavior as determined by a videotaped structured interview (VSI) at the end of 4.5 years. At that time, the treatment group had significantly lower Type A scores than the control group. The cumulative annualized total cardiac recurrence rate was 5.5% for the control group and 2.6% for the treatment group, a statistically significant difference. The cumulative cardiac death rate was 6.4% for the control group and 3.4% for the treatment group, a significant difference, at 3.5 years. Cumulative death rates at 4.5 years did not differ. Type A behavior was observed in 97.5% of the patients enrolled in the RCCP. Counseling appeared to have a significant and powerful effect on recurrent cardiac events. In addition to Type A-related differences, anger and depression also decreased (Mendes de Leon, Powell, & Kaplan, 1991).

A second study (Rahe, Ward, & Hayes, 1979) of patients who had recently experienced an MI used a group therapy treatment. In this study, 43 men and one woman were randomly assigned to control or treatment groups and were followed for 4 years. The members of the treatment group completed a 9-hour treatment program that included education about CHD and Type A behavior, behavior modification instruction, and emotional support. The group therapy began almost immediately following the MI. After 4 years, coronary morbidity and mortality were significantly lower in the treatment group than in the control group. It was also significantly more likely that members of the treatment group had returned to work compared to members of the control group. The members of the treatment group exhibited less Type A behavior at the end of the study than at the beginning. Members of the treatment group, however, did not remember the content of the educational sessions. The authors concluded that the supportive aspects of the therapeutic intervention were responsible for the differences in morbidity and mortality observed between the treatment and control groups.

These two intervention studies demonstrated that combination therapy can be effective at altering Type A behavior and reducing the progression of CHD, as demonstrated by lower cardiac morbidity and mortality in the treatment group. The two treatment approaches differed in the number of hours of intervention and the lag time between the MI and the beginning of the intervention. The therapy of less duration, beginning almost immediately after the MI (Rahe et al., 1979), resulted in comparable success to that of the therapy beginning 6 months after the MI (Friedman et al., 1986; Powell et al., 1984). In both studies, the interventions were conducted by physicians or psychologists or both. It would be reasonable for nurses to develop and use similar interventions.

The treatment studies that show the best efficacy were those employing a comprehensive approach. The current view of Type A behavior is broad and encompasses physiological, cognitive, behavioral, and social aspects of life. The treatment approach for altering Type A behavior and its subsequent cardiovascular consequences also must be comprehensive and seek to alter many components of the person's life. Friedman's (1996) book, *Type A Behavior: Its Diagnosis and Treatment,* provides an excellent summary of Type A behavior prevention and modification based on available research studies.

➤ CHILDREN AND TYPE A BEHAVIOR

The rationale for examining Type A behavior in children is twofold. The first goal is to try to understand the development of Type A behavior, and the second is to relate Type A behavior during childhood to subsequent development of CHD in adulthood. The MYTH (Table 15.1) was developed specifically to evaluate Type A behavior in children using behavioral criteria (Mathews & Angulo, 1980).

Type A behavior in children has been found to be related to their parents' behavior. The relationship between mothers' behavior and their preschool-age children's behavior was moderated by the degree of dissension in their families (Fukunishi, Saito, & Fujito, 1992). Boys' Type A behavior tended to decrease as dissension increased, whereas the

opposite was true for girls. Among slightly older children, Type A behavior in boys was related to their mothers' Type A behavior and that in girls was related to their fathers' Type A behavior (Forgays & Forgays, 1991). The relative contribution of genetic factors and environmental influences on Type A behavior in children was used to assess whether Type A behavior in children might potentially be modified. Studies of monozygotic (identical) and same-sex dizygotic (fraternal) twin pairs age 6 to 11 years (Meininger, Hayman, Coates, & Gallagher, 1988) and slightly older children (Meininger, Hayman, Coates, & Gallagher, 1998) revealed that genetics made a large contribution to Type A behavior, but that environment also plays a role. They concluded that the environmental contribution to Type A behavior was less than its contribution to other risk factors, such as serum cholesterol, triglycerides, and high-density lipoproteins. Despite this limitation, there is substantial potential for altering these risk factors in children. The authors also concluded that altering these risk factors in children might promote a healthy lifestyle among adolescents and adults, and that this possibility deserves serious attention. Currently, no longitudinal research has evaluated the relationship between childhood Type A behavior and CHD in adulthood.

➤ NURSING RESEARCH

Since 1982, nursing research has included Type A behavior in studies involving risk factors for CHD. The Cumulative Index for Nursing and Allied Health Index includes more than 200 references for Type A behavior. Nursing research has not focused on the development of Type A behavior as an independent construct but has evaluated it as one of many known risk factors in appropriate clinical populations. Nursing research has focused on Type A behavior and blood pressure, including transient changes (Sparacino et al., 1979), the effects of rate of speech (Thomas & Friedmann, 1990, 1994), and the blood pressure of inner-city black women (Smyth, Call, Hansell, Sparacino, & Strodtbeck, 1978; Smyth & Yarandi, 1994). In addition, Type A behavior and coping responses (Smyth & Yarandi, 1992), assessment of Type A behavior in children and adolescents (Brown & Tanner, 1990; Meininger et al., 1991); and the relative contributions of genetic and environmental factors to Type A behavior (Meininger et al., 1988) have been examined. One nursing study focused on Type B behavior (Thomas, 1986). The nursing research has been incorporated within the context of research addressing Type A behavior and CHD for each of the topics in the previous sections.

➤ CONCLUSION AND FUTURE RESEARCH

The preponderance of evidence supports the relationship between Structured Interview (SI) appraisal of Type A behavior and CHD morbidity and mortality. There is strongest evidence for a relationship between SI-assessed Type A behavior and atherosclerosis. Other measures of Type A behavior appear to be measuring separate but often related constructs. Currently, the videotaped SI is considered to be the "gold standard" for assessing Type A behavior. It appears that altering Type A behavior is effective in reducing CHD-associated risk. The preponderance of the research was conducted using middle-class men. Additional research is required to extend these findings to women, minorities, and diverse socioeconomic groups.

Two components of Type A behavior, speech stylistics and hostility, are thought to be the toxic components of the behavior pattern. There is ample evidence that rapid speech is characteristic of Type A behavior and that reducing rate of speech reduces cardiovascular reactivity, a suspected mechanism for the pathogenesis of CHD, even among Type A individuals. Hostility appears to be a separate construct from SI-assessed Type A behavior, although some aspects may be embedded within Type A behavior, especially when measured with the Jenkins Activity Survey (JAS). Hostility and other psychological constructs, such as anxiety and depression, also have been implicated in the development of and recovery from CHD. In addition to Type A behavior, hostility, depression, and anxiety are significant predictors of CHD incidence (Friedman, 1996; Matthews, 1988). The relative gains through interventions to address all these psychological factors as mechanisms to reduce incidence, slow progression, and decrease mortality from CHD deserve further investigation.

There is evidence that environmental factors influence Type A behavior development in children and that it is possible to alter Type A behavior in children before they reach adolescence. Currently, however, there are no data relating childhood Type A behavior as assessed with the MYTH to SI-assessed Type A behavior in adulthood or to CHD in adulthood. This area merits further investigation.

Because Type A behavior has been identified as a preventable risk factor for CHD and cardiovascular mortality (Review Panel, 1981), appropriate interventions to ameliorate it at the primary and secondary prevention stages have the potential to slow or stop the progression of CHD. Nurses can identify Type A behavior through behavioral evaluations such as the MYTH and the SI for children, adolescents, and adults before clinical signs of disease are apparent. Although research is necessary to document the utility of interventions for reducing CHD risk among Type A children, there is sufficient evidence that multicomponent interventions, including behavior modification and support, can reduce CHD-associated risk among adults. Nurses' interventions to support patients' health by modifying Type A behavior can impact CHD morbidity and mortality.

➤ REFERENCES

Anderson, N. B., Williams, R. B., Jr., Lane, J. D., Hanley, T., Simpson, S., & Houseworth, S. J. (1986).

Type A behavior, family history of hypertension and cardiovascular responsivity among black women. *Health Psychology, 5,* 393-406.

Audy, R. J. (1971). Measurement and diagnosis of health. In *Environmental essays on the planet as home.* Boston: Houghton Mifflin.

Barefoot, J. C., Dahlstrom, W. G., & Williams, R. B. (1983). Hostility, CHD incidence, and total mortality: A 25 year follow-up study of 255 physicians. *Psychosomatic Medicine, 45,* 59-63.

Barefoot, J. C., Dodge, K. A., Peterson, B. I., Dahlstrom, W. G., & Williams, R. B. (1989). The Cook-Medley Hostility Scale: Item content and ability to predict survival. *Psychosomatic Medicine, 51,* 46-57.

Blumenthal, J. A., Lake, J. D., & Williams, R. B. (1985, Summer). The inhibited power motive, Type A behavior and patterns of cardiovascular response during the structured interview and thematic apperception test. *Journal of Human Stress,* 82-92.

Booth-Kewley, S., & Friedman, H. S. (1987). Psychological predictors of heart disease: A quantitative review. *Psychological Bulletin, 101,* 343-362.

Bortner, R. W. (1969). A short rating scale as a potential measure of pattern A behavior. *Journal of Chronic Disease, 20,* 525-533.

Brown, M. S., & Tanner, C. (1990). Measurement of Type A behavior in preschoolers. *Nursing Research, 39,* 207-211.

Buselli, E. F., & Stuart, E. M. (1999). Influence of psychosocial factors and biopsychosocial interventions on outcomes after myocardial infarction. *Journal of Cardiovascular Nursing, 13,* 60-72.

Byrne, D. G., Rosenman, R. H., Schiller, E., & Chesney, M. A. (1985). Consistency and variation among instruments purporting to measure the Type A behavior pattern. *Psychosomatic Medicine, 47,* 242-260.

Cohen, J. B., & Reed, D. (1985). Type A behavior and coronary heart disease among Japanese men in Hawaii. *Journal of Behavioral Medicine, 8,* 343-352.

Contrada, R. J., & Krantz, D. S. (1988). Stress, reactivity, and Type A behavior: Current status and future directions. *Annals of Behavioral Medicine, 10,* 64-74.

Cook, W. W., & Medley, D. M. (1954). Proposed hostility and pharisaic-virtue scales for the MMPI. *Journal of Applied Psychology, 38,* 414-418.

Corse, C. D., Manuck, S. B., Cantwell, J. D., Giordani, B., & Matthews, K. A. (1982). Coronary prone behavior and cardiovascular response in persons with and without coronary heart disease. *Psychosomatic Medicine, 44,* 449-459.

DeBacker, G., Kornitzer, M., Kittel, F., & Dramaix, M. (1983). Behavior, stress, and psychosocial traits as risk factors. *Preventive Medicine, 12,* 32-36.

Dembroski, T. M., MacDougall, J. M., Costa, P. T., & Grandits, G. A. (1989). Components of hostility as predictors of sudden death and myocardial infarction in the multiple risk factor intervention trial. *Psychosomatic Medicine, 45,* 59-63.

Dembroski, T. M., MacDougall, J. M., Williams, Hanley, T. L., & Blumenthal, T. A. (1985). Components of Type A, hostility, and anger in relationship to angiographic findings. *Psychosomatic Medicine, 47,* 219-233.

Eaker, E. D., Abbot, R. D., & Kannel, W. B. (1989). Type A behavior and uncomplicated angina pectoris in men and women: The Framingham Study. *American Journal of Cardiology, 63,* 1042-1045.

Engle, G. L. (1977). The need for a new medical model: A challenge for biomedicine. *Science, 196,* 129-136.

Engle, G. L. (1980). The clinical application of the biopsychosocial model. *American Journal of Psychiatry, 137,* 535-544.

Engler, M. B., & Engler, M. M. (1995). Assessment of the cardiovascular effects of stress. *Journal of Cardiovascular Nursing, 10,* 51-63.

Forgays, D. K., & Forgays, D. G. (1991). Type A behavior within families: Parents and older adolescent children. *Journal of Behavioral Medicine, 14,* 325-339.

Frank, K. A., Heller, S. S., Kornfeld, D. S., Sporn, A. A., & Weiss, M. B. (1978). Type A behavior and coronary angiographic findings. *Journal of the American Medical Association, 240,* 761-763.

Fredrikson, M., & Blumenthal, J. A. (1992). Serum lipids, neuroendocrine and cardiovascular responses to stress in healthy Type A men. *Biological Psychology, 34,* 45-58.

French-Belgian Collaborative Group. (1982). Ischemic heart disease and psychological patterns: Prevalence and incidence studies in Belgium and France. *Advances in Cardiology, 29,* 25-31.

Friedman, M. (1969). *The pathogenesis of coronary artery disease.* New York: McGraw-Hill.

Friedman, M. (1996). *Type A behavior and its diagnosis and treatment.* New York: Plenum Press.

Friedman, M., & Rosenman, R. H. (1959). Association of specific overt behavior pattern with blood and cardiovascular findings. *Journal of the American Medical Association, 169,* 1286-1296.

Friedman, M., & Rosenman, R. (1974). *Type A behavior and your heart.* New York: Knopf.

Friedman, M., Thoresen, C. E., Gill, J. J., Ulmer, D., Powell, L. H., Price, V. A., Brown, B., Thompson, L., Rabin, D. D., Breall, W. S., Bourg, E., Levy, R., & Dixon, T. (1986). Alteration of Type A behavior and its effect on cardiac recurrences in postmyocardial infarction patients: Summary results of the recurrent coronary prevention project. *American Heart Journal, 112,* 653-665.

Friedmann, E., Thomas, S. A., Kulick-Ciuffo, D., Lynch, J. J., & Suginohara, M. (1982). The effects of normal and rapid speech on blood pressure. *Psychosomatic Medicine, 44,* 545-552.

Fukunishi, I., Saito, S., & Fujito, K. (1992). Influence of mother-child relationship on the development of the Type A behavior pattern. *Child Psychiatry and Human Development, 22,* 213-220.

Gill, J. J., Price, V. A., Friedman, M., Thorensen, C. E., Powell, L. H., Ulmer, D., Brown, B., & Drews, F. R. (1985). Reduction in Type A behavior in healthy middle aged American military officers. *American Heart Journal, 110,* 503-514.

Glass, D. C. (1977). *Behavior patterns, stress and coronary disease.* Hillsdale, NJ: Lawrence Erlbaum.

Haynes, S. G., & Feinleib, M. (1982). Type A behavior and the incidence of coronary heart disease in the Framingham Heart Study. In H. Denolin (Ed.), *Psychological problems before and after myocardial infarction. Advances in cardiology, 29* (pp. 85-94). Basel: Karger.

Haynes, S. G., Feinleib, M., Levine, S., Scotch, N., & Kannel, W. B. (1978a). The relationship of psychosocial factors to coronary heart disease in the Framingham Study II: Prevalence of coronary heart disease. *American Journal of Epidemiology, 107,* 384-402.

Haynes, S. G., Levine, S., Scotch, N., Feinleib, M., & Kannel, W. B. (1978b). The relationship of psychosocial factors to coronary heart disease in the Framingham Study I: Methods and risk factors. *American Journal of Epidemiology, 107,* 362-383.

Haynes, S. G., & Matthews, K. A. (1988). Review and methodological critique of recent studies on Type A behavior and cardiovascular disease. *Annals of Behavioral Medicine, 10,* 47-59.

Hearn, M. D., Murray, D. M., & Luepker, R. V. (1989). Hostility, coronary heart disease, and total mortality: A 33-year follow-up study of university students. *Journal of Behavioral Medicine, 12,* 105-121.

Jenkins, C. D. (1978). A comparative review of the interview and questionnaire methods in the assessment of coronary prone behavior pattern. In T. Dembroski, S. M. Weiss, J. Shields, S. Haynes, & M. Feinleib (Eds.), *Coronary prone behavior* (pp. 71-88). New York: Springer-Verlag.

Jenkins, C. D., Zyzanski, S. J., & Rosenman, R. H. (1971). Progress toward validation of a computer-scored test for the Type A coronary-prone behavior pattern. *Psychosomatic Medicine, 33,* 193-202.

Jenkins, C. D., Zyzanski, S. J., & Rosenman, R. H. (1979). *Jenkins Activity Survey Form C Manual.* New York: The Psychological Corporation.

Johnston, D. W., & Shaper, A. G. (1983). Type A behavior in British men: Reliability and intercorrelation of two measures. *Journal of Chronic Disease, 36,* 203-207.

Johnston, D. W. (1993). The current status of the coronary prone behaviour pattern. *Journal of the Royal Society of Medicine, 86,* 406-409.

Kawachi, I., Sparrow, D., Kubansky, L. B., Spiro, A., III, Vokonas, P. S., & Weiss, S. T. (1998). Prospective study of a self-report Type A scale and risk of coronary heart disease. *Circulation, 98,* 405-412.

Leon, G. R., Finn, S. E., Murray, D. M., & Bailey, J. M. (1988). Inability to predict cardiovascular disease from hostility scores or MMPI items related to Type A behavior. *Journal of Consulting and Clinical Psychology, 56,* 597-600.

Lindsey, A. M. (1982). Phenomena and physiological variables of relevance to nursing, review of a decade of work: Part I. *Western Journal of Nursing Research, 4,* 343-364.

MacDougall, J. M., Dembroski, T. M., Dimsdale, J. E., & Hackett, T. E. (1985). Components of Type A, hostility, and anger-in: Further relationships to angiographic findings. *Health Psychology, 4,* 137-152.

Matthews, K. A. (1982). Psychological perspectives on the Type A behavior pattern. *Psychological Bulletin, 91,* 293-323.

Matthews, K. A. (1986). *Handbook of stress, reactivity and cardiovascular disease.* New York: John Wiley.

Matthews, K. A. (1988). Coronary heart disease and Type A behaviors: Update on and alternative to the Booth-Kewley and Friedmann (1987) Quantitative Review. *Psychological Bulletin, 104,* 373-380.

Matthews, K. A., & Angulo, J. (1980). Measurement of Type A behavior in children: Assessment of children's competitiveness, impatience-anger, and aggression. *Child Development, 51,* 466-475.

Matthews, K. A., & Haynes, S. G. (1986). Type A behavior pattern and coronary disease risk update and critical evaluation. *American Journal of Epidemiology, 123,* 923-960.

McCranie, E. W., Watkins, L. O., Brandsma, J. M., & Sisson, B. D. (1985). Hostility, coronary heart disease (CHD) incidence, and total mortality: Lack of association in a 25-year follow-up study of 478 physicians. *Journal of Behavioral Medicine, 9,* 119-125.

Meininger, J. C., Hayman, L. L., Coates, P. M., & Gallagher, P. (1988). Genetics or environment? Type A behavior and cardiovascular risk factors in twin children. *Nursing Research, 37,* 341-346.

Meininger, J. C., Hayman, L. L., Coates, P. M., & Gallagher, P. (1998). Genetic and environmental influences on cardiovascular disease risk factors in adolescents. *Nursing Research, 47,* 11-18.

Meininger, J. C., Stashinko, E. S., & Hayman, L. L. (1991). Type A behavior in children: Psychometric properties of the Matthews Youth Test for Health. *Nursing Research, 40,* 221-227.

Mendes de Leon, C. F., Powell, L. H., & Kaplan, B. H. (1991). Change in coronary-prone behaviors in the recurrent coronary prevention project. *Psychosomatic Medicine, 53,* 407-419.

Muller, J. E., Abela, G. S., Nesto, R. W., & Tofler, G. H. (1994). Triggers, acute risk factors and vulnerable plaques: The lexicon of a new frontier. *Journal of the American College of Cardiology, 23,* 809-813.

Nunes, E. V., Frank, K. A., & Kornfeld, D. S. (1987). Psychological treatment for the Type A behavior pattern and for coronary heart disease: A meta-analysis of the literature. *Psychosomatic Medicine, 48,* 159-173.

Osler, W. (1910). The Lumleian lectures on angina pectoris. *Lancet, 1,* 697-702, 839-844, 973-977.

Powell, L. H., Friedman, M., Thoresen, C. E., Gill, B., & Ulmer, D. K. (1984). Can the Type A behavior pattern be altered? A second year report from the Recurrent Coronary Prevention Project. *Psychosomatic Medicine, 46,* 293-314.

Price, V. A. (1982). *Type A behavior pattern: A model for research and practice.* New York: Academic Press.

Ragland, D. R., & Brand, R. J. (1988). Type A behavior and mortality from coronary heart disease. *New England Journal of Medicine, 318,* 65-69.

Rahe, R. M., Ward, H. W., & Hayes, V. (1979). Brief group therapy in myocardial infarction rehabilitation. Three to four year follow-up of a controlled trial. *Psychosomatic Medicine, 41,* 229-242.

Review Panel on Coronary Prone Behavior and Coronary Heart Disease. (1981). Coronary-prone behavior and coronary heart disease: A critical review. *Circulation, 63,* 1199-1215.

Rosenman, R. H. (1978). The interview method of assessment of the coronary prone behavior pattern. In T. M. Dembroski, S. M. Weiss, J. L. Shields, S. G. Haynes, & M. Feinleib (Eds.), *Coronary prone behavior* (pp. 55-69). New York: Springer-Verlag.

Rosenman, R. H. (1983). Coronary-prone behavior pattern and coronary heart disease. Implications for the use of beta-blockers in primary prevention. In R. H. Rosenman (Ed.), *Psychosomatic risk factors and coronary heart disease. Indications for specific preventive therapy.* Bern: Huber.

Rosenman, R. H. (1993). Relationship of the Type A behavior pattern with coronary heart disease. In L. Goldenberger & S. Breznitz (Eds.), *Handbook of stress: Theoretical and clinical aspects* (2nd ed., pp. 449-476). New York: Free Press.

Rosenman, R. H., Brand, R. J., Jenkins, C. D., Friedman, M., Straus, R., & Wurm, M. (1975). Coronary heart diseases in the Western Collaborative Group Study: Final follow-up experience of 8½ years. *Journal of the American Medical Association, 233,* 872-877.

Rosenman, R. H., & Friedman, M. (1961). Association of specific behavior patterns in women with blood and cardiovascular findings. *Circulation, 24,* 1173-1184.

Rosenman, R. H., Friedman, M., Straus, R., Wurm, M., Kositchek, R., Hahn, W., & Werthessen, N. T. (1964). A predictive study of coronary heart disease: The Western Collaborative Group Study. *Journal of the American Medical Association, 189,* 15-22.

Roskies, E., Kearney, H., Spavak, M., Surkis, A., Cohen, C., & Gilman, S. (1979). Generalizability and durability of treatment effects in an intervention program for coronary prone (Type A) managers. *Journal of Behavioral Medicine, 2,* 195-207.

Scherwitz, L., Berton, K., & Leventhal, H. (1977). Type A assessment and interaction in the behavior pattern interview. *Psychosomatic Medicine, 39,* 229-240.

Scherwitz, L., & Canick, J. (1988). Self-reference and coronary heart disease risk. In B. K. Houston & C. R. Snyder (Eds.), *Type A behavior pattern: Research, theory, and intervention* (pp. 146-167). New York: John Wiley.

Schucker, B., & Jacobs, B. (1977). Assessment of behavioral risk for coronary disease by voice characteristics. *Psychosomatic Medicine, 39,* 219-228.

Shekelle, R. B., Gale, M., Ostfeld, A. M., & Paul, O. (1983). Hostility, risk of coronary heart disease, and mortality. *Psychosomatic Medicine, 45,* 109-114.

Siegman, A. W., Anderson, R. A., & Berger, T. (1990). The angry voice: Its effects on the experience of anger and cardiovascular reactivity. *Psychosomatic Medicine, 52,* 631-643.

Smyth, K., Call, J., Hansell, S., Sparacino, J., & Strodtbeck, F. L. (1978). Type A behavior pattern and hypertension among inner-city black women. *Nursing Research, 27,* 30-35.

Smyth, K. A., & Yarandi, H. N. (1992). A path model of type A and type B responses to coping and stress in employed black women. *Nursing Research, 41,* 260-265.

Smyth, K. A., & Yarandi, H. N. (1994). Relative risk of untreated hypertension in type-A employed African American women. *Journal of Human Hypertension, 8,* 89-93.

Sparacino, J., Hansell, S., & Smyth, K. (1979). Type A (coronary-prone) behavior and transient blood pressure change. *Nursing Research, 28,* 198-204.

Sprafka, J. M., Folsom, A. R., Burke, G. L., Hahn, L. P., & Pirie, P. (1990). Type A behavior and its association with cardiovascular risk. *Journal of Behavioral Medicine, 13,* 1-13.

Suarez, E. C., Williams, R. B., Jr., Kuhn, C. M., Zimmerman, E. H., & Schanberg, S. M. (1991). Biobehavioral basis of coronary-prone behavior in middle aged men. Part II: Serum cholesterol, the Type A behavior pattern, and hostility as interactive modulators of physiological reactivity. *Psychosomatic Medicine, 53,* 528-537.

Thomas, S. A., & DeKeyser, F. (1996). Hypertension. *Annual Review Nursing Research, 14,* 3-22.

Thomas, S. A., & Friedmann, E. (1990). Type A behavior and cardiovascular responses during verbalization in cardiac patients. *Nursing Research, 39,* 48-53.

Thomas, S. A., & Friedmann, E. (1994). The cardiovascular effects of rate of verbal communication. *Journal of Cardiovascular Nursing, 9,* 16-26.

Thomas, S. A., & Liehr, P. (1995). Cardiovascular reactivity during verbal communication: An emerging risk factor. *Journal of Cardiovascular Nursing, 9*(2), 1-11.

Thomas, S. A., Liehr, P., DeKeyser, F., & Friedmann, E. (1993). Nursing blood pressure research, 1980-1990: A biopsychosocial perspective. *Image, 25,* 157-164.

Thomas, S. P. (1986). A descriptive profile of Type B personality. *Image, 18,* 4-7.

Thoresen, C. E., Friedman, M., Gill, J. K., & Ulmer, D. K. (1982). Recurrent Coronary Prevention Project: Some preliminary findings. *Acta Medica Scandinavia, 660*(Suppl.), 172-192.

Williams, R. B., Jr., Hanley, T. L., Lee, K. L., Kong, Y., Blumenthal, J. A., & Whalen, R. E. (1980). Type A behavior, hostility, and coronary atherosclerosis. *Psychosomatic Medicine, 42,* 539-549.

Williams, R. B., Jr., Suarez, E. C., Kuhn, C. M., Zimmerman, E. A., & Schanberg, S. M. (1991). Biobehavioral basis of coronary-prone behavior in middle-aged men. Part I: Evidence for chronic SNS activation in Type As. *Psychosomatic Medicine, 53,* 517-527.

CHAPTER 16

The Acute Myocardial Infarction Coping Model

A Midrange Theory

Nancy R. Reynolds and Angelo A. Alonzo

T he Acute Myocardial Infarction Coping Model (Alonzo & Reynolds, 1996a, 1996b, 1997, 1998) provides a framework for understanding acute myocardial infarction (AMI) care-seeking behavior (see Figure 16.1). In this model, it is proposed that the relatively neglected areas of emotional response and social situation are key elements in understanding why individuals may delay seeking definitive health care services following the onset of life-threatening AMI symptoms. This chapter provides an overview of the origins and key elements of the model and an analysis of its utility for nursing research and practice.

➤ ORIGINS

It has been well established that to receive maximal benefit from thrombolytic therapies, individuals who are experiencing an AMI must obtain treatment rapidly. Prompt action not only reduces the mortality rate but also preserves heart function (Berger et al., 1994; Weaver et al., 1993). Even though the advantages of rapid AMI treatment are clear, the time from the onset of acute symptoms of AMI to definitive emergency care is often protracted, and individuals with a prior history of AMI or coronary artery disease (CAD) or both are particularly apt to extend care seeking (Bleeker et al., 1995; Bury et al., 1992; Kenyon, Ketterer, Gheorghiade, & Goldstein, 1991; Roth, Herling, & Vishlitzki, 1995; Wallbridge, Tweddel, Martin, & Cobbe, 1992). Although AMI care-seeking delay has been studied frequently, it is not well understood (Wielgosz & Nolan, 1991). Rather than examining the prehospital period as a time when the individual must actively cope with a difficult-to-assess acute health care crisis that is occurring in the midst of many interacting social, psychological, and cultural processes, researchers have often taken a more narrow clinical approach (Alonzo & Reynolds, 1998).

Research completed in nursing thus far demonstrates how difficult it may be for patients to accurately interpret their AMI symptoms and determine whether to seek care. For example, atypical presentation of cardiac symptoms (Lee, 1997; Lee, Bahler, Taylor, Alonzo, & Zeller, 1998), a mismatch between symptom expectations and actual symptoms experienced (Johnson & King, 1995; Scherck, 1997), and failure to experience or appraise symptoms as serious (Dempsey, Dracup, & Moser, 1995; Dracup & Moser, 1997; Reilly, Dracup, & Dattolo, 1994; Scherck, 1997) have been found to delay AMI care seeking. Although this research provides important insight, there has been minimal consideration of how emotional and social situational processes may influence AMI symptom interpretation and care-seeking behavior.

In the AMI coping model, the problem of extended care seeking during AMI is conceptualized within a broad inclusive theoretical framework that considers the multidimensional features of care seeking and coping and focuses specifically on the importance of emotions and the social situation. The four-phase model was inductively and deductively derived (Alonzo & Reynolds, 1996a, 1996b) from an analysis of empiric and theoretic literature, which concerns mainly self-regulation theory (Leventhal, 1980; Leventhal & Cameron, 1987) and Mead's (1938) conceptualization of the "act." The phases of the AMI coping model are in essence a synthesis of the two conceptualizations as applied to AMI coping. The "act" is a way of conceptualizing the primary structure of our ongoing, emergent social behavior (Mead, 1938). In the Self-Regulation Model, Leventhal and colleagues (Leventhal, 1980; Leventhal & Cameron, 1987) suggest a conceptualization similar to Mead's in which individuals cope with symptoms of illness within a self-regulative systems model. Both conceptualizations

emphasize that relevant self-monitoring information is processed over time.

Since its initial development (Alonzo & Reynolds, 1996a, 1996b), the AMI coping model has been further refined to consider in more detail the role of emotions and coping, the potential of posttraumatic stress disorder (PTSD), and related problems in response to the experience of AMI (Alonzo & Reynolds, 1997, 1998), and the influence of cumulative adversity (Alonzo, 1998, 1999).

➢ ELEMENTS OF THE AMI COPING MODEL

Coping

In the AMI coping model, the individual is viewed as an active problem solver who engages in conscious, and intentional, cognitive and behavioral efforts to manage specific external or internal demands or both that are appraised as taxing or exceeding the resources of the individual. This view is consistent with conceptions of coping described by Leventhal and Cameron (1987), Lazarus and Folkman (1984), and Mead (1938). In the AMI model, particular emphasis is placed on the relationship that the individual has with both internal and external environments, namely, his or her body and the surrounding socially defined situation as described by Ball (1972). Coping efforts are regarded as either problem focused or focused on emotional regulation (Leventhal & Cameron, 1987), where problem-solving efforts are viewed as attempts to do something constructive about stressful conditions and emotion-focused coping is viewed as an effort to regulate the emotional consequences of the stressful event. In both coping circumstances, internal biophysiological and emotional stressors produced by the experience of symptoms have exceeded the resources of the individual (Lazarus & Folkman, 1984) and become a taxing and potentially traumatic experience (Goldberger, 1983). The process of attempting to restore balance in the situation of an impending AMI is conceptualized in terms of four phases of coping (Figure 16.1): impulse and cognitive recognition, perception and covert action plan, overt manipulation, and assessment and consummation.

Phases of Coping

Phase I: Impulse and Cognitive Recognition

The primary substantive process of Phase I is symptom recognition and labeling. Phase I begins when the individual experiences a symptomatic impulse or stimuli that distinguishes itself from background expectancies (Alonzo, 1979) and that exceeds normal expectations in a manner compelling enough that it is not easily ignored. The labeling process requires that symptoms are placed within an understandable framework or, as Leventhal (Leventhal, 1980; Leventhal & Cameron, 1987) suggests, an illness representation—the cognitive structure by which individuals organize, analyze, and interpret information.

Memories are thought to be a significant aspect of illness representations. Memories reflect the individual's past experiences and include affective, emotional responses, such as those associated with AMI, and the more common abstract and conceptual information about symptoms and signs provided by health care professionals or associations (e.g., the American Heart Association's, 1992, warning symptoms of a heart attack). Illness representations involve beliefs about possible associated symptoms, the cause of the disease, how long it lasts, how it might be treated and cured, and likely sequelae (see Chapter 20, this volume).

Phase I ends when the individual has a tentative label or a hypothesis regarding the meaning of the symptoms and proceeds to address the demands of the symptom representation in terms of developing a coping strategy. Central to developing a strategy are knowledge, behaviors, and efforts to regulate emotional arousal (Alonzo & Reynolds, 1998).

Phase II: Perception and Covert Action Plan

The primary process in the second phase is covert construction, manipulation, and assessment of strategies to cope with symptoms. Covert coping means constructing a "line of action" (Blumer, 1969) directed toward establishing a stable relationship with symptoms and what Mead (1938) referred to as the "collapsed act," meaning that the individual engages in covert reflective analysis to determine how to achieve restoration of equilibrium.

In the case of symptoms, the individual examines his or her environment for possible causes, explanations, consequences, remedies, strategies, or all of these to make them stable and predictable. In this context, predictable and stable mean that symptoms will be lessened in intensity or frequency, made predictable in terms of their reoccurrence or being associated with a treatment regimen, brought below an acceptable threshold of attention or emotional arousal, or all of these. For Mead (1938), the collapsed act is a "subjective substitute for an objective reality" (p. 122) with which one anticipates having contact. In the current context, if the individual perceives signs and symptoms to be of a noncardiac, respiratory problem, his or her covert coping activities could include thinking about using an inhaler (if he or she is an asthma patient) or possibly calling a friend who sometimes complains of shortness of breath for information. Alternatively, if the individual is a cardiac patient, he or she may try to recall a prior cardiac event and mentally run through his or her past symptoms, problem solving, and resources, whether lay or medical.

As the result of symptoms and covert coping, the individual is now in a new and more sensitive relationship with his or her environments (biophysical, social situational, psychological or cognitive, and emotional). Covert action requires the use of knowledge and perceived behavioral resources immediately available to the individual, more distant

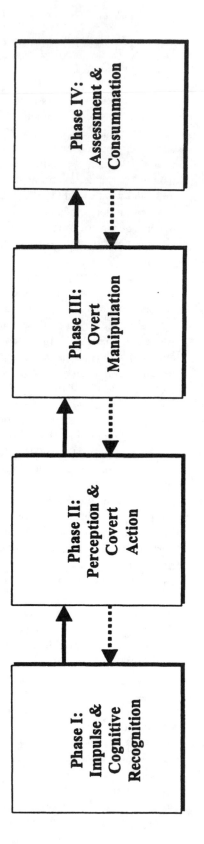

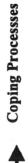

Figure 16.1. Phases of the Acute Myocardial Infarction (AMI) Coping Model

resources possessed by lay others, and the medical resources of physicians and other health care providers such as nurses.

Phase III: Overt Manipulation

Phase III is characterized by overt behavior, manipulation, and recursive reassessment. Manipulation is the locus of reality for Mead (Natanson, 1956) and can prove to be extremely time-consuming (Alonzo, 1980; Hartford, Karlson, Sjölin, Holmberg, & Herlitz, 1993). In essence, the coping line of action constructed covertly is now implemented, and in so doing the individual is constantly testing, revising, and reconstructing lines of action. As symptoms evolve, change, or reoccur, and if overt manipulation is not effective, the processes of impulse relabeling and covert actions are revisited and can occur simultaneously as the individual and lay others attempt to manipulate the environment to cope with the stressful event of symptoms and emotional arousal.

Covertly constructed behavioral strategies are overtly implemented to establish a predictable and stable relationship with the symptoms. As overt coping develops, the individual and lay others are constantly evaluating whether instrumental efforts and resources are effective, whether available information is accurate and consistent with their ongoing experiences and representations, and whether emotional and affective responses to symptoms and the emerging coping efforts are under control and, particularly for lay others, not blocking instrumental coping and assessment. If, in the course of behavioral coping, problems or additional impulses occur, the individual may return to Phases I and II to modify his or her illness representations, behavior, knowledge, or emotional regulation so that consummation can occur.

Following up on the prior respiratory example of Phase II, if the signs and symptoms are not responding to a respiratory regimen, the individual and those around him or her will return to Phases I and II to relabel signs and symptoms and to construct a new or mod-

ified strategy for coping with the signs and symptoms. The process is recursive in that it continues until some sense of stability or equilibrium is reached, whether clinically appropriate or not.

Phase IV: Assessment and Consummation

In Phase IV, or the consummatory phase, the primary process is the experience of fulfillment or restored equilibrium, fulfillment of covertly constructed strategies, and reduced emotional and affective arousal. Although the assessment and consummation phase conceptualizes the process of restored equilibrium, in a real sense it is an analytic point that is used to highlight the outcome of coping with a single discrete illness event that has occurred within the life course and flow of life course events (Alonzo, 1999). On consummation, the AMI event has been contained by available resources (e.g., stabilizing care obtained in the emergency department) and a measure of equilibrium achieved. In actuality, the individual and others will continue to cope with the consequences of an AMI for a long time.

Emotions and Coping

Each of the phases described previously combines the Meadian and Leventhal conceptions of how individuals cope with a traumatic, turbulent experience in a self-regulatory action scheme. Emotions are thought to have a particularly profound influence on AMI care-seeking behavior. Emotions are regarded as having an involuntary, compelling quality that is mediated through the individual's perception and the situational response to emotions (Safran & Greenberg, 1991). Emotions can be a product of genetically programmed states of arousal and socialized sentiments (Gordon, 1981) that are situationally connected and biophysically independent. At the fundamental organismic and biopsychological level of processing, there is a very basic primary, even primal, response to symptoms normally associated with AMI (e.g., chest pressure, discomfort or pain, left arm pain and tingling, gastrointestinal distress, shortness of breath, lightheadedness and dizziness, perspiration, and overwhelming dread). This may arouse fear, anxiety, or helplessness in the individual that can be quite independent of the socially defined situation. Thus, at an organismic or autonomic and hormonal level (Izard, 1993), symptoms of AMI have the potential to provide a turbulent, traumatic stimuli independent of the individual's constructive propensities. It is this independent stimuli and the arousal produced that are addressed by the AMI coping model. A fundamental assumption is that emotional arousal becomes objectified from the flow of ongoing experience and action. In this sense, the affect control theory (Heise, 1989; MacKinnon, 1994; Smith-Lovin, 1990) is consistent with what is proposed in the context of AMI. Emotional states are the product of the interaction between physiological arousal and cognition about the cause of the arousal. Leventhal (1980) argues, "The problem of the relationship of cognition to emotion should not be reduced to the issue of who is to rule, but how the pair interact to govern" (p. 193).

If we view individuals as being in social situations and assume they desire a stable social identity (Robinson & Smith-Lovin, 1992), then we can understand individuals' cognitive response to symptoms, especially if we assume the primacy of desiring to maintain social situational engagement and participation. MacKinnon (1994) aptly summarizes an appropriate basic understanding of responses to AMI: "[E]motions are episodic, situationally instigated, ephemeral affective experiences with physiological and cognitive components. . . . [Emotions] are cognitive signals, rich in affective meaning, that inform people how they are doing in establishing and validating situated identities in social interaction" (p. 31).

Integrating the strands of emotional conceptualizations from symbolic interaction inspired affect control theory, and Leventhal's (1980) emotion component of self-regulation theory, the convergent point appears to be that emotions are a consequence of a discrepancy between what the individual expects to occur, to experience, to be perceived as, or to engage in and what is actually experienced. In a sense, experiencing symptoms of AMI is a discrepancy in bodily and health expectations in situationally meaningful settings. In Leventhal's conceptualization, the violation of social and emotional schematic expectations is a "critical source of affective experiences and reactions" (p. 187). Emotions come from both the deviation from expectation and the specific meaning of the stimulus. Emotions are thus an evaluation of some part of the world in relation to oneself (Franks & McCarthy, 1989) or, as Hochschild (1990) suggests, in relation to bodily sensations. In a very real sense, symptoms of an AMI and their potential meaning and consequences represent a turbulent, traumatic stimuli that arouses in the individual, and those around him or her, a level of emotional responsiveness requiring an adaptive coping strategy to regain a sense of comfort, normality, or restored situational sentiments regarding the self.

Prior History of AMI and Emotional Coping

Interestingly, individuals with a prior history of AMI and coronary heart disease (CHD) do not tend to seek time-dependent medical care during subsequent episodes of acute coronary disease faster (and frequently do so more slowly) (Bleeker et al., 1995; Leitch, Birbara, Freedman, Wilcox, & Harris, 1989) than individuals who have not experienced a first AMI (Bleeker et al., 1995; Bury et al., 1992; Kenyon et al., 1991; Roth et al., 1995; Turi et al., 1986; Wallbridge et al., 1992). This is problematic because these individuals are at far greater risk for death (Gruppo Italiano per lo Studio Della Streptochinasi Nell'infarto Miocardico, 1992) and increased morbidity. One would expect that prior knowledge and emotional and behavioral experiences would enhance sensitivity and responsiveness to recurrent AMI symptoms; this is often not the case. When this phenomenon is considered within the framework described previously, a possible explanation can be derived.

Individuals with a history of ischemic heart disease have episodic or autobiographical memories (Leventhal & Cameron, 1987) of prior responses to and experiences with symptoms of AMI and CHD diagnostic procedures and their potential meanings and consequences. These experiences may interfere with and preclude expedient care seeking for the following reasons. First, individuals with preexistent disease may have an idiosyncratic illness representation. They may be more likely to mislabel symptoms and signs of subsequent AMIs (Hartford et al., 1993) and find difficulty determining whether they need care (Meischke, Ho, Eisenberg, Schaeffer, & Larsen, 1995), especially if new symptoms are not similar to previous ones (Johnson & King, 1995).

Second, those who have had an AMI and who have participated in cardiac rehabilitation may engage in longer periods of evaluation because the rehabilitation process may encourage a sense of optimism, efficacy, and invulnerability (Wielgosz, Nolan, Earp, Biro, & Wielgosz, 1988). Rehabilitation may contribute to what Weinstein (1988) terms an "optimistic bias," wherein cardiac patients erroneously believe that their own risk is less than that of others because of their participation. Weinstein further indicates that the source of this optimism could also be incorrect information, a need to sustain self-esteem and, as noted previously, to sustain situational participation, or both.

Third, some individuals (as many as 25%; Kutz, Garb, & David, 1988; Kutz, Shabiai, Solomon, Neumann, & David, 1994) may experience a form of Post-Traumatic Stress Disorder (PTSD) (Hanson, 1990) and/ or reactive and secondary alexithymia, a disorder characterized by psychic numbing and inability to process symptomatic information (Taylor, Bagby, & Parker, 1991; von Rad, 1984). The experience of an AMI may be similar in many respects to the reported experiences of assault, domestic abuse, and combat survivors and so on (Wilson, 1984). Individuals with PTSD demonstrate intrusion of past experiences, a desire to avoid stimuli associated with past experiences, increased psychological arousal or hypervigilance, and psychic numbing or ideational constriction (Horowitz, Wilner, & Alvarez, 1979).

There are three traumas of AMI that may contribute to PTSD-like symptoms or alexithymia or both. First is the primary trauma of the insult to the myocardium or heart muscle and related symptoms and signs. Social psychologically, there is the fright and overwhelming dread of the potential loss of life and of social control, of the breakdown of social situations, of a diminished continuity of life, and of future expectations and the assault on ones social identity across many domains. The outcome of an AMI may leave the individual with angina pectoris, or chest pain with exertion, and other disabilities. In addition, and a very significant part of medical treatment, are the relatively invasive experiences of coronary bypass surgery, angioplasty, angiography, pacemaker implantation, stress testing, and the numerous side effects of cardiac medications. In essence, the individual is now diagnosed as having a potentially fatal and life-threatening, possibly terminal, chronic disease.

Next, there are secondary traumas of experiences in accessing and using emergency medical services (EMS) or dialing 911, calling a physician, entering the emergency department (ED), and experiencing hospitalization. Over the long term, becoming a cardiac patient, going through cardiac rehabilitation, changing work and lifestyles, and experiencing repeated physician consultations and medical regimens can become part of the secondary trauma of AMI. Last, at the tertiary level, there are many stressful mini-events of being a patient in the modern health care system. These small but cumulative traumas are the administrative hassles associated with health insurance, workmen's compensation and other disability insurance, hospital and physician billing services, and, if eligible, Medicare and Medicaid.

Individuals who experience repeated traumas are particularly apt to demonstrate a range of maladaptive coping. Fullilove, Lown, and Fullilove (1992), for example, described a "spectrum of posttraumatic disturbances" ranging from anxiety and depression at one end of the spectrum to PTSD at the other. Similarly, Turner and Lloyd (1995) demonstrated that individuals who experienced the "cumulative adversity" of lifetime traumas are at risk for manifesting psychopathologies that, in the context of AMI, could interfere with effective coping. There is an increasing body of evidence linking AMI and depression (Fielding, 1991; Frasure-Smith, Lesperance, & Talajic, 1993). Geyer, Broer, Haltenhof, Buhler, and Merschbacher (1994) also found data to support the connection between adverse event frequency and severity and depression.

Considered within the AMI model of coping, it can be seen that emotion-focused coping impaired by PTSD-like symptomatology or alexithymia could inhibit a timely response to symptoms of AMI within a self-regulatory process. Whether the individual experiences the avoidance of PTSD or the numbness of reactive alexithymia, the result is a dissociative response that obstructs the application of knowledge or the use of problem-focused coping that might facilitate expeditious arrival at the ED during subsequent AMIs or other cardiac events. Furthermore, the traumatogenic potential of AMI may have implications for maladaptive coping during subsequent ischemic events and other comorbidities over the life course (Alonzo, 1998, 1999).

➤ IMPLICATIONS FOR PRACTICE

Consistent with the emphasis of nursing, the AMI coping model stresses the client perspective and the importance of the social situation. The model suggests that an understanding of the clients' response to the threat of AMI is ascertained by understanding their perceptions or implicit models of the threat that may be particularly influenced by prior experiences with the threat of AMI or other chronic health problems or both, priorities strongly influenced by the home context, and untoward emotional reaction.

As represented in Figure 16.2, this framework provides guidance for the development of intervention strategies to reduce care-seeking delay. This conceptualization suggests that if individuals in the midst of the potentially traumatic experience of AMI (particularly those with histories of AMI and CHD) are to call the EMS or arrive at hospital EDs sooner, interventions, whether at the individual or community level, should take into consideration three elements derived from self-regulation theory and the Meadian conceptualization of the act (Leventhal, 1980; Leventhal & Cameron, 1987; Mead, 1938). First, knowledge is needed by the individual and lay others to correctly label symptoms (typical and atypical) as indicative of an AMI. Second, it is necessary to provide feasible behaviors that individuals and lay others can engage in to access definitive medical care (e.g., dialing 911). Last, and perhaps most important, it is necessary to provide an understanding of, and skills to cope with, the primary emotional arousal in regard to the traumatic experience of AMI symptoms. It must be understood that the knowledge and behaviors necessary to obtain effective care may contribute to emotional arousal and paralyze timely action. Thus, the secondary and tertiary arousal engendered by knowledge and behaviors necessary to construct a strategy to cope with the acute AMI illness experience and potential consequences must be addressed.

Issues discussed previously are also relevant to the clinical setting in the early phases of clinical assessment. Although a certain amount of dissociative behavior may be beneficial in the early phases of AMI hospitalization (Croyle & Ditto, 1990; Esteve, Valdes, Riesco, Jodar, & de Flores, 1992; Flowers, 1992; Kenyon et al., 1991), continued anxiousness, depersonalization, and dissociation could be considered indicative of a form of reactive posttraumatic stress syndrome and cumulative adversity syndromes. This assessment would be especially appropriate among

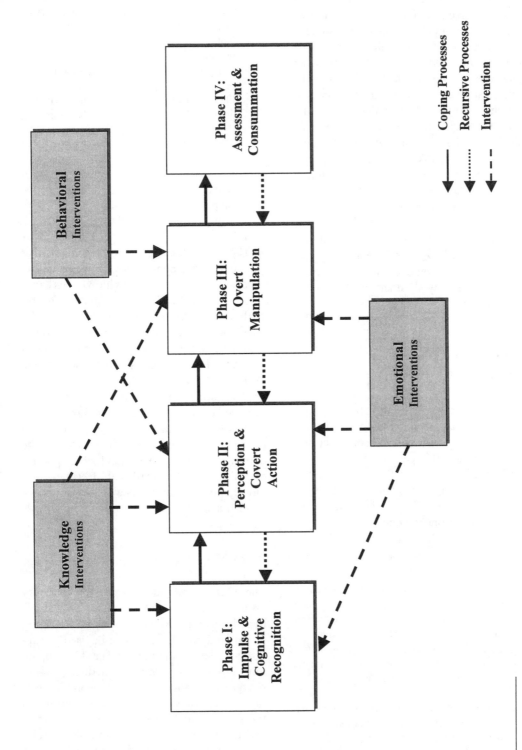

Figure 16.2. Phases of AMI Coping and Interventions

419

patients with a history of cardiovascular disease or other chronic diseases and those with comorbid psychosocial life course experiences. The pursuit of an agenda of systematic patient assessment or screening, and a logical extension into research, could be facilitated by the use of available and validated instruments designed to measure PTSD. Two instruments are currently available. The Mississippi PTSD scale provides a measure of the degree of PTSD in a civilian population (Vreven, Gudanowski, King, & King, 1995), and the Davidson Trauma Scale (Davidson, Book, & Colket, 1997) is suited to screening for PTSD and assessing severity and treatment outcomes when interventions are attempted. Assessing cumulative adversity can be accomplished by using Turner and Lloyd's (1995) scale of adverse events. These instruments are relatively short and easily administered and scored.

➤ IMPLICATIONS FOR RESEARCH

The model has not been directly tested. To date, support has been derived by systematic review of extant literature and empirical studies supporting self-regulation theory and the Meadian conception of the act (Alonzo & Reynolds, 1996a, 1996b, 1997, 1998). From the basic set of conceptualizations, the following propositions are derived:

1. The decision to seek AMI care is a process that occurs over time.
2. Patients and lay others are aware of and can recall their problem-solving and decision-making activities that contributed to their delayed or expeditious AMI care seeking.
3. Emotional responses in the form of fear, anxiety, or dissociation interfere with the use of AMI care-seeking knowledge and behavior.
4. Patients' responses to AMI symptoms will be affected by the social situation in which they initially occur. For example, individuals in the home versus the work environment will delay longer.

5. Individuals with a history of a prior AMI will be more likely to delay AMI care seeking as a consequence of (a) mislabeling AMI symptoms, (b) optimistic bias (if they participated in cardiac rehabilitation), or (c) AMI-related trauma and PTSD.
6. Individuals with a history of comorbidities or cumulative adversity or both will be more likely to delay AMI care seeking as a consequence of (a) mislabeling AMI symptoms, (b) emotional arousal (in the form of fear, anxiety, or dread), or (c) PTSD, or (d) all of these.
7. Knowledge, behaviors, and emotional interventions applied to strategic points in the care-seeking process will be more effective than general educational strategies.

The model lends itself to both qualitative and quantitative approaches to understanding the care-seeking behavior of individuals experiencing an AMI. That is, the model is useful with approaches that focus on the phenomenological experience of the individual client and with approaches that focus on understanding responses across individuals. To understand more fully why sociodemographic variables have not proved to be useful in understanding AMI care-seeking (Dracup et al., 1995), special attention should be given to important subgroups, such as women, the elderly (Turi et al., 1986), and ethnic and racial minorities (Maynard et al., 1991). As previously noted, individuals with a prior history of AMI also require special attention.

➤ SUMMARY

The AMI coping model is a midrange theory (Walker & Avant, 1995) from which testable hypotheses regarding AMI coping can be deduced, and new findings can be used to support and extend the theory. The AMI coping model was inductively and deductively derived from extant empiric and theoretic literature. The following are key assumptions of the model: (a) The individual is an active problem solver who engages in conscious, intentional cognitive and behavioral effort to manage specific external or internal demands or both that are appraised as taxing or exceeding the resources of the individual; (b) individuals desire a stable social situational identity; (c) emotions have an involuntary, compelling quality that is mediated through the individual's perception and situational responses; and (d) emotional arousal becomes objectified from the flow of ongoing experience and action. Key concepts in the model are coping, emotions, cumulative stress, and the phases of AMI coping—impulse and cognitive recognition, perception and covert action plan, overt manipulation, and assessment and consummation. These concepts are defined theoretically and to date have not been operationalized. Relational statements are described but have not been tested. The theory has fairly broad boundaries that have recently been expanded to consider the effects of cumulative adversity on AMI coping processes. The model is complex; it has the potential to be useful to nursing research and practice, however. Although aspects of the model are abstract and difficult to operationalize at this point, several components are testable.

Individuals experiencing symptoms of AMI are in the midst of a potentially traumatic, turbulent emotional experience. Although the advantages of rapid AMI treatment are clear, time from the onset of acute AMI symptoms to definitive emergency care is often protracted, and individuals with a prior history of AMI or CAD or both are particularly apt to delay care-seeking. In specifying emotional response and social reality as key elements, the AMI model of coping provides a health care framework for broadening our understanding of AMI care-seeking behavior.

➤ REFERENCES

Alonzo, A. A. (1979). Everyday illness behavior: A situational approach to health status deviations. *Social Science and Medicine, 13A,* 397-402.

Alonzo, A. A. (1980). Acute illness behavior: A conceptual exploration and specification. *Social Science and Medicine, 14A,* 515-526.

Alonzo, A. A. (1998, April). *The experience of chronic illness and post-traumatic stress disorder: Understanding coping behavior.* Paper presented at the an-

nual meeting of the Pacific Sociological Association, San Francisco.

Alonzo, A. A. (1999). Acute myocardial infarction and post-traumatic stress disorder: The consequences of cumulative adversity. *Journal of Cardiovascular Nursing, 13,* 33-45.

Alonzo, A. A., & Reynolds, N. R. (1996a). Emotions and care-seeking during acute myocardial infarction: A model for intervention. *International Journal of Sociology and Social Policy, 16,* 97-122.

Alonzo, A. A., & Reynolds, N. R. (1996b). Care-seeking during acute myocardial infarction: A model for intervention. *Research in the Sociology of Health Care, 13B,* 393-409.

Alonzo, A. A., & Reynolds, N. R. (1997). Responding to symptoms and signs of acute myocardial infarction: How do you educate the public? *Heart & Lung, 26,* 263-272.

Alonzo, A. A., & Reynolds, N. R. (1998). The structure of emotions during acute myocardial infarction. *Social Science & Medicine, 46,* 1099-1110.

American Heart Association. (1992). *Heart attack* [Pamphlet]. Dallas, TX: Author.

Ball, D. W. (1972). The definition of the situation: Some theoretical and methodological consequences of taking W. I. Thomas seriously. *Journal for the Theory of Social Behavior, 2,* 61-82.

Berger, P. B., Bell, M. R., Holmes, D. R., Gersh, B. J., Hopfenspirger, M., & Gibbons, R. (1994). Time to reperfusion with direct coronary angioplasty and thrombolytic therapy in acute myocardial infarction. *American Journal of Cardiology, 73,* 231-236.

Bleeker, J. K., Simons, M. L., Erdman, R. A. M., Leenders, C. M., Kruyssen, H. A. C. M., Lamers, L. M., & Van Der Does, E. (1995). Patient and doctor delay in acute myocardial infarction: A study of Rotterdam, the Netherlands. *British Journal of General Practice, 45,* 181-184.

Blumer, H. (1969). *Symbolic interaction: Perspective and method.* Englewood Cliffs, NJ: Prentice Hall.

Bury, G., Murphy, A. W., Power, R., Daly, S., Mehigan, C., & Walsh, J. P. (1992). Awareness of heart attack signals and cardiac risk markers amongst the general public in Dublin. *Irish Medical Journal, 85,* 90-91.

Croyle, R., & Ditto, P. H. (1990). Illness cognition and behavior: An experimental approach. *Journal of Behavioral Medicine, 13,* 31-52.

Davidson, J. R., Book, S. W., & Colket, J. T. (1997). Assessment of a new self-rating scale for posttraumatic stress disorder. *Psychological Medicine, 27,* 153-160.

Dempsey, S. J., Dracup, K., & Moser, D. K. (1995). Women's decision to seek care for symptoms of acute myocardial infarction. *Heart & Lung: The Journal of Acute and Critical Care, 24,* 444-456.

Dracup, K., & Moser, D. K. (1997). Beyond sociodemographics: Factors influencing the decision to seek treatment for symptoms of acute myocardial infarction. *Heart & Lung: The Journal of Acute and Critical Care, 26,* 253-262.

Dracup, K., Moser, D. K., Eisenberg, M., Meischke, H., Alonzo, A. A., & Braslow, A. (1995). Causes of delay in seeking treatment for heart attack symptoms. *Social Science & Medicine, 40,* 379-392.

Esteve, L. G., Valdes, M., Riesco, N., Jodar, I., & de Flores, T. (1992). Denial mechanisms in myocardial infarction: Their relations with psychological variables and short-term outcome. *Journal of Psychosomatic Research, 36,* 491-496.

Fielding, R. (1991). Depression and acute myocardial infarction: A review and reinterpretation. *Social Science and Medicine, 32,* 1017-1027.

Flowers, B. J. (1992). The cardiac denial of impact scale: A brief, self-report research measure. *Journal of Psychosomatic Research, 36,* 469-475.

Franks, D. D., & McCarthy, E. D. (Eds.). (1989). *The sociology of emotions: Original essays and research papers.* Greenwich, CT: JAI.

Frasure-Smith, N., Lesperance, F., & Talajic, M. (1993). Depression following myocardial infarction: Impact on 6-month survival. *Journal of the American Medical Association, 270,* 1819-1825.

Fullilove, M. T., Lown, A., & Fullilove, R. E. (1992). Crack 'hos and skeezers: Traumatic experiences of women crack users. *Journal of Sex Research, 29,* 275-287.

Geyer, S., Broer, M., Haltenhof, H., Buhler, K. E., & Merschbacher, U. (1994). The evaluation of life event data. *Journal of Psychosomatic Research, 38,* 823-835.

Goldberger, L. (1983). The concept and mechanisms of denial: A selective overview. In S. Breznitz (Ed.), *The denial of stress.* New York: International University Press.

Gordon, S. L. (1981). Sociology of sentiments and emotion. In M. Rosenberg & R. H. Turner (Eds.), *Social psychology sociological perspectives* (pp. 562-592). New York: Basic Books.

Gruppo Italiano per lo Studio Della Streptochinasi Nell'infarto Miocardico. (1992). Six-month survival in 20,891 patients with acute myocardial infarction randomized between alteplase and streptokinase with or without heparin. *European Heart Journal, 13,* 1692-1697.

Hanson, R. (1990). The psychological impact of sexual assault on women and children: A review. *Annals of Sex Research, 3,* 187-232.

Hartford, M., Karlson, B. W., Sjölin, M., Holmberg, S., & Herlitz, J. (1993). Symptoms, thoughts, and environmental factors in suspected acute myocardial infarction. *Heart and Lung, 22,* 64-70.

Heise, D. (1989). Effects of emotion displays on social identification. *Social Psychology Quarterly, 52,* 10-21.

Hochschild, A. R. (1990). Ideology and emotion management: A perspective and path for future research. In T. Kemper (Ed.), *Research agendas in the sociology of emotions.* Albany: State University of New York Press.

Horowitz, M., Wilner, N., & Alvarez, W. (1979). Impact of Event Scale: A measure of subjective stress. *Psychosomatic Medicine, 41,* 209-218.

Izard, C. (1993). Four systems for emotional activation: Cognitive and noncognitive processes. *Psychological Review, 100,* 68-90.

Johnson, J. A., & King, K. B. (1995). Influence of expectations about symptoms on delay in seeking treatment during a myocardial infarction. *American Journal of Critical Care, 4,* 29-35.

Kenyon, L. W., Ketterer, M. W., Gheorghiade, M., & Goldstein, S. (1991). Psychological factors related to prehospital delay during acute myocardial infarction. *Circulation, 84,* 1969-1976.

Kutz, I., Garb, R., & David, D. (1988). Post-traumatic stress disorder following myocardial infarction. *General Hospital Psychiatry, 10,* 169-176.

Kutz, I., Shabiai, H., Solomon, Z., Neumann, M., & David, D. (1994). Post-traumatic stress disorder in myocardial infarction patients: Prevalence study. *Israel Journal of Psychiatry and Related Sciences, 31,* 48-56.

Lazarus, R. S., & Folkman, S. (1984). *Stress, appraisal, and coping.* New York: Springer.

Lee, H. (1997). Typical and atypical clinical signs and symptoms of myocardial infarction and delayed seeking of professional care among blacks. *American Journal of Critical Care, 6,* 7-15.

Lee, H., Bahler, R., Taylor, A., Alonzo, A., & Zeller, R. A. (1998). Clinical symptoms of myocardial infarction and delayed treatment-seeking behavior in blacks and whites. *Journal of Applied Biobehavioral Research, 3,* 135-159.

Leitch, J. W., Birbara, T., Freedman, B., Wilcox, I., & Harris, P. J. (1989). Factors influencing the time from onset of chest pain to arrival at the hospital. *Medical Journal of Australia, 150,* 6-8.

Leventhal, H. (1980). Toward a comprehensive theory of emotion. *Advances in Experimental Social Psychology, 13,* 139-207.

Leventhal, H., & Cameron, L. (1987). Behavioral theories and the problem of compliance. *Patient Education and Counseling, 10,* 117-138.

MacKinnon, N. J. (1994). *Symbolic interactionism as affect control.* Albany: State University of New York Press.

Maynard, C., Litwin, P. E., Martin, J. S., Cerqueira, M., Kudenchuk, P. J., Ho, M. T., Kennedy, J. W., Cobb, L. A., Shaeffer, S. M., Hallstrom, A. P., & Weaver, W. D. (1991). Characteristics of black patients admitted to coronary care units in metropolitan Seattle: Results from the Myocardial Infarction Triage and Intervention Registry (MITI). *American Journal of Cardiology, 67,* 18-23.

Mead, G. H. (1938). *The philosophy of the act.* Chicago: University of Chicago Press.

Meischke, H., Ho, M. T., Eisenberg, M. S., Schaeffer, S. M., & Larsen, M. P. (1995). Reasons patients with chest pain delay or do not call 911. *Annals of Emergency Medicine, 25,* 193-197.

Natanson, M. (1956). *The social dynamics of George H. Mead.* Washington, DC: Public Affairs Press.

Reilly, A., Dracup, K., & Dattolo, J. (1994). Factors influencing prehospital delay in patients experiencing chest pain. *American Journal of Critical Care, 3,* 300-306.

Robinson, D., & Smith-Lovin, L. (1992). Selective interaction as a strategy for identity maintenance: An affect control model. *Social Psychology Quarterly, 55,* 12-28.

Roth, A., Herling, M., & Vishlitzki, V. (1995). The impact of "Shahal" (a new cardiac emergency service) on subscribers' requests for medical assistance: Characteristics and distribution of calls. *European Heart Journal, 16,* 129-133.

Safran, J., & Greenberg, L. (1991). *Emotion, psychotherapy, and change.* New York: Guilford.

Scherck, K. A. (1997). Recognizing a heart attack: The process of determining illness. *American Journal of Critical Care, 6,* 267-273.

Smith-Lovin, L. (1990). Emotion as the confirmation and disconfirmation of identity: An affect control model. In T. Kemper (Ed.), *Research agendas in the sociology of emotions.* Albany: State University of New York Press.

Taylor, G. J., Bagby, R. M., & Parker, J. D. A. (1991). The alexithymia construct: A potential paradigm for psychosomatic medicine. *Psychosomatics, 32,* 153-164.

Turi, Z. G., Stone, P. H., Muller, J. E., Parker, C., Rude, R. E., Raabe, D. E., Jaffe, A. S., Hartwell, T. D., Robertson, T. L., Braunwald, E., & the Milis Study Group. (1986). Implications for acute intervention related to time of hospital arrival in acute myocardial infraction. *American Journal of Cardiology, 58,* 203-209.

Turner, R. J., & Lloyd, D. A. (1995). Lifetime traumas and mental health: The significance of cumulative adversity. *Journal of Health and Social Behavior, 36,* 360-376.

von Rad, M. (1984). Alexithymia and symptom formation. *Psychotherapy and Psychosomatics, 42,* 80-89.

Vreven, D. L., Gudanowski, D. M., King, L. A., & King, D. W. (1995). The civilian version of the Mississippi PTSD scale: A psychometric evaluation. *Journal of Traumatic Stress, 8,* 91-99.

Walker, L. O., & Avant, K. C. (1995). *Strategies for theory construction in nursing* (3rd ed.). Norwalk, CT: Appleton & Lange.

Wallbridge, D. R., Tweddel, A. C., Martin, W., & Cobbe, S. M. (1992). The potential impact of patient self-referral on mortality in acute myocardial infarction. *Quarterly Journal of Medicine, 85,* 901-909.

Weaver, W. D., Cerqueira, M., Hallstrom, A. P., Litwin, P. E., Martin, J. S., Kudenchuk, P. J., & Eisenberg, M. (1993). Prehospital-initiated vs. hospital-initiated thrombolytic therapy. The myocardial infarction triage and intervention trial. *Journal of the American Medical Association, 270,* 1211-1216.

Weinstein, N. D. (1988). The precaution adoption process. *Health Psychology, 7,* 355-386.

Wielgosz, A. T. J., & Nolan, R. P. (1991). Understanding delay in response to symptoms of acute myocardial infarction: A compelling agenda. *Circulation, 84,* 2193-2195.

Wielgosz, A. T. J., Nolan, R. P., Earp, J. A., Biro, E., & Wielgosz, M. B. (1988). Reasons for patient's delay in response to symptoms of acute myocardial infarction. *CMAJ, 139,* 853-857.

Wilson, J. P. (1984). A comparative analysis of posttraumatic stress syndrome among individuals exposed to different stressor events. *Journal of Sociology and Social Welfare, 11,* 793-825.

CHAPTER 17

Hardiness

A Model of Commitment, Challenge, and Control

Marilyn Ford-Gilboe and Judith A. Cohen

n the 1960s, social psychologists began to focus their attention on psychosocial factors, such as personality and behavior, as contributors to the dynamic stress, coping, and health relationship. Kuo and Tsai (1986) wrote, "In contrast to personality theories that hold a passive, reactive view of man, theories proposed by existential psychologists accentuate the strenuous traits of authentic living: competence, appropriate striving, and productive orientation" (p. 137). With this worldview, Kobasa (1979) sought to determine the personality characteristics that helped some people remain healthy (despite high levels of stress) while others became ill. She proposed a constellation of three personality characteristics—control, commitment, and challenge. These aspects of hardiness were proposed to be fundamental aspects of authentic living. Development and examination of the hardiness construct evolved from a 7-year longitudinal study of male business

executives called the Chicago Stress Project (Maddi & Kobasa, 1984). In the original study, business executives were selected for study because it was believed that their leadership roles were very stressful and demanding, and it was clear that not everyone in these roles became ill.

Interestingly, nursing was specifically identified as an area in which there has been much interest in and study of hardiness. (Both a hardiness model and Health-Related Hardiness Scale were developed within the discipline [Pollock, 1986].) Three reasons for this unusual appeal were suggested by Ouelette (1993): Nursing (a) places a high premium on understanding people under stress and their potential to become ill, (b) is intrigued by positive and negative assumptions about personality, and (c) understands the need to recognize environmental demands or stressors placed on its clients.

➤ HISTORICAL EVOLUTION OF THE HARDINESS CONSTRUCT

The concept of hardiness evolved from existential psychology. It is considered that humans search for authenticity by creating personal meaning through self-reflection, decision making, and actions that promote personal growth. Stressful life events are inevitable challenges that provide opportunities for growth and the development of authenticity (Kobasa, 1979; Maddi & Kobasa, 1984). Drawing from previous work in the field (e.g., Antonovsky, 1979), Kobasa conceptualized hardiness as a constellation of three personality characteristics—control, commitment, and challenge—that were fundamental to authentic living. The control component of hardiness relates to a person's belief in his or her ability to influence or to manage life events. The opposite of control is powerlessness. The second component, commitment, refers to active engagement in daily living and having a clear purpose in life. The opposite of commitment is alienation. For the final component, challenge, change is considered as a normal part of living and an opportunity for growth and development. The opposite of challenge is threat. When combined, these three qualities form a personality style of stress resistance that Kobasa called hardiness (Kobasa, 1979, 1982; Maddi & Kobasa, 1984).

In addition to the direct (main) consequence of hardiness on health, both moderator (buffering) and mediator (indirect) effects have been proposed. The terms moderator and mediator, however, have been used interchangeably, leading to confusion about the conceptual role of hardiness in stress resistance (Jennings & Staggers, 1994). Maddi and Kobasa (1984) propose that hardiness has direct and indirect (mediating) effects on health outcomes. As a mediator of the relationship between stressful life events and health status, hardiness is thought to promote the use of social resources and to facilitate "transformational coping," an approach to managing stressful life events that results in less strain

and, ultimately, reduced illness and enhanced well-being.

Transformational coping involves changing stressful life events by altering them directly or by thinking about them optimistically. This is reflected in identifying new ways of managing situations, developing and carrying out a plan of action, and mobilizing resources. In contrast, "regressive coping" involves avoiding experiences with stressful life events and thinking about them pessimistically (Maddi & Kobasa, 1984). The effect of transformational coping on health status is further mediated by the health practices of the individual. Evidence to support both direct and mediating effects of hardiness on health status has been found in a variety of studies, whereas there is considerably less support for the buffering or moderating effects of this construct (Jennings & Staggers, 1994; Orr & Westman, 1990; Tartasky, 1993).

Although evidence for the effect of hardiness on health outcomes exists and the appeal of this concept is quite apparent, Kobasa's work has been highly criticized regarding several unresolved conceptual and methodological issues. Key concerns include (a) the question of applicability of the generic concept of hardiness (developed primarily from samples of male executives) to women, persons of lower socioeconomic status, and those with health problems; (b) whether hardiness is a single concept with three underlying components or three distinct concepts; (c) reliance on self-reports of health status in most studies—such reports may be inaccurate or biased; (d) unresolved measurement problems regarding the use of negatively worded indicators to measure the positive components of control, commitment, and challenge; (e) persistent psychometric problems for many different instruments used to measure hardiness and inconsistency in scoring of these measures; (f) inappropriate use of analysis of variance (ANOVA) and analysis of covariance (ANCOVA) for data analyses; and (g) the need to more fully address how hardiness develops or evolves over time, including the conditions under which it can be learned and modified (Funk, 1992; Funk & Houston, 1987; Huang, 1995; Hull, Van Treuren, & Virnelli, 1987; Jennings & Staggers, 1994; Low, 1996; Orr & Westman, 1990; Pollock, 1989a; Tartasky, 1993; Wagnild & Young, 1991). In-depth discussions of these issues are available in the works cited previously.

➤ HEALTH-RELATED HARDINESS

In an attempt to overcome some of the difficulties identified by critics of Kobasa's work, Pollock (1986), a nurse scientist, proposed the construct of health-related hardiness (HRH). Although conceptualization of HRH was derived from Kobasa's work, it differs from the more generic concept in two ways. First, Pollock proposes health-specific definitions of the three dimensions of hardiness that differ from Kobasa's more general conceptualizations. Commitment is defined as involvement in health-related activities appropriate for dealing with health stressors. Control refers to the use of ego resources to appraise, interpret, and respond to health stressors. Finally, challenge reflects reappraisal of the health stressors as potentially beneficial or rewarding rather than threatening or harmful (Pollock, 1989a).

Second, Pollock extended Kobasa's work by situating HRH within an adaptation framework synthesized from the works of Selye (1956), Lazarus (1966), and Roy (1976). The Adaptation to Chronic Illness Framework (Figure 17.1) provides a reference point for investigating human responses to chronic illness (Pollock, 1986, 1989a). Consistent with Roy's conceptual model, Pollock proposes that an individual's level of adaptation is a function of both the type and the severity of the focal stimuli (the chronic illness), contextual stimuli (other stressors in the situation), and residual stimuli (stressors from other life experiences, not clearly definable) (Pollock, 1989a). Furthermore, the impact of these stimuli on adaptation is dependent on the person's perception of the chronic illness. Thus, in Pollock's model, hardiness may affect ad-

aptation to chronic illness both directly and indirectly through its interaction with characteristics of the person and the health stressor (Pollock, 1989a).

Pollock's research has focused on examining contextual factors, including HRH, involvement in health promotion activities, coping style, use of social resources, and ability to tolerate stress as well as the perceived severity of chronic illness as mediators of the relationship between the stress engendered by chronic illness and both physiological and psychosocial adaptation (Pollock 1989a, 1993; Pollock, Christian, & Sands, 1990).

➤ FAMILY HARDINESS

Family hardiness, an emerging concept, extends Kobasa's concept of individual hardiness to the family system. Family hardiness, a strength that mediates the relationship between stressful life events and family adaptation, is proposed to consist of four components: (a) control—the family's sense of control over life events, (b) challenge—the family's perception of change as an opportunity to learn and grow, (c) commitment—the family's active orientation in adapting to stressful situations, and (d) confidence—the family's ability to endure life experiences with a sense of interest and meaning (McCubbin, McCubbin, & Thompson, 1991). Although the first three of these dimensions are conceptually similar to both hardiness and HRH, the confidence dimension is a unique aspect of family hardiness.

The concept of family hardiness was originally developed as part of the Family Stress, Coping, and Health Project at the University of Wisconsin-Madison. Within the Resiliency Model of Family Stress, Adjustment, and Adaptation (McCubbin & McCubbin, 1993), the most recent theory to evolve from this work, family hardiness is considered a resistance resource. Resistance resources are capabilities of the family that are drawn on to manage the stressor so that a crisis is averted and family adjustment is promoted

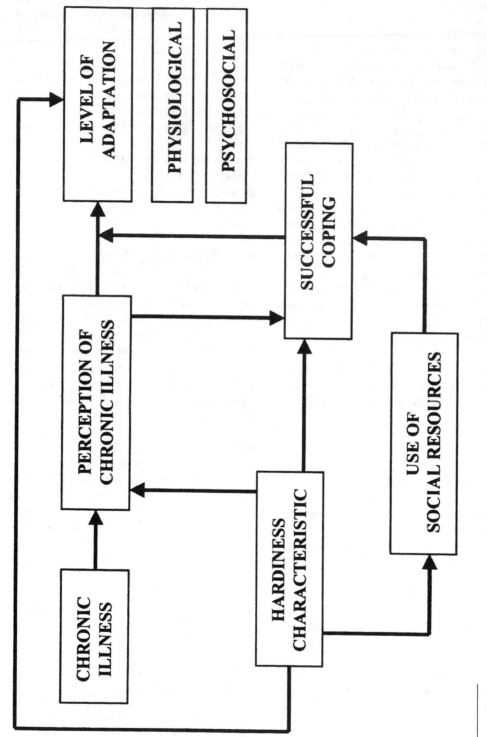

Figure 17.1. Adaptation to Chronic Illness Framework (adapted with permission from S. Pollock, "The Hardiness Characteristic: A Motivating Factor in Adaptation." *Advances in Nursing Science, 11*(2), 53-62. © 1989 Aspen Publishers)

(McCubbin & McCubbin, 1993). Thus, hardy families are more likely to be proactive in changing life events, to learn from them, and to incorporate these changes into their pattern of living (McCubbin et al., 1991). For a more detailed discussion of the Resiliency Model of Family Stress, Adjustment, and Adaptation, see Chapter 12 in this volume.

➢ MEASURES OF HARDINESS

The Hardiness Scale

Kobasa (1979) initially developed a composite scale composed of six subscales to measure the three components of hardiness. The Alienation From Self and the Alienation From Work scales (Maddi, Kobasa, & Hoover, 1979) were thought to measure commitment. The Security scale and the Cognitive Structure scale of the California Life Goals Evaluation Schedule (Hahn, 1966) assessed challenge. The Powerlessness scale of the Alienation Test (Maddi et al., 1979) and the Locus of Control scale (Rotter, Seeman, & Liverant, 1962) were used to determine control. (The Cognitive Structure scale was eliminated from the instrument after a factor analysis.)

The Hardiness composite measure has had several revisions, resulting in both short forms (20 and 36 items) and a long form (50 items) that are in current use. The second revision led to a 36-item measure based on factor analysis. Consistent with the approach used in the first measure, all of the 36 items are negatively worded. This 36-item short form has been most commonly used in studies conducted by nurse scientists (Johnson-Saylor, 1991; Lambert, Lambert, Klipple, & Mewshaw, 1989, 1990; Magnani, 1990).

In response to criticism about the use of negative indicators to consistently measure control, commitment, and challenge, the recent 50-item version of the Hardiness Scale contains both positive and negative indicators of the hardiness dimensions (Jennings &

Staggers, 1994). Although the development of this third version of the Hardiness Scale is difficult to trace, it has been used in nursing education research (Langemo, 1990; Pagana, 1990). A shortened, 20-item instrument has also been derived from Kobasa's original Hardiness Scale. This tool has been used to examine hardiness and perceived health of rural adults (Lee, 1991). The use of many different versions of Kobasa's tool has been identified as a limitation of her work; it makes comparisons of findings across studies very difficult (Tartasky, 1993).

There is little published information about the reliability or validity of Kobasa's early instruments. Investigators who used the measures have provided limited information. Internal consistency estimates for the initial instrument were in the acceptable range for both commitment ($\alpha = .79-.85$) and control ($\alpha = .88$) but unacceptably low for the challenge dimension ($\alpha = .41-.44$). Test-retest reliability was acceptable for all three components; the range was from .70 to .86 (Maddi et al., 1979).

Reliability estimates found in published studies in which various versions of Kobasa'a instruments have been used provide support for internal consistency of both the total hardiness scores and the commitment subscales ($\alpha = > .70$). For example, for the 36-item instrument, internal consistency has ranged from .72 to .81 for the total score (Lambert et al., 1989, 1990; McCranie, Lambert, & Lambert, 1987) and from .72 to .77 for the commitment subscale (Lambert et al., 1990; Lee, 1991). For the 50-item version, internal consistency was strong for both the total score ($\alpha = .85$) and the commitment subscale ($\alpha = .77$). Similar estimates have been obtained for the 20-item version ($\alpha = .81$ for total score and $\alpha = .72$ for commitment) (Lee, 1991).

Although internal consistency of both total hardiness scores and commitment subscales has been acceptable for each version, there has been more variation in the reliability of the control subscale for both the 36-item ($\alpha = .62-.72$) (Hull et al., 1987; Lambert et al.,

1990) and the 50-item versions ($\alpha = .65$). Reported internal consistency estimates for the challenge subscale have been unacceptably low for the 36-item version ($\alpha = .23-.51$) (Hull et al., 1987; Lambert et al., 1990) but higher for both the 20-item and the 50-item versions ($\alpha = .70$ and .65, respectively) (Jennings & Staggers, 1994).

Content validity has not been reported by Kobasa for any versions of the Hardiness Scale. Furthermore, in factor analyses conducted with various versions of the scale, both two- and three-factor solutions have been found. In subsequent testing, items have loaded inconsistently on the factors identified, suggesting problems with construct validity (Jennings & Staggers, 1994).

The Health-Related Hardiness Scale

The Health-Related Hardiness Scale (HRHS) was developed by Pollock (1986) to measure the presence of HRH in the chronically ill and is based on her theoretical definitions of control, commitment, and challenge. She believed that the three components of hardiness provided general resistance to stress, thereby improving adaptation to chronic illness (Pollock, 1986, 1989a). The HRHS uses a 6-point Likert-type format ranging from "strongly disagree" (1) to "strongly agree" (6).

The original scale contained 48 items— 30 from the Alienation scale (Maddi et al., 1979) and 18 from the Multidimensional Health Locus of Control scales (Wallston, Maides, & Wallston, 1978). Consistent with Kobasa's approach, Pollock initially measured hardiness with negative indicators. Through the phases of testing and development, the number of items on the HRH has changed several times to include 48 items (Pollock, 1986), 42 items (Pollock, 1989a), 40 items (Pollock, 1989a), 51 items (Pollock & Duffy, 1990; Pollock et al., 1990), and 34 items (Pollock & Duffy, 1990).

Beginning with the 42-item version of the HRHS, both positive and negative indicators of hardiness were included. Pollock (1989b) reported higher internal consistency ($\alpha = .80$ for total scale, $\alpha = .82$ for control, $\alpha = .74$ for commitment, and $\alpha = .65$ for challenge) for this version than that reported for Kobasa's Hardiness Scale. Internal consistency reliability estimates for each subsequent version of the HRHS have been in the acceptable range ($\alpha = > .70$) for both the total and subscale scores (Jennings & Staggers, 1994).

The most recent version of the HRHS is the result of factor analysis of the previous 51-item scale using data from 389 persons with chronic illnesses who were part of two larger studies. The resulting 34-item scale contains two moderately correlated factors ($r = .36$) that share 14% of common variance. Factor 1 contains 20 items representing challenge (13 items) and commitment (7 items). Factor 2 is composed of 14 control items. These findings are consistent with the dialogue in which the dimensionality of hardiness has been questioned (Funk & Houston, 1987; Hull et al., 1987; Wagnild & Young, 1991). The 34-item version of the HRH is more internally consistent than previous versions ($\alpha = .91$ for total score, and $\alpha = .87$ for each subscale). Test-retest reliability coefficients during a 6-month interval were reported as $\alpha = .76$ for the total score, $\alpha = .74$ for challenge or commitment, and $\alpha = .78$ for control (Pollock & Duffy, 1990).

Predictive validity of the HRHS has been demonstrated through significant, positive correlations with measures of (a) perceived health status ($r = .28$), (b) engagement in health promotion activities ($r = .23$), (c) use of social support ($r = .45$), and (d) physiological adaptation ($r = .45$) (Pollock 1989a, 1989b). Unlike Kobasa's measures, predictive validity of the challenge subscale of the HRHS has also been demonstrated (Jennings & Staggers, 1994). Evidence of convergent validity of the HRHS has been found through a significant moderate correlation ($r = .54$) between the HRH and Kobasa's Hardiness Scale, suggesting that these measures tap similar, but not identical, concepts (Pollock, 1989b).

Family Hardiness Index

The Family Hardiness Index (FHI) is a 20-item summated rating scale developed to measure the concept of family hardiness—a stress-resistance resource of families. This instrument is one of many developed by McCubbin et al. (1991) as part of their ongoing research program (i.e., the Family Stress, Coping, and Health Project). Because family hardiness is a characteristic of the family unit, items are framed from a "we" rather than "I" orientation. Items are arranged in four subscales that reflect the theoretical dimensions of family hardiness: (a) co-oriented commitment—the family's sense of its strengths, dependability, and ability to work together (8 items); (b) challenge—the family's efforts to be innovative, active, and to learn from experiences (5 items); (c) control—the family's sense of being in control of family life rather than being driven by outside forces (3 items); and (d) confidence—the family's sense of being able to plan ahead and their ability to endure hardships with interest and meaningfulness (4 items). Respondents are asked to rate how well each statement reflects their families using a 4-point Likert-type scale format (*false* = 0, *mostly false* = 1, *mostly true* = 2, and *true* = 4). Nine negatively worded items must be reverse scored. Total and subscale scores are obtained by summing applicable items. Higher scores reflects higher degrees of family hardiness (McCubbin et al., 1991).

Initial testing of the FHI was completed with a sample of 304 nonclinical families at various stages of the family life cycle. Internal consistency was $\alpha = .82$ for the total score and ranged from .73 to .82 for the subscales. In subsequent studies conducted with families with a chronically ill member, internal consistency ranged from .76 to .85 for the total score (Carey, Oberst, McCubbin, & Hughes, 1991;

Donnelly, 1994; Failla & Jones, 1991; Munkres, Oberst, & Hughes, 1992; Oberst, Hughes, Chang, & McCubbin, 1991). Subscale reliabilities reported in two of these studies ranged from .47 to .79 (Donnelly, 1994; Failla & Jones, 1991).

As evidence of concurrent validity of the FHI, positive correlations between total FHI scores and measures of family flexibility ($r = .22$), family time and routines ($r = .23$), and quality of family life ($r = .20$) were reported by the developers (McCubbin et al., 1991). The magnitude of these correlations provides weak support for concurrent validity of the FHI. Stronger evidence, however, has been provided by a substantial correlation ($r = .67$) between the FHI and the Family Functioning Style Scale (Trivette, Dunst, Deal, Hammer, & Propst, 1990).

Construct validity of the FHI was supported through a factor analysis of the 20 items. As hypothesized, the 20 items loaded cleanly on the four predicted factors with item loadings of .51 and higher (McCubbin et al., 1991).

➤ NURSING RESEARCH INVESTIGATING HEALTH-RELATED HARDINESS

The parameters of the literature search for this review included an examination of the Cumulative Index for Nursing and Allied Health Literature (January 1983 to December 1998) using the keyword "hardiness" and a manual search for the years 1980-1983. Articles were included if they were research reports published in American or Canadian journals in which a nurse was the primary author. In all, 29 articles were identified in which nurse researchers investigated the relationships between hardiness and other variables in diverse populations, including hardiness and health status of healthy persons (Conrad, Riedel, & Gibbs, 1990; Johnson-Saylor, 1991; Lee, 1991; Magnani, 1990; Nicholas, 1993), self-care agency of caregivers (Schott-Baer, Fisher, & Gregory, 1995), work stress and burnout in nurses (Boyle, Grap, Younger, & Thornby, 1991; Collins, 1996; Duquette, Kerouac, Sandhu, Ducharme, & Saulnier, 1995; Keane, Ducette, & Alder, 1985; Lambert & Lambert, 1993; Langemo, 1990; McCranie et al., 1987; Rich & Rich, 1987; Simoni & Paterson, 1997; Topf, 1989), nursing students' appraisal of clinical education (Pagana, 1990), and adaptation to illness (Carson & Green, 1992; Cataldo, 1993; Goodwin, 1988; Hamner, 1996; Lambert et al., 1989; Narsavage & Weaver, 1994; Nicholas & Webster, 1993; Oberst et al., 1991; Pollock, 1986, 1989b; Pollock et al., 1990; Ross, 1991). In three articles, a related concept, family hardiness, was examined in caregivers (Carey et al., 1991), cancer patients (Oberst et al., 1991), and families of children with developmental disabilities (Failla & Jones, 1991).

The 13 research articles that examined hardiness and adaptation to illness used a variety of conceptual frameworks. Although Pollock's (1986, 1989a) Adaptation to Chronic Illness Model was the most often used, it was applied in only 4 studies. Other guiding frameworks included Lazarus's model of stress and coping ($n = 1$), Roy's Adaptation Model ($n = 2$), Viktor Frankl's existential theory ($n = 1$), and a combination of stress-depression theory, Pollock's concept of HRH, and the concept of death attitudes ($n = 1$). No specific hardiness framework was identified in 4 of the studies. In the majority (9/13) of the studies, small samples ranging from 30 to 99 participants were used. Three studies used samples of 100 to 125, and 1 study employed a large sample of 289 participants. Participants included persons living with a variety of chronic illnesses: diabetes (Pollock, 1986, 1989b, 1990; Ross, 1991), heart disease or hypertension (Pollock, 1986, 1990), chronic obstructive pulmonary disease (Narsavage & Weaver, 1994), rheumatoid arthritis (Lambert et al., 1989, 1990; Pollock, 1991), renal disease (Goodwin, 1988), multiple sclerosis (Pollock, 1990), cancer, HIV, AIDS-related complex, and AIDS (Carson &

Green, 1992; Nicholas & Webster, 1993; Oberst et al., 1991), and depression (Cataldo, 1993). Although Kobasa's (1979) original work on hardiness was almost exclusively conducted with essentially healthy men, both genders were represented in these clinical samples. Generally, men reported higher levels of hardiness than women. All studies used quantitative research methodology, and most employed correlational designs. Statistical analyses were conducted using correlations, ANOVA, ANCOVA, multiple regression, and discriminant function analysis.

Empirical Support for Pollock's Model

Overall, there is fairly consistent support for Pollock's conceptualization of hardiness. In considering the direct effect of hardiness on adaptation, significant correlations between total hardiness and measures of physiological or psychological adaptation or both were found in all but 1 of the 8 studies in which this relationship was examined. This one study (Goodwin, 1988) reported a low correlation using a very small sample size ($N = 35$), thus leaving room for speculation about the adequacy of statistical power. These findings were upheld regardless of severity of illness in one study (Lambert et al., 1989). In a synthesis of findings from 5 studies, Pollock (1993) reported differences in the pattern of relationships between hardiness and two different types of adaptation (physiological and psychosocial) by diagnosis, although relationships between hardiness and adaptation were found in only three of the four diagnostic groups studied. These findings suggest that hardiness may exert a direct effect on adaptation to chronic illness across diagnostic groups, but that the type of adaptation may vary and be an important consideration.

The relationships found between each of the three dimensions of hardiness and adaptation have been less consistent than the relationships found between overall hardiness and adaptation. These inconsistent findings are a reminder of the continued debate regarding the dimensional structure of hardiness. It has been suggested that hardiness is not a unitary concept and that the dimensions of hardiness need better explication, definition, and measurement (Huang, 1995; Jennings & Staggers, 1994; Tartasky, 1993).

Support for the indirect (mediating) effect of hardiness on adaptation has been provided by significant correlations between hardiness and a variety of intervening variables, including coping, participation in patient education programs, health promotion activities, and social support. In a secondary analysis of data from five samples of persons with chronic illnesses, 34% of the variance in psychosocial adaptation and 21% of the variance in physiological adaptation were accounted for by two different sets of mediating variables (Pollock, 1993). Hardiness and health promotion activities were the only two variables to significantly predict adaptation in both the physiological and the psychological domains. Specifically, involvement in health promotion activities was positively related to physiological adaptation in those with diabetes, multiple sclerosis, and hypertension but not in those with rheumatoid arthritis. Health promotion activities, however, were positively related to psychological adaptation for all groups (Pollock, 1993). In addition to these two variables, perception of disability and ability to tolerate stress predicted psychosocial adaptation in those with diabetes and rheumatoid arthritis, whereas diagnosis and duration of illness predicted physiological adaptation across diagnostic groups. Significant relationships have also been found between HRH and social support in persons with HIV (Nicholas & Webster, 1993) and rheumatoid arthritis (Lambert et al., 1989, 1990).

Stage of Theory Development

The Adaptation to Chronic Illness Model, an elaboration of Roy's Adaptation Model for chronic illness, has provided direction for a program of nursing research aimed at identifying predictors of adaptation to chronic ill-

ness and determining whether relationships between variables differ by diagnostic group (Pollock, 1993). Theoretical and operational levels of the theory have been specified and modified based on research findings. The theory is testable and of moderate scope. Support for hypothesized relationships between theory concepts has been found in studies of persons living with different chronic illnesses (Pollock, 1993). Although the theory was developed to predict adaptation to chronic illness, theory-testing approaches have been based primarily on correlation and its derivatives. Thus, the level of evidence available provides support for the explanatory value of this theory. More definitive theory testing using path analysis or structural equation modeling or both needs to be undertaken to firmly establish the Adaptation to Chronic Illness Model as a predictive theory that could lead to intervention.

➤ IMPLICATIONS FOR RESEARCH AND PRACTICE

With nursing's increasing interest in quality of life, health promotion, and coping with stress, hardiness will continue to have much meaning for its' research and practice. Several theoretical, measurement, and design limitations need to be addressed in future research, however.

Theoretical concerns regarding the definition of hardiness remain unresolved. It is unclear how Kobasa (1979) determined the dimensions of hardiness and whether these dimensions fully capture the essence of hardiness. Pollock's (1986) concept of HRH and subsequent research have been based on Kobasa's work, thereby perpetuating the problem of conceptual imprecision. Given the lack of clarity regarding the construct and the ensuing debate regarding its unidimensionality versus multidimensionality, qualitative studies focused on describing the essence of hardiness and identifying its underlying structure could contribute greatly to resolving current theoretical debates. Findings from qualitative studies would also be useful in differentiating hardiness from other concepts and in developing or refining, or both, the quantitative measures of the concept. Formal concept clarification is essential if the role of hardiness as a stress-resistance resource is to be fully captured and understood.

In reviewing the literature, it is evident that, although some investigators defined hardiness using Kobasa's definition, the HRHS, a measure of health-related hardiness, was used to collect data. The fit between conceptual and operational definitions is an important consideration. Kobasa's instrument is best used to measure the generic concept of hardiness, whereas the HRHS taps health-related hardiness and is best used with individuals who are ill.

With the exception of Pollock's program of research that has examined the chronically ill over time, most studies investigating hardiness have been cross-sectional in nature. Research that explores how hardiness develops and changes over time in relationship to other salient variables is needed. Maddi and Kobasa (1991) examined the conditions in early life that lead to the development of hardiness. They found that family atmosphere rather than socioeconomic background leads to a sense of commitment, control, and challenge. Supportive early interventions that demonstrate encouragement and acceptance of children by parents build commitment. Children who feel supported view themselves and the world in a positive and worthwhile way. Early environments permitting mastery build control. When children attempt and accomplish moderately difficult tasks (more difficult than what they can easily perform), they gain a sense of mastery and success and an ability to influence events. Finally, "rich" environments build challenge. Parents who encourage children to view change as interesting and an opportunity for growth help their children to feel challenged rather than threatened.

Future research needs to examine environmental characteristics and stimuli necessary for facilitating hardiness during middle childhood and adolescence and, ultimately,

how coworkers, employers, or mentors can affect the maintenance or enhancement of hardiness in adults. The following are other questions that need to be addressed concerning the development of hardiness: Is there more than one pattern of hardiness depending on where one is in life span development? To what extent is hardiness a relatively stable personality trait or the result of individual context? Can hardiness be taught? If so, how can this best be accomplished, and who should do it? What role can nursing play in the development of HRH?

Also, previous research has mostly used correlational designs, with data being analyzed through ANOVA or ANCOVA. Future research needs to test both Kobasa's and Pollock's models using more advanced methods of statistical analysis, such as path analysis or structural equation modeling.

Pollock (1989a) wrote that "once nurse scientists understand the effects of hardiness and how it promotes health and adaptation in both well individuals and those with health problems, the implications for nursing practice will be limitless" (p. 53). The value of developing and testing interventions aimed at enhancing hardiness for persons learning to cope with the stress of their illnesses is particularly relevant for nursing (Lambert et al., 1989; Pollock, 1993). At a time of increasing focus on technology and dehumanization within the health care system, attention by nurses to the uniqueness of individuals and their needs is absolutely critical. Different kinds of educational or health programs may have to be developed for different levels of hardiness to facilitate adaptation to illness and to enhance quality of life. There is a concomitant need for experimental studies to test interventions aimed at the development of hardiness. If this can be demonstrated, the effect of such interventions on adaptational outcomes and cost could be studied.

Kobasa specifically cites nursing as a "special case" in the study of hardiness. She notes (as quoted in Ouellette, 1993, p. 85), "The attention to hardiness has much to do with nurses' attempts to explicate their distinctive identity as health care professionals." Nurses place a high premium on identifying people who do well in coping with stress, the body-mind-spirit connection, and the need to recognize how the environment and its stressors impact people. At a time when nurses perceive that they have lost control over their practice and over their ability to care for people in a manner reflecting the professional values to which they are committed, the construct of hardiness remains a quintessential focus for the discipline.

➤ REFERENCES

Antonovsky, A. (1979). *Health, stress and coping.* San Francisco: Jossey-Bass.

Boyle, A., Grap, M., Younger, J., & Thornby, D. (1991). Personality hardiness, ways of coping, social support and burnout in critical care nurses. *Journal of Advanced Nursing, 16,* 850-857.

Carey, P., Oberst, M., McCubbin, M., & Hughes, S. (1991). Appraisal and caregiving burden in family members caring for patients receiving chemotherapy. *Oncology Nursing Forum, 18,* 1341-1348.

Carson, V., & Green, H. (1992). Spiritual well-being: A predictor of hardiness in patients with acquired immunodeficiency syndrome. *Journal of Professional Nursing, 8*(4), 209-220.

Cataldo, J. K. (1993). Hardiness and depression in the institutionalized elderly. *Applied Nursing Research, 6*(2), 89-91.

Collins, M. A. (1996). The relation of work stress, hardiness, and burnout among full-time hospital staff nurses. *Journal of Nursing Staff Development, 12*(2), 81-85.

Conrad, K., Riedel, J., & Gibbs, J. (1990). Effect of work site health promotion programs on employee absenteeism. *AAOHN Journal, 38*(12), 573-580.

Donnelly, E. (1994). Parents of children with asthma: An examination of family hardiness, family stressors and family functioning. *Journal of Pediatric Nursing, 9*(6), 398-408.

Duquette, A., Kerouac, S., Sandhu, B. K., Ducharme, F., & Saulnier, P. (1995). Psychosocial determinants of burnout in geriatric nursing. *International Journal of Nursing Studies, 32*(5), 443-456.

Failla, S., & Jones, L. C. (1991). Families of children with developmental disabilities: An examination of family hardiness. *Research in Nursing and Health, 14,* 41-49.

Funk, S. C., & Houston, B. K. (1987). A critical analysis of the hardiness scale's validity and utility. *Journal of Personality and Social Psychology, 53,* 572-578.

Goodwin, S. (1988). Hardiness and psychosocial adjustment in hemodialysis clients. *ANNA Journal, 15*(4), 211-216.

Hahn, M. (1966). *California life goals evaluation schedule.* Palo Alto, CA: Western Psychological Services.

Hamner, J. B. (1996). Preliminary testing of a proposition from the Roy adaptation model. *Image: Journal of Nursing Scholarship, 28*(3), 215-220.

Huang, C. (1995). Hardiness and stress: A critical review. *Maternal-Child Nursing Journal, 23*(3), 82-89.

Hull, J. G., Van Treuren, R. R., & Virnelli, S. (1987). Hardiness and health: A critique and alternative approach. *Journal of Personality and Social Psychology, 53,* 518-530.

Jennings, B. M., & Staggers, N. (1994). A critical analysis of hardiness. *Nursing Research, 43*(5), 274-281.

Johnson-Saylor, M. (1991). Psychosocial predictors of healthy behavior in women. *Journal of Advanced Nursing, 16,* 1164-1171.

Keane, A., Ducette, J., & Alder, D. (1985). Stress in ICU and non-ICU nurses. *Nursing Research, 34*(4), 231-236.

Kobasa, S. (1979). Stressful life events, personality and health: An inquiry into hardiness. *Journal of Personality and Social Psychology, 37,* 1-11.

Kobasa, S. (1982). Commitment and coping in stress resistance among lawyers. *Journal of Personality and Social Psychology, 42*(4), 707-717.

Kuo, W. H., & Tsai, Y. M. (1986). Social networking, hardiness, and immigrant's mental health. *Journal of Health and Social Behavior, 27,* 133-149.

Lambert, C., & Lambert, V. (1993). Relationships among faculty practice involvement, perception of role stress and psychological hardiness of nurse educators. *Journal of Nursing Education, 32,* 171-179.

Lambert, V., Lambert, C., Klipple, G., & Mewshaw, E. (1989). Social support, hardiness, and psychological well-being in women with arthritis. *Image: Journal of Nursing Scholarship, 21*(3), 128-131.

Lambert, V., Lambert, C., Klipple, G., & Mewshaw, E. (1990). Relationships among hardiness, social support, severity of illness, and psychological well-being in women with rheumatoid arthritis. *Health Care for Women International, 11,* 159-173.

Langemo, D. (1990). Impact of work stress in female nurse educator. *Image: Journal of Nursing Scholarship, 22*(3), 159-162.

Lazarus, R. S. (1966). *Psychological stress and the coping process.* New York: McGraw-Hill.

Lee, H. (1991). Relationship of hardiness and current life events to perceived health in rural adults. *Research in Nursing and Health, 14,* 351-359.

Low, J. (1996). The concept of hardiness: A brief but critical commentary. *Journal of Advanced Nursing, 24,* 588-590.

Maddi, S., & Kobasa, S. (1984). *The hardy executive: Health under stress.* Chicago: Dorsey.

Maddi, S., & Kobasa, S. (1991). The development of hardiness. In A. Monat & R. Lazarus (Eds.), *Stress and coping: An anthology* (pp. 245-257). New York: Columbia University Press.

Maddi, S., Kobasa, S., & Hoover, M. (1979). An alienation test. *Journal of Humanistic Psychology, 19,* 73-76.

Magnani, L. (1990). Hardiness, self-perceived health and activity among independently functioning older adults. *Scholarly Inquiry for Nursing Practice, 4*(3), 171-183.

McCranie, E., Lambert, V., & Lambert, C. (1987). Work stress, hardiness, and burnout among hospital staff nurses. *Nursing Research, 36*(6), 374-378.

McCubbin, M., & McCubbin, H. (1993). Families, coping and illness: The resiliency model of family stress, adjustment and adaptation. In C. Danielson, B. Hamel-Bissell, & P. Winstead-Fry (Eds.), *Families, health & illness: Perspectives on coping and intervention* (pp. 21-63). St. Louis, MO: C. V. Mosby.

McCubbin, M., McCubbin, H., & Thompson, A. (1991). Family hardiness index. In H. I. McCubbin & A. Thompson (Eds.), *Family assessment inventories for research and practice* (2nd ed., pp. 127-133). Madison: University of Wisconsin System.

Munkres, A., Oberst, M., & Hughes, S. (1992). Appraisal of illness, symptom distress, self-care burden and mood states in patients receiving chemotherapy for initial and recurrent cancer. *Oncology Nursing Forum, 19*(8), 1201-1209.

Narsavage, G. L., & Weaver, T. E. (1994). Physiologic status, coping, and hardiness as predictors of outcomes in chronic obstructive pulmonary disease. *Nursing Research, 43*(2), 90-94.

Nicholas, P. K. (1993). Hardiness, self-care practices and perceived health status in older adults. *Journal of Advanced Nursing, 18*(7), 1085-1094.

Nicholas, P. K., & Webster, A. (1993). Hardiness and social support in human immunodeficiency virus. *Applied Nursing Research, 6*(3), 132-135.

Oberst, M., Hughes, S., Chang, A., & McCubbin, M. (1991). Self-care burden, stress appraisal and mood among persons receiving radiotherapy. *Cancer Nursing, 14*(2), 71-78.

Orr, E., & Westman, M. (1990). Does hardiness moderate stress and how? A review. In M. Rosenbaum (Ed.), *Learned resourcefulness: On coping skills, self-control and adaptive behavior* (pp. 64-94). New York: Springer.

Ouelette, S. C. (1993). Inquiries into hardiness. In L. Goldberger & S. Breznitz (Eds.), *Handbook of stress: Theoretical and clinical aspects* (2nd ed., pp. 77-100). New York: Free Press.

Pagana, K. (1990). The relationship of hardiness and social support to student appraisal of stress in an initial clinical nursing situation. *Journal of Nursing Education, 29*(6), 255-261.

Pollock, S. (1986). Human responses to chronic illness: Physiologic and psychosocial adaptation. *Nursing Research, 35*(2), 90-96.

Pollock, S. (1989a). The hardiness characteristic: A motivating factor in adaptation. *Advances in Nursing Science, 11*(2), 53-62.

Pollock, S. (1989b). Adaptive responses to diabetes mellitus. *Western Journal of Nursing Research, 11*(3), 265-280.

Pollock, S. (1993). Adaptation to chronic illness: A program of research for testing nursing theory. *Nursing Science Quarterly, 6*(2), 86-92.

Pollock, S., Christian, B., & Sands, D. (1990). Responses to chronic illness: Analysis of psychological and physiological adaptation. *Nursing Research, 39,* 300-304.

Pollock, S., & Duffy, M. (1990). The health-related hardiness scale: Development and psychometric analysis. *Nursing Research, 39*(4), 218-222.

Rich, V., & Rich, A. (1987). Personality hardiness and burnout in female staff nurses. *Image: Journal of Nursing Scholarship, 19*(2), 63-66.

Ross, M. (1991). Hardiness and compliance in elderly patients with diabetes. *Diabetic Educator, 17*(5), 372-375.

Rotter, J. B., Seeman, M., & Liverant, S. (1962). Internal vs. external locus of control of reinforcement: A major variable in behavior therapy. In N. F. Washburne (Ed.), *Decisions, values, and groups* (pp. 473-516). London: Pergamon.

Roy, C. (1976). *Introduction to nursing: An adaptation model.* Englewood Cliffs, NJ: Prentice Hall.

Schott-Baer, D., Fisher, L., & Gregory, C. (1995). Dependent care, care-giver burden, hardiness, and self—Care agency of caregivers. *Cancer Nursing, 18*(4), 299-305.

Selye, H. (1956). *The stress of life.* New York: McGraw-Hill.

Simoni, P. S., & Paterson, J. J. (1997). Hardiness, coping, and burnout in the nursing workplace. *Journal of Professional Nursing, 13,* 178-185.

Tartasky, D. S. (1993). Hardiness: Conceptual and methodological issues. *Image: Journal of Nursing Scholarship, 25*(3), 225-229.

Topf, M. (1989). Personality, hardiness, occupational stress, and burnout in critical care nurses. *Research in Nursing and Health, 12,* 179-186.

Trivette, C., Dunst, C., Deal, A., Hammer, A., & Propst, S. (1990). Assessing family strengths and family functioning style. *Topics in Early Childhood Special Education, 10,* 16-35.

Wagnild, G., & Young, H. (1991). Another look at hardiness. *Image: Journal of Nursing Scholarship, 23*(4), 257-259.

Wallston, K., Maides, S., & Wallston, B. (1978). Health-related information seeking as a function of health-related locus of control and health value. *Journal of Research in Personality, 10,* 215-222.

CHAPTER 18

Hope and Hopelessness

Edith D. Hunt Raleigh

ascination with the phenomenon of hope dates back to the Bible. Hope for a better future and salvation is a hallmark of the Scriptures. St. Paul characterized hope as the essence of faith: "But hope that is seen is no hope at all. Who hopes for what he already has? But if we hope for what we do not yet have, we wait for it patiently" (Romans 8: 24-25, New International Version). A 17-century Dutch philosopher and theologian, Baruch de Spinoza (as cited in Bernard, 1977), defined hope as a joy that comes from past or future images when something is in doubt. In the late 20th century, theoretical and scientific interest in the concept of hope has developed among investigators and clinicians in psychology, medicine, and nursing.

Although there are a variety of conceptualizations of hope, there is agreement on the essential characteristics of the concept. Hope, a factor in coping, is future oriented and considered to be multidimensional by most theorists. It enables an individual to cope with a stressful situation by expecting a positive out-come. Because a positive outcome is expected, the individual is motivated to act in the face of uncertainty. There are differences in conceptualizations with regard to whether hope has both state and trait components, whether it exists on a continuum with hopelessness, and whether it is an antecedent, a strategy, or an outcome of coping (Raleigh & Boehm, 1994).

Hope is rarely discussed without considering hopelessness and vice versa; the relationship between these concepts is rarely explicated, however. In the psychology literature, many authors have linked hopelessness with negative emotions. Some, such as Beck (1963, 1967) and Bernard (1977), identify hopelessness as a core characteristic of depression and suicidal behavior (Alloy, Abramson, Metalsky, & Hartlage, 1988; Beck, Kovacs, & Weissman, 1975; Beck, Weissman, Lester, & Trexler, 1974; Minkoff, Bergman, Beck, & Beck, 1973). In fact, Bernard hypothesized that hope, like depression, may originate from "heredity, physiology and health, environment, and personal and individual orientation—especially the orientation of responsibility" (p. 285). Other authors consider hope and hopelessness to be related but nonlinear concepts (Farran, Herth, & Popovich, 1995) and to exist simultaneously in the same individual (Dufault & Martocchio, 1985). Still others think hope and hopelessness are on a continuum (McGee, 1984; Stotland, 1969). As the various models of hope are examined, these differences will be presented.

The literature search in preparation for the writing of this chapter included books and research and theoretical articles published from 1965 to 1998 by psychologists, physicians, and nurses. Computer and hand searches using Medline and the Cumulative Index for Nursing and Allied Health Literature were used to identify publications with the words "hope" or "hopelessness" in the title or conceptual framework. The focus of the review is nursing models and research; seminal works in psychology were included for background purposes, however. To be included in this review, research articles needed to identify the specific hope model used; therefore, many articles are omitted from this review. Forty-two publications met the review criteria.

Psychologists and physicians presented the earliest explorations of hope in the literature. Later, nurses joined the discussion. The oldest models can be attributed to psychologists, predominately Lynch (1965) and Stotland (1969). Although Lynch and other theorists are frequently mentioned as background for research, Stotland's model is most often cited as the conceptual framework. In addition, instruments to measure hope have been developed using Stotland's model. Consequently, I have selected it for detailed discussion.

➤ MODELS OF HOPE IN PSYCHOLOGY

With the exception of Stotland (1969), the earliest theorists focused their efforts on developing a definition of hope and offering a few propositions without producing an empirically adequate model. Lynch (1965) considered hope to be "the very heart and center of a human being. It is the best resource of man, always there on the inside, making everything possible when he is in action, or waiting to be illuminated when he is ill" (p. 31). He defined hope as the fundamental knowledge that a difficult situation can be worked out and that goals can be reached. Imagining and wishing are not possible for the hopeless. Hopelessness prevents one from imagining beyond the present.

Melges and Bowlby (1969) proposed that "hope and hopelessness reflect a person's estimate of the probability of his achieving certain goals" (p. 690). The individual determines the probability relative to past successes and failures with similar goals. If there is an expectation of success in meeting goals through one's plans of action, hope exists. If failure is predicted, hopelessness exists. Thus, Melges and Bowlby described hope and hopelessness as opposite expectations and self-efficacy as a fundamental component of self-esteem and a major element in determining whether one feels hopeful or hopeless. Hope encompasses goals that are short term or long term and may involve hopefulness about short-term goals simultaneously with hopelessness about long-term goals.

Stotland's Model of Hope

The publication of Ezra Stotland's book, *The Psychology of Hope* (1969), revolutionized the discussions regarding the concept of hope. Prior to this book, many investigators considered hope and hopelessness to be vague and indistinct concepts that prohibited quantification and systematic study. Through a review of the literature, Stotland developed a theory that portrays hope as an expectation of future goal attainment that is mediated by the importance of the goal for the individual and motivates action to achieve the goal. Expectation of goal attainment and importance of the goal are determinants of motivation. The greater the expectation and the greater the importance of the goal to the individual, the greater will be the effort to achieve the goal. If the goal is important and the individual perceives a low probability of attaining it, anxiety will be experienced. Because there is motivation to avoid anxiety, the greater the anxiety, the more the individual will be motivated to escape it. Hope is a component of adaptive action in a difficult situation, and hopelessness is a factor in maladaptive behavior.

Because Stotland's (1969) model operationalized hope for the first time, many investigators have used it to develop instruments to measure hope and as a framework for their research. In the following sections, brief descriptions of the instruments that have been developed using Stotland's model are provided, and studies that have used the instruments are mentioned. The discussion ends with an analysis of the model. This pattern will be used throughout this chapter. The descriptions are necessarily brief and limited to instruments that use the models described. A summary of published instruments (including those not linked to a model discussed in this chapter) is presented in Table 18.1. For in-depth discussion of instruments and relevant research, refer to *Hope and Hopelessness: Critical Clinical Constructs* (Farran, Herth, et al., 1995).

Instruments Based on Stotland's Model of Hope

Beck Hopelessness Scale. This scale (Beck et al., 1974) is based on Stotland's (1969) conceptualization of hope in that it operationalizes negative expectancies into three dimensions of hopelessness: (a) affective, (b) motivational, and (c) cognitive. It consists of 20 true-false items scored 0 or 1 and summed (range 0-20). Both positive and negative items are used with positive items reverse scored. Higher scores indicate higher levels of hopelessness. The Beck Hopelessness Scale (BHS) was tested with 294 patients hospitalized for recent suicide attempts. A high level of internal consistency was demonstrated (Table 18.1), and concurrent validity was supported by a significant correlation be-

tween clinical ratings of hopelessness and BHS scores. Construct validity was established by the confirmation of hypotheses in several studies (Beck et al., 1974; Minkoff et al., 1973; Vatz, Winig, & Beck, 1969). The BHS has found much use, most notably as a measure of divergent validity for other instruments. It is unidimensional although simple to administer, and it has well-established reliability and validity.

The Hope Scale. This scale (Erickson, Post, & Paige, 1975) was the first to be based on Stotland's (1969) conceptualization of hope. It consists of 20 future goals "common in our society" (p. 324). In the first section, subjects rate the importance of each goal on a 7-point scale. In the second section of the scale, subjects rate the same items on a 0 to 100 scale of probability of occurrence. The scale was tested for stability with psychiatric patients (Table 18.1). Construct validity was assessed through hypotheses tested as described later. The Hope Scale focuses on one dimension of hope and has limited applicability to use in diverse populations because the goals are common for individuals in adulthood through midlife. The scales of 1 to 7 and 0 to 100 are cumbersome and difficult for subjects.

Stoner Hope Scale. Conceptualizations for the Stoner Hope Scale (SHS; Stoner, 1982) include works by Stotland (1969), Lynch (1965), and Marcel (1967). It is a revision of the Hope Scale (Erickson et al., 1975) and consists of 30 goals, 10 for each domain (Global, Interpersonal, and Intrapersonal). Both the importance and the probability sections have a 4-point scale, and scores are obtained by multiplying the probability score by the importance score for each goal. Summing the products for the appropriate items produces the subscale scores and total hope score. Divergent validity was assessed with the BHS producing a significant negative correlation (Table 18.1). A high level of internal consistency was also reported. Although developed to be a multidimensional scale, the SHS has not undergone factor analysis. It is

(text continued on page 443)

TABLE 18.1 Selected Measures for the Phenomenon of Hope

Measure and Author	Variable(s) Measured	Brief Description	Reliability	Validity	Populations Initially Studied
Hopelessness Scale (Beck, Weissman, Lester, & Trexler, 1974)	Hopelessness based on Stotland's (1969) conceptualization	20 true-false items scored 0 or 1 and summed; possible range, 0-20	Internal consistency: Cronbach's alpha = .93	Predictive: support for hypothesized relationships	Hospitalized suicidal patients (N = 294)
Hope Scale (Erickson, Post, & Paige, 1975)	Hope using Stotland's (1969) conceptualization of expectation of goal attainment	20 goals common in our society rated on importance (1; 7-point scale) and probability of occurrence (P; 100-point scale)	Stability: test-retest (1 week); (1) r = .79 and (P) r = 78	Predictive: support for hypothesized relationships	Undergraduate college students (N = 140); male psychiatric patients (N = 100)
Stoner Hope Scale (Stoner, 1982)	Hope using Stotland's (1969) conceptualization and adapted from the Hope Scale (Erickson et al., 1975)	30 goals, 10 each domain: global, interpersonal, intrapersonal; 4-point scale for importance and 4-point scale for probability of occurrence; possible total score = 480	Internal consistency: Cronbach's alpha = .93	Divergent: Hopelessness Scale correlation = –.47	Cancer patients (N = 58)
Hopelessness Scale for Children (Kazdin, French, Unis, Esveldt-Dawson, & Sherick, 1983)	Hopelessness using Stotland's (1969) conceptualization and adapted from the Hopelessness Scale	17 true-false items; score range, 0-17	Internal consistency: Cronbach's alpha = .75	Predictive: support of hypothesized findings	Psychiatric inpatient children (N = 66)
Hope Index (Staats, 1989)	Hope using Stotland's (1969) and Beck's (1967) conceptualizations	16 goal statements rated 0-5; degree of desire and expectation for goal; possible scores, 0-400; two subscales: self, other	Internal consistency: Cronbach's alpha = .86 Stability: test-retest (3½-9 weeks) r = .60	Concurrent criterion-related: satisfaction with life = .41; optimism = .37 Divergent: Hopelessness Scale –.47 Construct: factor analysis supported two factors (subscales)	Undergraduate students (N = 234) Healthy adults in community (N = 303)

Instrument	Conceptual Basis	Description	Reliability	Validity	Sample
Snyder Hope Scale (Snyder et al., 1991)	Hope based on Stotland's (1969) work	12 items on a 4-point scale; possible scores, 12-48	Internal consistency: Cronbach's alpha = .71-76 Stability: test-retest (8 weeks) r = .73, (3-week) r = .85	Criterion-related with self-esteem (r = .58), expectancy for success (r = .55), life experience (r = .54), and life orientation (r = .60) Divergent: Hopelessness Scale r = -.51	Healthy adults and adults with psychiatric illnesses (N = 2,753)
Multidimensional Hope Scale (Raleigh & Boehm, 1994)	Hope based on Stotland's (1969) work	Adapted from Stoner Hope Scale (Stoner, 1982); 37 items on 4-point scale for importance and 4-point scale for probability of occurrence of goal; weighted probability score; possible range, -222 to 222 Six subscales: civic interest, health, spirituality, self-actualization, resource to others, social support	Internal consistency: Cronbach's alpha, total scale = .95; subscales = .77-92 Stability: (2-week) r = .82	Construct: factor analysis confirmed six factors (subscales) Divergent: Hopelessness Scale r = -.45	Adults with chronic conditions in the community (N = 450)
Miller Hope Scale (Miller & Powers, 1988)	Hope using theological, philosophical, psychological, socioanthropological, biological, and nursing literature	40 items on a 5-point scale; possible scores, 40-200 Three subscales: satisfaction with self, others, and life; avoidance of hope threats; anticipation of a future	Stability: test-retest (2-week) r = .82 Internal consistency: Cronbach's alpha = .93; subscales = .82-.91	Divergent: Hopelessness Scale correlation = -.54 Criterion-related: psychological well-being = .71; existential well-being = .82 Construct: factor analysis supported three factors (subscales)	College students (N = 522)
Hopefulness Scale for Adolescents (Hinds & Gattuso, 1991)	Hope using Hinds's (1984) conceptualization of hope	24-Item visual analog scale; possible scores, 0-2,400; consists of two alternate forms	Internal consistency: Cronbach's alpha = .76-94	Construct: reported claimed but no findings published	Healthy, acutely ill, and chronically ill adolescents (N = 400)

(continued)

TABLE 18.1 Continued

Scale	Concept/Definition	Items	Reliability	Validity	Sample
Herth Hope Scale (HHS; Herth, 1991)	Hope using Dufault and Martocchio model	30 items rated on a 4-point summated scale; possible scores, 0-90. Subscales: temporality and future, positive readiness and expectancy, interconnectedness	Internal consistency: Cronbach's alpha = .75-89. Stability: test-retest (3 weeks) r = .89-.91	Construct: factor analysis supported three hypothesized factors (see subscales)	Pretest with adult cancer patients (N = 60). Healthy adults (N = 185), elderly in community (N = 40), elderly widow(er)s (N = 75)
Herth Hope Index (Herth, 1992)	Hope using Dufault and Martocchio model	Shortened version of the HHS. 12 items on a 4-point scale; three subscales of HHS	Internal consistency: Cronbach's alpha = .94-.98. Stability: (2-week) r = .91	Concurrent criterion-related with HHS r = .92. Construct: factor analysis confirmed three factors (subscales)	Acutely ill, chronically ill, and terminally ill adults (N = 172)
Gottschalk Hope Scale (Gottschalk, 1974)	Hope = a measure of optimism that a favorable outcome is likely to occur	Content analysis of 5-minute speech samples; scale has seven categories weighted 1 or -1	Interrater reliability: Cronbach's alpha = .85	Predictive: Studies demonstrated significant differences in mental health crisis group versus normative adult group	Psychiatric outpatients (N = 68)
Hope Index Scale (Obayuwana et al., 1982)	Hope using an aggregation of theories and concepts found in literature	60 yes-no items; score range, 0-500	Internal consistency: Kuder-Richardson's formula 20 = .61	Divergent: Hopelessness Scale correlation = -.88	Graduate students (N = 150). Psychiatric patients (N = 150)
Geriatric Hopelessness Scale (Fry, 1984)	Hopelessness derived from interviews with subclinically depressed elderly adults	30 true-false items; score range, 0-30	Internal consistency: Cronbach's alpha = .69-.71. Spearman-Brown split-half reliability = .70-.73	Construct: factor analysis supported four factors. Predictive: support for hypothesized relationships with depression and self-esteem	Older adults in the community (N = 78)
Nowotny Hope Scale (Nowotny, 1989)	Hope using psychological, theological, psychiatric, and nursing literature	29 items on a 4-point scale (reduced from 47 items). Six subscales: active involvement, confidence, relates to others, spiritual beliefs, comes from within, future is possible	Internal consistency: Cronbach's alpha, total scale = .90; subscales = .51-75	Divergent: Hopelessness Scale = -.47. Construct: factor analysis confirmed six factors (subscales)	Healthy adults (N = 156). Cancer patients (N = 150)

limited by the scoring system that produces the same score for a goal that is important as that for one that is not as important when the probabilities are reversed.

Hopelessness Scale for Children. The BHS was the model for the development of the Hopelessness Scale for Children (HSC; Kazdin, French, Unis, Esveldt-Dawson, & Sherick, 1983). The BHS was reworked to be appropriate for children 6 years of age or older. It contains 17 dichotomous (true-false) items with scores that range from 0 to 17 (higher scores mean greater hopelessness). A high level of internal consistency was demonstrated (Table 18.1) With a sample of 66 psychiatric inpatient children, validity was established with moderate to high correlations between hopelessness and lower self-esteem and greater severity of depression. As with the BHS, this scale is unidimensional. In addition, there is a need to explore the relationship between hope and developmental level. The HSC may have some limitation for young children because of reading level.

Hope Index. The conceptual framework for Staats's (1989) Hope Index (HI) is derived from Stotland's (1969) and Beck's (1967) work. The 16 goal statements of the HI are rated by respondents on a 6-point scale for degree of desire for the goal and degree of expectation for attaining the goal. Eight of the goals are "personally-focused" and 8 are "other-focused." A score is obtained by multiplying the desire score by the expectation score and summing the 16 items. The higher the score, the higher the level of hope. Internal consistency is adequate, and stability is moderate (Table 18.1). Concurrent criterion-related validity was also demonstrated to be moderate. Divergent validity was assessed by a significantly negative correlation with the BHS. Factor analysis supported the two subscales of self and other. The HI is consistent with its conceptual framework. Although the HI is brief, the instructions and appearance are somewhat complex and limit its use.

Snyder Hope Scale. Another tool based on Stotland's (1969) work, the Snyder Hope Scale (SNHS; Snyder et al., 1991), consists of 12 items on a 4-point scale. Four items assess goal-directed determination, 4 assess planning ways to achieve the goal, and 4 are fillers. In samples of healthy adults and adults with psychiatric illnesses, internal consistency and stability were evaluated (Table 18.1). Concurrent validity was established with positive correlations between SNHS and measures of self-esteem, expectancy for success, life experience, and life orientation. Divergent validity was assessed by a negative correlation with the BHS. The SNHS is promising as a clinical measure because of its brevity and simplicity. It is limited in its dimensions because it is confined to rational goals and omits relational or spiritual goals.

Multidimensional Hope Scale. This scale (Raleigh & Boehm, 1994) was adapted from the SHS and is based on Stotland's (1969) theory of hope. It consists of 37 items on 4-point scales for importance of the goal and perceived probability of occurrence. A weighted probability score for each item, which makes zero the midpoint (score $- 2.5 =$ weighted score), is multiplied by each importance score. Subscale scores and total hope scores are produced by summation of the cross-products for each item. The Multidimensional Hope Scale (MDHS) was tested with community-based adults with chronic conditions. High levels of internal consistency and stability were demonstrated (Table 18.1). Divergent validity was established by a correlation with the BHS. Factor analysis resulted in a six-factor solution. These six factors comprise the subscales of civic interest, health, spirituality, self-actualization, social support, and resource to others. The MDHS expands to include dimensions not assessed by some other instruments. Its usefulness in the clinical setting is limited due to its length and complexity in scoring.

Research That Used Stotland's Model

The literature search resulted in several studies that were based on Stotland's (1969) model. The proposed relationship between hopefulness and mental health has been supported by studies involving hospitalized psychiatric patients and college students (Erickson et al., 1975) in which significant relationships were found between lower levels of hope and psychopathology and greater anxiety. Similarly, in community-based older adults (Farran & McCann, 1989; Farran & Popovich, 1990) and geropsychiatric inpatients (Farran, Wiken, & Fidler, 1995), the best predictors of hope were mental health, social support, physical health, and activities of daily living. In addition, hope has been positively related to social function and morale (Rideout & Montemuro, 1986).

Stotland's (1969) model of hope has also been used in studies of populations with physical illnesses. In support of Stotland's (1969) proposition that hope is a component of adaptive action, significant positive relationships have been found between the level of hope and the level of coping (Herth, 1989) and strong religious convictions (Brandt, 1987; Herth, 1989; Raleigh, 1992) in adult patients with cancer and other chronic conditions. Unpredictability has been found to be inversely related to hopefulness and motivation (Mishel, Hostetter, King, & Graham, 1984; Staples & Jeffrey, 1997); that is, the greater the unpredictability of a situation, the less the expectation of achievement (or hope) and motivation to act. Support for Stotland's proposition that increased anxiety motivates the individual to try to escape it was found in studies of individuals with a variety of chronic conditions, including cancer (Raleigh, 1992) and geropsychiatric inpatients (Farran, Wiken, et al., 1995). Strategies for improving hopefulness reported by participants included keeping active, participating in religious activities, thinking about other things, and talking with others—all means of distracting one from the source of anxiety.

Researchers have found no significant differences in level of hope based on phase of illness in adults with cancer (Ballard, Green, McCaa, & Logsdon, 1997; Brandt, 1987; Raleigh, 1992; Stoner & Keampfer, 1985). This may suggest no support for the proposition that hope is perceived probability of goal attainment; it may be a function of what the patient perceives as the goal, however. Raleigh (1992) found that patients at different stages of illness reported hopes with different timelines. Those who were terminally ill tended to focus on hopes in the short term; nevertheless, they considered themselves very hopeful.

Analysis of Stotland's Model of Hope

Stotland's (1969) model of hope has been widely used and tested by nurse researchers and psychologists, leading to significant support for many relationships in the model. According to Walker and Avant (1995), "A theory is an internally consistent group of relational statements that presents a systematic view about a phenomenon and that is useful for description, explanation, prediction, and/or control" (p. 26). Stotland's model of hope provides an understanding of the concept that meets these requirements. The model is logically adequate in that predictions can be and have been made from it. Several researchers have tested these predictions, and they make sense and there are no obvious logical fallacies. Stotland's model has proved to be useful. It has been used to develop several measures of hope and hopelessness, and it has been used by many researchers as a conceptual framework. It is broadly generalizable to various populations and situations as demonstrated by the variety of research it has generated. It also has parsimony in that it can be described using few concepts and relationships, but it is broad in its application. If the theory is to be empirically testable, the components of the model must have operational definitions (Fawcett, 1984). Stotland initiated the study of hope by being the first to operationalize it. As a result, many studies have been conducted that demonstrate that the model also has empirical adequacy.

➤ MODELS OF HOPE IN NURSING

The concept of hope has immediate application for nursing practice. In the process of caring for the whole individual, the presence or absence of hopefulness is evident to the nurse. Anecdotally, nurses report instances in which hopefulness or hopelessness appeared to impact the client outcome. The North American Nursing Diagnosis Association (NANDA) recognizes the nursing diagnosis of hopelessness, which is defined as "a state in which an individual sees limited or no alternatives or personal choices available and is unable to mobilize energy on his/her behalf" (Kim, McFarland, & McLane, 1997, p. 41). Conceptualizations of hopefulness and hopelessness began to appear in the nursing literature long before NANDA developed hopelessness as a diagnosis. Two of the earliest nurse authors in this area were Travelbee (1971) and Lange (1978). In the early 1980s, nurses began to use hope models in their research.

Travelbee (1971) addressed hope and hopelessness in discussing the critical care nurse's role. She proposed that "hope is something halfway between knowing and willing" (p. 161) what will happen in the future. It suggests solutions to problems, imparts security in this knowledge, and generates energy that produces motivation to act. On the basis of this definition, Travelbee advocated for the nurse's role in fostering hopefulness in patients. Lange (1978) described the concept of hope and differentiated it from similar concepts of wishing, expectation, and optimism. A model of hope began to take form in nursing with Lange's explication of the hope structure as a process for maintaining hope. Soon after, nurses began to develop and test their models, beginning with Miller (1983). These models are presented in the following sections. Models with supporting subsequent research are detailed in greater depth. Nursing

models without subsequent research are listed in the Appendix for further reference.

Miller's Model of Hope

Miller (1983, 1992) states that hope is a complex multidimensional construct. It is more than goal attainment; it encompasses a state of being. It involves a confident expectation of an ongoing good state or liberation from a difficult situation. Hope exists at three levels that are depicted in Figure 18.1. The first level focuses on superficial wishes, is characterized by shallow optimism, requires little psychic energy to maintain, and produces no despair when it is not actualized. The second level focuses on hoping for relationships, self-improvement, and personal accomplishments and involves greater psychic energy than the first level. If these hopes are not actualized, anxiety results. The third level is related to a desire for relief from suffering, personal trial, or entrapment and involves a total dedication of psychic energy. If the individual perceives that relief is not impending, deep despair or giving up occur.

Miller and Powers (1988) identified 11 essential elements of hope from interviews of critically ill patients. Mutuality and affiliation pertain to interpersonal relationships and the experience of unconditional love. Sense of the possible involves a global attitude that there is potential in life. Avoidance of absolutizing entails allowing flexibility in one's expectations and avoiding an all-or-nothing attitude. Anticipation embraces the confident expectation of some future good combined with acceptance of the need to patiently wait. Establishing and achieving goals are the "objects of one dimension of hope" (p. 418). Psychologic well-being and coping are factors that empower the individual to have the necessary psychic energy. Purpose and meaning in life give the individual something to live for and to receive a sense of satisfaction with life. Freedom is the ability to recognize that the individual can impact an outcome and maintain a positive attitude. Reality surveillance involves cognitive tasks designed to obtain in-

LEVELS OF HOPE

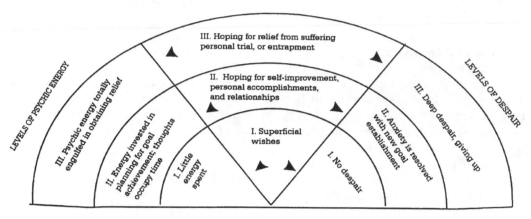

Figure 18.1. Levels of Hope, Despair, and Psychic Energy (From *Coping With Chronic Illness: Overcoming Powerlessness* [p. 415] by J. F. Miller, 1992, Philadelphia: F. A. Davis. Copyright © 1992 [2nd ed.] by F. A. Davis Co. Reprinted with permission.)

formation that confirms the reality of the hope. Optimism is essential for hope. Finally, mental and physical activation encompasses energy that is used to counteract apathy of despair. Miller (1992) proposes that hope may be inspired by others and presents a model that focuses on nursing strategies designed to inspire hope. These are discussed later.

Instrument Based on Miller's Model of Hope

Miller Hope Scale. The Miller Hope Scale (MHS; Miller & Powers, 1988) was derived from Miller's conceptualization of hope. It contains 40 items that are rated on a 5-point scale. Higher scores indicate higher hope. Some items are reverse scored to avoid response set. A high level of internal consistency and stability were demonstrated in a sample of college students (Table 18.1). Criterion-related concurrent validity was assessed by correlations with measures of psychological well-being and existential well-being. Divergent validity was assessed with the BHS. Factor analysis resulted in a three-factor solution: Factor I, satisfaction with self, others, and life; Factor II, avoidance of

hope threats; and Factor III, anticipation of a future. The MHS has been used in numerous studies with adequate to excellent psychometric properties reported (Beckerman & Northrop, 1996; Foote, Piazza, Holcombe, Paul, & Daffin, 1990), and it has been translated into several languages. It may be limited in its clinical use by its length. The items are conceptually consistent with the model.

Research That Used Miller's Hope Model

Many studies have used the MHS as the measure of hope, but most of these used a conceptual framework related to other variables, such as uncertainty, and are therefore not included in this review (Brackney & Westman, 1992; Fehring, Miller, & Shaw, 1997; Irvin & Acton, 1997; McGill & Paul, 1993; Zorn & Johnson, 1997). In addition, some research used Miller's hope model as the conceptual framework but focused on the Hope-Despair model by Miller, a model of hope-inspiring strategies. These are discussed later.

The finding of lower scores on the MHS for a sample of elderly adults living in a long-term care facility compared to those of the young, healthy population used by Miller and Powers (1988) in their original psychometric testing (Beckerman & Northrop, 1996) supports the importance of mutuality and affiliation and establishing and achieving goals in hopefulness. These elements of hope are also supported by the finding of a significant positive correlation between the MHS factor avoidance of hope threats and social support (Hirth & Stewart, 1994).

The roles of psychological well-being and coping in hope are supported by findings of a significant positive correlation between hope and caregiver well-being (Irvin & Acton, 1997). In addition, hope was shown to be a mediator of the relationship between stress and well-being. Although significant positive correlations were found between hope and education and financial status in one study of the elderly (McGill & Paul, 1993), there was no correlation with education in another study (Mishel et al., 1984). Higher education and income would be expected to increase sense of well-being and avoidance of hope threats.

Support for the roles of purpose and meaning in life and mutuality and affiliation can be found in significant positive correlations between religious well-being or intrinsic religiosity and hope (Fehring et al., 1997; Zorn & Johnson, 1997) and self-esteem and social support and hope (Foote et al., 1990). Furthermore, hope accounted for 31% of the variance in religious well-being, the only significant predictor in this study.

A negative correlation between hope and external locus of control suggests that the perception of chance associated with external locus of control reduces perceptions of the ability to attain relief from a personal trial or suffering (Brackney & Westman, 1992). No relationship was found between hope or hopelessness and the measure of internal locus of control.

Analysis of Miller's Model of Hope

Miller's (1983, 1992) model of hope focuses on definitions of concepts related to hope, with a few statements of relationships among the concepts. This reduces its ability to explain, predict, or control phenomena. The sparseness of relational statements also hinders the model's logical adequacy in that relationships cannot be diagrammed (Walker & Avant, 1995). Miller's model has proved to have limited usefulness to researchers who used the MHS but chose to use another conceptual framework. It is broadly generalizable to many populations and situations and has been used with various groups, including college students (Miller & Powers, 1988), elderly (Beckerman & Northrup, 1996; Fehring et al., 1997), the chronically ill (Hirth & Stewart, 1994; Miller, 1992), the critically ill (Miller, 1989), and their spouses (Patel, 1996). It lacks parsimony in that it uses many concepts and unclear relationships. Miller has developed an operational definition of hope that lends itself to testing. As a result, many studies have been conducted that use the MHS to operationalize hope, but its empirical adequacy has not been demonstrated.

Self-Sustaining Process Model

Hinds and Martin (1988) used the grounded theory approach to develop a definition of hope and the Self-Sustaining Process model. Grounded theory approach is an inductive research technique first described by Glaser and Strauss (1967). A theory evolves from the research process that involves formulation, testing, and redevelopment of propositions.

According to Hinds (1984, 1988a), hope, for adolescents, is defined as "the degree to which an adolescent believes that a personal tomorrow exists" (1984, p. 360). There are four hierarchical levels of believing in this model: (a) forced effort, (b) personal possibilities, (c) expectation of a better tomorrow, and (d) anticipation of a personal future. With forced effort, the adolescent exhibits a more positive attitude that is artificial. Personal possibilities refers to the adolescent's belief that second chances exist for the self. A general positive future orientation is characteristic of expectation of a better tomorrow, and a specific positive future orientation is evident in anticipation of a personal future.

Hinds and Martin (1988) conceptualized the Self-Sustaining Process by which adolescents help themselves achieve hopefulness during their illness experience. This process involves four sequential phases; each phase has specific strategies associated with it (Figure 18.2).

The first phase of the Self-Sustaining Process is cognitive discomfort (T_1), the degree to which mental uneasiness is experienced related to disheartening or negative thoughts. The second phase is distraction (T_2), in which the negative thoughts are replaced with neutral or positive thoughts and conditions through cognitive and behavioral activities. The third phase is cognitive comfort (T_3), which encompasses the experience of solace, lifted spirits, and consideration of future possibilities. The fourth phase is personal competence (T_4), in which adolescents view themselves as "resilient, resourceful, and adaptable in the face of serious health threats" (Hinds & Martin, 1988, p. 339). Movement through the process is indicated by a plus sign in Figure 18.2.

Hinds and Martin (1988) concluded that the Self-Sustaining Process is variable in that it can occur in minutes or weeks. Some phases take longer than others and may be bypassed. They also found positive relationships among the concepts (e.g., greater cognitive discomfort relates to more attempts at distraction). Also, behaviors and attitudes of others, including nurses, can influence the adolescent's movement through the process.

Instrument Based on the Self-Sustaining Process Model

Hopefulness Scale for Adolescents. The Hopefulness Scale for Adolescents (HSA; Hinds & Gattuso, 1991) is a 24-item visual analog scale based on Hinds's (1984) conceptualization of hope and was developed from statements made by adolescents in her grounded theory work. According to Hinds, hope is the extent to which an adolescent expects a positive future. An open-ended ques-

tion at the end of the scale asks adolescents to identify specific, hoped-for goals. Then, the researcher estimates the probability of attaining the hoped-for goals. Scores can range from 0 to 2,400. The higher scores indicate higher hopefulness.

The authors constructed two alternate forms because of the volatility of hopefulness and the need to take repeated measurements on the same individual. Comparability of the forms was assessed statistically but not specified (Hinds & Gattuso, 1991). Internal consistencies for the instrument are moderate to high (Table 18.1). Although construct validity assessment has been reported, no specific findings have been published. The HSA is the only scale designed for adolescents and that has alternate forms. It is relatively easy to administer. It is limited, however, to rational thought and relational dimensions of hope.

Research That Used the Self-Sustaining Process Model

Three studies were found that used the Self-Sustaining Process model and the HSA. Two support the importance of the perception that others have hope for the individual as described in the Self-Sustaining Process. The third study (Connelly, 1998) examined the relationship between adolescent pregnancy status and hopefulness and found none; hope scores for the sample were not reported, however. A longitudinal, correlational study of 25 adolescents receiving treatment for substance abuse (Hinds, 1988b) found a positive correlation between hope and adolescents' perception of degree of caring by the nurses. Another study of 99 high school students found that hopefulness helps to explain the relationship between perceived social support and general well-being (Yarcheski, Scoloveno, & Mahon, 1994). These researchers surmised that greater social support fosters adolescent hopefulness or the "comforting life-sustaining belief that a personal and positive future exists" (Hinds, 1984, p. 3), which contributes to general well-being. Much additional research is needed to support the adequacy of this model.

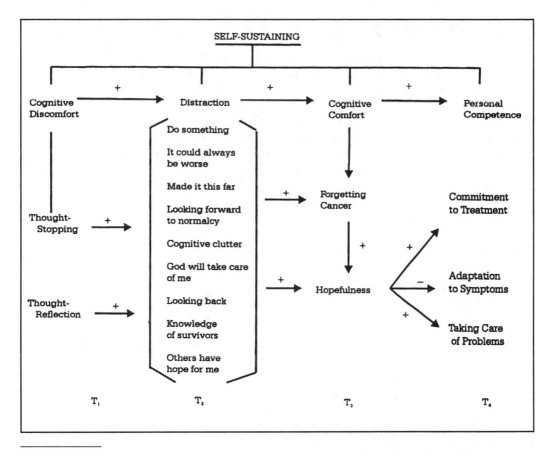

Figure 18.2. The Substantive Theory: Categories, Core Concepts, and the Central Organizing Construct (T_1-T_4 are time frames) (from "Hopefulness and the Self-Sustaining Process in Adolescents With Cancer," by P. S. Hinds and J. Martin, 1988, *Nursing Research, 37*(6), p. 337. Copyright © 1988 by AJN. Reprinted with permission of Lippincott, Williams & Wilkins.)

Analysis of the Self-Sustaining Process Model

The Self-Sustaining Process (Hinds & Martin, 1988) provides an understanding of hopefulness in adolescents that shows promise for description, explanation, prediction, and control. The model is logically adequate in that relationships are clear and predictions can be made from it (Walker & Avant, 1995). This model may prove to be useful in a narrow population of adolescents. It has been used to develop a measure of hope, although it has not been used widely as a conceptual framework. It is narrowly generalizable to the adolescent population, and it has parsimony in that it can be described using relatively few concepts

and relationships. The Self-Sustaining Process model operationalizes hope for the adolescent and should stimulate more research to test its empirical adequacy.

Dufault and Martocchio's Model of Hope

Dufault and Martocchio (1985) also used the grounded theory approach to develop a conceptualization of hope. The researchers described their methodology as "participant observation in multiple settings" (pp. 379-380). Hope is defined as "a *multidimensional dynamic life force characterized by a confident* yet *uncertain* expectation of achieving a future *good* which, to the hoping person, is *realistically* possible and *personally significant*" (p. 380). Dufault and Martocchio describe hope as a process and not as a trait. It has two spheres and six common dimensions (Figure 18.3).

The spheres are generalized hope and particularized hope. Generalized hope relates to a sense of an indeterminate future good. Dufault and Martocchio (1985) note that "generalized hope protects against despair when a person is deprived of particular hopes, and preserves or restores the meaningfulness of life—past, present, and future—in circumstances of all kinds" (p. 380). Particularized hope focuses on a specific hope object that "may be concrete or abstract, explicitly stated or implied" (p. 380) and stimulates coping with obstacles and strategies for attaining the hope object.

Dufault and Martocchio (1985) described the following dimensions of hope: affective, cognitive, behavioral, affiliative, temporal, and contextual. The affective dimension focuses on "sensations and emotions that are part of the hoping process" (p. 382). It involves feelings of confidence, uncertainty, and personal significance about the outcome. The cognitive dimension focuses on "the processes by which individuals wish, imagine, wonder, perceive, think, remember, learn, generalize, interpret, and judge in relation to hope" (p. 384). The behavioral dimension focuses on "the action orientation of the hoping person in relation to hope" (p. 385). Actions taken may be those designed to directly achieve a hope or those motivated by, but do not directly affect, the desired outcome, such as praying or following religious customs. The affiliative dimension focuses on "the hoping person's sense of relatedness or involvement beyond self as it bears upon hope" (p. 386). This dimension pertains to relationships with people and God and may be expressed as a reliance on or receptivity to help from others. The temporal dimension focuses on "the hoping person's experience of time (past, present, and future) in relation to hopes and hoping. Hope is directed toward a future good, but past and present are also involved in

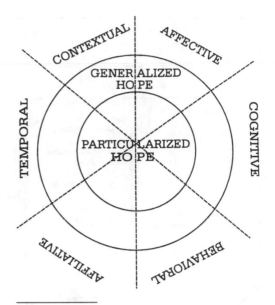

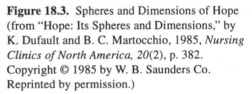

Figure 18.3. Spheres and Dimensions of Hope (from "Hope: Its Spheres and Dimensions," by K. Dufault and B. C. Martocchio, 1985, *Nursing Clinics of North America, 20*(2), p. 382. Copyright © 1985 by W. B. Saunders Co. Reprinted by permission.)

the hoping process" (p. 387). The contextual dimension focuses on "those life situations that surround, influence, and are a part of persons' hope. In a sense, the contexts serve as the circumstances that occasion hope, the opportunity for the hoping process to be activated, or as a situation for testing hope" (p. 388).

Dufault and Martocchio (1985) do not consider hope and hopelessness to be polar opposites on a continuum. Individuals may be hopeful for one outcome and hopeless in relation to another outcome. The multidimensionality and process orientation of hope ensure that there is always hope for something.

Instruments Based on Dufault and Martocchio's Model of Hope

Herth Hope Scale. The Herth Hope Scale (HHS; Herth, 1991) consists of 30 positive and negative items contained in three subscales: temporality and future, positive readiness and expectancy, and interconnectedness. The HHS is a 4-point summated rating scale with higher scores indicating higher levels of hope. Internal consistency and stability were moderately high (Table 18.1). Factor analysis supported the three hypothesized factors. Divergent validity was assessed with the BHS. The HHS is truly multidimensional, including relational, rational, spiritual, and experiential elements of hope. It is limited by its length for use in clinical settings but is easily administered.

Herth Hope Index. The Herth Hope Index (HHI; Herth, 1992) was adapted from the HHS and designed to be used in the clinical setting. This shortened version consists of 12 items developed from items on the HHS that are in a 4-point scale with a higher score indicating higher levels of hope. Internal consistency and stability were high (Table 18.1). Correlation between the HHS and the HHI was .92. Factor analysis with varimax rotation resulted in a three-factor solution consistent with the HHS. The HHI contains all the dimensions and assets of the HHS, but it is a brief version that can be used in clinical settings.

Research That Used Dufault and Martocchio's Model of Hope

Because few relationships are proposed in Dufault and Martocchio's (1985) model of hope, research using this model tends to focus on confirming variables that can be related to hope. Thus, researchers are using an inductive method to add to the model. Significant positive relationships have been found between higher level of hope and level of coping response, strong faith, and no interference with family role responsibilities in a sample of adult cancer patients (Herth, 1991). This offers initial confirmation of the role of these variables in hopefulness. In a sample of elderly widows or widowers, Herth (1990a) also found a positive relationship between level of hope and the use of positive coping styles identified by Jalowiec (1987) as confrontive,

optimistic, palliative, supportant, and self-reliant. A significant negative relationship was found between level of hope and negative coping styles: evasive, emotive, and fatalistic. These findings support the positive role particularized hope plays in coping. Herth found a significant positive relationship between level of hope and level of grief resolution, which can be a result of effective coping. Hope accounted for 79% of the variance in grief resolution.

Research has also resulted in a greater understanding of the temporal dimension. Interviews of healthy older adults revealed differences in focus and future orientation of hope "based on age, place of residence, health status, and functional ability" (Herth, 1993, p. 146). Consistent with other studies based on Stotland's model of hope (Ballard et al., 1997; Raleigh, 1992; Stoner & Keampfer, 1985), extent of illness was not found to be related to level of hope in a sample of adult cancer patients (Herth, 1991). These findings support the explanation that hope is directed toward a future good regardless of the context.

Analysis of Dufault and Martocchio's Model of Hope

Dufault and Martocchio's (1985) model of hope defines the elements of hope but presents few relational statements. As with Miller's model of hope, this reduces its ability to explain, predict, or control phenomena and hinders the model's logical adequacy (Walker & Avant, 1995). The proposed relationship between hope and coping has proven to have usefulness to researchers who have developed measures of hope or used it as a conceptual framework for their studies or both. It is broadly generalizable to many populations and situations and has been used with various groups ranging from healthy elderly to individuals with cancer. It lacks parsimony in that it uses many concepts and few relationships are clear. Dufault and Martocchio have developed an operational definition of hope that has resulted in instrument development and testing. Due to the limited number of studies using this model, empirical adequacy has not been demonstrated.

➤ IMPLICATIONS FOR THEORY, PRACTICE, AND RESEARCH

Hope and Coping

Although it may be obvious to all but the casual observer that hope and coping are interrelated concepts, the literature does not consistently address the existence or nature of this relationship. Often, hope is described as a coping strategy (Bruhn, 1984; Korner, 1970; Lazarus & Folkman, 1984; Raleigh & Boehm, 1994), but it may also be described as an antecedent to coping (Dufault & Martocchio, 1985; Owen, 1989; Weisman, 1979) or as an outcome of coping (Engel, 1968; Farran & McCann, 1989). In fact, hope may have a role in all three aspects of coping. As an antecedent, hope influences how the individual perceives the situation that may be a challenge or threat to goals. As a coping strategy, hope enables the individual to appraise the situation as a challenge rather than a threat and to muster problem-focused or emotional-focused resources (Farran, Herth, et al., 1995). Finally, as an outcome, hope results from the use of coping strategies, such as prayer and interpersonal interaction (Raleigh, 1992). Hopelessness, however, occurs when coping becomes ineffective (Farran, Herth, et al., 1995; Stotland, 1969).

Some research supports hope as a coping strategy. In a study of adolescents with cancer, Hinds (1988b) found that participants reported using two strategies, forgetting cancer and hopefulness, to achieve cognitive comfort, which is part of the larger coping process. Other research suggests that hope is an outcome of using coping mechanisms. In a study of 45 individuals with chronic conditions, Raleigh (1992) found that participants reported using strategies to maintain hope such as physical activity, religious activities, mental distraction, or interaction with others. Herth (1989) found that hope and coping re-

sponses were related in a study of 120 cancer patients and suggested that fostering hope in the cancer patient is important for the coping response. The Coping Process Nursing Model developed by Herth depicts hope and coping resources as equal components in the coping process that affect the coping response either positively or negatively. These findings suggest that additional discussion of and research on the relationship between hope and coping are essential.

Nursing Practice Implications

Intuitively and anecdotally, nurses understand the important roles that hope plays in achieving and maintaining wellness and that hopelessness plays in illness and death. Evidence to support these assumptions is accumulating. Numerous studies have indicated the role of hopelessness in psychopathology (Beck et al., 1975; Beck, Steer, Kovacs, & Garrison, 1985; Farran & Popovich, 1990; Minkoff et al., 1973). Schmale and Iker (1971) documented a relationship between hopelessness and the occurrence of cervical carcinoma. Scientists documented a correlation between hope and immune system function (Udelman, 1982; Udelman & Udelman, 1985), but research in this area has not continued. Because of the promising results of Udelman's study, additional research in this area is warranted. In addition, studies have shown that nurses are sources of hope for their clients (Dufault, 1981; Herth, 1990a, 1990b, 1993; Hinds, 1988b; Miller, 1989; Raleigh, 1992). Because of increasing evidence and the position of influence that nurses have in relation to patients and their families, nurses must be proactive in supporting hope in clients. Various strategies, based on theory or descriptive research, have been proposed.

An understanding of strategies for fostering hope begins with identifying those reportedly used by clients. Several studies (Herth, 1990b, 1993; Miller, 1989; Patel, 1996; Raleigh, 1992) have demonstrated fairly consistent findings with regard to activities that individuals report that they use, although the order of use varies according to health status. Subjects include the terminally, critically, and chronically ill as well as healthy adults. Common categories of hope-fostering strategies include (a) cognitive strategies that restructure threatening information to make it less threatening, (b) purposeful activities, (c) conviction that a positive outcome is possible, (d) maintaining a worldview that life has meaning and growth results from struggles, (e) spiritual beliefs and practices that transcend suffering, (f) a relationship with caregivers who convey positive messages and faith in the patient, (g) relationships with loved ones, (h) a sense of being in control, (i) maintaining goals (small or large and short or long term), (j) distraction, (k) humor or lightheartedness, (l) uplifting memories, or all of these (Herth, 1990a, 1993, 1995; Patel, 1996; Raleigh, 1992; Wake & Miller, 1992). In addition, some studies (Herth, 1990a; Miller, 1989) listed threats to hope identified by these patients. Hopes were threatened when the patient sensed a physical setback, abandonment and isolation, negative hospital experiences, or a devaluation of his or her personhood.

Interventions to foster hope have been proposed by nurses. Common ones include (a) providing comfort and pain relief (Herth, 1995; Johnson, Dahlen, & Roberts, 1997), (b) facilitating relationships with family and health care providers (Herth, 1995; Kim, 1989), (c) assisting to define and redefine hopes (Herth, 1995; Johnson et al., 1997), (d) facilitating an expression of spirituality (Herth, 1995), and (e) encouraging awareness of small positive aspects of a situation (Herth, 1995; Johnson et al., 1997). Herth's (1995) study of 141 hospice and home health care nurses found that nurses rated similar interventions as useful and effective for terminally and chronically ill patients. Providing pain control and comfort was reported by both groups of nurses as most useful and most effective. Both groups also rated connectedness with others very highly.

Miller (1992) developed a model (Figure 18.4) that summarizes the types of nursing strategies that may be useful to foster hope in patients. These strategies relate to several of the critical elements of hope described in her conceptual model. Nurses may foster hope through the affiliative dimension by promoting sustaining relationships and connectedness with others. Nurses can also enhance patients' sense of control or support them, if necessary, to temporarily relinquish control. Nurses can use a life-promoting interpersonal framework by maintaining a positive focus that emphasizes the patient's potential for recovery or adaptation or both. Expanding the patient's and family's coping repertoire and supporting the patient's reality surveillance will also foster hopes. Finally, nurses should provide assistance with identifying or revising goals or both and supporting and encouraging the patient's relationship with God or a meaningful Higher Being.

Nurses have been reticent to conduct intervention studies related to hope-fostering strategies. This may be explained by the focus on development of conceptual frameworks and instruments to accurately measure hope, but it is more likely that this reticence derives from the difficulty in isolating hope from so many other confounding variables, such as coping effectiveness and self-esteem. Much nursing research has focused on determining the relationships between hope and these other variables. It is time, however, for nurses to address this issue.

Implications for Research

In examining the level of theory development for the concepts of hope and hopelessness, it is apparent that, although much theorizing has occurred, there has not been much empirical testing of the theories and models. Even though investigators routinely identify the conceptual framework for their studies, they seldom address whether the study findings support or are related to the aspects of the model. Efforts have focused on determining relationships that exist between hope and other concepts without examining how these concepts relate to the conceptual framework of the study.

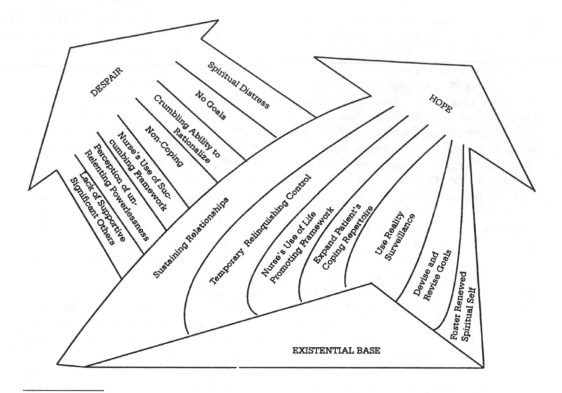

Figure 18.4. Hope-Despair Model (from *Coping With Chronic Illness: Overcoming Powerlessness* [p. 425] by J. F. Miller, 1992, Philadelphia: F. A. Davis. Copyright © 1992 [2nd ed.] by F. A. Davis Co. Reprinted with permission.)

This lack of focus on specific theory testing may be explained by the fact that much of the theory regarding hope in the nursing literature is in the concept development stage (Walker & Avant, 1995). In an effort to determine relational statements, nursing research focuses on finding relationships between hope and other concepts. Although the interest in hope has geometrically increased in the past two decades, the research has been broad and unfocused. Some studies have used nursing hope models as conceptual frameworks, but many other studies have used a variety of concepts other than hope as the framework. There is a distinct need for nurses to attend to the purposeful building of theory around the concept of hope. In addition, research needs to focus on the testing of strategies used and reported by nurses for fostering hope. Interventions based on theory and suggested by the research literature should be tested for their empirical effectiveness with a variety of patient populations.

➤ CONCLUSION

Hope is a concept that is extremely important in understanding the coping process. Although several models of hope have been proposed, the role of hope in the coping process is not clearly understood. Hope models need additional testing and, specifically, the relationship between hope and the coping process needs to be more carefully examined. In addition, interventions need to be related to current theories and tested for effectiveness. There is much work to be done in relation to the concept of hope. To paraphrase St. Paul, "the harvest is plenty and the workers are few."

APPENDIX Nursing Models of Hope Without Additional Testing

Model and Author	Method	Definition of Hope	Propositions and Statements
Travelbee's (1971) model of hope	Review of theological, philosophical, psychological, and nursing literature	"Hope is something halfway between knowing and willing what will happen in the future" (p. 161).	Hope suggests solutions to problems, imparts security in this knowledge, and generates energy that produces motivation to act. Hope is the opposite of despair and transcends the situation.
Lange's (1978) model of hope	Review of philosophical, psychological, and medical literature	The model states that the definition of hope is elusive. It differentiates hope from wishing, expectation, and optimism.	Hope structure is a process for maintaining hope that consists of affective components (faith-doubt continuum) and cognitive functions (selected information that will sustain hope). There are four tasks of hoping: reality surveillance, encouragement, worrying, and mourning. Hope and hopelessness are opposites on a continuum.
McGee's (1984) model of hope	Adaptation of Stotland's (1969) model of hope	Operational definition: stimulus for action exists (problem, unmet need, or goal). "The responses to the stimulus may include feelings, thoughts, expectancies, or actions regarding a state of being that is desired and needed but not currently experienced." The response is based on "the perceived importance of the goal, perceived solutions to the problem, and calculated probabilities for successful action" (p. 36).	The level of hopefulness is proportional to the perceived probability of attaining the goal and the perceived importance of the goal. Extent of action to achieve the goal is proportional to the expectation of achievement and the nearness of the goal. Hope and hopelessness are polar opposites on a continuum. Hope is both a state and a trait.
Hope in Persons With Cancer (Owen, 1989)	Grounded theory: interviews with six oncology clinical nurse specialists	Hope is a dynamic process. The hopeful person is "innately equipped with positive personal attributes that, despite the circumstances, enable uplifting feelings and thoughts to be found, thereby creating a hopeful state" (p. 78). Hope consists of six subthemes: goal setting, positive personal attributes, future redefinition, meaning in life, peace, and energy.	The ability to redefine goals contributes to the ability to remain hopeful during changing circumstances or prognosis. Hopeful patients acknowledge the reality of diagnosis or prognosis and put it in perspective to be able to cope with the impact on lives.

(continued)

APPENDIX Continued

Model and Author	Method	Definition of Hope	Propositions and Statements
			Family and meaning of life events, and not time, define the future of hopeful patients.
			Finding meaning in life supports hope.
			Hopeful patients maintain an inner peace.
			Hopeful patients give and receive emotional and physical energy.
Dialectic of Maintaining Hope (Ersek, 1992)	Grounded theory: interviews with 20 adults who underwent bone marrow transplant	This model uses Dufault and Martocchio's definition of hope as a "multidimensional, dynamic life force that focuses on positive expectations of the future and is influenced by others" (p. 883).	The process of maintaining hope consists of dealing with it and keeping it in its place. Dealing with it is "the process of confronting the negative possibilities inherent in the illness experience and allowing the full range of thoughts, behaviors, and emotions resulting from the recognition" (p. 884). Keeping it in its place is "the process of managing the impact of the disease and its treatment by controlling one's response to the disease and therapy" (p. 885).

➤ REFERENCES

Alloy, L. B., Abramson, L. Y., Metalsky, G. I., & Hartlage, S. (1988). The hopelessness theory of depression: Attributional aspects. *British Journal of Clinical Psychology, 27*, 5-21.

Ballard, A., Green, A. B., McCaa, A., & Logsdon, M. C. (1997). A comparison of the level of hope in patients with newly diagnosed and recurrent cancer. *Oncology Nursing Forum, 24*, 899-904.

Beck, A. T. (1963). Thinking and depression. *Archives in General Psychiatry, 9*, 324-333.

Beck, A. T. (1967). *Depression: Clinical, experimental, and theoretical aspects.* New York: Harper & Row.

Beck, A. T., Kovacs, M., & Weissman, A. (1975). Hopelessness and suicidal behavior. *Journal of the American Medical Association, 234*, 1146-1149.

Beck, A. T., Steer, R. A., Kovacs, M., & Garrison, B. (1985). Hopelessness and eventual suicide: A 10-year prospective study of patients hospitalized with suicidal ideation. *American Journal of Psychiatry, 142*, 559-563.

Beck, A. T., Weissman, A., Lester, D., & Trexler, L. (1974). The measurement of pessimism: The hopelessness scale. *Journal of Consulting and Clinical Psychology, 42*, 861-865.

Beckerman, A., & Northrop, C. (1996). Hope, chronic illness and the elderly. *Journal of Gerontological Nursing, 22*(5), 19-25.

Bernard, H. W. (1977). Hope vs. hopelessness. *Humanitas, 13*, 283-290.

Brackney, B., & Westman, A. (1992). Relationships among hope psychosocial development, and focus locus of control. *Psychological Reports, 70*, 864-866.

Brandt, B. T. (1987). The relationship between hopelessness and selected variables in women receiving chemotherapy for breast cancer. *Oncology Nursing Forum, 12*(2), 35-39.

Bruhn, J. G. (1984). Therapeutic value of hope. *Southern Medical Journal, 77*(2), 215-219.

Connelly, C. D. (1998). Hopefulness, self-esteem, and perceived social support among pregnant and nonpregnant adolescents. *Western Journal of Nursing Research, 20,* 195-209.

Dufault, K. (1981). *Hope in elderly persons with cancer.* Unpublished doctoral dissertation, Case Western Reserve University, Cleveland, OH.

Dufault, K., & Martocchio, B. C. (1985). Hope: Its spheres and dimensions. *Nursing Clinics of North America, 20,* 379-391.

Engel, G. L. (1968). A life setting conducive to illness: The giving up-given up complex. *Annals of Internal Medicine, 69,* 293-300.

Erickson, R. C., Post, R. D., & Paige, A. B. (1975). Hope as a psychiatric variable. *Journal of Clinical Psychology, 31,* 324-330.

Ersek, M. (1992). The process of maintaining hope in adults undergoing bone marrow transplantation. *Oncology Nursing Forum, 19,* 883-889.

Farran, C. J., Herth, K. A., & Popovich, J. M. (1995). *Hope and hopelessness.* Thousand Oaks, CA: Sage.

Farran, C. J., & McCann, J. (1989). Longitudinal analysis of hope in community-based older adults. *Archives of Psychiatric Nursing, 3,* 272-276.

Farran, C. J., & Popovich, J. M. (1990). Hope: A relevant concept for geriatric psychiatry. *Archives of Psychiatric Nursing, 4,* 124-130.

Farran, C. J., Wiken, C. S., & Fidler, R. (1995). A study of hope in geriatric patients. *Journal of Nursing Science, 1*(1/2), 16-26.

Fawcett, J. (1984). The metaparadigm of nursing: Present status and future refinements. *Image, 16,* 84-87.

Fehring, R. J., Miller, J. F., & Shaw, C. (1997). Spiritual well-being, religiosity, hope, depression, and other mood states in elderly people coping with cancer. *Oncology Nursing Forum, 24,* 663-671.

Foote, A., Piazza, D., Holcombe, J., Paul, P., & Daffin, P. (1990). Hope, self-esteem, and social support in persons with multiple sclerosis. *Journal of Neuroscience Nursing, 22,* 155-159.

Fry, P. (1984). Development of a geriatric scale of hopelessness: Implications for counseling and intervention with the depressed elderly. *Journal of Counseling Psychology, 31,* 322-331.

Glaser, B. G., & Strauss, A. (1967). *The discovery of grounded theory: Strategies for qualitative research.* Chicago: Aldine.

Gottschalk, L. (1974). A hope scale applicable to verbal samples. *Archives of General Psychiatry, 30,* 779-785.

Herth, K. A. (1989). The relationship between level of hope and level of coping response and other variables in patients with cancer. *Oncology Nursing Forum, 16,* 67-72.

Herth, K. A. (1990a). Relationship of hope, coping styles, concurrent losses, and setting to grief resolution in the elderly widow(er). *Research in Nursing & Health, 13,* 109-117.

Herth, K. A. (1990b). Fostering hope in terminally ill people. *Journal of Advanced Nursing, 15,* 1250-1259.

Herth, K. A. (1991). Development and refinement of an instrument to measure hope. *Scholarly Inquiry for Nursing Practice: An International Journal, 5,* 39-56.

Herth, K. A. (1992). Abbreviated instrument to measure hope: Development and psychometric evaluation. *Journal of Advanced Nursing, 17,* 1251-1259.

Herth, K. A. (1993). Hope in older adults in community and institutional settings. *Issues in Mental Health Nursing, 14,* 139-156.

Herth, K. A. (1995). Engendering hope in the chronically and terminally ill: Nursing interventions. *American Journal of Hospice and Palliative Care, 12*(5), 31-39.

Hinds, P. S. (1984). Inducing a definition of hope through the use of grounded theory methodology. *Journal of Advanced Nursing, 9,* 357-362.

Hinds, P. S. (1988a). Adolescent hopefulness in illness and health. *Advances in Nursing Science, 10,* 79-88.

Hinds, P. S. (1988b). The relationship of nurses' caring behaviors with hopefulness and health care outcomes in adolescents. *Archives of Psychiatric Nursing, 2,* 21-29.

Hinds, P. S., & Gattuso, J. (1991). Measuring hopefulness in adolescents. *Journal of Pediatric Oncology Nursing, 8,* 92-94.

Hinds, P. S., & Martin, J. (1988). Hopefulness and the self-sustaining process in adolescents with cancer. *Nursing Research, 37,* 336-340.

Hirth, A. M., & Stewart, M. J. (1994). Hope and social support as coping resources for adults waiting for cardiac transplantation. *Canadian Journal of Nursing Research, 26*(3), 31-48.

Irvin, B. L., & Acton, G. J. (1997). Stress, hope, and well-being of women caring for family members with Alzheimer's disease. *Holistic Nursing Practice, 11*(2), 69-79.

Jalowiec, A. (1987). *Jalowiec Coping Scale (revised).* Unpublished manuscript, University of Illinois, Chicago.

Johnson, L. H., Dahlen, R., & Roberts, S. L. (1997). Supporting hope in congestive heart failure patients. *Dimensions of Critical Care Nursing, 16,* 65-78.

Kazdin, A., French, N., Unis, A., Esveldt-Dawson, K., & Sherick, R. (1983). Hopelessness, depression, and suicidal intent among psychiatrically disturbed inpatient children. *Journal of Consulting and Clinical Psychology, 51,* 504-510.

Kim, J. J., McFarland, G. K., & McLane, A. M. (1997). *Pocket guide to nursing diagnosis* (7th ed.). St. Louis, MO: C. V. Mosby.

Kim, R. S. (1989). Hope as a mode of coping in amyotrophic lateral sclerosis. *Journal of Neuroscience Nursing, 21,* 342-347.

Korner, I. N. (1970). Hope as a method of coping. *Journal of Consulting and Clinical Psychology, 34,* 134-139.

Lange, S. P. (1978). Hope. In C. E. Carlson & B. Blackwell (Eds.), *Behavioral concepts and nursing interventions* (2nd ed., pp. 171-190). Philadelphia: J. B. Lippincott.

Lazarus, R., & Folkman, S. (1984). *Stress, appraisal and coping.* New York: Springer.

Lynch, W. F. (1965). *Images of hope: Imagination as the healer of the hopeless.* Notre Dame, IN: University of Notre Dame Press.

Marcel, G. (1967). Desire and hope. In N. Lawrence & D. O'Conner (Eds.), *Readings in existential phenomenology.* Englewood Cliffs, NJ: Prentice Hall.

McGee, R. F. (1984). Hope: A factor influencing crisis resolution. *Advances in Nursing Science, 6*(4), 34-44.

McGill, F. S., & Paul, P. B. (1993). Functional status and hope in elderly people with and without cancer. *Oncology Nursing Forum, 20,* 1207-1213.

Melges, F. T., & Bowlby, J. (1969). Types of hopelessness in psychopathological process. *Archives of General Psychiatry, 20,* 690-699.

Miller, J. F. (1983). *Coping with chronic illness: Overcoming powerlessness.* Philadelphia: F. A. Davis.

Miller, J. F. (1989). Hope-inspiring strategies of the critically ill. *Applied Nursing Research, 2,* 23-29.

Miller, J. F. (1992). *Coping with chronic illness: Overcoming powerlessness* (2nd ed.). Philadelphia: F. A. Davis.

Miller, J. F., & Powers, M. (1988). Development of an instrument to measure hope. *Nursing Research, 37,* 6-10.

Minkoff, K., Bergman, E., Beck, A. T., & Beck, R. (1973). Hopelessness, depression and attempted suicide. *American Journal of Psychiatry, 130,* 455-459.

Mishel, M., Hostetter, T., King, B., & Graham, V. (1984). Predictors of psychosocial adjustment in patients newly diagnosed with gynecological cancer. *Cancer Nursing, 7,* 291-299.

Nowotny, M. (1989). Assessment of hope in patients with cancer: Development of an instrument. *Oncology Nursing Forum, 16,* 57-61.

Obayuwana, A., Collins, J., Carter, A., Rao, M., Mathura, C., & Wilson, S. (1982). Hope Index Scale: An instrument for the objective assessment of hope. *Journal of the National Medical Association, 74,* 761-765.

Owen, D. C. (1989). Nurses' perspectives on the meaning of hope in patients with cancer: A qualitative study. *Oncology Nursing Forum, 16,* 75-79.

Patel, C. T. C. (1996). Hope-inspiring strategies of spouses of critically ill adults. *Journal of Holistic Nursing, 14,* 44-65.

Raleigh, E. D. (1992). Sources of hope in chronic illness. *Oncology Nursing Forum, 19*(3), 443-448.

Raleigh, E. D., & Boehm, S. B. (1994). Development of the multidimensional hope scale. *Journal of Nursing Measurement, 2,* 155-167.

Rideout, E., & Montemuro, M. (1986). Hope, morale, and adaptation in patients with chronic heart failure. *Journal of Advanced Nursing, 11,* 429-438.

Schmale, A. H., & Iker, H. P. (1971). Hopelessness as a predictor of cervical cancer. *Social Science and Medicine, 5,* 95-100.

Snyder, C., Harris, C., Anderson, J., Holleran, S., Irving, L., Sigmon, S., Yoshinobu, L., Gibb, J., Langelle, C., & Harney, P. (1991). The will and the ways: Development and validation of an individual-differences measure of hope. *Journal of Personality and Social Psychology, 60,* 570-585.

Staats, S. (1989). Hope: A comparison of two self-report measures for adults. *Journal of Personality Assessment, 53,* 366-375.

Staples, P., & Jeffrey, J. (1997). Quality of life, hope, and uncertainty of cardiac patients and their spouses before coronary artery bypass surgery. *Canadian Journal of Cardiovascular Nursing, 8,* 7-16.

Stoner, M. H. (1982). Hope and cancer patients. *Dissertation Abstracts International, 43,* 1983B-2592B. (University Microfilms No. 83-12, 243)

Stoner, M. H., & Keampfer, S. H., (1985). Recalled life expectancy information, phase of illness and hope in cancer patients. *Research in Nursing & Health, 8,* 269-274.

Stotland, E. (1969). *The psychology of hope.* San Francisco: Jossey-Bass.

Travelbee, J. (1971). Hopelessness. In J. Travelbee (Ed.), *Interpersonal aspects of nursing* (pp. 159-177). Philadelphia: F. A. Davis.

Udelman, D. L. (1982). Stress and immunity. *Psychotherapy Psychosomatics, 37,* 176-184.

Udelman, D. L., & Udelman, H. D. (1985). A preliminary report on anti-depressant therapy and its effects on hope and immunity. *Social Science and Medicine, 20,* 1069-1072.

Vatz, K., Winig, G., & Beck, A. T. (1969). *Pessimism and a sense of future time constriction as cognitive distortions in depression.* Unpublished manuscript, University of Pennsylvania, Philadelphia.

Wake, M. M., & Miller, J. F. (1992). Treating hopelessness. *Clinical Nursing Research, 1,* 347-365.

Walker, L. O., & Avant, K. C. (1995). *Strategies for theory construction in nursing* (3rd ed.). Norwalk, CT: Appleton & Lange.

Weisman, A. D. (1979). *Coping with cancer.* New York: McGraw-Hill.

Yarcheski, A., Scoloveno, M. A., & Mahon, N. E. (1994). Social support and well-being in adoles-cents: The mediating role of hopefulness. *Nursing Research, 43,* 288-292.

Zorn, C. R., & Johnson, M. T. (1997). Religious well-be-ing in noninstitutionalized elderly women. *Health Care for Women International, 18,* 209-219.

CHAPTER 19

Locus of Control, Perceived Control, and Learned Helplessness

JoAnn B. Ruiz-Bueno

Encounters with health care and illness are considered to be stressful situations. Nurses' knowledge and intimate interactions with patients make them the logical interventionists to reduce distress. Florence Nightingale (1860/1969) noted nursing's responsibility when she wrote, "If you knew how unreasonably sick people suffer from reasonable causes of distress, you would take more pains about these things" (p. 104). Control, by various definitions, can make predictions about potential responses to health and illness situations and can provide strategies to assist patients in coping with these situations or, by its perceived or actual absence, can interfere with coping. The purpose of this chapter is to sort out these various control constructs by describing the theoretical development of each type of control and to provide empirical evidence of the usefulness of the theory that has evolved.

An individual's perception of his or her ability to exercise direction in or over situations and events predicts and impacts almost every facet of life. Skinner (1995) maintains that perceived control is a robust predictor of one's behavior, motivation, performance, and emotion. It can predict success or failure in very diverse domains of life, ranging from school performance to coping with health-related stress and aversive events. For nursing, we are most concerned with its relationship with health and illness, and for the purposes of this chapter, we are concerned with its moderating effect on coping with stressors.

Various investigators have defined the construct of control differently (Kofta, Weary, & Sedek, 1998; Rotter, 1966, 1975; Skinner, 1995; Thompson, 1981; Wallston, Wallston, & DeVellis, 1978). There is no single clear, specific, inclusive, and agreed on definition. In general, *control* refers to one's perception of one's ability to alter a situation, response, or outcome related to a stimulus or all three, and it includes the potential for an inverse relationship.

This chapter focuses on four of the most popular control constructs used in nursing investigations and their application in the discipline of nursing as we examine stress and coping: (a) locus of control (LOC), (b) health locus of control (HLOC), (c) personal control (PC), and (d) learned helplessness (LH). Health locus of control will be addressed separately from LOC because of its slightly different orientation, which makes it of particular relevance to nursing investigations. Using a literature review as the approach to content, a computer and hand search in the Cumulative Index for Nursing and Allied Health Literature was performed. The limitations imposed on the first search were (a) research article and (b) English language. This search yielded 634 LOC entries, 24 HLOC entries, 593 PC articles, and 21 LH entries. When these were further limited to key nursing journals, 261 entries related to at least one of the four constructs were identified (LOC, 120; HLOC, 23; PC, 97; and LH, 21). The author's expert knowledge of the field led to additional resources. Control related to nurses/occupational, nursing students, and nonhealth or nonillness variables were eliminated. Because the focus of this book is stress and coping, articles that included a measure of stress and/or coping in relation to control are included in the tables presented in this chapter.

A second computer search was conducted in psychology. Limits imposed on this search were human studies, English language, and journal articles. This search yielded 14,870 articles (LOC, 9,191; HLOC, 2,733; PC, 936; and LH, 2,010). Selected key and classic studies are included in this review.

Most investigators agree that the four control constructs (LOC, HLOC, PC, and LH) had their origins in psychology's social learning theory of personality (Bandura, 1977; Rotter, 1954, 1960). Social learning theory integrates stimulus-response (reinforcement) theory and cognitive theory. It includes four classes of variables: behaviors, expectancies, reinforcements, and psychological situations (Rotter, 1975).

Behaviors are a person's actions. The potential for a behavior to occur in any psychological situation is determined by the expectation that a behavior will lead to a particular outcome and by the perceived value of the reinforcement(s) or reward(s). In social learning theory, when an individual perceives two psychological situations to be similar, then his or her expectations for a similar reinforcement generalize from the first situation to the next similar situation (Rotter, 1975).

➤ LOCUS OF CONTROL THEORY

Theory Development

Julian Rotter (1966, 1975) is credited with proposing locus of control as a construct that refines predictions of how reinforcements change expectancies. He proposed that a test of an individual's beliefs in the forces (within self and outside of self) that were responsible for outcomes would be useful in predicting behavior that led to outcomes in a multitude of situations. The test he constructed, the Rotter (1966) Internal-External (I-E) Locus of Control Scale, originated from the general theoretical framework of social learning theory (Rotter, 1954, 1960). It is based on the following concepts. *Generalized expectancies* for a specific type of reinforcement to occur are spread across situations that are perceived as similar and thus are major determinants of behavior potential. Building on this concept of reinforcement, control is categorized as either internal or external. *Internal control* refers to the degree that one believes that reinforcements are contingent on one's own behavior or a belief that it is a stable characteristic. *External control* refers to the degree that one believes that an event is either unpredictable or under the control of fate, luck, chance, or powerful others. Although other operationalizations of the LOC construct have been developed, it continues to be measured primarily with Rotter's (1966) I-E Scale. Lefcourt (1976, 1981) and Phares (1976) provide detailed reviews of LOC research and its applications in psychology and samples of other LOC instruments, whereas Oberle (1991) reviewed LOC and health-related research.

Rotter's (1966) I-E Scale used forced choice questions, and the scores on the two subscales are distributed along a continuum rather than yielding a typology of control (Rotter, 1975). Locus of control as it was originally conceived continues to be used today. Rotter (1990) related the heuristic value of LOC to four propositions that include the importance of (a) having a precise definition of the construct, (b) embedding the construct in a broader theory of behavior, (c) measuring the construct with instruments derived from psychological theory, and (d) disseminating knowledge (publication). A sampling of LOC instruments that have been developed to measure the four control constructs is provided in Table 19.1. Locus of control is considered a midrange theory (Walker & Avant, 1995).

It must be remembered that LOC is a broadly defined construct that should be applied in measuring relatively stable, cross-sectional individual differences rather than fixed traits or types, and its value is for general predictions (Rotter, 1990). Therefore, it is not an appropriate measure for all situations, particularly in very specific situations in which a more narrowly defined construct is needed.

Lazarus and Folkman (1984) noted that in stress and coping research, LOC's greatest predictive value has been in highly ambiguous situations, in which one's general belief about control serves as a resource to moderate the appraisal of new or novel stimuli. When the situation is not highly ambiguous, situational characteristics may be more useful in judging controllability.

Much of the investigation of LOC, including health-related studies, has been conducted within its parent discipline (psychology) (Krause, 1985; Rotter, 1990). As noted earlier, the initial on-line search revealed 9,191 entries in this area. Investigations of LOC in relation to stress and coping that support Lazarus and Folkman's (1984) view have also emerged. One example is Auerbach, Kendall, Cutter, and Levitt's (1976) investigation of the interaction of LOC and preparatory information (sensation information) on adjustment during dental surgery. Dental surgery can be viewed as an unambiguous and highly specific (rather than general) situation. In this study of adults, no interaction between LOC and the intervention was found.

Locus of Control and Nursing Knowledge

Most of the major theories of nursing do not include LOC as a major construct. An exception is Pender's (1982) early Health Promotion Model. She described stress *à la* Selye (1977) as the nonspecific response to demands made on the body. Control was an important component of this model. The need for control was described as crucial to personal competence throughout the life span. Lack of competency could lead to frustration and powerlessness. She used Rotter's (1954) social learning theory and LOC (Rotter, 1966) in her model. In this model, internal control results in assertive behavior to shape the environment for the support of growth and self-actualization. Internal control is necessary to view one's own behavior as affecting current and future health outcomes and as a motivator that leads one to engage in health promotion and health protection activities and to assume responsibility for one's own health. In contrast, she describes the externally controlled person as one who responds more readily to role modeling, or to suggestions from others, for engaging in health-promoting and -protecting activities. Pender's Health Promotion Model is considered a midrange theory (Walker & Avant, 1995).

Pender's (1987, 1996) revised model shifted in theoretical orientation from LOC to a model integrating constructs from expectancy value theory and social cognitive theory (namely, perceived control) to better address

TABLE 19.1 Selected Measures for the Control Construct

Measure and Author	Category of Control Measured	Description	Reliability	Validity	Populations Studied
Internal-External Locus of Control Scale (Rotter, 1966)	Internal-external locus of control	20-item forced-choice format	.72-.78	Construct validity	Psychology students and prisoners
Levenson (1973)	Multidimensional locus of control: internality, powerful others, chance	Three 8-item Likert-type scales	.67 .82 .79	.08 .74 .78	Functionally psychotic and neurotic patients
Nowicki-Strickland Locus of Control Scale for Children (Nowicki & Strickland, 1973)	Internal-external locus of control	40-Item, yes-no format	.63-.71	.63-.81	School-children
Multidimensional Health Locus of Control Scale (Wallston, Wallston, & DeVellis, 1978)	Health locus of control	Three 6-item Likert-type scales	.75-.81	.50-.73	Students
Client Control Q-Sort (Dennis, 1987)	Belief of importance of hospital events and situation control	45 items, crossing types of control with hospitalization events	.48-.90	.98	Medical and surgical military patients
Multidimensional Health Locus of Control Types (Rock, Meyerowitz, Maisto, & Wallston, 1987)	Health locus of control types	Three 6-item Likert-type scales	.85	.89	Undergraduate and graduate students
Learned Helplessness Scale (Quinless & Nelson, 1988)	Learned helplessness	20-item Likert-type scales	.79 .82 .92 .94	Content and face validity	Undergradute students Oncology patients Hemodialysis patients Spinal cord injury patients

nursing's holistic perspective. Her model also addresses stress and coping from the prospective of Lazarus and Folkman (1984). The relationship between selected components of Pender's model and LOC has been studied in older persons (Duffy, 1993; Speake, Cowart, & Pellet, 1989), midlife women (Duffy, 1988; Gillis & Perry, 1991), and coronary artery disease patients (Fleetwood & Packa, 1991). All these studies reported significant positive relationships between LOC and the components studied.

The general value of the LOC construct in nursing has been as a predictor variable (Kelly, 1995; LaMontagne, 1987; Pellino & Oberst, 1992; Wells, 1994). Findings have been inconsistent in some studies (Chang, 1979; Kelly, 1995). The major reason for these mixed results may be that LOC, which has been a successful predictor in general situations, has also been assumed to be reliable in very specific situations.

Locus of Control and Nursing Research

Studies of the LOC construct in nursing have reported findings similar to those of Auerbach and colleagues (1976), who determined that LOC may not be a useful predictor in very specific situations. An example is Chang's (1979) study of the institutionalized elderly. She investigated the relationship between LOC, trust (described as a generalized expectancy), situational control (patient's perception of control in activities of daily living), and morale (as an outcome measure of adaptation). In this study of subjects' adaptation to living in a nursing home (a very specific situation), situational control was a better predictor of morale than LOC.

Several other nursing investigations of the LOC association with health and illness variables with seemingly contradictory findings are noteworthy. These studies focused on various health-seeking behaviors. Balsmeyer (1984) used Rotter's (1966) I-E Scale in her early study of hypertensives. She found that internally oriented hypertensive participants were more involved in health-seeking behavior as demonstrated by greater adherence to keeping clinic appointments. In a contrasting study, Saltzer and Saltzer (1987) investigated LOC and health-seeking behaviors. They followed Rotter's (1975) recommendation that specific measures of LOC would be more useful in clinical situations in which one is seeking specific predictions about behavior. Using an investigator-developed Acne Locus of Control Scale (derived from Rotter's I-E Scale), the researchers found that the health behavior of those seeking medical care was associated with a higher external LOC. Huckstadt (1987) also used a specific measure of LOC related to drinking. In this study, differences in LOC were found between alcoholics, recovering alcoholics, and nonalcoholics. Alcoholics scored least internally, recovering

alcoholics scored more internally than alcoholics, and nonalcoholics scored more internally than either of the other two groups.

The variation in internal versus external LOC results may be related to many factors. Adhering to a regimen of care (appointments) for chronic conditions such as hypertension can be interpreted differently from the initial seeking of care for an acute condition such as acne. Another factor might be the use of a general versus a specific instrument to measure LOC.

Many studies have explored the relationship between LOC and stress and health outcome variables. Similar to studies that did not measure a stress or coping variable or both, results have been mixed. Studies including a stress or coping variable or both along with LOC are summarized in Table 19.2. These are arranged chronologically. With one exception (Wells, 1994), nursing studies with a stress or health outcome focus used a stress/coping/adaptation framework and a variety of LOC measures, including different scales used to measure LOC and also LOC scales used specifically for pain and for children. None of the studies in Table 19.2 used Rotter's I-E Scale. Chronologically, there appears to be an increasing effort to match the instrument to the population and problem. Convenience sampling was used in all of the studies, and sample sizes were 100 or less. With these major limitations, generalizations are not possible. There appears to be some support for LOC as a predictor of coping style in children (LaMontagne, 1987), pain and mood (Pellino & Oberst, 1992), distress and disability in chronic pain sufferers (Wells, 1994), and parental stress (Kelly, 1995). It may not be a predictor of morale (Chang, 1979).

Locus of Control and Implications for Nursing Research

The studies reported in Table 19.2 provide support for the need for more studies before predictions can be made about the association between LOC and either health-seeking

TABLE 19.2 Selected Nursing Studies That Investigated Locus of Control (LOC) and Stress and/or Coping Outcomes

Author	LOC Instrument	General Theoretical Framework	Sample	Related Findings
Chang (1979)	Levenson LOC Scales (Levenson, 1973) Reliability = .08-.78 Variability = .67-.79	Adaptation theory Learning theory	30 elderly residents in four skilled nursing facilities	LOC not a predictor of morale; situational control strongest predictor of morale
LaMontagne (1987)	Nowicki-Strickland Locus of Control Scale for Children (Nowicki & Strickland, 1973) Reliability = .63-.71 Variability = .63-.81	Stress and coping	42 children hospitalized to have surgery	Active copers significantly more internal than either avoidant or combination copers
Pellino and Oberst (1992)	Levenson Locus of Control Scales (Levenson, 1974) Reliability = .08-.78 Variability = .67-.79	Stress and coping	40 outpatient back pain patients	Perception of internal control of pain predictor of mood and pain
Wells (1994)	Pain-Related Control Scale and Pain-Related Self-Statements Scale (Flor & Turk, 1988) Reliability = .77-.92 Variability = .61-.66	Expectancy for control of reinforcement	71 patients with chronic nonmalignancy pain	Relationship of control beliefs to distress and disability in chronic pain supported
Kelly (1995)	Parental Health Beliefs Scale (Tinsley & Holtgrave, 1989) Reliability = .96 Variability = .72	Stress adaptation model	47 adolescent mother-infant dyads	Significant correlations between parent stress and both internal LOC and powerful other LOC; correlations between parenting stress and chance LOC not significant

NOTE: All studies reported use of nonprobability sampling techniques except that by Chang (1979), in which the sampling technique was not reported.

behaviors or specific diagnostic conditions. To date, the construct of LOC has been most valuable in prediction, and it is probably not amenable to nursing intervention because of its relative stability (Rotter, 1990) and because internal control is partially a product of maturational development (LaMontagne & Hepworth, 1991). One of the basic assumptions is that LOC concerns individual differences in beliefs that develop over time and that are relatively stable; thus, altering them may be a difficult process.

In the context of stress and coping, the importance of the congruence among variable definition, theoretical underpinnings, and appropriateness of the measurement, as well as consideration of the situational context, must be emphasized. Incongruence among these factors can influence the outcome of the study and its usefulness in terms of predicting the moderating effect of LOC on the stress and/or health outcomes.

➤ HEALTH LOCUS OF CONTROL

Because LOC had not been a reliable predictor of health-related behavior, an expansion of theory to include health outcomes was undertaken by Wallston and colleagues (1978). Health locus of control, as it became known, was originally thought of as a unidimensional construct and was developed to improve the predictive power of LOC measures in specific situations. The authors later expanded this conceptualization to a multidimensional construct. Rather than measuring generalized LOC beliefs, the Multidimensional Health Locus of Control (MHLC) scales (Wallston et al., 1978) were developed to assess specific beliefs about control over health. Locus of control is described as a relatively stable individual difference (Rotter, 1990). In contrast, the MHLC is based on the assumption that one can be internally or externally controlled or both at any given time, depending on the situation. With the MHLC, the LOC concepts are measured with two external scales (chance and powerful others) and one internal scale. Differences between Wallston et al.'s and Rotter's instruments are further represented by a significant change in measurement technique. Rotter's I-E Locus of Control Scale uses questions with forced-choice responses, whereas the MHLC uses questions with Likert-type scales. Health locus of control is considered a midrange theory (Walker & Avant, 1995).

In health psychology research, HLOC has become one of the most frequently assessed variables (Rock, Meyerowitz, Maisto, & Wallston, 1987). Investigations have reported inconsistent and only modest findings with the use of the MHLC instrument, however. Wallston and Wallston (1982) offer the explanation that the pattern of responses across the three MHLC scales may be more meaningful than any individual scores. They suggest categorizing subjects into one of the following eight types based on their pattern of response: (a) pure internal, (b) pure powerful others external, (c) pure chance external, (d) double external, (e) believer in control, (f) yea-sayer, (g) nay-sayer, and (h) Type VI (which is undefined).

Wallston and Wallston's (1982) suggestion to categorize subjects to identify these patterns of response was followed in an investigation by Rock and colleagues (1987). They conducted a study designed to discover clusters. Analysis of data led to a reduction in the number of types from the suggested eight to six: (a) pure internal, (b) double external, (c) pure chance, (d) yea-sayer, (e) nay-sayer, and (f) believer in control. A second study was then conducted to assess the reliability, validity, and clinical utility of the six clinical types (Rock et al., 1987). Only two of the nursing studies included in this review (Saudia, Kinney, Brown, & Young-Ward, 1991; Waller & Bates, 1992) included classification of subjects into these typologies as a part of data analysis. Patterns of response across the MHLC scales (Wallston et al., 1978) provide untapped potential for knowledge development, which could demonstrate the usefulness of health-related LOC in nursing and appropriate situations for application.

Health Locus of Control and Nursing Research

Some nursing studies explored HLOC in a variety of contexts—for example, studies of potentially stressful encounters without a stress or coping outcome variable or both. Study variables included healthy elders (Waller & Bates, 1992), preventive health behaviors (Zindler-Wernet & Weiss, 1987), and the specific diagnoses of tuberculosis (Healy, 1997), diabetes (Meize-Grochowski, 1989), and HIV-positive (Ragsdale, Kotarba, Morrow, & Yarbrough, 1995). Another study investigated the stability of HLOC over time in a hospital setting (Halfens, 1995).

Other studies measuring both HLOC and one or more stress or coping variables or both are summarized in Table 19.3. In this group of HLOC studies, there tends to be larger sample sizes (most were 100 or more). The predominant theoretical frameworks are stress and coping (Dodd, Dibble, & Thomas, 1993; Kuehn & Winters, 1994; Saudia et al., 1991; Younger, Marsh, & Grap, 1995) or Pender's (1982) Health Promotion Model, which includes stress management (Duffy, 1988, 1993; Speake et al., 1989). One study used Bandura's (1977) social learning theory (Waller & Bates, 1992). All studies used the MHLC scales without modifications, except for the study by Dodd et al. (1993), which used scales adapted for use with cancer patients.

In summary, MHLC scores have shown value as predictors of health responsibility, nutrition, and stress management (Duffy, 1988). A modified version of the MHLC adapted for cancer patients was not a predictor of the number of coping strategies recorded by chemotherapy outpatients (Dodd et al., 1993). Health locus of control subscales were found to be associated with higher stress management scores (Speake et al., 1989) and good health practices including stress management (Duffy, 1993; Waller & Bates, 1992). It should be noted that all these studies used nonprobability sampling techniques.

Health Locus of Control and Implications for Nursing Research

Health locus of control as a moderator of the stress-health outcome linkage has great potential for nursing research and theory development. As with LOC, studies of HLOC have been mostly descriptive in nature. These studies are useful for expanding knowledge about predictor variables. In the stress-health outcome context, several studies have explored the relationship between HLOC and coping (Dodd et al., 1993; Kuehn & Winters, 1994; Saudia et al., 1991). No studies were

found that addressed the potentially moderating effect of HLOC on the appraisal of stress. Because nursing research has focused on HLOC for many years, it should now focus on the interaction effects with other stress and coping variables, including interventions.

Another area of research potential is the patterns of responses on the MHLC and the typology that resulted from Rock and colleagues' (1987) studies. Although two studies included an analysis of data for determining specific types, the relationship of these types to other variables was not addressed. Additional studies are needed to explore and interpret this categorization more thoroughly. This is an area that appears to have been overlooked by researchers, even though it has potential for knowledge development and may relate to future interventions.

➤ PERSONAL OR PERCEIVED CONTROL

Theory Development

In the section on LOC, a brief review was given for the development of the concept of control as it emerged from social learning theory (Rotter, 1954, 1960). The broadly defined construct of LOC, which measures relatively stable cross-sectional individual differences, was followed by discussion of the multidimensional construct of HLOC, which is specific to the health care setting. The latter construct is based on the assumption that one can be internally or externally controlled or both at any given time, depending on the situation, specifically in relation to health.

For personal control (PC), rather than viewing control as a relatively stable personality disposition with elements residing both within oneself and in the environment, it is viewed as resting within the individual. This view was further developed by Rodin (1990), who described personal control as arising from one's need to be a causal agent in one's own world. Skinner (1995) described control as a basic need for competence, Kofta and colleagues (1998) described PC as perception of the self as a source of causation. These descriptions are congruent with the concept of perceived control as a moderator of the stress-health outcome linkage and the transition from the use of social learning theory to the use of a variety of control perspectives. Use of varied theories has led to differing definitions of control and a search for appropriate instruments to measure it.

Personal or Perceived Control and Nursing Knowledge

The referent descriptions of PC have been varied and broad. In an effort to be more specific, a variety of typologies have been proposed by different researchers, including Averill (1973), Lewis (1987), Miller (1979), and Thompson (1981). Miller's typology is limited to behavioral control categories and so is not discussed here.

Averill's Typology of Control

Averill (1973) can be credited with clarifying the meaning of the concept of personal control over aversive stimuli by distinguishing among three different types of PC that have emerged from a variety of studies: (a) behavioral control, (b) cognitive control, and (c) decisional control. Early studies using this typology included applying electrical shock in a laboratory setting (Cornelius & Averill, 1980). *Behavioral control* is defined as the availability and use of an action that directly influences or modifies the objective characteristics of an aversive or threatening event. An example is allowing subjects to modify the time of onset or the intensity of electrical shock. *Cognitive control* refers to the way an individual interprets a potentially harmful encounter. There are two types of cognitive control: information gain and appraisal. An example of information gain is obtaining information about the predictability, such as a

warning signal, of an aversive event. An illustration of appraisal is giving information (e.g., sensory information) that allows the person to search for clues about potential harm, thus altering the meaning associated with an upcoming aversive event. *Decisional control* allows the individual to either choose the action he or she wants to take or to agree with the course of action that must be taken. An example is influencing the extent to which subjects believe they agree with or are a part of an experience, even though it might be painful or aversive (Averill, 1973; Cornelius & Averill, 1980). This typology has been especially useful in nursing as a guide for designing potential interventions and is considered a midrange theory (Walker & Avant, 1995).

Thompson's Typology of Control

Thompson (1981) presented a very general definition of control as "the belief that one has at one's disposal a response that can influence the aversiveness of an event" (p. 89). She believed that Averill's (1973) typology was unsatisfactory, mainly because she disagreed with his definition of cognitive control and because of questions about the usefulness of decisional control. She proposed a new four-category typology. In her typology, behavioral control is defined as the person's belief that an action is available that is capable of affecting the aversiveness of an event by terminating it, making it less intense or less probable, or by changing its timing or duration. An example is the freedom to reposition the body during a procedure to reduce discomfort that is associated with the procedure. Cognitive control refers to the belief that one has a mental strategy available that can affect the unpleasantness of the event. Examples are avoidant strategies (e.g., ignore, disassociate, distract, or deny). Information, rather than being a component of cognitive control, is included in the Thompson typology as a category of variables capable of generating feelings of control. *Information,* in a variety of forms, refers to a communication to the

TABLE 19.3 Selected Nursing Studies That Investigate Health Locus of Control (HLOC) and Stress and/or Coping Outcomes

Author	Health Locus of Control Instrument	General Theoretical Framework	Sample	Related Findings
Duffy (1988)	Multidimensional Health Locus of Control (MHLC; Wallston, Wallston, & DeVellis, 1978) Reliability = .75-.81 Variability = .50-.73	Health Promotion Model	262 university faculty and staff women	Predictor Set 1 (including chance LOC) was a predictor of health responsibility, nutrition, and stress management.
Speake, Cowart, and Pellet (1989)	MHLC (Wallston et al., 1978) Reliability = .75-.81 Variability = .50-.73	Health Promotion Model	297 elder volunteers	Higher scores on internal and powerful others subscales and positive perceptions of past health were associated with higher stress management scores.
Saudia, Kinney, Brown, and Young-Ward (1991)	MHLC (Wallston et al., 1978) Reliability = .75-.81 Variability = .50-.73	Combined stress appraisal and coping, social learning theory, and systems-in-change model	100 patients before cardiac surgery	No relationship was found between health locus of control and helpfulness of prayer as a coping mechanism.[a]
Waller and Bates (1992)	MHLC (Wallston et al., 1978) Reliability = .75-.81 Variability = .50-.73	Social learning theory	57 elder volunteers	Health elders had internal health locus of control, high generalized self-efficacy, and good health practices (stress management).[a]
Dodd, Dibble, and Thomas (1993)	Cancer Health Locus of Control Scale (Dickson, Dodd, Carrieri, & Levenson, 1985) Reliability = .48-.63 Variability = .33-.42	Coping, self-care, family systems	64 patients initiating chemotherapy	LOC was not a predictor of the number of coping strategies recorded by chemotherapy outpatients.
Duffy (1993)	MHLC (Wallston et al., 1978) Reliability = .75-.81 Variability = .50-.73	Health Promotion Model	477 volunteer elders	Healthy elders with high self-esteem and internal locus of control and older married elders with higher income and internal locus of control were more likely to report frequent practice of stress management.
Kuehn and Winters (1994)	MHLC (Wallston et al., 1978) Reliability = .75-.81 Variability = .50-.73	Stress and coping	125 aging postpolio survivors	Higher internal LOC was associated with more coping resources than chance or powerful other LOC.

NOTE: All studies used nonprobability sampling techniques.
a. Included analysis of typologies (Rock, Meyerowitz, Maisto, & Wallston, 1987).

person who is facing an aversive event. Examples of information include a warning signal preceding an aversive event (temporal information) or information about the characteristics of an event (such as typical sensations, procedural information, or causes of a disease). *Retrospective control* refers to the attribution of responsibility to oneself, thus asserting control over and preserving one's sense of personal influence. An example is a victim blaming himself or herself for an accident (Thompson, 1981).

Thompson's (1981) typology of control was not used in the theoretical framework of any of the nursing studies reviewed. Information about the sensations one might expect during an aversive event, however, was widely studied in nursing by Johnson and colleagues (Fuller, Endress, & Johnson, 1978; Johnson, 1973; Johnson, Christman, & Stitt, 1985; Johnson, Fuller, Endress, & Rice, 1978; Johnson, Kirchhoff, & Endress, 1975; Johnson, Rice, Fuller, & Endress, 1978). Thompson (1981) cited their research as support for considering information interventions as a separate category from cognitive control. Examples from these studies include information about typical sensations that reduced arousal during aversive events, such as ischemic pain (Johnson, 1973), cast removal in children (Johnson et al., 1975), and pelvic examination (Fuller et al., 1978).

Lewis's Integrative Typology of Control

Acknowledging that the construct of control is seldom defined, and that it is generally thought of as unidimensional, Lewis (1987) pointed out the theoretical importance of organizing an integrative typology. This typology considers the complexity of the multidimensionality of control. The five types of control that were suggested were based on the assumption that higher levels of control resulted in determinants of changed health outcomes. Lewis presented the following conceptual definitions:

(1) Processual control is the participation by the individual in discussions or decisions affecting the event, the response, the outcome, or the environmental context. (2) Contingency control is the individual's perception that his or her response to the event controls the outcome state of the individual. (3) Cognitive control is the individual's intellectual management of the event so as to reduce its perceived threatening properties. (4) Behavioral control is the actual alteration of the objective qualities of the event by the individual's own behavior. (5) Existential control is the individual's imposition of meaning and purpose on an event so as to decrease its perceived threatening properties. (p. 299)

Personal or Perceived Control and Nursing Research

Only one nursing study was found that used Lewis's (1987) typology of control (Vallerand & Ferrell, 1995). These researchers used this typology to organize data in a qualitative study of perceptions of control in cancer patients using individual members of patient-family caregiver-home-care nurse triads. Each type was described in relation to pain, and numerous interview data were reported that reflected the individual types.

None of the nursing literature reviewed used either Miller's (1979) or Thompson's (1981) typologies of control. Averill's (1973) typology was used in one of the studies (Dennis, 1990). Two studies used decisional control without relating it to a specific theoretical framework. The remainder of the studies in Table 19.4 used various definitions and measures of personal or perceived control.

Although several studies (Bowsher & Gerlach, 1990; Dennis, 1990) used social learning theory, both stress and coping theory and control theory were used in others (Szabo & Srtang, 1999; Topf, 1992) as theoretical frameworks. Three studies (Chen & Snyder, 1996; Montbriand, 1995; Mosher & Dracup, 1995) were atheoretical. Two studies were ethnographic; one of these used planned behavior (McBride, 1993), and the other was atheoretical but alluded to an element of control (Montbriand, 1995) as the organizing framework. An additional study, based on Lazarus and Folkman's (1984) cognitive-phenomenological theory of stress, explored the relationship between perceived control, perceived threat, and negatively toned emotions (Cordes, 1998).

Personal or Perceived Control and Implications for Nursing Research

It is evident from the diverse interpretations and measurement techniques that the construct of personal or perceived control is complex and multidimensional. Although attempts have been made to structure this phenomenon by the use of typologies, these are neither as inclusive nor as widely accepted as one would assume. The most complete body of knowledge in any area of PC is from the works of Johnson and colleagues (Fuller et al., 1978; Johnson et al., 1975, 1985; Johnson, Fuller, et al., 1978; Johnson, Rice, et al., 1978). In these studies, sensation information was used as an intervention in a wide variety of aversive encounters to reduce stress. Although these early studies are not discussed in this chapter in detail, they are in the realm of common nursing knowledge. They serve as an example of a theory-based, carefully planned, and ongoing program of study of the stress phenomenon using relevant theory-based instruments. Johnson's work is discussed in more detail in Chapter 10.

➤ LEARNED HELPLESSNESS

Theory Development

Learned helplessness (LH) is a special case of personal control. The construct originated in animal research, in which dogs were repeatedly exposed to an aversive stimulus over which they had little or no control and from which they could not escape. After failing to escape, they stopped trying. Later, when an escape was possible, they failed to learn new behavior leading to escape. This type of behavior was not seen in dogs that were exposed to controllable aversive stimuli or in a control group (Seligman & Maier, 1967). Learned helplessness was first offered as an explanation for human depression (Seligman, 1975). When later studies did not consistently support this explanation, the LH model was reformulated based on attribution theory, and a framework was devised that categorized how individuals assigned blame for uncontrollable events (Abramson, Seligman, & Teasdale, 1978). This framework includes three dimensions of attributions that individuals make for their helplessness: (a) universal versus personal, in which the LH attributional style is on an external-internal continuum; (b) global versus specific, in which the attributional style continuum can vary from a wide range of situations to a very narrow range of situations; and (c) stable versus unstable attributions, in which the deficits occur consistently over time or not. This categorization provided an explanation for why some individuals are more likely than others to develop LH (Abramson et al., 1978).

Stoner (1985) cited the lack of a valid and reliable instrument to measure LH in the clinical setting as one of the major problems hindering research in this area. In 1988, Quinless and Nelson developed an instrument to measure LH. Additional information about this instrument is found in Table 19.1. The measure is based on a model previously described (Abramson et al., 1978).

Learned Helplessness and Nursing Knowledge

Learned helplessness has been recognized as particularly relevant for nursing practice and research. Murphy (1982) traced the development of LH as a theory and detailed some specific clinical applications within psy-

TABLE 19.4 Selected Nursing Studies that Investigated Personal/Perceived Control and Stress and/or Coping Outcomes

Author	Control Instrument (and Variable)	General Theoretical Framework	Sample	Control-Related Findings
Dennis (1990)	Client Control Q-Set (Dennis, 1987) Reliability = .48-.90 Variability = .98	Social learning theory Personal control	30 medical and surgical inpatients (nonprobability)	Instrument identified activities that contribute to sense of control.
Bowsher and Gerlach (1990)	Desired Control Measure (Reid, Ziegler, Sangster, Haas-Hawkings, & Riusech, 1979) Reliability = .73-.80 Variability = .37-.38	Social learning theory	302 nursing home elders (nonprobability)	Personal control was a predictor of psychological well-being.
Wallston et al. (1991)	Investigator-developed Perceived Control Scale Reliability = .75	Control theory	74 chemotherapy patients (random assignment)	T1 choice, no-choice intervention and desire for control had no effect on perceived control. T2,3 choice group reported less helplessness than no-choice group.
Topf (1992)	Investigator-devised questionnaire item	Stress and coping Personal control	105 females in simulated hospital environment (nonprobability)	Personal control over sound levels was not significant in facilitating better sleep.
McBride (1993)	Ethnographic content analysis	Control theory	32 chronic obstructive pulmonary disease (COPD) patients (nonprobability)	Qualitative: Perceived control may influence decision making in COPD patients.
Montbriand (1995)	Ethnographic content analysis	Control theory (integrated)	300 cancer patients (nonprobability)	The study explored the desire to have or give away control: use of alternative therapies as control mechanism or sign of inability to cope.
Mosher and Dracup (1995)	Investigator-developed Control Attitude Scales Reliability = .62-.89 Variability = .58	Stress and coping	229 recovering cardiac event patients (nonprobability)	High control subjects reported less anxiety and better psychosocial adjustment than low control subjects.
Vallerand and Ferrell (1995)	Interview data	Typology of control	30 subjects (10 patient-caregiver-nurse triads) (nonprobability)	Perception of control by individual triad members was related to the five categories in Lewis's (1987) typology.
Chen and Snyder (1996)	Satisfaction with nursing home control subscale (Kirchbaum, Ryden, & Snyder, 1994)	Personal control	57 elderly nursing home residents (nonprobability)	Personal control was a predictor of satisfaction with care.

(continued)

TABLE 19.4 Continued

| Wallhagen and Brod (1997) | Researcher-designed interview questionnaire (two items) | Control theory | 101 Parkinson's disease patients (nonprobability) | Patient's perceived control over symptoms was significantly associated with both caregiver and patient well-being. |
| Szabo and Stang (1999) | Secondary analysis of qualitative data | Stress and coping | 21 family caregivers of dementia patients (nonprobability) | Maintaining or lacking control were related to how caregivers coped with their caregiving situations. |

chiatric and mental health nursing that are based on the work of Abramson et al. (1978). These include such interventions as introduce strategies that may be useful in reducing the aversiveness of an aversive outcome, changing the expectation of outcome from uncontrollable to controllable in appropriate situations, and changing internal, stable, and global attributions to external, unstable, and specific attributions. Stoner (1985) also reviewed the evolution of LH and its relevance in a particular patient population—cancer patients. Table 19.5 summarizes nursing studies of LH that include stress and/or coping variables.

Learned Helplessness and Nursing Research

Issues as diverse as distress over divorce, spousal battering, perceptions of depression, and depression in the elderly have been investigated by employing the concept of learned helplessness. Several studies have used the construct of LH to focus on women's relationships with their partners. Barron (1987) conducted her study before a specific instrument to measure LH had been developed. She explored the relationships among self-esteem, emotional distress, and women's causal explanations for divorce. Divorce is considered one of the most stressful of women's life experiences. Causal explanations were defined by LOC dimensions. In this study, emotional distress was related to causal explanations described as internal, stable, and global, and it occurred only in those women who believed they were helpless in preventing the marriage from ending. Barron's study offered support for LH theory. In Campbell's (1989) study, the learned helplessness model and the grief model were compared in relation to explaining women's response to battering. Battered women were compared with nonbattered women. The relationship between depression and physical symptoms supported the grief model and the relationship between self-care agency and self-esteem supported the learned helplessness model. Both models had significant explanatory power, with approximately 65% of the variance explained. Using depression as the sole outcome variable, both models were nearly equal in explanatory power.

Rydholm and Pauling (1991) explored and contrasted feelings of helplessness in a group of 10 hemodialysis patients and a group of 10 peritoneal dialysis patients. The newly developed Learned Helplessness Scale (Quinless & Nelson, 1988) was used to measure helplessness. Although both groups reported a moderately high perception of helplessness, hemodialysis patients had higher perceived helplessness scores than the peritoneal dialysis patients. The authors suggested that because hemodialysis patients were in the hospital setting, they might feel more controlled by others. In these patients, interventions to increase PC might alter feelings of helplessness.

TABLE 19.5 Selected Nursing Studies That Investigated Learned Helplessness and Stress and/or Coping Outcomes

Author	Measurement of Learned Helplessness	General Theoretical Framework	Sample	Related Findings
Lewis (1982)	Rosenberg's Self-Esteem Scale (Rosenberg, 1962) Purpose-in-Life Test (Crumbaugh, 1968)	Social learning theory Learned Helplessness	57 late-stage cancer patients	Greater control over life was associated with higher levels of self-esteem, lower levels of anxiety, and more purpose in life.
Barron (1987)	Women's Attribution to Divorce Questionnaire (Barron, 1987) Tennessee Self-Concept Scale (Fitts, 1972) Reliability = .61-.92 Variability = construct	Stress and coping Attribution theory	36 women ending first marriage	Learned helplessness model a predictor of emotional distress.
Campbell (1989)	Tennessee Self-Concept Scale (Fitts, 1972) Reliability = .61-.92 Variability = construct Beck Depression Inventory (Beck, 1972) Denyes Self-Care Agency Instrument (Denyes, 1980) Reliability = .70-.90 Variability = construct	Grief model Learned helplessness model	97 battered women 96 nonbattered controls	Battered women had more frequent and severe symptoms of stress and tried more solutions to relationship problems than nonbattered controls. Both grief and learned helplessness models had significant explanatory power.
Rydholm and Pauling (1991)	Learned Helplessness Scale (Quinless & Nelson, 1988) Reliability = .79-.94 Variability = content, face	Stress and coping theory	20 dialysis patients (10 hemodialysis and 10 peritoneal dialysis) (nonprobability)	Hemodialysis patients were more likely to experience feelings of helplessness than peritoneal dialysis patients.
Barder, Slimmer, and LeSage (1994)	Learned helplessness and instrumental helplessness subscales of Multiscore Depression Inventory (Berndt, Petzel, & Berndt, 1980)	Learned helplessness theory	140 elderly in acute, rehabilitation, and long-term health care settings (nonprobability)	Elders in long-term care setting were more vulnerable to experiencing learned helplessness and mood disturbance (depression) than those in acute or rehabilitation settings.

NOTE: All studies used nonprobability sampling techniques.

Barder, Slimmer, and LeSage (1994) investigated depression in the elderly. In their study, depression was better explained by the original LH theory that linked LH and depression than by the LH theory related to attributions about cause.

Learned Helplessness and Implications for Nursing Research

Learned helplessness has not been extensively studied within the discipline of nursing, particularly in relation to stress and coping (Table 19.5). Patients who receive nursing care may be at risk for developing LH because they may either be placed in an environment in which they have little or no control or face a diagnosis that is progressive and uncontrollable. Identifying patients most at risk, and developing interventions to increase their control may alter their feelings of learned helplessness. For this research discipline, exploration of a construct with great potential for altering stress-health outcomes in specific patients and environments is just beginning.

➤ CONTROL CONSTRUCTS ACROSS CULTURES

Nursing studies investigating control constructs have also been conducted in a number of different cultures. These include Australia, the United States, Wales, Austria, The Netherlands, and Norway, and among Vietnamese immigrants.

Australia

Phenomenological interviews were the methodology used by Gaskill, Henderson, and Fraser (1997). They explored the feelings of isolation in bone marrow transplant recipients. Striving to take charge, which was interpreted as patients' attempts to maintain control in this unique situation, emerged as a major theme in this study.

United States

A cross-cultural study was conducted by Hanson (1997) to explore cigarette smoking in African American, Puerto Rican, and non-Hispanic white teenage females. Using a three-item perceived behavioral scale to measured subjects' ability to control their own smoking, Hanson reported that in all three cultural groups perceived behavioral control had significant direct effects on smoking intention. Those with higher levels of personal control had higher intentions to quit.

Wales

In a qualitative study of persons recovering from lower limb fracture, Griffiths and Jordan (1998) found that seeking control (appraising and coping) was used as coping mechanisms during the convalescent period.

Austria

In a study of insulin pump recipients, Meize-Grochowski (1989) used a German translation of the MHLC (Wallston et al., 1978). Data were analyzed and subjects were classified according to Wallston and Wallston's (1982) typology. The majority were classified as believers in control (they scored high on internal HLOC and powerful others HLOC and low on chance LOC). The Austrian group was also compared on the subscales with a similar group in the United States. The difference between the groups on the powerful others subscale was significant, with the Austrian group scoring higher than the United States group.

The Netherlands

Hemophilia patients were studied by Triemstra and colleagues (1998), who explored the relationship between a variety of variables, including health beliefs about control (LOC) and well-being. Subjects with an internal LOC perceived hemophilia to be less serious than subjects with an external LOC.

In another study, HLOC was measured at three points in time in surgical patients. Halfens (1995) used the Dutch MHLC translated from Wallston et al.'s (1978) MHLC. In this Dutch sample, there was a significant increase in powerful others HLOC from preadmission to during hospital stay and a significant decrease after discharge.

Norway

Haldorsen, Indahl, and Ursin (1998) and Haldorsen, Wormgoor, Bjorholt, and Ursin (1998) included HLOC for patients who were on medical leave for low back pain in their two studies. In the first study, a light program of mobilization was administered 6 to 8 weeks into their sick leave. Internal HLOC, as a dominant component of a set of variables, was a predictor of not returning to work by 12 months after treatment. In the second study, a moderate program of mobilization was administered 6 to 8 hours per day on subjects who had been on sick leave for low back pain for at least 8 weeks. In this group of subjects, the association between psychological factors and not returning to work was not significant.

Vietnamese Immigrants

Healy (1997) used a dichotomized MHLC form written in Vietnamese, modified from Wallston et al.'s (1978) MHLC scales. Tuberculosis patients of both genders scored high on internal LOC, chance LOC, and powerful other LOC. Men, however, scored significantly higher than did women on the latter scale. Culture was used to explain this gender difference.

➤ SUMMARY

This chapter traced four important control constructs as moderators of the stress-health outcome linkage: LOC, HLOC, PC, and LH.

The roots of control theory lie in social learning theory (Rotter, 1954, 1960). Locus of control as a predictor in general situations was discussed. This was extended to HLOC, a multidimensional construct designed to increase the predictive ability in health-related situations and to increase applicability in both nursing research and nursing practice. In this review, two important instruments were reported. The first, the Multidimensional Health Locus of Control Scale (Wallston et al., 1978), has become widely used in nursing investigations (Table 19.3). The second, the Learned Helplessness Scale (Quinless & Nelson, 1988), is becoming recognized as an important instrument in the investigation of LH. Repeated studies in diverse samples have contributed reliability information.

The vast majority of studies discussed in this chapter have been descriptive or correlational. Describing and predicting are only the initial steps toward designing and applying nursing interventions to positively influence health.

The body of knowledge generated by Johnson and colleagues (Fuller et al., 1978; Johnson et al., 1975, 1985; Johnson, Fuller, et al., 1978; Johnson, Rice, et al., 1978) using sensation information as an intervention was developed as an ongoing research program. There is little evidence of this type of sustained study in other areas of control or LH literature in nursing. The following general conclusions can be made:

1. Locus of control is a relatively stable predictor in very general situations.
2. Both HLOC and LH have potential for nursing research and practice, but not enough is known about the constructs. Repeated, related, and sustained investigation is needed before their potential for nursing practice can be realized.
3. Personal control, although the most attractive construct as a guide to intervention, remains the most problematic construct. The nature of the construct continues to be nebulous, resulting in diverse theories, measure-

ments, and explanations. The development of various typologies has helped to clarify this problem. Much more knowledge about these typologies and their influence in moderating stress-health outcomes is needed, however.

4. In investigations related to these (or any) constructs, careful attention needs to be paid to matching the theoretical framework with the construct definitions and the instruments used to measure them.

5. Cultural differences may play an important role in all control constructs, and investigations among and between cultures need to be conducted.

➤ REFERENCES

Abramson, L. Y., Seligman, M. P. E., & Teasdale, J. D. (1978). Learned helplessness in humans: Critique and reformulation. *Journal of Abnormal Psychology, 87,* 49-74.

Auerbach, S. M., Kendall, P. C., Cutter, H. F., & Levitt, N. R. (1976). Anxiety, locus of control, type of preparatory information, and adjustment to dental surgery. *Journal of Consulting and Clinical Psychology, 44,* 809-818.

Averill, J. R. (1973). Personal control over aversive stimuli and its relationship to stress. *Psychological Bulletin, 50,* 296-303.

Balsmeyer, B. (1984). Locus of control and the use of strategies to promote self-care. *Journal of Community Health Nursing, 1,* 171-179.

Bandura, A. (1977). Self-efficacy: Toward a unifying theory of behavioral change. *Psychological Review, 84,* 191-215.

Barder, L., Slimmer, L., & LeSage, J. (1994). Depression and issues of control among elderly people in health care settings. *Journal of Advanced Nursing, 20,* 597-604.

Barron, C. R. (1987). Women's causal explanations of divorce: Relationships to self-esteem and emotional distress. *Research in Nursing & Health, 10,* 345-353.

Beck, A. T. (1972). *Depression: Causes and treatment.* Philadelphia: University of Pennsylvania Press.

Berndt, D., Petzel, T., & Berndt, S. (1980). Development and initial evaluation of a multiscore depression inventory. *Journal of Personality Assessment, 44,* 396-403.

Bowsher, J. E., & Gerlach, M. J. (1990). Personal control and other determinants of psychological well-being in nursing home elders. *Scholarly Inquiry for Nursing Practice: An International Journal, 4,* 91-107.

Campbell, J. C. (1989). The test of two explanatory models of women's responses to battering. *Nursing Research, 38,* 18-24.

Chang, B. L. (1979). Locus of control, trust, situational control and morale of the elderly. *International Journal of Nursing Studies, 16,* 169-181.

Chen, K., & Snyder, M. (1996). Perception of personal control and satisfaction with care among nursing home elders. *Perspectives, 20,* 16-19.

Cordes, D. (1998). *Perceived control, perceived threat, and negatively-toned emotions in women two to twelve weeks post-cardiac event.* Unpublished manuscript, Indiana University-Purdue University at Indianapolis School of Nursing, Indianapolis.

Cornelius, R. R., & Averill, J. R. (1980). The influence of various types of control on psychophysiological stress reactions. *Journal of Research in Personality, 14,* 503-517.

Crumbaugh, J. D. (1971). Cross-validation of purpose-in-life test based on Frankl's concepts. *Journal of Individual Psychology, 24,* 74-81.

Dennis, K. E. (1987). Dimensions of client control. *Nursing Research, 36,* 151-156.

Dennis, K. E. (1990). Patients' control and the information imperative: Clarification and confirmation. *Nursing Research, 39*(3), 162-166.

Denyes, M. J. (1980). Development of an instrument to measure self-care agency in adolescents. *Dissertation Abstracts International, 40,* 1716-B. (University Microfilms No. 80-25, 672)

Dickson, A. C., Dodd, M. J., Carrieri, V., & Levenson, H. (1985). Comparison of a cancer-specific locus of control and the Multidimensional Health Locus of Control scales in chemotherapy patients. *Oncology Nursing Forum, 12,* 49-54.

Dodd, M. J., Dibble, S. L., & Thomas, M. L. (1993). Predictors of concerns and coping strategies of cancer chemotherapy outpatients. *Applied Nursing Research, 6,* 2-7.

Duffy, M. E. (1988). Determinants of health promotion on midlife women. *Nursing Research, 37,* 358-362.

Duffy, M. E. (1993). Determinants of health-promoting lifestyles in older persons. *Image: The Journal of Nursing Scholarship, 25,* 23-28.

Fitts, F. H. (1972). *The self concept and behavior: Overview and supplement.* Los Angeles: Western Psychological Services.

Fleetwood, J., & Packa, D. R. (1991). Determinants of health-promoting behaviors in adults. *Cardiovascular Nursing, 5,* 67-79.

Flor, H., & Turk, D. C. (1988). Chronic back pain and rheumatoid arthritis: Predicting pain and disability from cognitive variables. *Journal of Behavioral Medicine, 11,* 251-265.

Fuller, S. S., Endress, M. P., & Johnson, J. E. (1978). The effects of cognitive and behavioral control on coping with an aversive health examination. *Journal of Human Stress, 4,* 18-25.

Gaskill, D., Henderson, A., & Fraser, M. (1997). Exploring the everyday world of the patient in isolation. *Oncology Nursing Forum, 24,* 695-700.

Gillis, A., & Perry, A. (1991). The relationships between physical activity and health promoting behaviors in mid-life women. *Journal of Advanced Nursing, 16,* 299-310.

Griffiths, H., & Jordan, S. (1998). Thinking of the future and walking back to normal: An exploratory study of patients' experiences during recovery from lower limb fracture. *Journal of Advanced Nursing, 28,* 1276-1288.

Haldorsen, E. M. H., Indahl, A., & Ursin, H. (1998). Patients with low back pain not returning to work: A 12-month follow-up study. *Spine, 23,* 1202-1208.

Haldorsen, E. M. H., Wormgoor, M. E. A., Bjorholt, P. G., & Ursin, H. (1998). Predictors for outcome of a functional restoration program for low back pain patients—A 12-month follow-up study. *European Journal of Physical Medicine and Rehabilitation, 4,* 103-109.

Halfens, R. J. G. (1995). Effect of hospital stay on health locus-of-control beliefs. *Western Journal of Nursing Research, 17,* 156-167.

Hanson, M. J. S. (1997). The theory of planned behavior applied to cigarette smoking in African-American, Puerto Rican, and non-Hispanic white teenage females. *Nursing Research, 46,* 155-162.

Healy, E. J. (1997). Health locus-of-control beliefs in Vietnamese clients with latent tuberculosis. *Nursing Connections, 10,* 39-46.

Huckstadt, A. (1987). Locus of control among alcoholics, recovering alcoholics, and non-alcoholics. *Research in Nursing & Health, 10,* 23-28.

Johnson, J. E. (1973). Effects of accurate expectations about sensations on the sensory and distress components of pain. *Journal of Personality and Social Psychology, 27,* 261-275.

Johnson, J. E., Christman, N. J., & Stitt, C. (1985). Personal control interventions: Short- and long-term effects on surgical patients. *Research in Nursing and Health, 8,* 131-145.

Johnson, J. E., Fuller, S. S., Endress, M. P., & Rice, V. H. (1978). Altering patients' responses to surgery: An extension and replication. *Research in Nursing and Health, 1,* 111-113.

Johnson, J. E., Kirchhoff, K. T., & Endress, M. P. (1975). Altering children's distress behavior during orthopedic cast removal. *Nursing Research, 24,* 404-410.

Johnson, J. E., Rice, V. H., Fuller, S. S., & Endress, M. P. (1978). Sensory information, instructions in a coping strategy, and recovery from surgery. *Research in Nursing and Health, 1,* 4-17.

Kelly, L. E. (1995). Adolescent mothers: What factors relate to level of preventive health care sought for their infants? *Journal of Pediatric Nursing, 10,* 105-113.

Kirchbaum, K., Ryden, M. B., & Snyder, M. (1994). *Satisfaction with Nursing Home Questionnaire.* Unpublished manuscript, University of Minnesota, School of Nursing, Minneapolis.

Kofta, M., Weary, G., & Sedek, G. (1998). Part I: The person as an agent of control. In M. Kofta, G. Weary, & G. Sedek (Eds.), *Personal control in action: Cognitive and motivational mechanisms* (pp. 1-3). New York: Plenum.

Krause, N. (1985, Spring). Stress, control beliefs, and psychological distress: The problem of response bias. *Journal of Human Stress,* pp. 11-19.

Kuehn, A. F., & Winters, R. K. V. (1994). A study of symptom distress, health locus of control, and coping resources of aging post-polio survivors. *Image: The Journal of Nursing Scholarship, 26,* 325-331.

LaMontagne, L. L. (1987). Children's preoperative coping: Replication and extension. *Nursing Research, 36,* 163-167.

LaMontagne, L. L., & Hepworth, J. T. (1991). Issues in the measurement of children's locus of control. *Western Journal of Nursing Research, 13,* 67-83.

Lazarus, R. S., & Folkman, S. (1984). *Stress, appraisal, and coping.* New York: Springer.

Lefcourt, H. M. (1976). *Locus of control. Current trends in theory and research.* New York: John Wiley.

Lefcourt, H. M. (Ed.). (1981). *Research with the locus of control construct: Volume 1. Assessment methods.* New York: Academic Press.

Levenson, H. (1973). Multidimensional locus of control in psychiatric patients. *Journal of Consulting and Clinical Psychology, 41,* 397-404.

Levenson, H. (1974). Activism and powerful others: Distinctions within the concept of internal-external control. *Journal of Personality Assessment, 38,* 377-383.

Lewis, F. M. (1982). Experienced personal control and quality of life in late-stage cancer patients. *Nursing Research, 31,* 113-119.

Lewis, F. M. (1987). The concept of control: A typology and health-related variables. *Advances in Health Education and Promotion, 2,* 277-309.

McBride, S. (1993). Perceived control in patients with chronic obstructive pulmonary disease. *Western Journal of Nursing Research, 15,* 456-464.

Mcizc-Grochowski, A. R. (1989). Health locus of control and glycosylated haemoglobin concentrations of implantable insulin pump recipients in Austria. *Journal of Advanced Nursing, 15,* 804-807.

Miller, S. M. (1979). Controllability and human stress: Method, evidence and theory. *Behaviour Research and Therapy, 17,* 287-304.

Montbriand, M. J. (1995). Alternative therapies as control behaviours used by cancer patients. *Journal of Advanced Nursing, 22,* 646-654.

Mosher, D. K., & Dracup, K. (1995). Psychosocial recovery from a cardiac event: The influence of perceived control. *Heart & Lung, 24,* 273-280.

Murphy, S. A. (1982). Learned helplessness: From concept to comprehension. *Perspectives in Psychiatric Care, 20,* 27-32.

Nightingale, F. (1969). *Notes on nursing: What it is and what it is not.* New York: Dover. (Original work published 1860)

Nowicki, S., Jr., & Strickland, B. (1973). A locus of control scale for children. *Journal of Consulting and Clinical Psychology, 40,* 148-154.

Oberle, K. (1991). A decade of research in locus of control: What have we learned? *Journal of Advanced Nursing, 16,* 800-806.

Pellino, T. A., & Oberst, M. T. (1992). Perception of control and appraisal of illness in chronic low back pain. *Orthopaedic Nursing, 11,* 22-26, 106.

Pender, N. J. (1982). *Health promotion in nursing practice.* Norwalk, CT: Appleton-Century-Crofts.

Pender, N. J. (1987). *Health promotion in nursing practice* (2nd ed.). Norwalk, CT: Appleton & Lange.

Pender, N. J. (1996). *Health promotion in nursing practice* (3rd ed.). Stamford, CT: Appleton & Lange.

Phares, E. J. (1976). *Locus of control in personality.* Morristown, NJ: General Learning Press.

Quinless, F. W., & Nelson, M. A. M. (1988). Development of a measure of learned helplessness. *Nursing Research, 37,* 11-15.

Ragsdale, K., Kotarba, J. A., Morrow, J. R., Jr., & Yarbrough, S. (1995). Health locus of control among HIV-positive indigent women. *Journal of the Association of Nurses in AIDS Care, 6,* 29-36.

Reid, D. W., Ziegler, M., Sangster, S., Haas-Hawkings, G., & Riusech, R. (1979). *The Desired Control Measure.* Unpublished manuscript.

Rock, D. L., Meyerowitz, B. E., Maisto, S. A., & Wallston, K. A. (1987). The derivation and validation of six multidimensional health locus of control scale clusters. *Research in Nursing and Health, 19,* 185-195.

Rodin, J. (1990). Control by any other name: Definitions, concepts, and processes. In J. Rodin, C. Schooler, & K. Schaie (Eds.), *Self directness: Cause and effects throughout the life course* (pp. 1-17). Hillsdale, NJ: Lawrence Erlbaum.

Rosenberg, M. (1962). Self-esteem and concern with public affairs. *Public Opinion Quarterly, 26,* 201-211.

Rotter, J. B. (1954). *Social learning and clinical psychology.* Englewood Cliffs, NJ: Prentice Hall.

Rotter, J. B. (1960). Some implications of a social learning theory for the prediction of goal directed behavior from testing procedures. *Psychological Review, 67,* 301-316.

Rotter, J. B. (1966). Generalized expectancies for internal versus external control of reinforcement. *Psychological Monographs: General and Applied, 80,* 1-26.

Rotter, J. B. (1975). Some problems and misconceptions related to the construct of internal versus external control of reinforcement. *Journal of Clinical and Consulting Psychology, 43,* 56-67.

Rotter, J. B. (1990). Internal versus external control of reinforcement. A case history of a variable. *American Psychologist, 45,* 489-493.

Rydholm, L., & Pauling, J. (1991). Contrasting feelings of helplessness in peritoneal and hemodialysis patients: A pilot study. *ANNA Journal, 18,* 183-184.

Saltzer, E. B., & Saltzer, E. I. (1987). Internal control and health: Which comes first? *Western Journal of Nursing Research, 9,* 542-554.

Saudia, T. L., Kinney, M. R., Brown, K. C., & Young-Ward, L. (1991). Health locus of control and helpfulness of prayer. *Heart & Lung: Journal of Critical Care, 20,* 60-65.

Seligman, M. E. P. (1975). *Helplessness: On depression, development, and death.* San Francisco: Freeman.

Seligman, M. E. P., & Maier, F. F. (1967). Failure to escape traumatic shock. *Journal of Experimental Psychology, 74,* 1-9.

Selye, H. (1977). Introduction. In D. Wheatly (Ed.), *Stress and the heart.* New York: Raven Press.

Skinner, E. A. (1995). *Perceived control, motivation, & coping.* Thousand Oaks, CA: Sage.

Speake, D. L., Cowart, M. E., & Pellet, K. (1989). Health perceptions and lifestyles of the elderly. *Research in Nursing & Health, 12,* 93-100.

Stoner, C. (1985). Learned helplessness: Analysis and application. *Oncology Nursing Forum, 12,* 31-35.

Szabo, V., & Strang, V. R. (1999). Experiencing control in caregiving. *Image: Journal of Nursing Scholarship, 31,* 71-75.

Thompson, S. C. (1981). Will it hurt less if I can control it? A complex answer to a simple question. *Psychological Bulletin, 90,* 89-101.

Tinsley, B., & Holtgrave, D. (1989). Maternal health locus of control beliefs, utilization of childhood preventive health services, and infant health. *Journal of Developmental and Behavioral Pediatrics, 10,* 236-241.

Topf, M. (1992). Effects of personal control over hospital noise on sleep. *Research in Nursing and Health, 15,* 19-25.

Triemstra, A. H. M., Van der Ploeg, H. M., Smit, C., Briet, E., Ader, H. J., & Rosendaal, F. R. (1998). Well-being of haemophilia patient: A model for direct and indirect effects of medical parameters on the physical and psychosocial functioning. *Social Science & Medicine, 47,* 581-593.

Vallerand, A. H., & Ferrell, B. R. (1995). Issues of control in patients with cancer pain. *Western Journal of Nursing Research, 17,* 467-483.

Walker, L. O., & Avant, K. C. (1995). *Strategies for theory construction in nursing* (3rd ed.). Norwalk, CT: Appleton & Lange.

Waller, K. V., & Bates, R. C. (1992). Health locus of control and self-efficacy beliefs in a health elderly sample. *American Journal of Health Promotion, 6,* 302-309.

Wallhagen, M. I., & Brod, M. (1997). Perceived control and well-being in Parkinson's disease. *Western Journal of Nursing Research, 19,* 11-31.

Wallston, K. A., Smith, R. A. P., King, J. E., Smith, M. S., Rye, P., & Burish, T. G. (1991). Desire for control and choice of antiemetic treatment for cancer chemotherapy. *Western Journal of Nursing Research, 13,* 12-29.

Wallston, K. A., & Wallston, B. S. (1982). Who is responsible for your health? The construct of health locus of control. In G. Sanders & J. Suls (Eds.), *Social psychology of health and illness* (pp. 65-95). Hillsdale, NJ: Lawrence Erlbaum.

Wallston, K. A., Wallston, B. S., & DeVellis, R. (1978). Development of the multidimensional health locus of control (MHLC) scales. *Health Education Monographs, 6,* 161-170.

Wells, N. (1994). Perceived control of pain: Relation to distress and disability. *Research in Nursing and Health, 17,* 295-302.

Younger, J., Marsh, K. J., & Grap, M. J. (1995). The relationship of health locus of control and cardiac rehabilitation to mastery of illness-related stress. *Journal of Advanced Nursing, 22,* 294-299.

Zindler-Wernet, P., & Weiss, S. J. (1987). Health locus of control and preventive health behavior. *Western Journal of Nursing Research, 9,* 160-179.

CHAPTER 20

Self-Regulation

The Commonsense Model of Illness Representation

Nancy R. Reynolds and Angelo A. Alonzo

*S*elf-regulation is a term that has been used broadly to refer to the voluntary control of a variety of physiological, psychological, and behavioral processes for coping and appraisal (Carver & Scheier, 1982, 1996). As applied in cognitive-behavioral models—for example, self-efficacy theory (Bandura, 1996), control theory (Carver & Scheier, 1982), and the Commonsense Model of Illness Representation (Leventhal, Meyer, & Nerenz, 1980)—self-regulation is used with reference to an adaptive process in which self-monitoring and reliance on perceptual appraisal or feedback is used as a guide for behavior. As such, self-regulation theory has been useful in broadening our understanding of the dynamic factors involved in many health behaviors. Self-regulation theories are advantageous in that they identify specific stages of cognition, action, and appraisal of perceptual feedback and emphasize the evolution of cognitions over time

(Baumeister & Heatherton, 1996; Cameron & Leventhal, 1995; Weinstein, 1993).

This chapter provides an overview of Leventhal and colleagues' (Diefenbach & Leventhal, 1996; Leventhal, 1986; Leventhal et al., 1997; Leventhal & Cameron, 1987; Leventhal, Diefenbach, & Leventhal, 1992; Leventhal, Nerenz, & Steele, 1984) self-regulation model of health and illness behavior, a review on how it has been tested, and an analysis of its utility in nursing. The self-regulatory model of Leventhal and colleagues, the Commonsense Model of Illness Representation, provides a particularly useful framework for nursing research (Johnson & King, 1985) and practice. Consistent with a focus in nursing, this model provides a framework for understanding the role of symptoms and emotions regarding a variety of health behaviors and places emphasis on patients' perceptions of their illnesses. Individuals are posited to have lay, commonsense ideas about their

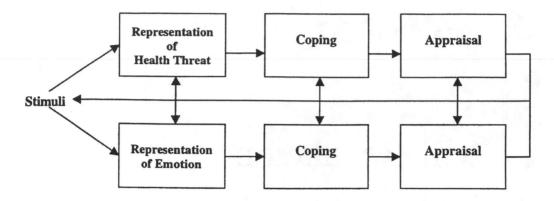

Figure 20.1. Commonsense Model of Illness Representation

health that guide how they cope with health and illness problems as they develop.

➤ FEATURES OF THE MODEL

The commonsense model (Cameron & Leventhal, 1995; Diefenbach & Leventhal, 1996; Leventhal, 1986; Leventhal et al., 1984, 1992, 1997; Leventhal & Cameron, 1987) is an information-processing model in which health-related behaviors are viewed as being heavily influenced by the patient's own definition or representation of an illness threat (Figure 20.1). The representations do not necessarily conform to scientific views, but they guide coping activities.

Development of the model initially emerged from a series of studies of fear communications that were conducted in the late 1960s by Leventhal and colleagues (Diefenbach & Leventhal, 1996; Leventhal, 1970). In these studies, high-fear messages were found to be more effective in changing attitudes toward a recommended health action in comparison to low-fear messages. Changes in attitudes, however, were found to be rather short lived, lasting only 24 to 48 hours, following exposure to the fear messages. Additional data showed that actions, such as getting a protective immunization or stopping smoking, occurred only when the participants exposed

to the fear messages also received a second message that facilitated the development of an action plan.

Neither the fear messages alone nor the action plans alone, however, resulted in action. Because the combination of action plan and fear message (whether high or low) produced action over a period of days and sometimes weeks, and because subjective feelings of fear and fear-induced attitude change faded within 48 hours, the researchers concluded that the action plan was linked not to fear but to some changed way of thinking about or representing the health threat. The realization that the health threat representation in combination with the action plan was the determining factor for subsequent coping actions led to a series of other studies designed to define the nature of the representation. The Commonsense Model of Illness Representation developed through this research (Diefenbach & Leventhal, 1996; Leventhal et al., 1997).

In the commonsense model, the individual is conceptualized as an active problem solver who is engages in parallel processing of two responses: the perceived reality of a health threat and the emotional reaction to this threat (Diefenbach & Leventhal, 1996). Individuals are thought to be motivated to regulate or minimize their health-related risks and act to reduce these health threats in ways consistent with their perceptions of them. The model is based on four basic assumptions (Leventhal et al., 1984).

Active Processing

It is assumed that behavior and experience are constructed by an underlying information-processing system that integrates current stimulus information with both innate and acquired codes or memories. An individual's experience of the world and its objects, emotional reaction to them, and coping reactions are created and organized by this processing system on a moment-by-moment basis (Leventhal et al., 1984).

Parallel Processing

The processing of information involves two parallel processing pathways. One pathway is primarily a conceptual, deliberative system that involves semantic knowledge (derived from culture), controlled, abstract processing, and procedural plans for coping with a health problem. The other is primarily emotional—a concrete, automatic system that involves episodic memories (derived from personal experiences) and perceptual, experiential processing, such as somatic sensations, feelings of fear, and impulsive coping responses. The two pathways interact as the individual responds to a health and illness experience. The interaction of the two pathways has important implications for the processing of symptoms and sensations. Emotions are thought, in essence, to create or influence the climate in which symptoms are processed. They can both influence symptom interpretation and generate additional symptoms that, when incorporated into the person's representation, influence coping and appraisal. Therefore, internal and external cues of health threat activate conceptual, reasoned efforts to understand and control the health threat. They also elicit concrete, emotional responses and efforts to control these emotions (Leventhal et al., 1984, 1997).

Stages in Processing

The processing system is assumed to operate in three stages: representation, coping, and appraisal (Leventhal et al., 1984).

Representation

The first stage creates the definition or the representation of the health threat and the emotion accompanying it. According to the model, both external and internal stimuli invoke illness representations, the cognitive structures by which individuals organize, analyze, and interpret information (both internal and external) and give it meaning. Many sources of information can contribute to an illness representation, including bodily symptoms and sensations, memories of past symptoms and illness experiences, interactions with others (including significant others and health care providers), and media sources.

When an individual experiences a stimulus (e.g., a person experiences an internal sensation or symptom or learns of an asymptomatic illness during a medical checkup), a process of interpretation is brought into play. The individual analyzes the stimulus and seeks an understandable explanation, the representation. An illness representation is thought to involve five distinct dimensions: identity, timeline, cause, controllability, and consequences. The identity dimension includes a disease label and the individual's ideas about the somatic representation of that disease (e.g., the location, extent, and feel of the symptoms). The timeline connects the stimulus to an expected time frame or expected duration of the illness (e.g., whether the stimulus is acute, chronic, or cyclic). The causal component is the individual's conceptions about the probable cause. The perceived controllability of the stimulus refers to the individual's conceptions about whether the stimulus or illness is responsive to self- and/or professional intervention. Finally, the perceived consequences are the anticipated repercussions of the stimulus or illness (conceptions about the short- and long-term outcomes of the illness in terms of personal experiences, economic hardship, or emotional upheaval).

Coping

The second stage, coping, involves the development and execution of response plans or procedures for coping with the representation. The categorization of a stimulus, its meaning, will shape the selection and performance of a coping strategy. Although an array of coping responses may be available to the individual, one's representation determines how one copes. The selection of a coping procedure (e.g., to take medications) is determined by conceptions about the nature of the illness threat.

Appraisal

In the third stage, appraisal, the patient evaluates the efficacy of the coping strategy. Of primary concern is whether or not coping responses have moved the individual closer or farther from desired outcomes specified by the representation. Information from the appraisal stage feeds back into the prior stages. If the patient appraises a particular coping effort as being ineffective, then this might result in the selection of an alternative coping strategy or even a change in the representation of the illness. Thus, the model is dynamic, with continuous, recursive feedback among the stages of the processing system. Each adaptive episode alters the underlying memory structures and thereby changes subsequent episodes.

Hierarchical Processing

The processing system is thought to be hierarchically organized, ranging from a very simple concrete level of processing to a highly abstract level. The simplest level of processing includes automatic mechanisms that make use of concrete stimulus features, whereas the most abstract levels make use of conceptual processes such as language, judgment, and synthesis of information. Inconsistencies can occur between concrete and abstract aspects of the illness experience. For example, a patient may be told that a treatment such as antiretroviral therapy is killing a virus and improving chances for survival, but the patient may actually feel worse because of the medication side effects. The abstract information that the patient's condition is improving is inconsistent with the concrete experience of signs and symptoms that the patient is having connected with the side effects of the therapy. Depending on his or her interpretation of this discrepancy, the patient may then alter his or her coping strategies accordingly to achieve greater consistency (Leventhal et al., 1984).

➢ USE AND TESTING OF THE MODEL IN NURSING AND RELATED DISCIPLINES

Many studies have tested or used (implicitly or explicitly) the Leventhal self-regulatory model as an organizing framework. Because of the complexity of the model, no one piece of research has addressed all facets of the model, but rather a host of research has focused on different aspects of the framework. The research summarized here addresses three primary content areas: (a) illness representations, (b) representations and associations with health behaviors, and (c) cognitive-behavioral self-regulatory interventions.

Illness Representations

Early work (Leventhal & Nerenz, 1982; Leventhal et al., 1984) led to the notion that illness representations contain many discrete dimensions. Since this early work, many researchers have explored illness representations of many different population groups. Illnesses include hypertension (Baumann & Leventhal, 1985; Meyer, Leventhal, & Gutmann, 1985), myocardial infarction (Petrie & Weinman, 1997), diabetes (Hamera et al., 1988; Hampson, 1997; O'Connell et al., 1984), pressure sores (Sebern, 1996), schizophrenia (Hamera, Peterson, Handley, Plumlee,

& Frank-Ragan, 1991), chronic fatigue syndrome (Moss-Morris, 1997), and conditions involving chronic pain (Jenson & Karoly, 1992; Morley & Wilkinson, 1995).

Studies exploring the illness representations of various population groups vary in emphasis, methodology, and terminology; it has been repeatedly shown, however, that people do hold cognitive representations of their illnesses. Furthermore, studies on the structure of illness representations have supported the five dimensions noted earlier (identity, timeline, cause, controllability, and consequences) by which experiences of illnesses are cognitively organized (Lau & Hartman, 1983; Scharloo & Kaptein, 1997; Skelton & Croyle, 1991). To date, most studies have been restricted to the assessment of one or two dimensions of the model, with little work done to examine the relationships among dimensions (Scharloo & Kaptein, 1997). Furthermore, although there is considerable support for the five dimensions of representation, there is increasing awareness that each of these components is subject to further differentiation and that there are other processes that need to be considered (Leventhal et al., 1997; Weinman & Petrie, 1997). For example, in addition to assessing individuals' illness representations, there is a need to understand people's views about their treatment (Horne, 1997).

Representations and Associations With Health Behaviors

Other research has linked illness representations with many health and illness outcomes. Researchers have shown, for example, that the implicit model held by a patient relates to his or her propensity to seek care. A case in point is the work completed by Lau, Bernard, and Hartman (1989), who found that the propensity to seek care was more likely for people who held strong representations of "identity" and "cure."

In a study of care-seeking behavior during the acute phase of myocardial infarction, Petrie and Weinman (1997) found the identity component of representations to be important. Less delay was associated with a higher degree of family history and correspondence of symptoms experienced with classic symptoms that are regarded as critical (e.g., breathlessness and pain).

In other research of persons across the life span, Leventhal and Crouch (1997) found changes in patterns of help seeking and health care utilization as people age. They concluded that these changes are not a direct effect of aging but a reflection of age-related modifications in the way that symptoms are perceived and evaluated as people age. These modifications in perception tend to result in more benign attributions and possible delays in help seeking. They found, however, that an increased sense of vulnerability combined with the need to reduce health risks and conserve personal resources moved older people toward higher levels of most preventive behaviors and better adherence to treatment.

The concept of representation has also been used to study other aspects of adherence. For example, Meyer et al. (1985) found that beliefs regarding "timeline" are related to how long a person remains in active treatment for hypertension. Research has also shown that representations about symptoms are powerful determinants of other adherence behavior. For example, it has been shown that people with diabetes hold beliefs about which of their symptoms are related to alterations in blood glucose. Although often inaccurate, it has been demonstrated that these representations are nonetheless used to guide decisions about behaviors such as diet and exercise (Baumann & Leventhal, 1985; Hamera et al., 1988; O'Connell, Hamera, Schorfheide, & Guthrie, 1990). Horne (1997), in a study of medication adherence, was able to discern how different patient representations about medications influenced treatment nonadherence. Interestingly, he found that medication nonadherence does not appear to be associated with the belief that medicines are unnecessary or ineffective. The majority of patients agreed that their present and future health depended on medicines. Many patients, however, held a view of medication by which their beliefs about necessity and efficacy were tempered by concerns about the potential for harm. These patients were less adherent.

Research has also linked representations with other health behaviors. Zimmerman and Olson (1994), for example, found individuals' perceptions concerning HIV timeline and identity, as well as self-efficacy, were significant predictors of risk behavior change.

Although a significant amount of work demonstrates that illness representations influence coping mechanisms, consensus has not been reached regarding which representations are the most salient in moving an individual toward a particular coping strategy in particular circumstances. There is evidence that some consistent relations exist between different illness perception dimensions and different health outcomes. In a review of 101 studies published between 1985 and 1995, Scharloo and Kaptein (1997) concluded that favorable outcomes appear to be associated with (a) high scores on "internal control," (b) high accuracy ratings on "identity" and "causes," (c) a belief that the illness will be intermittent or discontinuous, and (d) a low level of perceived disability or seriousness of the illness. To date, however, there has been limited study of the interaction between the five dimensions or exploration of the interplay of emotional processes.

Cognitive-Behavioral Self-Regulatory Interventions

Although not extensive, the current body of intervention literature supports the conceptualizations in the commonsense model, but additional validation is necessary. Although studies have examined the effect of psychoeducational interventions on cognitive and behavioral factors (Pimm, 1997), relatively few studies have directly manipulated cognitions or coping behaviors to investigate whether they mediate the therapeutic benefits of psychoeducational interventions (Leventhal et al., 1997). Although the model suggests that appropriate restructuring of the person's illness representation is necessary if self-regula-

tion of undesirable stimuli, such as pain or emotional distress, is to be improved, this may involve a fair degree of complexity. For example, Parker et al. (1984) presented rheumatoid arthritis patients with a 7-hour educational program. Although patients' knowledge about the disease increased, the intervention group reported more pain and disability than the control group. Although enhancing knowledge, the researchers concluded that the intervention may also have had a negative influence on illness cognitions by highlighting the salience of pain and the possible negative effects of rheumatoid arthritis.

To date, the most extensive intervention research guided by self-regulation theory has been completed by nursing researcher Jean E. Johnson and colleagues (Johnson, 1996; Johnson, Fieler, Wlasowicz, Mitchell, & Jones, 1997; Johnson, Fuller, Endress, & Rice, 1978; Johnson & King, 1985; Johnson, Lauver, & Nail, 1989; Johnson, Nail, Lauver, King, & Keys, 1988; Leventhal & Johnson, 1983). Some of Johnson's early work was completed in collaboration with Leventhal (Johnson & Leventhal, 1974; Leventhal & Johnson, 1983). Although her ongoing work shares many of the assumptions of the commonsense model, Johnson has developed an independent line of research that is focused on how patients cope with a specific procedure or treatment as part of the total illness experience as opposed to Leventhal's more inclusive approach.

In a series of studies, Johnson and colleagues (Johnson, 1996; Johnson, Fuller, et al., 1978; Johnson & King, 1985; Johnson et al., 1988, 1989, 1997) examined the effects of preparatory information that contains particular content: descriptions of the concrete, objective features of an impending experience. The concrete objective features of an event have four dimensions: (a) physical sensations (e.g., what is felt, heard, tasted, smelled, and seen), (b) temporal features (e.g., sequence and duration of events), (c) environmental features (e.g., people involved and characteristics of the setting), and (d) causes of the sensations. It is proposed that when preparatory information contains descriptions of the concrete, objective features of an impending treatment, problem-solving coping will be fostered that results in reduced disruption to patients' usual activities and better patient psychosocial outcomes. It is reasoned that when patients expect to experience the unambiguous, concrete, objective features, they will monitor their experience for the absence or presence of these features. Attention is focused on the concrete, objective aspects of the experience, and coping is focused on problem solving and direct actions. Because this coping process is often effective, patients are thus able to minimize the amount of disruption to their usual life activities (Johnson et al., 1997; Leventhal & Johnson, 1983).

Johnson and colleagues (Johnson, 1996; Johnson et al., 1997) investigated the effects of concrete, objective preparatory informational interventions on mood and disruption of usual life activities of patients coping with radiation therapy for breast or prostate cancer. It was found that patients who received the concrete, objective information were better able to maintain usual activities during and following treatment. Mood, however, was enhanced only among persons identified as having the personality characteristic of generally pessimistic expectations.

The self-regulatory model provides a fertile framework for guiding the development of intervention strategies for nursing. Work to date, however, clearly indicates that the design of effective interventions may likely involve considerable intricacy.

➤ MEASUREMENT

A variety of methodologies have been used to assess illness representations (Leventhal & Nerenz, 1985; Scharloo & Kaptein, 1997; Weinman, Petrie, Moss-Morris, & Horne, 1996). No gold standard has emerged (Weinman & Petrie, 1997). Researchers have commonly used semistructured or open-ended interview approaches to obtain data on illness representations (Leventhal & Nerenz, 1985; Scharloo & Kaptein, 1997; Weinman et al., 1996). (See Table 20.1.)

Various standardized instruments have also been employed or developed to measure illness representations (Table 20.1). Typically, only one or two illness representation dimensions have been measured with any given instrument (Scharloo & Kaptein, 1997). For example, representations consistent with the dimension of control have been assessed with the Multidimensional Health Locus of Control Scales (Andrykowski & Brady, 1994; Fowers, 1994), whereas the Pain Beliefs and Perceptions Inventory has been used to measure cause and timeline (Herda, Siegeris, & Basler, 1994; Williams, Robinson, & Geisser, 1994). Although conceptually consistent with the Leventhal model, the development of these instruments was not guided by precepts in the model. Other instruments that have been developed have drawn explicitly from the Leventhal model but have been developed to elicit illness representations of a particular diagnostic group. For example, the Personal Models of Diabetes Interview (Hampson, Glasgow, & Toobert, 1990) was designed to determine a wide range of beliefs of diabetic patients, including the five components of illness representations. Similarly, Horne and Weinman (1995) developed an instrument, the Beliefs About Medicines Questionnaire, that is specific to the measurement of beliefs about medication representations (Horne, 1997).

The theoretically based Illness Perception Questionnaire (IPQ; Weinman et al., 1996) enables researchers to assess each of the five cognitive representations of illness (identity, timeline, cause, controllability, and consequences) across population groups and lends itself to the study of interactions among the variables. The IPQ was specifically developed to assess the five cognitive dimensions of illness representation as described by Leventhal et al. (Diefenbach & Leventhal, 1996; Leventhal, 1986; Leventhal & Cameron, 1987; Leventhal et al., 1984, 1992, 1997). The instrument consists of five sub-scales, one for each of the attributes (identity, timeline, cause, controllability, and consequences). Identity is measured using a list of 15 symptoms. Timeline, controllability and cure, and consequences are measured using a

TABLE 20.1 Summary of Measures[a]

Dimension	Measure
Representations	Semistructured or open-ended interview
	Personal Models of Diabetes Interview (Hampson, Glasgow, & Toobert, 1990)
	Beliefs About Medicines Questionnaire (Horne & Weinman, 1995)
	Illness Perception Questionnaire (Weinman, Petrie, Moss-Morris, & Horne, 1996)
Coping	Carolina Self-Regulation Inventory (Massey & Pesut, 1991)
	Ways of Coping Checklist (Lazarus & Folkman, 1984)

a. For an extensive review of representation measures, see Scharloo and Kaptein (1997).

34-item, Likert-type scale. The IPQ has been used with a variety of chronic illnesses and has been found to be internally consistent and reliable (Weinman et al., 1996). This approach seems promising (Moss-Morris, 1997; Petrie & Weinman, 1997). Studies comparing the reliability and validity of this measure with those of others have not been completed, however.

Researchers have also used a variety of instruments to assess self-regulatory coping mechanisms. The Carolina Self-Regulation Inventory (Massey & Pesut, 1991) was developed to enable nurse clinicians and researchers to assess patient response to self-regulation interventions. Others have used the Ways of Coping Checklist (Lazarus & Folkman, 1984). Such scales are subject to criticisms of having a limited range of coping factors and a bias toward coping as positively valenced, and they are based on the assumption that persons are necessarily conscious of their coping processes (Leventhal, Suls, & Leventhal, 1993; Leventhal et al., 1997).

➤ **IMPLICATIONS FOR THEORY, PRACTICE, AND RESEARCH**

The commonsense model has the potential to advance knowledge development in many

ways. Consistent with the emphasis of nursing, the focal point of the model is the patient. The model suggests that an understanding of patients' responses to health threats is obtained by understanding their perceptions or implicit models of the threats they face. Particular emphasis is placed on the significance of the patient's interpretation of symptoms and on the individual as an active participant in the health care process.

This model provides a strong paradigm for integrating findings from diverse lines of research, and it can guide new research in nursing (Keller, Ward, & Baumann, 1989; Ward, 1993). The model has been used by nurses to guide the development of conceptual models and exploration of a broad range of health and illness experiences, including self-care processes (Keller et al., 1989), cardiac delay (the Acute Myocardial Infarction Coping Model; Alonzo & Reynolds, 1998), recovery from illness episodes (Massey & Pesut, 1991), diabetic adherence (Hamera et al., 1988; O'Connell et al., 1984), responses to diabetes (Newbern, 1990), functioning in schizophrenia (Hamera et al., 1991), cancer and cancer therapies (Johnson, 1996; Johnson et al., 1997; Ward, Leventhal, Easterling, Luchterhand, & Love, 1991; Ward, Leventhal, & Love, 1988), pressure ulcers (Sebern, 1996), genital herpes (Keller, Jadack, & Mims, 1991), and recovery from surgery

(Johnson, Fuller, et al., 1978; Johnson, Rice, Fuller, & Endress, 1978).

The model lends itself to different approaches to understanding the patient. It is useful with approaches that focus on the phenomenological experience of the individual patient and with designs that focus on understanding responses across individuals. Nursing studies have employed the model to facilitate an understanding of how patients adjust to illness using either qualitative (Manton, 1994; Newbern, 1990) or quantitative (Barevick & Johnson, 1990; Keller et al., 1991) methods .

Although considerable support has been rendered for some of the major precepts of the model, this review of the literature raises several issues and limitations. First, there is support for the five cognitive dimensions of representation. There is increasing awareness, however, that other processes need to be incorporated or the current dimensions need further delineation or both (Horne, 1997; Leventhal et al., 1997; Weinman & Petrie, 1997). For example, in addition to assessing illness perceptions, there is a need to understand people's views about the treatment or advice they have been given. Furthermore, previous research indicates that certain patterns of illness representations may be associated with better psychological and physical outcomes. To date, however, little research has tested which combinations of illness representations are the most important in determining behavior and adjustment. Although there is support for links between illness representations and coping behaviors, few data are available about how particular coping strategies are selected (Leventhal et al., 1997). This knowledge is important to guide development of effective intervention strategies.

The commonsense model has not been widely used to guide nursing practice explicitly, but several aspects appear to be used implicitly (Garvin, Huston, & Baker, 1992). Research by Johnson and colleagues (Johnson, 1996; Johnson & King, 1985; Johnson et al., 1988, 1989, 1997; Leventhal & Johnson,

1983) provides a foundation for the development of preparatory information interventions in nursing. It has also been suggested that patients' implicit models should routinely be explored as part of providing information to patients and families (Keller et al., 1989; Ward, 1993). This would enable delivery of information to the patient that is congruent with, rather than antithetical to, the patient's own representations. Implicit belief systems, however, may be difficult to uncover because patients may not realize that they hold these beliefs or, if they are recognized, patients may hide them because they do not conform to medical beliefs (Lowery, 1993). Furthermore, although it is clear that illness representations are important determinants of outcome and adjustment in chronic illness, it has not been established that they can effectively change illness beliefs to positively impact outcomes (Leventhal et al., 1997). Clearly there is considerable complexity in illness representations that needs to be further addressed.

Other questions remain about the cognitive and emotional processes involved in people's representations of health and illness. Leventhal et al. (1997) stressed the importance of enhancing an understanding of self-regulatory processes within the social and cultural contexts in which they occur. Additional work is needed to integrate the influence of social system variables. The interaction of emotional with cognitive factors also needs to be delineated in more detail. It is not clear if the pathways are truly separate and interacting or fused together (Leventhal et al., 1997).

Finally, there is a need for studies that compare the reliability and validity of different instruments that measure illness representations to provide researchers with a basis for choosing appropriately.

➤ SUMMARY

The Commonsense Model of Illness Representation provides a useful framework for broadening our understanding of the dynamic factors involved in the stress of health and illness behaviors. The model is particularly useful for knowledge development in nursing because it places emphasis on the role of symptoms and emotions regarding a variety of health behaviors, and it places emphasis on patients' perceptions of their illnesses.

➤ REFERENCES

Alonzo, A. A., & Reynolds, N. R. (1998). The structure of emotions during acute myocardial infarction: A model of coping. *Social Science and Medicine, 46*, 1099-1110.

Andrykowski, M. A., & Brady, M. J. (1994). Health locus of control and psychological distress in cancer patients: Interactive effects of context. *Journal of Behavioral Medicine, 17,* 439-458.

Bandura, A. (1996). Failures in self-regulation: Energy depletion or selective disengagement? *Psychological Inquiry, 7,* 2024.

Barevick, A. M., & Johnson, J. E. (1990). Preference for information and involvement, information seeking and emotional responses of women undergoing colposcopy. *Research in Nursing & Health, 13,* 17.

Baumann, L., & Leventhal, H. (1985). I can tell when my blood pressure is up: Can't I? *Health Psychology, 4,* 203-218.

Baumeister, R. F., & Heatherton, T. F. (1996). Self-regulation failure: An overview. *Psychological Inquiry, 7,* 115.

Cameron, L. D., & Leventhal, H. (1995). Vulnerability beliefs, symptom experiences, and the processing of health threat information: A self-regulatory perspective. *Journal of Applied Social Psychology, 25,* 1859-1883.

Carver, C. S., & Scheier, M. F. (1982). Control theory: A useful conceptual framework for personality, social, clinical, and health psychology. *Psychological Bulletin, 92,* 111-135.

Carver, C. S., & Scheier, M. F. (1996). Self-regulation and its failures. *Psychological Inquiry, 7,* 32-40.

Diefenbach, M. A., & Leventhal, H. (1996). The Commonsense Model of Illness Representation: Theoretical and practical considerations. *Journal of Social Distress and the Homeless, 5,* 11-38.

Fowers, B. J. (1994). Perceived control, illness status, stress, and adjustment to cardiac illness. *Journal of Psychology, 128,* 567-576.

Garvin, B. J., Huston, G. P., & Baker, C. F. (1992). Information used by nurses to prepare patients for a stressful event. *Applied Nursing Research, 5,* 158-163.

Hamera, E., Cassmeyer, V., O'Connell, K. A., Weldon, G. T., Knapp, T. M., & Kyner, J. L. (1988). Self-reg-

ulation in individuals with Type II diabetes. *Nursing Research, 37*(6), 363-367.

Hamera, E. K., Peterson, K. A., Handley, S. M., Plumlee, A. A., & Frank-Ragan, E. (1991). Patient self-regulation and functioning in schizophrenia. *Hospital & Community Psychiatry, 42*(6), 630-631.

Hampson, S. E. (1997). Illness representations and the self-management of diabetes. In K. J. Petrie & J. A. Weinman (Eds.), *Perceptions of health & illness* (pp. 323-349). Amsterdam: Harwood Academic.

Hampson, S. E., Glasgow, R. E., & Toobert, D. J. (1990). Personal models of diabetes and their relations to self-care activities. *Health Psychology, 9,* 632-646.

Herda, C. A., Siegeris, K., & Basler, H. D. (1994). The Pain Beliefs and Perceptions Inventory: Further evidence for a 4-factor structure. *Pain, 57,* 85-90.

Horne, R. (1997). Representations of medication and treatment: Advances in theory and measurement. In K. J. Petrie & J. A. Weinman (Eds.), *Perceptions of health & illness.* Amsterdam: Harwood Academic.

Horne, R., & Weinman, J. (1995). The Beliefs About Medicines Questionnaire (BMQ). In *Proceedings of the Special Group in Health Psychology.* Leicester, UK: British Psychological Society.

Jenson, M. P., & Karoly, P. (1992). Pain-specific beliefs, perceived symptom severity and adjustment to chronic pain. *Journal of Consulting and Clinical Psychology, 59,* 431-438.

Johnson, J. E. (1996). Coping with radiation therapy: Optimism and the effect of preparatory interventions. *Research in Nursing and Health, 19,* 2-12.

Johnson, J. E., Fieler, V. K., Wlasowicz, G. S., Mitchell, M. L., & Jones, L. S. (1997). The effects of nursing care guided by self-regulation theory on coping with radiation therapy. *Oncology Nursing Forum, 24*(6), 1041-1050.

Johnson, J. E., Fuller, S. S., Endress, M. P., & Rice, V. H. (1978). Altering patient's responses to surgery: An extension and replication. *Research in Nursing and Health, 1,* 111-121.

Johnson, J. E., & King, K. B. (1985). Influence of expectations about symptoms on delay in seeking treatment during myocardial infarction. *American Journal of Critical Care, 4,* 29-35.

Johnson, J. E., Lauver, D. R., & Nail, L. M. (1989). Process of coping with radiation therapy. *Journal of Consulting and Clinical Psychology, 57,* 358-364.

Johnson, J. E., & Leventhal, H. (1974). Effects of accurate expectations and behavioral instructions on reaction during a noxious medical examination. *Journal of Personality and Social Psychology, 29,* 710-718.

Johnson, J. E., Nail, L. M., Lauver, D. R., King, K. B., & Keys, H. (1988). Reducing the negative impact of radiation therapy on functional status. *Cancer, 61,* 46-51.

Johnson, J. E., Rice, V. H., Fuller, S. S., & Endress, M. P. (1978). Sensory information, instruction in coping strategy, and recovery from surgery. *Research in Nursing & Health, 1,* 4-7.

Keller, M., Jadack, R., & Mims, F. (1991). Perceived stressors and coping responses in persons with recurrent genital herpes. *Research in Nursing and Health, 14,* 421-430.

Keller, M. L., Ward, S., & Baumann, L. J. (1989). Processes of self-care: Monitoring sensations and symptoms. *Advances in Nursing Science, 12,* 54-66.

Lau, R., Bernard, T., & Hartman, K. (1989). Further exploration of common-sense representations of common illnesses. *Health Psychology, 2,* 195-219.

Lau, R. R., & Hartman, K. A. (1983). Common sense representations of common illnesses. *Health Psychology, 2,* 167-185.

Lazarus, R. S., & Folkman, S. (1984). *Stress, appraisal, and coping.* New York: Springer.

Leventhal, E. A., & Crouch, M. (1997). Are there differences in perceptions of illness across the life span? In K. J. Petrie & J. A. Weinman (Eds.), *Perceptions of health & illness.* Amsterdam: Harwood Academic.

Leventhal, E. A., Suls, J., & Leventhal, H. (1993). Hierarchical analysis of coping: Evidence from life-span studies. In H. W. Krohne (Ed.), *Attention and avoidance: Strategies in coping with aversiveness* (pp. 71-99). Seattle: Hogrefe & Huber.

Leventhal, H. (1970). Findings and theory in the study of fear communications. In L. Berkowitz (Ed.), *Advances in experimental social psychology* (Vol. 5, pp. 120-186). New York: Academic Press.

Leventhal, H. (1986). Symptom reporting: A focus on process. In S. McHugh & T. M. Vallis (Eds.), *Illness behavior: A multidisciplinary model* (pp. 219-237). New York: Plenum.

Leventhal, H., Benyamini, Y., Brownlee, S., Diefenbach, M., Leventhal, E. A., Patrick-Miller, L., & Robitaille, C. (1997). Illness representations: Theoretical foundations. In K. J. Petrie & J. A. Weinman (Eds.), *Perceptions of health and illness* (pp. 19-45). Amsterdam: Harwood Academic.

Leventhal, H., & Cameron, L. (1987). Behavioral theories and the problem of compliance. *Patient Education and Counseling, 10,* 117-138.

Leventhal, H., Diefenbach, M., & Leventhal, E. A. (1992). Illness cognition: Using common sense to understand treatment adherence and affect cognition interactions. *Cognitive Therapy and Research, 16,* 143-163.

Leventhal, H., & Johnson, J. E. (1983). Laboratory and field experimentation: Development of a theory of self-regulation. In P. J. Wooldridge, M. H. Schmitt, J. K. Skipper, & R. C. Lenarde (Eds.), *Behavioral science and nursing theory.* St. Louis, MO: C. V. Mosby.

Leventhal, H. D., Meyer, D., & Nerenz, D. (1980). The commonsense representation of illness danger. In S. Rachman (Ed.), *Contributions to medical psychology* (Vol. 2, pp. 7-31). Oxford, UK: Pergamon.

Leventhal, H., & Nerenz, D. (1982). Representations on threat and the control of stress. In D. Meichenbaum & M. Jaremko (Eds.), *Stress prevention and management: A cognitive behavioral approach.* New York: Plenum.

Leventhal, H., & Nerenz, D. (1985). The assessment of illness cognition. In P. Karoly (Ed.), *Measurement strategies in health psychology* (pp. 517-555). New York: John Wiley.

Leventhal, H. L., Nerenz, D. R., & Steele, D. J. (1984). Illness representations and coping with health threats. In A. Baum, S. E. Taylor, & J. E. Singer (Eds.), *Handbook of psychology and health* (pp. 219-252). Hillsdale, NJ: Lawrence Erlbaum.

Lowery, B. J. (1993). Response to "The Common Sense Model: An organizing framework for knowledge development in nursing." *Scholarly Inquiry for Nursing Practice: An International Journal, 7,* 91-94.

Manton, A. P. (1994). *Making the decision to seek care for a non-urgent illness: A qualitative study.* Unpublished doctoral dissertation, University of Rhode Island, Kingston.

Massey, J. A., & Pesut, D. J. (1991). Self-regulation strategies of adults. *Western Journal of Nursing Research, 13*(5), 627-634.

Meyer, D., Leventhal, H., & Gutmann, M. (1985). Common sense models of illness: The example of hypertension. *Health Psychology, 4,* 115-135.

Morley, S., & Wilkinson, L. (1995). The Pain Beliefs and Perceptions Inventory: A British replication. *Pain, 61,* 427-433.

Moss-Morris, R. (1997). The role of illness cognitions and coping in the aetiology and maintenance of chronic fatigue syndrome (CFS). In K. J. Petrie & J. A. Weinman (Eds.), *Perceptions of health & illness* (pp. 441-463). Amsterdam: Harwood Academic.

Newbern, V. B. (1990). Application of self-regulation theory to the year of denouement for an insulin-dependent diabetic. *Holistic Nursing Practice, 5,* 36-44.

O'Connell, K., Hamera, E., Schorfheide, A., & Guthrie, D. (1990). Symptom beliefs and actual blood glucose in Type II diabetes. *Research in Nursing and Health, 13,* 145-151.

O'Connell, K. A., Hamera, E. K., Knapp, T. M., Cassmeyer, V. L., Eaks, G. A., & Fox, M. A. (1984). Symptom use and self-regulation in type II diabetes. *Advances in Nursing Science, 6*(3), 19-28.

Parker, J. C., Singsen, B. H., Hewett, J. E., Walker, S. E., Hazelwood, S. E., Hall, P. J., Holsten, D. J., & Rodon, C. M. (1984). Educating patients with rheumatoid arthritis: A prospective analysis. *Archives of Physical Medicine Rehabilitation, 65,* 771-774.

Petrie, K. J., & Weinman, J. A. (1997). Illness representations and recovery from myocardial infarction. In K. J. Petrie & J. A. Weinman (Eds.), *Perceptions of health & illness* (pp. 441-463). Amsterdam: Harwood Academic.

Pimm, T. J. (1997). Self-regulation and psych-educational interventions for rheumatic disease. In K. J. Petrie & J. A. Weinman (Eds.), *Perceptions of health & illness* (pp. 349-379). Amsterdam: Harwood Academic.

Scharloo, M., & Kaptein, A. (1997). Measurement of illness perceptions in patients with chronic somatic illnesses: A review. In K. J. Petrie & J. A. Weinman (Eds.), *Perceptions of health & illness.* Amsterdam: Harwood Academic.

Sebern, M. D. (1996). Explication of the construct of shared care and the prevention of pressure ulcers in home health care. *Research in Nursing & Health, 19,* 183-192.

Skelton, J. A., & Croyle, R. T. (Eds.). (1991). *Mental representation in health and illness.* New York: Springer-Verlag.

Ward, S., Leventhal, H., Easterling, D., Luchterhand, C., & Love, R. (1991). Social support, self-esteem, and communication in patients receiving chemotherapy. *Journal of Psychosocial Oncology, 9,* 95-116.

Ward, S., Leventhal, H., & Love, R. (1988). Repression revisited: Tactics used in coping with a severe health threat. *Personality & Social Psychology Bulletin, 14,* 735-756.

Ward, S. E. (1993). The commonsense model: An organizing framework for knowledge development in nursing. *Scholarly Inquiry for Nursing Practice, 7*(2), 79-90.

Weinman, J., Petrie, K. J., Moss-Morris, R., & Horne, R. (1996). The Illness Perception Questionnaire: A new method for assessing the cognitive representation of illness. *Psychology and Health, 11,* 431-445.

Weinman, J. A., & Petrie, K. J. (1997). Perceptions of health and illness. In J. A. Weinman & K. J. Petrie (Eds.), *Perceptions of health & illness* (pp. 1-19). Amsterdam: Harwood Academic.

Weinstein, N. D. (1993). Testing four competing theories of health-protective behavior. *Health Psychology, 12,* 324-333.

Williams, D. A., Robinson, M. E., & Geisser, M. E. (1994). Pain beliefs: Assessment and utility. *Pain, 59,* 71-78.

Zimmerman, R. S., & Olson, K. (1994). AIDS-related risk behavior and behavior change in a sexually active, heterosexual sample: A test of three models of prevention. *AIDS Education & Prevention, 6,* 189-204.

CHAPTER 21

Stress, Self-Efficacy, and Health

Debra Siela and Ann W. Wieseke

ith the rapidly evolving health care system and the imperative emphasis on self-care, professional nurses are seeking theories that helps explain initiation and maintenance of health behaviors that can be used to guide nursing practice. Research has shown that the deleterious effects of some illnesses can be slowed, the risk of some illnesses decreased, and psychological and physical well-being increased by participating in self-care health behaviors.

One construct that addresses the factors involved in initiation and maintenance of self-care behavior is self-efficacy, derived from Bandura's broader social cognitive theory (SCT) (Bandura, 1977, 1989). Self-efficacy is becoming widely recognized by nurses as a concept that has theoretical and practical application related to initiation and maintenance of self-care health behaviors, including those behaviors related to stress and coping. Behavior is proposed to be a function of the subjective value of an outcome, the subjective probability that a particular behavior will achieve the valued outcome in a specific situation, and the individual's efficacy expectations in relation to performance of the behavior.

Searches of Medline and the Cumulative Index for Nursing and Allied Health Literature show that self-efficacy was first referenced in 1977. An increasing emphasis on self-efficacy in relation to self-care health behavior is evidenced by the number of publications (1,294) in the literature in the past two decades. The majority (936) of the studies were published in the past 6 years. Nurse researchers, in particular, have used the concept of self-efficacy, as defined by Bandura, more frequently in the past decade as evidenced by 95 published studies. A majority of the studies have used either Bandura's SCT (65 studies) or Pender's Health Promotion Model (30 studies) which includes self-efficacy (Tillet, 1998) as a framework. The Health Promotion Model, rooted in Bandura's SCT, recognizes the importance of cognitive-perceptual factors such as self-efficacy and modifying factors that influence the occurrence of health-promoting behaviors. Both frameworks identify that the individual is self-determining in relation to behavior.

The first section of this chapter provides an overview of the SCT. The second contains a review of self-efficacy research literature, and the third section presents an overview of the Health Promotion Model and related self-efficacy research. Research from both nursing and other disciplines is discussed. The fourth section describes the development of self-efficacy instruments, and the final section discusses implications for nursing research and practice related to self-efficacy. The research is limited to that related to health behavior published in the past two decades. Only studies that referenced the concept of self-efficacy as interpreted by Bandura were reviewed. There were 172 studies that met the review criteria, and half of these were conducted by nurse researchers. The largest number of studies completed by nursing professionals were related to health behavior of clients with cardiovascular disorders. The majority reviewed used descriptive, correlational designs rather than a predictive design. Methodological concerns limit generalizability of findings and contributions to nursing knowledge and practice in many of the studies.

➤ SOCIAL COGNITIVE THEORY

Bandura reconceptualized the social learning theory (SLT) to formulate a middle-range theory, the SCT, as a framework for analyzing human motivation, thought, and action. According to the tenets of SLT, environment affects behavior; behavior, however, does not affect the environment (Bandura, 1986). In the reformulation, Bandura proposed that there was a reciprocal relationship between environment and behavior. This relationship or reciprocal determinism and self-efficacy thus became the core of the SCT.

The SCT involves understanding how human cognitions, actions, motivations, and emotions affect one another reciprocally (Bandura, 1986). The theory asserts that people are self-reflective and self-regulative and can mold their environment because of these attributes. Individuals can change their environment in this way because they are able to symbolize their thoughts and experiences, which are then internalized in their cognitive processes.

Through symbolic interactions, individuals create models of experience in their cognitive processes. The created models are then used to test hypothetical courses of action, to predict outcomes, and as a framework to communicate these experiences to others (Bandura, 1986). People perform behaviors that are purposive or goal directed because they have a previous model based on their symbolizing capacity (Bandura, 1986). People develop standards for behavior and evaluate behaviors against these standards. According to the SCT, individuals are able to analyze their own thoughts, experiences, and behaviors. When people use self-reflection, they create the cognitive base, perceptions of self-efficacy, for self-regulation or control of subsequent behaviors.

Self-Efficacy and Triadic Reciprocality

In 1989, Bandura broadened the principle of reciprocal determinism to that of triadic reciprocality. Triadic reciprocality added the interaction of inner personal factors to the previously conceptualized interaction of environmental and behavioral factors. Inner personal factors include cognition, emotion, and biological events. On the basis of triadic determinism, the original definition of self-efficacy—one's belief in one's ability to perform a specific behavior or set of behaviors required to produce an outcome—was changed to include beliefs about the individual's capability to exercise control over events that affect his or her life (Bandura, 1977, 1989). Self-efficacy then referred to perceptions that evolve initially from the interactions of inner personal factors (particularly cognitive factors) with behavior, environmental events, and

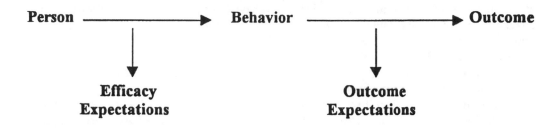

Figure 21.1. Self-Efficacy (from A. Bandura, "Self-Efficacy: Toward a Unifying Theory of Behavioral Change." *Psychological Review, 84,* 191-215. Copyright © 1977 by the American Psychological Association. Reprinted with permission.)

other inner personal factors (Bandura, 1986). The three factors of environmental events, inner personal events, and behavior may not directly interact, and they may not affect each other simultaneously or with equal strength. People respond cognitively, behaviorally, and emotionally to environmental events. Through cognition, people exert control over (self-regulate) their behavior or emotions in response to environmental events. Self-regulation involves self-appraisal of one's abilities. The process of self-appraisal leads to the development of efficacy expectations and outcome expectations that are synthesized into perceptions of self-efficacy that help determine whether an individual ultimately initiates or maintains a specific behavior or both.

Self-efficacy, as noted previously, is determined by efficacy expectations and outcome expectations (Bandura, 1986) (see Figure 21.1). *Efficacy expectations* are beliefs about one's ability to perform the behavior that will produce an expected outcome. *Outcome expectations* are the beliefs that engaging in a certain behavior or behaviors will result in a specific outcome.

Dimensions of Efficacy Expectations

Efficacy expectations can be assessed on three dimensions: (a) magnitude, (b) strength, and (c) generality. Magnitude of efficacy expectations refers to the ordering of tasks by difficulty level. People may have high efficacy expectations at lower levels of difficulty and lower efficacy expectations at higher levels of difficulty. Strength of efficacy expectations refers to a judgment of the certainty one has of the ability to perform a certain behavior. Most research on self-efficacy has measured only the strength dimension when assessing efficacy expectations (Holden, 1991; O'Leary, 1985; Strecher, DeVillis, Becker, & Rosenstock, 1986).

Generality of efficacy expectations refers to the extent to which efficacy expectations about a specific behavior and its related outcome generalize to other situations. Bandura (1986) initially proposed that self-efficacy beliefs were situation specific and were not generalizable. In 1991, however, he broadened the concept, stating that generalization can occur if other situations are similar in social structure so that development of skills or behaviors covaries (Bandura, 1991).

Sources of Efficacy Information

Not only does the nursing profession need to recognize the dimensions of efficacy expectations but also an understanding of the sources of efficacy information must be acquired to enable application of the theory to nursing practice. Efficacy expectations evolve from cognitive appraisal of information about previous performance accomplishments, vicarious experiences, verbal persuasion, and autonomic arousal found within the personal, behavioral, and environmental factors of a situation (Bandura, 1982). High levels of efficacy expectations will not result in performance of a desired behavior if deficits are present in an individual's perceived capabilities as identified through cognitive appraisal of information available from these sources. Given perceptions of adequate skills, resources, and incentives, efficacy expectations are a major determinant of behavior choice, amount of effort, and persistence with a behavior (Bandura, 1986).

Mastery, one source of efficacy information and also called enactive attainment, originates from an individual's personal experiences (Bandura, 1982). Mastery is attained after successfully performing the given behavior many times. Many people believe that this is the most persuasive of all sources of efficacy information in determining positive perceptions of self-efficacy for a behavior.

Vicarious learning or modeling is another source of efficacy information. When people see or visualize others with similar attributes performing a behavior successfully, they perceive that they too are able to perform the behavior successfully.

A third source of efficacy information is verbal persuasion. Verbal persuasion is the act of trying to talk someone into believing that they possess the ability to successfully perform a desired behavior (Bandura, 1986). The effectiveness of this source depends on the perceived expertness, trustworthiness, and attractiveness of the source (Petty & Cacioppo, 1981). This source of efficacy information is not as effective for increasing efficacy expectations as mastery or vicarious experiences (Bandura, 1986).

The physiological state of the individual, autonomic arousal, is the fourth source of efficacy information. The information about physiologic state includes that of somatic arousal in stressful situations, such as fear, fatigue, shortness of breath, and pain (Bandura, 1986). People with high somatic arousal tend to have low self-efficacy for performing certain behaviors.

Summary of Social Cognitive Theory

The SCT proposes that the influences of environmental events, behavior, and inner personal factors interact with each other in a reciprocal fashion (Bandura, 1989). Inner personal factors include cognition, emotion, and biologic events. Through cognition, people are able to self-reflect, appraising thoughts, experiences, and behaviors. When people self-reflect, they create the cognitive base for self-regulation or control of subsequent behaviors. Self-reflection leads to perceptions of self-efficacy.

Self-efficacy is defined as beliefs about the capability to exercise control over events that affect the individual's life (Bandura, 1989). For the individual to judge capability to perform a behavior, he or she must examine the information from sources of efficacy information, including enactive attainment, vicarious experience, verbal persuasion, and autonomic arousal. Bandura (1986) wrote that behavior initiation and maintenance are determined by perceptions of self-efficacy that evolve from efficacy and outcome expectations. Efficacy expectations are beliefs about one's ability to engage or execute a given behavior that will result in an expected outcome. Outcome expectations are the beliefs that engaging in a certain behavior or behaviors will result in a specific result. Efficacy expectations vary on the three dimensions of magnitude, strength, and generality.

Critical Examination of Social Cognitive Theory

The SCT, formulated through a process of deduction for the purpose of explaining behavior initiation, change, and maintenance, is useful in nursing practice. The theory emphasizes variables thought to influence health behaviors. Understanding how the health care consumer can be motivated to initiate and sustain behaviors that will promote health or maintain health is a priority for nursing. The SCT is logical and simple to comprehend, with reciprocal relationships between variables clearly identified and linked with performance of purposive, goal-directed behavior. The content of the theory provides insights and adds useful information to the body of nursing knowledge. The theory is parsimonious, although it deals with complex phenomena related to human behavior. The process of reciprocal determinism is easy to understand and is generalizable across diverse populations (Dzewaltowski, Noble, & Shaw, 1990; Waller & Bates, 1992; Wieseke, 1991), although the original research involved only adult phobics as subjects (Bandura, 1977). The theory can be applied to nursing practice and health education because teaching and learning involve behavioral initiation, change, and maintenance. The SCT provides a framework for nursing research that critically analyzes and manipulates variables embedded within the theory, providing a basis for nursing interventions and further research. The theory is testable and has been supported through research both within and outside the domain of health behavior. Measurement of the variables in the SCT, however, is complicated by the interchangeable use of terms such as self-inducements and self-incentives for motivation. Efficacy expectations are also referred to as self-efficacy, perceived self-efficacy, and perceived competence, despite Bandura's (1986) definitions. Outcome expectations are referred to as anticipated consequences. Semantic consistency and clarity would enhance communication, understanding, and application of the theory. A related problem concerns the lack of operational definitions for some concepts found within the SCT.

Bandura (1986) stated that efficacy expectations vary across three dimensions of magnitude, generality, and strength; no clear guidelines were provided to facilitate consistent measurement of these dimensions across studies, however. As a result, studies have used a variety of methods for measuring efficacy expectations. For example, efficacy expectations have been measured by means of Likert-type items (Desharnais, Bouillon, & Godin, 1986) and by identifying the percentage of confidence (0-100%) for performing increasingly difficult levels of a behavior (Hilgenkamp, 1987). Variations in scales even occur within methodological types. For example, a 1-item Likert-type response format was applied to measure self-efficacy in one study (Gortner et al., 1988), whereas another study employed a tool with 17 Likert-type items (Waller, Crow, Sands, & Becker, 1988).

Clearing-Sky (1986) and Hilgenkamp (1987) measured the dimensions magnitude and strength in relation to exercise behavior. Subjects were asked to identify the percentage of confidence they had about whether they could successfully perform a specific exercise task (measured by distance arranged in increasing values) and the percentage of confidence they had that they would continue to do the exercise program after the course in which they were enrolled had ended. Generality of efficacy expectations was not assessed.

Dzewaltowski et al. (1990) used a different approach and asked subjects to report their exact percentage of confidence in performing an exercise activity three times per week during four different time frames despite any disconfirming experiences. The only dimension of efficacy expectations assessed was that of strength.

Waller et al. (1988) assessed efficacy expectations using a Likert-type format. Generalization of efficacy expectations was measured in relation to a variety of health promotion behaviors; magnitude and strength dimensions, however, were not measured.

The previously mentioned studies illustrate the different methodologies and interpretations employed to investigate efficacy expectations. Consistent measures are needed to enable valid comparisons across studies and generalization of results to other populations.

► RELATIONSHIP OF SELF-EFFICACY TO STRESS AND COPING PROCESS

Although no research directly compares Bandura's self-efficacy concept to the concepts of stress and coping as proposed by Lazarus and Folkman (1984), both theorists report a relationship between the two concepts. Bandura (1997) states that according to the SCT, stress reactions in people occur because of a low sense of self-efficacy to exercise control over unpleasant threats and disturbing environmental demands. If people believe they can control (high self-efficacy) a threat or stressor, they are not negatively emotionally aroused, and they are able to use coping strategies effectively. If people believe they cannot control their environment, they experience stress and cannot function adequately. Bandura agreed with Lazarus and Folkman (1984) that the most important stressors with which humans have to cope involve psychological threats. Bandura, however, believes that the intensity of reactions to stress are directly related to levels of self-efficacy for coping rather than the actual threat and environmental variables.

Similar to Bandura's propositions, Lazarus and Folkman state that part of secondary appraisal of a threat is the probability that a given coping option will accomplish what it is supposed to accomplish and the probability that one can apply a particular coping strategy or set of strategies effectively. Lazarus and Folkman note that there is a parallel between the concept of situational appraisals and control and self-efficacy. They indicate that efficacy expectations as identified by Bandura affect the extent to which a person feels threatened and, thus, direct coping behavior. Lazarus and Folkman propose that efficacy expectations are part of secondary appraisal, which includes a total evaluation of alternative coping options that affect emotions and coping.

Bandura (1995) discussed the relationship of threat and self-efficacy, stating that people's beliefs in their coping capabilities affect how much stress and depression they experience in threatening or difficult situations as well as their level of motivation to perform a specific behavior. Efficacy beliefs affect vigilance toward potential threats and how they are perceived and cognitively processed. People who believe, due to low self-efficacy, that potential threats are unmanageable may perceive many aspects of their environment and life as perilous, perpetuating coping deficiencies. Severity of possible threats is exaggerated, and they worry about things that rarely happen. Bandura and Lazarus and Folkman agree that low self-efficacy for managing threat produces greater stress and impairs level of functioning.

Bandura and Lazarus and Folkman concur that when people perceive outcomes are difficult they use cognitive coping strategies and restructure the cognitive meaning of the outcomes. If recurring difficult situations are uncontrollable, people resort to cognitive coping strategies designed to lessen their stress.

Lazarus (1991) identified two concepts that overlap with self-efficacy and are involved in the appraisal process: coping potential and future expectations. Coping potential and future expectations incorporate appraisal of potential environmental response to a coping action. These appraisals help determine the coping strategies chosen to decrease stress and negative emotional arousal.

Bandura (1997) suggests using coping strategies to meet the challenge of maintaining the quality of life with chronic disease or the aftermath of serious illness by the exercise of control over emotional distress associated with such conditions. Active involvement in purposeful activities is a good coping strategy when appraising and managing distress, feelings of despair, and emptiness in chronic disease states. The theorists agree that these strategies include more positive reappraisals of one's life situation, reordering one's lifestyle priorities, controlling perturbing ideation, alleviating stress by cognitive means, and seeking social support.

Lazarus and Folkman (1991) note that the main component in coping effectiveness is whether or not the choice of coping strategy is appropriate in a stressful situation. They agree with Bandura that the major criterion for coping effectiveness is the extent to which an outcome is within the person's control. If the outcome is within the person's control, problem-focused forms of coping that are intended to achieve the desired outcome are appropriate, and emotion-focused forms of coping may inhibit coping effectiveness. If the outcome is not perceived to be within the person's control, emotion-focused forms of coping that promote reduction of stress are appropriate.

In conclusion, self-efficacy and stress and coping are strongly related. Secondary appraisal, situational appraisal, coping potential, and future expectations as discussed by Lazarus are intimately intertwined with efficacy expectations and outcome expectations as discussed by Bandura. Research focused on stress and coping and self-efficacy has addressed health behaviors. Bandura and Lazarus note that health behaviors can be effective coping strategies for managing stressful situations.

➤ SELF-EFFICACY AND HEALTH BEHAVIOR RESEARCH

The following sections summarize information reported in meta-analyses of self-efficacy research and provide examples of studies that addressed the relationships of both efficacy expectations and outcome expectations in relation to self-efficacy, health behavior, and stress and coping. Next, a discussion of research related to specific health concerns from the perspectives of both nursing and other disciplines is provided.

Self-efficacy has been studied extensively for its role in initiation, change, and maintenance of health behaviors in both well and ill populations. Holden (1991), O'Leary, (1985), and Strecher et al. (1986) reviewed self-efficacy research studies grouped by health concerns. Health concerns addressed included cardiac rehabilitation, chronic lung disease, cigarette smoking, weight control, eating disorders, alcohol abuse, adherence to medical regimens, pain, management of depression, stress management, and contraceptive behavior.

O'Leary (1985) examined several studies on self-efficacy and health outcomes such as smoking cessation. O'Leary found that high levels of self-efficacy were associated with increased adherence to medical regimens, especially when the individual recognized the perceived health threat and the desired outcomes of related health behaviors.

Strecher et al. (1986) reviewed studies that examined self-efficacy in relation to cigarette smoking, weight control, contraceptive behavior, alcohol abuse, and exercise. All studies indicated that self-efficacy consistently predicted short- and long-term success in initiating and maintaining health behavior. Most important, as proposed by Bandura (1986), in studies that measured both efficacy and outcome expectations self-efficacy was an even stronger predictor of health behavior.

Holden (1991) performed a meta-analysis on 56 studies examining the relationship between self-efficacy and health behaviors and found that self-efficacy consistently predicted health-related behavioral outcomes. The analysis revealed a statistically significant negative correlation between observed effect sizes and the length of time from the individual's self-efficacy appraisal to actual performance of the behavior. Holden also concluded that self-efficacy was not merely a component of other general constructs regarding the self, such as self-esteem or locus of control, but also a uniquely predictive construct. In addition, Holden found that self-efficacy predicted a variety of behavioral outcomes, including those related to cigarette smoking, pain, weight loss, exercise, and dental care. Interestingly, the relationship was much weaker for weight loss and pain-related behavioral outcomes—a phenomenon that needs additional investigation.

Hofstetter et al. (1990) examined self-efficacy and the relationship between efficacy and outcome expectations. The sample for the study consisted of 2,053 male and female residents selected from the population of San Diego, California. Variables measured included self-efficacy, modeling, social support, benefits, knowledge about exercise, normative beliefs, medical history, exercise history, heart-healthy diet habits, smoking, body mass index, education, and sex—all variables identified as pertinent in the SCT. Results of the study revealed that self-efficacy was not unidimensional but rather multidimensional as well as highly domain specific. The researchers found that outcome expectations were distinct from efficacy expectations. As indicated by Bandura (1986), if the individual does not desire the outcome, measuring efficacy expectations is of little relevance.

Grembowski et al. investigated self-efficacy and health behavior among older adults who were enrollees of a Medicare program (N = 2,524). They found that adults with higher self-efficacy for health behaviors based on efficacy expectations, including those related to exercise, dietary fat intake, weight control, alcohol intake, and smoking, have better functional, mental, and self-rated health than those with lower self-efficacy. Outcome expectations were correlated negatively with perceived health risks, suggesting that outcome expectations may have some influence on the initiation and achievement of behavior change in older adults. Outcome expectations, however, were not related significantly to health status, providing support for the SCT's assumption that outcome expectations may be dependent partially on self-efficacy. The study provided support for the assumptions, including triadic reciprocality, of the SCT.

If only efficacy expectations are measured, results may not be as valid, reliable, and applicable as results from studies that measure both efficacy and outcome expectations. Findings will also be more accurate if researchers first determine whether the individual desires the specified outcome and then measure efficacy expectations for being able to perform the necessary behaviors to achieve that outcome. If the outcome is not desired, efficacy expectations for performing the pertinent behaviors to achieve the outcome will be low.

Cardiovascular Disease

The majority of nursing self-efficacy research studies have been conducted on clients with cardiovascular disease (Allen, Becker, & Swank, 1990; Burns, Camaione, Froman, & Clark, 1998; Carroll, 1995; Clark & Dodge, 1999; Gillis et al., 1993; Gulanick, 1991; Shuster & Waldron, 1991; Schuster, Wright, & Tomich, 1995; Sullivan, LaCroix, Russo, & Kathon, 1998; Thomas, 1993; Vidmar & Robinson, 1994). Results showed that high levels of self-efficacy were related to and predictive of exercise activity, adherence to cardiac rehabilitation regimens, improved social and physical function, and increased exercise tolerance.

Schuster and Waldron (1991) conducted a longitudinal exploratory study to investigate gender differences in anxiety, self-efficacy, activity tolerance, and adherence in cardiac rehabilitation patients with diagnosed coronary artery disease (N = 101). Results of the study indicated that on enrollment in a cardiac rehabilitation program, women were significantly less self-efficacious, more anxious, and less able to tolerate physical activity than men. Although not statistically significant, the data revealed that women attended the cardiac rehabilitation sessions less regularly than did men. These findings are congruent with those of Verbrugge (1985), who found that females showed higher morbidity for both acute and chronic diseases, restricted activities more because of health problems, and spent more days in bed than men. The researchers recommended that before entry to cardiac rehabilitation, assessments should be made of self-efficacy, anxiety, activity tolerance, and adherence to individualize rehabilitation strategies, facilitate attainment of rehabilitation goals, and promote adherence to the program. Schuster and Waldron also suggested that results related to adherence may reflect a phenomenon identified by Bandura (1986) in that both too much and too little self-efficacy may be related to the absence or decreased performance of physical activity. High self-efficacy of men and low self-efficacy of women may both have hindered adherence to the program. No other studies in the reviewed literature were found to support this assumption, however. A question can be asked as to why males and females respond in different ways to cardiac experiences. Also, why do their responses, although opposite, sometimes result in the same behavioral outcomes?

Schuster et al. (1995) conducted a subsequent study to explore gender differences in the behavioral outcomes of postoperative coronary artery bypass graft (CABG) surgery patients ($N = 73$) in home programs compared to those in structured cardiac rehabilitation programs. No significant differences were found over time between home and structured programs for males and females on self-efficacy, length of time before return to work, diet adherence, smoking cessation, and medication adherence. Self-efficacy for physical activity and knowledge did significantly increase over time, regardless of the type of program or gender. The researchers concluded that self-efficacy related to the ability to endure exercise and complete activities of daily living improved over time as physical status improved. Additional research needs to be conducted to examine the relationships between and predictability of study variables in relation to physical activity, especially self-efficacy.

In another study of clients in cardiac rehabilitation, Vidmar and Robinson (1994) examined the relationship between self-efficacy and exercise compliance. Significant positive relationships were found between total self-efficacy and exercise compliance, exercise barriers, and exercise behavior. Individuals who perceived many barriers to exercise tended to exercise at a higher level to overcome barriers. Exercise barriers efficacy was found to be the most significant predictor of exercise behavior. Research must be performed to determine if subjects who respond in this way interpret overcoming barriers as a challenge rather than a threat. On the basis of the findings, the researchers recommended that to increase self-efficacy and exercise compliance strategies related to the sources of self-efficacy information should be implemented, such as (a) offering a variety of exercise modalities, (b) educating about use of equipment and physiologic responses to exercise, (c) allowing individuals to take part in structured activities when desired as a means to increase motivation by observing others exercising, (d) providing verbal encouragement, (e) suggesting alterations in exercise regimens, and (f) recommending counseling regarding setting and attaining goals. They also suggested that self-efficacy be reinforced regularly during long-term treatment regimens, such as dietary changes, smoking cessation, and stress management.

Carroll (1995) evaluated self-efficacy, self-care agency, and self-care and recovery behaviors at four points in time in elderly people after CABG surgery. Results revealed that self-efficacy increased during the recovery period, as did self-care agency and the ability to perform self-care and recovery behaviors. Women were found to be less self-efficacious before surgery, at discharge, and at 6 weeks after surgery than men. By 12 weeks after surgery, however, men and women reported equal self-efficacy. Women obviously increased their self-efficacy more than men during the 12 weeks after surgery. In addition, self-efficacy was found to be a mediator between self-care agency and self-care and recovery behaviors of walking, climbing stairs, and general activities. No explanation for gender differences was offered, and additionally research must be conducted to explore this issue. Carroll suggested that reported increased self-efficacy, increased self-care agency, and improved activity performance might be influenced by the physiologic recovery because recovery provides physiologic arousal efficacy information. In addition, Carroll suggested that nurses provide coaching and guidance to the patients. Coaching should include encouraging performance of self-care behaviors in a supportive environment before discharge, assisting with setting and supporting realistic daily goals of performance, and mandatory attendance at an educational offering before discharge. These coaching strategies lead to increased self-efficacy because they use all sources of efficacy information.

Allen et al. (1990) investigated self-efficacy and functional status after CABG surgery. The longitudinal study involved 125 male patients. Women were purposely excluded from the study because they constituted only 19% of all CABG surgeries and because potential gender differences might confound results. Self-efficacy was found to be a significant and independent predictor of 6-month postoperative physical activity and social and leisure activity. Men with higher self-efficacy performed more physical, social, and leisure activities. Self-efficacy was a better predictor of functional status than disease severity, functional capacity, comorbidity, or preoperative functioning. On the basis of study results, attempts should be made to increase self-efficacy in cardiac rehabilitation programs.

In summary, self-efficacy has been shown to be a strong predictor of functional outcomes and physical activity in people who have cardiac illness or are post-CABG. Clearly, more research is needed involving women because the results predominantly reflect the reporting of men. Additional research must examine self-efficacy over time, across cultures, and across interventions.

Pulmonary Disease

Self-efficacy in patients with pulmonary disease is another area of health behavior research (Atkins, Kaplan, Timms, Reinsch, & Lofback, 1984; Devins & Edwards, 1988; Gormley, Carrieri-Kohlman, Douglas, & Stulbarg, 1993; Kaplan, Ries, Prewitt, & Eakin,

1994; Scherer & Schmieder, 1997; Toshima, Kaplan, & Ries, 1990, 1992). Nurses have performed relatively few studies of self-efficacy in pulmonary disease. High levels of self-efficacy have been shown to be associated with enhanced symptom management, decreased perceptions of dyspnea, improved functional status, and increased exercise and increased exercise tolerance.

Atkins et al. (1984) examined efficacy expectations of patients with chronic obstructive pulmonary disease (COPD) in a walking program. The researchers also investigated the relationship between locus of control and self-efficacy. The sample included 22 men and 38 women with moderate to severe COPD as determined by forced expiratory volume in 1 second (FEV_1) percent predicted. Researchers measured efficacy expectations after the exercise prescription was given and 3 months later. Statistically significant differences were found in distance walked and exercise tolerance in participants who were in the experimental treatment groups compared to those in the control group at the end of 3 months. Those in treatment groups walked farther and tolerated the activity better. Results suggested that interventions based on sources of efficacy information, particularly mastery and verbal persuasion, improved self-efficacy in walking in adults with COPD, as proposed in the SCT. In addition, Atkins et al. reported that health locus of control had a weaker relationship with walking and behavior change during the 3 months. These findings support Bandura's assumption that self-efficacy, because it is behavior specific, is more predictive of a health behavior than the more general concept of health locus of control.

Another study examined self-efficacy in 119 patients (32 women and 87 men) with stable COPD who were undergoing pulmonary rehabilitation. Researchers measured exercise endurance, quality of well-being, depression, and self-efficacy (Toshima et al., 1990, 1992). Participants were assigned either to an education control group that received exercise training or to an education control group that did not receive exercise training. After 6 months, the exercise training group had a significant increase in exercise tolerance. Although self-efficacy in walking did improve from baseline, in contrast to findings of Schuster et al. (1995), it was not a significant change. Members of the exercise training group, who initially had higher self-efficacy scores for treadmill walking, demonstrated the greatest endurance on the treadmill. Toshima et al. asserted that physiological feedback was a strong source of efficacy information for people with COPD because they experience discomfort, such as dyspnea and fatigue, with activity and sometimes even at rest, creating a negative autonomic feedback. When people with COPD perceive aversive autonomic feedback while attempting behaviors such as exercise, this autonomic source of efficacy information may limit efficacy expectations and subsequently self-efficacy. Thus, if people with COPD are helped to experience a more positive autonomic state or are able to avoid focusing on negative autonomic feedback, they may perceive a greater degree of self-efficacy. Another consideration is that women and men may experience not only their disease symptoms but also exercise treatment differently.

Devins and Edwards (1988) conducted a study of self-efficacy and smoking reduction in COPD patients. Participants (27 men and 21 women) had smoked for at least 15 years and were currently smoking at least 10 cigarettes a day. Through an educational process, study participants were exposed to the various behavioral techniques used to reduce smoking. Participants were then asked to rate the perceived effectiveness of each technique, thus measuring their outcome expectations. The strength of efficacy expectations was measured by rating their confidence in being able to perform each of the smoking-cessation techniques. The researchers also measured motivation to stop smoking using a motivational index and a smoking index. At 1 month and 3 months post-original testing and educational sessions, self-efficacy was the only significant predictor of reduced smoking. Measuring both efficacy and outcome expectations specific to a behavior, as Bandura (1986) did,

yielded information about the multidimensional concept of self-efficacy, thus enhancing the generalizability of study findings.

In 1993, Gormley et al. examined treadmill self-efficacy and walking performance in 52 patients with COPD. FEV_1 percentage predicted was lower in men than women before interventions started. Subjects were randomly assigned to a monitored exercise group or a coached exercise group. Self-efficacy was defined as the level that corresponded to the highest treadmill speed and grade for which participants had the greatest confidence. Results showed that both self-efficacy and walking performance increased significantly over time for both groups; there were no significant differences between the two groups, however.

Gormley et al. (1993) suggested that through the efficacy information of mastery by exercise, the dyspnea-inactivity-dyspnea cycle for the COPD patients was interrupted. In addition, participants were probably inactive because aversive autonomic feedback, such as dyspnea and fatigue, decreased confidence in the ability to perform exercise activity. Interestingly, this supposition was supported because most of the participants consistently underestimated their ability to exercise. Gormley et al. stated that the reason there were no differences between the groups in self-efficacy is that both groups exercised in a safe, monitored setting with a nurse present. The presence of the nurse was enough to increase self-efficacy and security even in participants who were only monitored and received no coaching. Both groups were provided mastery experiences for their exercise, the strongest source of efficacy information. Another important finding was that women increased their self-efficacy significantly more than did men, as also occurred in the Carroll (1995) study. In the beginning, women reported lower self-efficacy than men, even when they reported better walking performance. The researchers suggested that women focused more on their uncomfortable autonomic state than did men during the initial exercise test—thus the initial low level of self-efficacy. In addition, past experiences and socialization may have influenced the women's perceptions. Many of the women were of the generation in which women were taught that they were not capable of great physical tasks—thus the lower self-efficacy for physical tasks. The researchers recommended that clinicians assess self-efficacy related to exercise in all COPD patients, especially women, attending pulmonary rehabilitation programs. By recognizing patients with lower self-efficacy, strategies could then be used to improve both self-efficacy and walking performance.

Kaplan et al. (1994) investigated the relationships of self-efficacy to FEV_1, diffusing capacity for carbon monoxide (DL_{CO}; measures how well the lung transfers gas from inspired air to blood), VO_2 max (standard measure of exercise tolerance, maximum oxygen uptake), and arterial oxygen level as predictors of mortality among 129 patients (32 women and 87 men) with COPD. Self-efficacy was measured with an instrument that asked subjects to rate their expectations for walking progressively longer distances for longer periods of time. Results indicated that self-efficacy for walking was a significant predictor of survival, as were FEV_1, VO_2 max, and DL_{CO}. The pO_2 was not a significant predictor of survival. Statistical analysis, however, revealed that FEV_1 accounted for the greatest amount of variance in the prediction of survival. The researchers noted that self-reports of self-efficacy could compete favorably with physiologic measures to predict mortality in COPD patients. They proposed that efficacy expectations in COPD patients were affected by the seriousness of the underlying illness producing an aversive autonomic state.

Scherer and Schmieder (1997) investigated the effect of a pulmonary rehabilitation program on self-efficacy and the ability to manage or avoid breathing difficulty in certain situations. Results indicated that self-efficacy increased significantly over time from pretest to posttest at 1 month but decreased slightly at 6 months post-outpatient pulmonary rehabilitation (OPR) in relation to managing or avoiding breathing difficulty associated with physi-

cal exertion. Higher scores on the COPD Self-Efficacy Scale (CSES) indicated greater confidence in the ability to manage or avoid breathing difficulty and were correlated with lower scores of perceived dyspnea. Self-efficacy was still greater at 6 months post-OPR than before OPR; therefore, periodic reinforcement or review sessions are recommended to maintain high levels of self-efficacy. Interestingly, in contrast to the findings of Gormley et al. (1993), the researchers reported no significant differences between men and women on pre- and postprogram scores on the CSES, Dyspnea Scale, and 12-minute distance.

In summary, multiple studies involving subjects with COPD have provided support for predictive relationships between self-efficacy and symptom management, exercise tolerance, and endurance. These relationships have been shown to be strong even in the face of other factors such as inclement weather. Additional studies must be conducted across a wider section of subjects and situations to develop reliable valid instruments for measuring self-efficacy in COPD patients.

Physical Activity

The relationship between physical activity and self-efficacy is an area of research that has been investigated only to a limited extent by nurses but to a much greater extent by other professionals (Bosscher & Van Der, 1995; Courneya & McAuley, 1994; Godin & Shephard, 1985; Kingery & Glasglow, 1989; McAuley, 1994; McAuley, Courneya, & Lettunich, 1991; Parkatti, Deeg, Bosscher, & Launer, 1998). The following discussion provides a sample of the self-efficacy research that has been completed and that provided support for a positive relationship, even a predictive relationship, between self-efficacy and physical activity.

Godin and Shephard (1985) conducted a study on gender differences in perceived physical self-efficacy among older individuals. Data analysis revealed significant differences between men and women in total physical self-efficacy and perceived physical ability, with women having lower scores. No significant differences were found based on age. Godin and Shephard suggested that gender differences in self-efficacy, and therefore actual physical activity, were due to sociocultural influences of a particular era rather than biological differences. The differences in self-efficacy levels need to be identified and incorporated into design and implementation of programs to enhance physical activity of older adults.

McAuley et al. (1991) examined the effects of acute (single-graded exercise test) and long-term (structured exercise program) exercise on perceptions of personal efficacy with respect to physical capabilities. Results revealed that men had significantly higher sit-up self-efficacy than women at both times. The researchers suggested that the difference in sit-up self-efficacy was a physiologic advantage that men had over women because men were leaner and took longer to reach the targeted heart rate. Both men and women increased bicycle and walk and jog self-efficacy during the 20-week time period, with the levels of self-efficacy equal across genders at 20 weeks. Women, however, actually had greater increases in self-efficacy levels because their levels were lower initially for the three physical activities than those of the men. Interestingly, men had more bicycle self-efficacy than women at baseline and Time 2. McAuley et al. suggested that gender differences at baseline in sit-up, bicycle, and walk and jog self-efficacy were related to beliefs about physical abilities based on past physical experiences and different sociocultural upbringing of men and women.

Diabetes Management

A limited number of studies have explored the relationship between self-efficacy and diabetes management (Davis, 1997; Holcomb et al., 1998; Hurley & Shea, 1992; Kingery & Glasglow, 1989; Leonard, Skay, &

Rheinberger, 1998; Padgett, 1991; Skelly, Marshall, Haughly, Davis, & Dunford, 1995; Wang, Wang, & Lin, 1998). Examples of research that provides evidence of a positive relationship between levels of self-efficacy and health promotive behaviors in diabetes management are presented here.

Skelly et al. (1995) assessed the influence of perceptions of self-efficacy and confidence in outcomes related to diabetes self-care regimens in a sample of 118 middle-aged, inner-city African American women. At the time of the initial interview, subjects reported high levels of self-efficacy about self-care related to medications and glucose monitoring but not diet or exercise. At Time 2, self-efficacy levels had increased for all the behaviors; they were still lower for diet and exercise, however, as evidenced by less adherence for these behaviors. Additional research needs to be conducted on this phenomenon.

The Insulin Management Diabetes Self-Efficacy Scale and the Diabetes Self-Care Scale were used by Hurley and Shea (1992) in a study examining diabetes management behaviors in a sample of 142 adults who self-administered insulin. Subjects had high levels of self-efficacy at both times, and strong positive correlations were found between self-efficacy and self-care behaviors of general diabetes management and diet control. There was also a strong positive correlation between insulin self-efficacy beliefs and self-care. Higher levels of self-efficacy enabled individuals to optimize self-care skills. The provided personal mastery experiences, vicarious experiences available, verbal persuasion, and emotional support provided by the nurses in the safe hospital environment enhanced self-efficacy and improved the likelihood of self-care behavior for diabetes management.

Kingery and Glasgow (1989) examined self-efficacy and outcome expectations in the self-regulation of non-insulin-dependent diabetes mellitus. The sample consisted of 127 diabetic outpatients (85 women and 42 men). The researchers found that exercise self-efficacy was a more significant predictor of exercise levels in women than in men. They found, however, that outcome expectations were a more significant predictor of exercise levels for men than for women. Kingery and Glasgow suggested that different educational strategies need to be used for men and women to increase self-efficacy with subsequent improved exercise levels for diabetes management. Women may need assistance in increasing self-efficacy related to exercise skills, whereas men may need increased self-efficacy to increase understanding of the importance of exercise for diabetes management.

Rheumatoid Arthritis

Few studies have supported self-efficacy as a mediator of health outcomes for individuals diagnosed with rheumatoid arthritis (Barlow, 1998; Lorig, Chastain, Ung, Shoor, & Holman, 1989; Riemsma et al., 1998). Lorig et al. explored this relationship in an experimental study involving 144 adults measured by the Beck Depression Scale. Self-efficacy was measured using the Arthritis Self-Efficacy Scale developed by the researchers that contained three subscales related to pain, function, and other symptoms (fatigue, activity regulation, and depression). Subjects who received the intervention significantly increased self-efficacy levels and decreased levels of depression and pain. Function improved, possibly because of the increase in self-efficacy.

Psychosocial Concerns

Self-efficacy has been shown to be related to adjustment in cancer patients (Beckham, Burker, Lytle, Feldman, & Costakis, 1997), maternal depression and child temperament (Gross, Conrad, Fogg, & Wothke, 1994), psychological distress and problem-focused coping (Sharts-Hopko, Regan-Kubinski, Lincoln, & Heverly, 1996), adaptation in battered women (Varvaro & Palmer, 1993), stress and coping in early psychosis (MacDonald, Pica, McDonald, Hayes,

& Baglioni, 1998), coping with labor (Lowe, 1991), decreasing mental frailty in at-risk elders (McDougall & Balver, 1998), functional ability and depression after elective total hip replacement surgery (Kurlowicz, 1998), and distress and adjustment in Mexican American college students (Solberg & Villarreal, 1997). Overall, high levels of self-efficacy were negatively correlated with depression, mental frailty, and stress and positively correlated with enhanced coping and adaptation as well as health outcomes (less fatigue and pain).

Many of the studies used instruments designed by the researchers to be behavior specific, as did Varvaro and Palmer (1993). Varvaro and Palmer developed the Self-Efficacy Scale for Battered Women to assess self-efficacy needs of and develop treatment plans for abused women ($N = 43$) who presented to the emergency room. The women were found to have low levels of self-efficacy for asking for help, shrugging off self-doubts, saying what they think, and feeling without fear. Subjects were found to have a need for information on abuse, safety, and self-empowerment to decrease fear and promote adaptive psychosocial functioning. Individualized treatment plans were developed with components that addressed the sources of efficacy information. These components included providing the women with abuse information and information on where and how to get help, helping them create a plan for safety, and helping them identify, create, and practice coping skills. When assessing 8 of the subjects after they attended an educational support group for battered women for 12 weeks in which the intervention plan was implemented, the researchers found a significant increase in self-efficacy. The increase in self-efficacy was translated by the subjects into better control over their lives.

Preventive Behaviors

Self-efficacy has been investigated in two areas of behavior that are considered preventive and promotive in nature. Self-efficacy has been found to be predictive of behavior related to obtaining regular mammograms (Allen, Sorensen, Stoddard, Colditz, & Peterson, 1998) and breast self-examination (Gonzalez, 1990). In addition, self-efficacy has been shown to be related to condom use by college students (Brafford & Beck, 1991) and black adolescent women (Jemmott & Jemmott, 1992), safe sex behaviors (Cecil & Pinkerton, 1998; Goldman & Harlow, 1993; Kalichman, Roffman, Picciano, & Bolan, 1998), and AIDS preventive behaviors among 10th-grade students (Kasen, Vaughan, & Walter, 1992) and female drug users (Brown, 1998). Researchers have developed behavior-specific self-efficacy scales, with most measuring only the strength dimension.

For example, high levels of self-efficacy were found to be positively correlated with performance of breast self-examination when Mexican American subjects, who attended a local health clinic, were given guidance and training that were sensitive to cultural needs (Gonzalez, 1990). High levels of self-efficacy were positively associated with frequency of breast self-examination, supporting the proposition that self-examination was central to the behavior. Gonzalez suggested that to increase self-efficacy in relation to a specific behavior, the nurse must carefully assess cultural and language variables and use gathered data to help individualize care plans and optimize health outcomes.

Smoking Cessation

Studies have demonstrated a predictive relationship between self-efficacy and smoking cessation (De Vries, Mudde, Dijkstra, & Willemsen, 1998; Kowalski, 1997; Pohl, Martinelli, & Antonakos, 1998). Kowalski, for example, explored self-efficacy in relation to smoking cessation behaviors and adherence in 75 adult subjects at the beginning of a smoking cessation program and 3 months after completion of the program. Self-efficacy scores at the beginning of the program significantly predicted whether or not subjects

would be smoking 3 months after completion of the program. Subjects with higher self-efficacy scores at the beginning were more likely to stop smoking and maintain the status of nonsmoker 3 months after completion of the program. Kowalski suggested that believing that one could stop smoking forever influences the level of motivation, energy, and commitment necessary to break the habit.

In summary, research has provided support for the assumptions of the SCT in the areas of health behavior. Additional research must be conducted to assess the impact of additional environmental, behavioral, and inner personal factors on self-efficacy and subsequently on health behavior. In addition, research needs to be conducted that examines the relationships between self-efficacy, stress and coping, and health behaviors, with the end result being the design of effective interventions.

➤ OVERVIEW OF THE HEALTH PROMOTION MODEL

A theory base supported by research is a necessity for professional nursing practice. A search for a theory to guide nursing research and practice containing the existing accepted definition of self-efficacy led to the Health Promotion Model (HPM). One of the first models was developed by Pender (1982), who identified that the primary focus of nursing care should be helping the individual toward optimal health, well-being, and self-actualization rather than just disease prevention.

The HPM was developed by Pender to explain and predict the behavior of individuals related to health promotion (Lusk, Ronis, Kerr, & Atwood, 1994). The model is rooted in Bandura's (1977) social learning theory, (now called the social cognitive theory), which recognizes the importance of cognitive-perceptual factors and modifying factors that influence the occurrence of health-promoting behaviors. The model is based on the following assumptions: (a) The individual has a drive toward health, (b) the individual's personal definition of health has more importance than that of others, and (c) the individual person is the focus of the model (Tillet, 1998). The model can guide nursing practice and research that aims to enhance the individual's ability to perform behaviors that help prevent and manage disease and, most important, promote health (Pender, Barkauskas, Hayman, Rice, & Anderson, 1992; Tillet, 1998.

The model identifies individual characteristics and experiences that directly affect behavior-specific cognitions and affect. Individual characteristics and experiences that are considered modifying factors include demographic characteristics, body composition and weight, expectations, health-promoting behavior options available in the environment, and prior experiences with health actions. Cognitive-perceptual factors portrayed in the model are defined as motivational mechanisms related to health promotion behaviors and are portrayed as amenable to change. Cognitive-perceptual factors include the importance of health to the individual, perceived control of health, perceived self-efficacy, personal definition of health, perceived health status, and perceived benefits and barriers to health-promoting behaviors. Behavior-specific cognitions interact with each other to create a commitment to a plan of action and directly influence health-promoting behavior. In addition, the behavioral outcome is directly affected by the commitment to a plan of action and immediate competing demands and preferences. Competing demands refer to conflicts for which the individual has low control, and competing preferences include alternate behaviors associated with high personal control.

The HPM assumes that those who value health are more likely to perform behaviors that will enhance their health. Perceived control related to this performance and outcome combined with a strong belief that the behavior is possible, a high perception of perceived benefits, and low perceived barriers to such behaviors influence the likelihood that the individual will perform the behaviors. Interpersonal influences on behavior (family, peers, and providers), norms and support, and behavior models, as well as situational influences (options, demand and preference characteristics, and aesthetics), help determine the likelihood of performance of health-enhancing behaviors. The professional nurse applying the HPM, completing a thorough assessment to identify positive and negative variables, can design interventions to enhance the likelihood that the individual will perform health-promoting behaviors. A comprehensive discussion of the HPM, research using the model, and the relationships among the model's concepts are in Chapter 13.

➣ SELF-EFFICACY INSTRUMENT DEVELOPMENT

Many instruments have been developed to measure self-efficacy in relation to health behaviors. Some of the instruments measure only the strength dimension of efficacy expectations. Conner and Norman (1995) suggested that to truly measure self-efficacy a scale must assess risk perception, outcome expectancy, and all dimensions of efficacy expectations. The researchers suggested that outcome expectancy statements should be worded as "if-then" statements, whereas efficacy expectations statements should be worded as confidence statements. They also suggested that self-efficacy scales should include positive and negative outcomes. Self-efficacy instruments, some of which apply the guidelines suggested by Conner and Norman, include Cardiac Diet Self-Efficacy and Cardiac Exercise Self-Efficacy instruments (Hickey, Owen, & Froman, 1992); Knowledge, Attitude, and Self-Efficacy Asthma Questionnaire (Wigal et al., 1993); COPD Self-Efficacy Scale (Wigal, Creer, & Kotses, 1991); Self-Efficacy Scale (Sherer et al., 1982); Self-Efficacy Scale for Battered Women (Varvaro & Palmer, 1993); Maternal Self-Efficacy Scale (Gross et al., 1994); Cancer Self-Efficacy Scale (Beckham et al., 1997); Long-Term Medication Behaviour

Self-Efficacy Scale (De Geest, Abraham, Gemoets, & Evers, 1994); Epilepsy Self-Efficacy Scale (Dilorio, Faherty, & Manteuffel, 1992); Headache Self-Efficacy Scale (Martin, Holroyd, & Rokicki, 1993); Preoperative Self-Efficacy Scale (Oetker & Taunton, 1994); General Perceived Self-Efficacy Scale (Schwarzer & Jerusalem, 1995); Osteoporosis Self-Efficacy Scale (Horan, Kim, Gendler, Froman, & Patel, 1998); Hormone Replacement Therapy Self-Efficacy Scale (Ali, 1998); and the Insulin Management Diabetes Self-Efficacy Scale (Hurley, 1990). Examination of the instruments reveals a variety of methodologies used to measure self-efficacy; most, however, use a Likert-type format. Even within this format, however, different descriptors are used, including very confident to not at all confident, strongly agree to strongly disagree, and very likely to very unlikely. In addition, the scales do not all measure both outcome and efficacy expectations or all three dimensions of efficacy expectations.

Hurley (1990) provides a good example of self-efficacy instrument development. The Insulin Management Diabetes Self-Efficacy Scale was designed to assess and identify individuals who would benefit from individualized care in addition to traditional diabetes health education. The 28-item instrument also could be used as an outcome measure of postdiabetes education. Items on the instrument were borrowed from other instruments and created by the researcher to reflect self-efficacy in relation to diabetes activities of daily living. Items contained action words that were not outcomes, contained only one behavior, used positive or negative wording related to ability, used the word diabetic as an adjective and not a noun, contained descriptors of varied situational variables, and used the term "insulin" rather than "medication." Strength and magnitude of efficacy expectations were measured in different items. Generalizability does not appear to be addressed by the scale. Behaviors measured included general, diet, exercise, foot care, monitoring, insulin administration, and detecting, preventing, or treating high and low blood glucose reactions. Ten items were negatively phrased. Subjects were asked to respond to each behavioral item using a Likert-type scale with a possible score of strongly agree (1) to strongly disagree (6).

Validity and reliability have been tested in more than eight studies with inpatients or outpatients or both. Sample sizes have ranged from 5 to more than 127. Expert review, exploratory factor analysis, and convergent validity have provided support for construct and content validity of the instrument. Reliability was confirmed by Cronbach's alpha statistic, test-retest stability, and interrater reliability assessment. The majority of the self-efficacy instruments have not been tested as extensively as the Insulin Management Self-Efficacy Scale, and such testing needs to be completed to be able to use findings when designing, implementing, and evaluating interventions to enhance self-efficacy and health behavior.

➤ IMPLICATIONS OF SELF-EFFICACY

Bandura (1986) stated that behavior is influenced by self-efficacy as based on perceived efficacy expectations and outcome expectations. These evolve from cognitive appraisal of the sources of information found within the inner personal, behavioral, and environmental components of a situation as also reported by Lazarus. Self-efficacy has been associated with and has predicted behavioral choice, behavioral change, initiation of behavior, behavioral elimination, the amount of effort expended to perform a behavior, and persistence of a variety of health behaviors. High levels of self-efficacy were revealed to (a) enhance smoking cessation behaviors, increasing length of abstinence and decreasing risk of relapse; (b) enhance weight management; (c) increase control of eating disorders and decrease risk of relapse; (d) increase pain tolerance and enhance pain management behaviors; (e) increase adherence to medical regimens; (f) be instrumental in the control of addictive behaviors; (g) increase exercise activity during and after cardiac and pulmonary rehabilitation; (h) enhance the effects of health education; (i) improve stress management; and (j) increase performance of health promotion behaviors in general. Support has been found for generalization of self-efficacy to similar situations and behaviors.

Interventions designed to produce behavioral change have been found to be more effective if the assumptions of the SCT are incorporated in their design and implementation. Interventions evolving from the mastery source of information, such as participatory exercise classes with individuals with similar characteristics and experiences grouped together, are the most potent in influencing self-efficacy and related behavior. Mastery is achieved more quickly if behaviors are broken down into components and each component is addressed in a logical manner separately, possibly mastering from simple to complex. Verbal persuasion and emotional arousal appear to be the most common methods of intervention to increase self-efficacy and improve health behaviors. Health education and public advertisements, although not as effective sources of information as mastery, are appropriate for helping identify barriers, benefits, and consequences of a behavior while identifying desired outcomes. In addition, research has shown that to maintain a behavioral change, reinforcement must be provided intermittently as appropriate for the behavior being addressed. Verbal persuasion and emotional arousal are excellent sources of information for reinforcement.

Additional research using conceptual and operational definitions consistent with the SCT must be conducted to support the reliability, validity, and applicability of the theory to nursing practice and research in the areas of health behavior and stress and coping. More research needs to be completed that addresses outcome expectations and all three dimensions of efficacy expectations to evaluate the multidimensional character of self-efficacy. Most studies have not addressed all four sources of efficacy information involved in cognitive appraisal and subsequent behavior. Research also must be conducted to develop reliable, valid instruments that can be used, or modified for use, across behavioral categories and populations. Items on a self-efficacy instrument need to reflect the four sources of efficacy information and three dimensions of efficacy expectations as well as outcome expectations. Specific positive and negative consequences of a behavior need to be identified within the instrument. Ideally, the individual would identify expected outcomes because these must be relevant to the individual in a specific situation to be cognitively appraised in relation to efficacy expectations and actual behavioral performance.

➤ REFERENCES

Ali, N. (1998). The hormone replacement therapy self-efficacy scale. *Journal of Advanced Nursing, 28*(5), 1115-1119.

Allen, J., Becker, D., & Swank, R. (1990). Factors related to functional status after coronary artery bypass surgery. *Heart & Lung, 19*(4), 337-343.

Allen, J., Sorensen, G., Stoddard, A., Colditz, G., & Peterson, K. (1998). Intention to have a mammogram in the past. *Health Education Behavior, 25*(4), 474-488.

Atkins, C., Kaplan, R., Timms, R., Reinsch, S., & Lofback, K. (1984). Behavioral exercise programs in the management of chronic obstructive pulmonary disease. *Journal of Counseling and Clinical Psychology, 52*(4), 591-603.

Bandura, A. (1977). Self-efficacy: Toward a unifying theory of behavioral change. *Psychological Review, 84,* 191-215.

Bandura, A. (1982). Self-efficacy mechanism in a human agency. *American Psychologist, 37,* 122-147.

Bandura, A. (1986). *Social foundations of thought and action: A social cognitive theory.* Englewood Cliffs, NJ: Prentice Hall.

Bandura, A. (1989). Human agency in social cognitive theory. *American Psychologist, 44*(9), 1175-1184.

Bandura, A. (1991). Self-efficacy mechanism in physiological activation and health-promoting behavior. In J. Madden (Ed.), *Neurobiology of learning, emotion and affect* (pp. 229-270). New York: Raven Press.

Bandura, A. (1995). Exercise of personal and collective efficacy in changing societies. In A. Bandura (Ed.), *Self-efficacy in changing societies* (pp. 1-45). New York: Cambridge University Press.

Bandura, A. (1997). *Self-efficacy: The exercise of control.* New York: Freeman.

Barlow, J. (1998). Understanding exercise in the context of chronic disease: An exploratory investigation of self-efficacy. *Perception and Motor Skills, 87*(2), 439-446.

Beckham, J., Burker, E., Lytle, B., Feldman, M., & Costakis, M. (1997). Self-efficacy and adjustment in cancer patients: A preliminary report. *Behavioral Medicine, 23*(3), 138-142.

Bosscher, R., & Van Der, H. (1995). Physical performance and physical self-efficacy in the elderly. *Journal of Aging & Health, 7*(4), 459-475.

Brafford, L., & Beck, K. (1991). Development and validation of a condom self-efficacy scale for college students. *College Health, 39,* 219-225.

Brown, E. (1998). Female injecting drug users: Human immunodeficiency virus risk behavior and intervention needs. *Journal of Professional Nursing, 14*(6), 361-369.

Burns, K., Camaione, D., Froman, R., & Clark, B. (1998). Predictors of referral to cardiac rehabilitation. *Clinical Nursing Research, 7*(2), 1054-1077.

Carroll, D. (1995). The importance of self-efficacy expectations in elderly patients recovering from coronary artery bypass surgery. *Heart & Lung, 24,* 50-59.

Cecil, H., & Pinkerton, S. (1998). Reliability and validity of a self-efficacy instrument for protective sexual behaviors. *Journal of American College Health, 47*(3), 113-121.

Clark, N., & Dodge, J. (1999). Exploring self-efficacy as a predictor of disease management. *Health Education & Behavior, 26,* 1090-1981.

Clearing-Sky, M. (1986). *A path analysis of the biopsychosocial variables related to exercise performance and adherence.* Unpublished doctoral dissertation, Michigan State University, East Lansing.

Conner, M., & Norman, P. (1995). *Predicting health behaviour: Research and practice with social cognition models* (pp. 163-196). Buckingham, UK: Open University Press.

Courneya, K., & McAuley, E. (1994). Are there different determinants of the frequency, intensity, and duration of physical activity? *Behavioral Medicine, 20*(2), 84-90.

Davis, J. (1997). *The relationship between self-efficacy of diabetes management and health-promoting behaviors.* Unpublished manuscript.

De Geest, S., Abraham, I., Gemoets, H., & Evers, G. (1994). Development of the Long-Term Behaviour Self-Efficacy Scale: Qualitative study for item development. *Journal of Advanced Nursing, 19,* 233-238.

Desharnais, R., Bouillon, J., & Godin, G. (1986). Self-efficacy and outcome expectations as determinants of exercise adherence. *Psychological Reports, 59,* 1155-1159.

Devins, G., & Edwards, P. (1988). Self-efficacy and smoking reduction in chronic obstructive pulmonary disease. *Behavior Research Therapy, 26*(2), 127-135.

De Vries, H., Mudde, A., Dijkstra, A., & Willemsen, M. (1998). Differential beliefs, perceived social influences, and self-efficacy expectations among smokers in various motivational phases. *Previews in Medicine, 27*(5), 681-689.

Dilorio, C., Faherty, B., & Manteuffel, B. (1992). The development and testing of an instrument to measure self-efficacy in individuals with epilepsy. *Journal of Neuroscience Nursing, 24,* 9-13.

Dzewaltowski, D., Noble, J., & Shaw, J. (1990). Physical activity participation: Social cognitive theory versus the theories of reasoned action and planned behavior. *Journal of Sport & Exercise Psychology, 12,* 388-405.

Gillis, C., Gortner, S., Hauck, W., Shinn, J., Sparacino, P., & Tompkins, C. (1993). A randomized clinical trial of nursing care for recovery from cardiac surgery. *Heart & Lung, 22*(2), 125-133.

Godin, G., & Shephard, R. (1985). Gender differences in perceived self-efficacy among older individuals. *Perceptual and Motor Skills, 60,* 599-602.

Goldman, J., & Harlow, L. (1993). Self-perception variables that mediate AIDS preventive behavior in college students. *Health Psychology, 12*(6), 489-498.

Gonzalez, J. (1990). Factors relating to frequency of breast self-examination among low-income Mexican-American women. *Cancer Nursing, 13*(3), 134-142.

Gormley, J., Carrieri-Kohlman, V., Douglas, M., & Stulbarg, M. (1993). Treadmill self-efficacy and walking performance in patients with COPD. *Journal of Cardiopulmonary Rehabilitation, 13,* 424-431.

Gortner, S., Gilliss, C., Shinn, J., Sparacino, P., Rankin, S., Leavitt, M., Price, M., & Hudes, M. (1988). Improving recovery following cardiac surgery: A randomized clinical trial. *Journal of Advanced Nursing, 13,* 649-661.

Grembowski, D., Patrick, D., Diehr, P., Durham, M., Beresford, S., Kay, E., & Hecht, J. (1993). Self-efficacy and health behavior among older adults. *Journal of Health and Social Behavior, 34,* 89-104.

Gross, D., Conrad, B., Fogg, L., & Wothke, W. (1994). A longitudinal model of maternal self-efficacy, depression, and difficulty temperament during toddlerhood. *Research in Nursing and Health, 17,* 207-215.

Gulanick, M. (1991). Is phase 2 cardiac rehabilitation necessary for early recovery of patients with cardiac disease? A randomized, control study. *Heart & Lung, 20,* 9-15.

Hickey, M., Owen, S., & Froman, R. (1992). Instrument development: Cardiac diet and exercise self-efficacy. *Nursing Research, 41*(6), 347-351.

Hilgenkamp, K. (1987). *The role of self-efficacy in various stages of exercise involvement among novice female runners.* Unpublished doctoral dissertation, University of Nebraska, Lincoln.

Hofstetter, C., Sallis, J., Hovell, M., Byron, M., Jones, S., Rummani, S., Scott, K., Wagers, R., & Weiss, D. (1990). Some health dimensions of self-efficacy: Analysis of theoretical specificity. *Social Medicine, 31*(9), 1051-1056.

Holcomb, J., Lira, J., Kingery, P., Smith, D., Lane, D., & Goodway, J. (1998). Evaluation of Jump into Action: A program to reduce the risk of non-insulin dependent diabetes mellitus in school children on the Texas-Mexico border. *Journal of School Health, 68*(7), 282-288.

Holden, G. (1991). The relationship of self-efficacy appraisals to subsequent health related outcomes: A meta-analysis. *Social Work in Health Care, 16,* 53-93.

Horan, M., Kim, K., Gendler, P., Froman, R., & Patel, M. (1998). Development and evaluation of the Osteoporosis Self-Efficacy Scale. *Research in Nursing and Health, 21*(5), 395-403.

Hurley, A. (1990). Measuring self care ability in patients with diabetes: The Insulin Management Diabetes Self-Efficacy Scale. In O. Strickland & C. Waltz (Eds.), *Measurement of nursing outcomes* (pp. 28-44). New York: Springer.

Hurley, A., & Shea, C. (1992). Self-efficacy: Strategy for enhancing diabetes self-care. *The Diabetes Educator, 18*(2), 146-150.

Jemmott, L., & Jemmott, J. (1992). Increasing condom-use intentions among sexually active black adolescent women. *Nursing Research, 41*(5), 273-279.

Kalichman, S., Roffman, R., Picciano, J., & Bolan, M. (1998). Risk for HIV infection among bisexual men seeking HIV-prevention services and risks posed to their female partners. *Health Psychology, 17*(4), 320-327.

Kaplan, R., Ries, A., Prewitt, L., & Eakin, E. (1994). Self-efficacy expectations predict survival for patients with chronic obstructive pulmonary disease. *Health Psychology, 13*(4), 366-368.

Kasen, S., Vaughan, R., & Walter, H. (1992). Self-efficacy and AIDS preventive behaviors among tenth grade students. *Health Education Quarterly, 19*(2), 187-202.

Kearney, B., & Fleischer, B. (1995). Development of an instrument to measure exercise of self-care agency. *Research in Nursing and Health, 2,* 25-34.

Kingery, P., & Glasglow, R. (1989). Self-efficacy and outcome expectations in the self-regulation of non-insulin dependent diabetes mellitus. *Health Education, 20*(7), 13-19.

Kowalski, S. (1997). Self-esteem and self-efficacy as predictors of success in smoking cessation. *Journal of Holistic Nursing, 15*(2), 128-142.

Kurlowicz, L. (1998). Perceived self-efficacy, functional ability, and depressive symptoms in older elective surgery patients. *Nursing Research, 47*(4), 219-226.

Lazarus, R. (1991). *Emotion & adaptation.* New York: Oxford University Press.

Lazarus, R., & Folkman, S. (1984). *Stress, appraisal, and coping.* New York: Springer.

Lazarus, R., & Folkman, S. (1991). The concept of coping. In A. Monet & R. Lazarus (Eds.), *Stress and coping: An anthology* (pp. 189-227). New York: Columbia University Press.

Leonard, B., Skay, C., & Rheinberger, N. (1998). Self-management development in children and adolescents with the role of maternal self-efficacy and conflict. *Journal of Pediatric Nursing, 13*(4), 224-233.

Lorig, K., Chastain, R., Ung, E., Shoor, S., & Holman, H. (1989). Development and evaluation of a scale to measure perceived self-efficacy in people with arthritis. *Arthritis and Rheumatism, 32,* 37-44.

Lowe, N. (1991). Maternal confidence in coping with labor. *Journal of Obstetrics, Gynecology, & Neonatal Nursing, 20*(6), 457-463.

Lusk, S., Ronis, D., Kerr, M., & Atwood, J. (1994). Test of the Health Promotion Model as a causal model of worker's use of hearing protection. *Nursing Research, 43*(3), 151-157.

MacDonald, E., Pica, S., McDonald, S., Hayes, R., & Baglioni, A. (1998). Stress and coping in early psychosis: Role of symptoms, self-efficacy, and social support in coping with stress. *British Journal of Psychiatry, 172*(Suppl. 33), 122-127.

Martin, N., Holroyd, K., & Rokicki, M. (1993). The Headache Self-Efficacy Scale: Adaptation to recurrent headaches. *Headache, 33,* 244-248.

McAuley, E. (1994). Self-efficacy and intrinsic motivation in exercising middle-aged adults. *Journal of Applied Gerontology, 13*(4), 355-370.

McAuley, E., Courneya, K., & Lettunich, J. (1991). Effects of acute and long-term exercise on self-efficacy responses in sedentary, middle-aged males and females. *The Gerontologist, 31*(4), 534-542.

McDougall, G., & Balver, J. (1998). Decreasing mental frailty in at-risk elders. *Geriatric Nursing, 19*(4), 222-224.

Oetker, S., & Taunton, R. (1994). Evaluation of a Self-Efficacy Scale for Preoperative Patients. *American Operating Room Nurse Journal, 60,* 43-50.

O'Leary, A. (1985). Self-efficacy and health. *Behavioral Research and Therapy, 23*(4), 437-451.

Parkatti, T., Deeg, D., Bosscher, R., & Launer, L. (1998). Physical activity and self-rated health among 55 to 89 year old Dutch people. *Journal of Aging & Health, 10*(3), 311-326.

Pender, N. J. (1982). *Health promotion in nursing practice.* Norwalk, CT: Appleton-Century-Croft.

Pender, N., Barkauskas, V., Hayman, L., Rice, V., & Anderson, E. (1992). Health promotion and disease prevention: Toward excellence in nursing practice and education. *Nursing Outlook, 40*(3), 106-112.

Petty, R., & Cacioppo, J. (1981). *Attitudes and persuasion: Classic and contemporary approaches.* Dubuque, IA: William C. Brown.

Pohl, J., Martinelli, A., & Antonakos, C. (1998). Predictors of participation in a smoking cessation intervention group among low-income women. *Addictive Behaviors, 23*(5), 699-704.

Riemsma, R., Rasker, J., Taal, E., Griep, E., Wouters, J., & Wiegman, O. (1998). Fatigue in rheumatoid arthritis: The role of self-efficacy and problematic social support. *British Journal of Rheumatology, 37*(10), 1042-1046.

Scherer, Y., & Schmieder, L. (1997). The effect of a pulmonary rehabilitation program on self-efficacy, perception of dyspnea, and physical endurance. *Heart & Lung, 26,* 15-22.

Schuster, P. (1988). *Instrument development for psychosocial variables correlated with contingency contracting and adherence.* Unpublished manuscript.

Schuster, P., & Waldron, J. (1991). Gender differences in cardiac rehabilitation patients. *Rehabilitation Nursing, 16*(5), 248-253.

Schuster, P., Wright, C., & Tomich, P. (1995). Gender differences in the outcomes of participants in home programs compared to those in structured cardiac rehabilitation programs. *Rehabilitation Nursing, 20*(2), 93-101.

Schwarzer, R., & Jerusalem, M. (1995). Generalized Self-Efficacy Scale. In J. Weinman, S. Wright, & M. Johnstone (Eds.), *Measures in health psychology: A user's portfolio. Causal and control beliefs* (pp. 35-37). Windsor, UK: NFER-NELSON.

Sharts-Hopko, N., Regan-Kubinski, M., Lincoln, P., & Heverly, M. (1996). Problem-focused coping in HIV infected mothers in relation to self-efficacy, uncertainty, social support, and psychological distress. *Image: Journal of Nursing Scholarship, 28*(2), 107-111.

Sherer, M., Maddux, J., Mercandate, B., Prentice-Dunn, S., Jacobs, B., & Rogers, R. (1982). The Self-Efficacy Scale: Construction and validation. *Psychological Reports, 51,* 663-671.

Skelly, A., Marshall, J., Haughey, B., Davis, P., & Dunford, R. (1995). Self-efficacy and confidence in outcomes as determinants of self-care practices in inner city, African-American women with insulin-dependent diabetes. *The Diabetic Educator, 21,* 38-46.

Solberg, V., & Villarreal, P. (1997). Examination of self-efficacy, social support, and stress. *Hispanic Journal of Behavioral Sciences, 19*(2), 182-193.

Strecher, V., DeVillis, B., Becker, M., & Rosenstock, I. (1986). The role of self-efficacy in achieving health behavior change. *Health Education Quarterly, 13,* 72-91.

Sullivan, M., LaCroix, A., Russo, J., & Kathon, W. (1998). Self-efficacy and self-reported functional status in coronary heart disease: A six month prospective study. *Psychosomatic Medicine, 60*(4), 473-478.

Thomas, J. (1993). Cardiac inpatient education: The impact of educational methodology on self-efficacy. *Journal of Cardiopulmonary Rehabilitation, 13,* 398-405.

Tillet, L. (1998). The Health Promotion Model. In A. Marriner-Tomey & M. Raile Allegood (Eds.), *Nursing theorists and their work* (pp. 529-537). St. Louis, MO: C. V. Mosby/Year Book.

Toshima, M., Kaplan, R., & Ries, A. (1990). Experimental evaluation of rehabilitation in chronic obstructive pulmonary disease: Short-term effects on exercise endurance and health status. *Health Psychology, 9*(3), 237-252.

Toshima, M., Kaplan, R., & Ries, A. (1992). Self-efficacy expectancies in chronic obstructive pulmonary disease rehabilitation. In R. Schwarzer (Ed.), *Self-efficacy: Thought control of action* (pp. 325-354). Washington, DC: Hemisphere.

Varvaro, F., & Palmer, M. (1993). Promotion of adaptation in battered women: A self-efficacy approach. *Journal of the American Academy of Nurse Practitioners, 5*(6), 264-270.

Verbrugge, L. (1985). Gender and health: An update on hypotheses and evidence. *Journal of Health and Social Behavior, 26,* 156-182.

Vidmar, P., & Robinson, L. (1994). The relationship between self-efficacy and exercise compliance in a cardiac population. *Journal of Cardiopulmonary Rehabilitation, 14,* 246-254.

Waller, K., & Bates, R. (1992). Health locus of control and self-efficacy beliefs in a health elderly sample. *American Journal of Health Promotion, 6*(4), 302-309.

Waller, P., Crow, C., Sands, D., & Becker, H. (1988). Health related attitudes and health promoting behaviors: Differences between health fair attenders and a community comparison group. *American Journal of Health Promotion, 3,* 17-24.

Wang, J., Wang, R., & Lin, C. (1998). Self-care behaviors, self-efficacy, and social support effect on the glycemic control of patients newly diagnosed with non-insulin dependent diabetes mellitus. *Kao Hsuing I Hsueh Ko Hseuh Tsa Chih, 14*(12), 807-815.

Wieseke, A. (1991). *Self-care attributes and correlates identified by individuals with chronic disease.* Unpublished manuscript.

Wigal, J., Creer, T., & Kotses, H. (1991). The COPD Self-Efficacy Scale. *Chest, 99*(5), 1193-1196.

Wigal, J., Stout, C., Brandon, M., Winder, J., McConnaughy, K., Creer, T., & Kotses, H. (1993). The Knowledge, Attitude, and Self-Efficacy Asthma Questionnaire. *Chest, 104,* 1144-1148.

Chapter 22

Stress, Uncertainty, and Health

Cecilia R. Barron

U ncertainty is part of life and is believed to be inherent in the stress, coping, and illness experience (Babrow, Kasch, & Ford, 1998) when persons lack an adequate explanatory framework for understanding their situations and predicting outcomes (Yoshida, 1997). As such, uncertainty is of interest to nursing. A search of the Cumulative Index for Nursing and Allied Health Literature (CINAHL) database using the word "uncertainty" for the time period 1982 through May 1998 yielded 1,056 records. The majority of studies have investigated uncertainty in acute or chronic illness using one of Mishel's (1981, 1988, 1990) conceptualizations or one of Mishel's (1983a, 1983b; Mishel & Epstein, 1990) questionnaires for assessing uncertainty or both, or they have interpreted qualitative findings with reference to Mishel's writings.

The concept of uncertainty is central to understanding various aspects of the stress, coping, and illness experience, including diagnosis (Fillion, Lemyre, Mandeville, & Piché, 1996) and treatment phases (Christ-

man, 1990; Mishel & Sorenson, 1991) as well as living with chronic illness (Hilton, 1988; Lugton, 1997). Also, the literature on uncertainty is not limited to the patient but also includes friends and family members (Dickerson, 1998; Theobald, 1997). Moreover, uncertainty is the central concept in the theory of uncertainty in illness related to acute (Mishel, 1981, 1988) and chronic (Mishel, 1990) illness and is implicit in self-regulation models of coping with the illness experience (Johnson, Fieler, Jones, Wlasowicz, & Mitchell, 1997; Leventhal, Diefenbach, & Leventhal, 1992).

In addition to a search of the CINAHL database, the Medline and PsychInfo databases were searched from 1982 through May 1998 to ensure that sources pertaining to the concept of uncertainty and with significant implications for nursing were identified. Medline and PsycInfo identified 5,098 and 3,013 records, respectively. There were duplications across databases, however, because of the overlap in journals from which they abstract. Because of the sheer volume of litera-

517

ture on uncertainty, articles earmarked by the searches and accessible for review were delimited by the following criteria: (a) The articles were written in English; (b) uncertainty articles were published in nursing journals, or the articles in nonnursing journals were deemed to have significant implications for the understanding of uncertainty by nursing; and (c) research articles directly measured uncertainty, or uncertainty as a major concept emerging from the data. Because of the prominence of Mishel's conceptualizations in the nursing literature, the evolution and description of the theory of uncertainty in illness related to acute (Mishel, 1981, 1988) and chronic (Mishel, 1990) illness is presented here, followed by a review of the uncertainty research.

➤ UNCERTAINTY IN ILLNESS

Mishel's Theory of Uncertainty in Illness

Acute Illness

According to Mishel (1984, 1988), *uncertainty* is the inability to determine the meaning of illness-related events and occurs when insufficient cues prevent the person from adequately structuring or categorizing an event, thus inhibiting the person's ability to predict outcomes adequately. The first pictorial representation, the Model of Perceived Uncertainty in Illness, focused on uncertainty related to acute illness (Mishel, 1981). The conceptualization was based on a cognitive appraisal model and incorporated many conceptual ideas from the writings of Lazarus (Lazarus, 1974; Lazarus & Folkman, 1984) and other theorists, such as Moos and Tsu (1977), Norton (1975), and Wyler (1974). According to the model, factors within the person and characteristics of the stimuli influence the person's perception of illness-related events. When stimuli are perceived as uncertain, the person is unable to subjectively evaluate the illness, treatment, and hospitalization

events. Lack of a cognitive structure of the illness and related events hinders the person from adequately appraising the situation, thus influencing subsequent decision making. Events perceived as uncertain are appraised as threatening and necessitate coping with the uncertainty. Stress occurs when the person is unable to resolve the uncertainty. Therefore, Mishel's (1981) original model conceptualized uncertainty as negative.

Development of the Mishel Uncertainty in Illness Scale (MUIS; Mishel, 1981) facilitated research on this concept, which in turn contributed to the revision of the model (Mishel, 1988). The focus of the revised model remained on uncertainty during acute illness or downward illness trajectory (Mishel, 1988) in patients undergoing active medical treatment (Mishel, 1988, 1995). Key concepts of the model include stimuli frame, cognitive capacity, and structure providers as antecedents to uncertainty; inference and illusion as part of the appraisal process; coping; and adaptation. A diagram of Mishel's (1988) modified model is shown in Figure 22.1. The major changes in the model included (a) the use of the word "uncertainty" within the pictorial representation, (b) adaptation as the major outcome of coping with uncertainty, (c) uncertainty appraised as an opportunity or a "danger" (as either positive or negative), (d) greater elaboration of stimuli characteristics, and (e) the addition of resources (structure providers).

According to the revised model (Mishel, 1988), *stimuli frame* refers to characteristics of the stimulus as perceived by the individual and consists of three components: symptom pattern, event familiarity, and event congruency. Uncertainty is likely to be present when the person perceives (a) inconsistency in symptoms to form a pattern (symptom pattern), (b) the environment as sufficiently novel (event familiarity), and (c) little or no congruency between expectations and experiences in the illness-treatment situation (event congruency).

Cognitive capacity refers to the ability to process information. This capacity includes

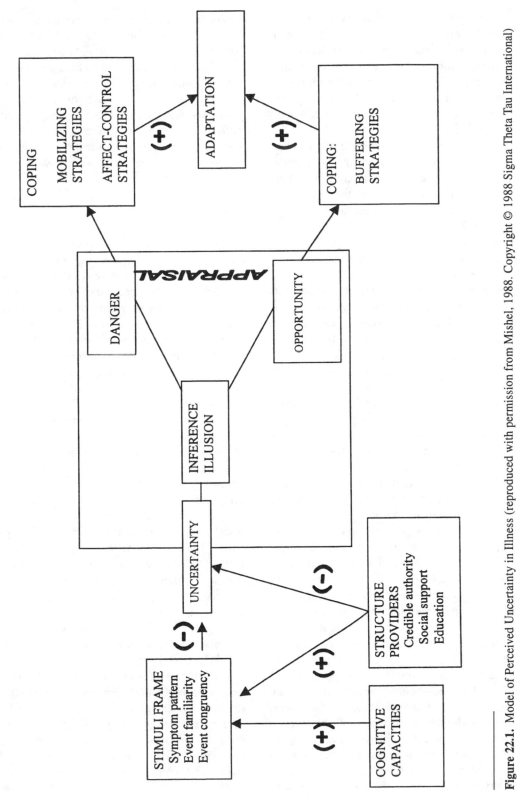

Figure 22.1. Model of Perceived Uncertainty in Illness (reproduced with permission from Mishel, 1988. Copyright © 1988 Sigma Theta Tau International)

the ability to attend to information. Pain, medication, nutrition, and perceptions that the environment is dangerous may influence the person's ability to attend to information (Mishel, 1988). Moreover, information overload, as well as the disease process such as dementia, also may influence attention, encoding, and recall.

Structure providers are the available resources for assistance with interpretation of the stimuli frame and include credible authority (trust and confidence in the health care provider), social support (availability of individuals for assistance), and education. Education contributes to the knowledge base from which relevant cognitive maps are developed and used for comparison with current illness-treatment stimuli. It provides the person with the ability to modulate the uncertainty (Mishel, 1988). Structure providers directly reduce uncertainty and indirectly reduce it through the stimuli frame components.

Appraisal in uncertainty involves the processes of inference and illusion. *Inferences* refer to general beliefs about the self and one's interaction with the environment (Mishel, 1988) and to the evaluation of uncertainty based on related situations from the past (Mishel, 1990). Personality dispositions, such as learned resourcefulness, sense of mastery, and locus of control, may affect the development of inferences (Mishel, 1988) by influencing perceptions and interpretations of current stimuli that are then encoded into memory. *Illusions* refer to beliefs arising from uncertainty and generally reflect a positive outlook. Significant others and health care providers may help the person maintain hope by fostering illusions. Inferences and illusions result in appraisals of danger or opportunity. Mishel (1988) emphasizes the experience of uncertainty as neutral until it is appraised.

When uncertainty is appraised as a danger, coping is initiated to reduce the uncertainty and to manage the emotions through mobilizing and affect-management strategies. When uncertainty is appraised as an opportunity, coping is initiated to maintain uncertainty so as to sustain the belief in a positive outcome. Buffering methods are used to block the input of new stimuli that could alter the person's appraisal of uncertainty as an opportunity. Buffering strategies include avoidance, selective inattention to information, minimization of threatening information, and the reordering of priorities. Effective coping via buffering, mobilizing, affect-control strategies, or all three promotes adaptation. Adaptation serves as the outcome to effective coping with uncertainty.

Chronic Illness

The original theory of uncertainty in illness (Mishel, 1981), and the modification (Mishel, 1988), were developed and tested primarily within the context of acute illness or downward illness trajectory and did not address (a) the experience of living with uncertainty within the context of chronic illness or a treatable acute phase with probable recurrence; (b) the nonlinear impact of antecedent variables on the appraisal of uncertainty across time; and (c) the possibility that growth or increased complexity, as opposed to adaptation, may be the desired outcome state (Mishel, 1990). Moreover, contrary to the original theory that postulates opportunity appraisals only in situations characterized by a high probability of negative consequences (i.e., downward trajectory), uncertainty was found to be appraised as opportunity in long-term chronic illness without a downward trajectory (Mishel & Murdaugh, 1987). In response to these problems, Mishel (1990) reconceptualized the theory for use in chronic illness. The reconceptualization assumes those persons with chronic illness are receiving maintenance treatment for their condition (Mishel, 1990, 1995).

The theory of uncertainty in (chronic) illness incorporates the following characteristics (Mishel, 1990): (a) As an open system, the person interchanges energy with the environment; (b) the person can change over time; (c) the person's appraisal of uncertainty is not static but evolves over time; and (d) the desired state may not be equilibrium but rather increased complexity. On the basis of insights obtained from chaos theory (Pool, 1989), uncertainty in illness was viewed as beginning in one part of the human system and having the potential to spread to the entire system. The more uncertainty spreads, the greater the likelihood that it will invade significant aspects of the person's life and jeopardize the stability of the personal system. Continual and pervasive uncertainty can destroy the cognitive structures that give meaning, which in turn promotes disorganization (Mishel, 1990).

When instability in the personal system reaches a critical threshold, the person is propelled toward a new state characterized by a higher-order, more complex orientation toward life. Structure providers, previous life experiences, and the person's physiological status influence the formation of a new life orientation. The new worldview being constructed is characterized by probabilistic and conditional thinking and necessitates the person's acceptance of uncertainty as inherent in life. The person gradually moves from an uncertainty appraisal of danger to an appraisal of opportunity.

Because the new orientation toward life is fragile, the person needs assistance from the environment to support the necessary cognitive restructuring. The process of reevaluation of uncertainty can be blocked or prolonged when (a) the person does not interact with potential social resources, (b) structure providers do not support the person's probabilitic or conditional view of life, (c) the provider's approach to the provision of health care communicates an overt or covert devaluation of the probabilistic view, and (d) the person's role responsibilities compete with the psychological work necessary for structuring of the new value system.

In response to a critical review (Mast, 1995) of the research on adult uncertainty in illness, Mishel (1995) emphasized that the two conceptualizations (Mishel, 1988, 1990) are not interchangeable. Whereas the first conceptualization (Mishel, 1988) addresses persons receiving active medical treatment for the acute phase of an illness, the second conceptualization (Mishel, 1990) addresses persons receiving maintenance treatment for stabilization of a long-term illness (Mishel, 1995). Therefore, studies addressing one conceptualization cannot be interpreted in terms of the other. Mishel (1990) cautioned, however, that the theory was reconceptualized "not to disregard the existing theoretical statements and linkages but to expand them to account for a perspective of growth and self-organization" as an outcome of coping with uncertainty in chronic illness (p. 258).

➤ MEASURES OF UNCERTAINTY

Mishel's Uncertainty in Illness Scales

Mishel's uncertainty questionnaires are the primary paper-and-pencil tools used to assess uncertainty in illness (Mishel, 1981, 1983a, 1983b, 1984; Mishel & Epstein, 1990). Her original work on instrument development began with the MUIS (Mishel, 1981). The 30-item scale was constructed to examine uncertainty in adults undergoing treatment for an active disease process. The MUIS uses a 5-point, Likert-type format and has undergone several revisions as a result of multiple psychometric evaluations. Versions range from 28 to 34 items and yield two to four factors: (a) ambiguity of illness cues, (b) complexity related to cues about the treatment and the system of care, (c) inconsistency related to information received, and (d) unpredictability of illness outcomes from illness and treatment cues. Factor reliabilities range from .71 to .91 and are strongest for ambiguity and complexity (Mishel & Epstein, 1990).

Diagnostic-specific versions of the uncertainty scale have been developed to enhance clinical application of the questionnaires to specific diagnostic groups (Mishel, 1983a). Persons with various health problems, such as cardiovascular and lupus patients, completed the MUIS, and cluster analyses were used to develop the diagnostic-specific versions. The specific diagnostic version is administered together with the MUIS to allow for comparison across diagnostic entities.

Whereas the MUIS was designed for use with hospitalized adults, a 28-item community version (MUIS-C) is used for nonhospitalized adults. The community version may be used by family members of the nonhospitalized chronically ill (Mishel & Epstein, 1990). A 34-item Parents' Perception of Uncertainty Scale (PPUS) (Mishel, 1983b) was used to evaluate the degree of uncertainty perceived by parents of an ill child and can be modified for use by a spouse or relative of an ill family member.

The MUIS has been translated into Swedish, German, Chinese, Egyptian, Thai, Korean, and Hebrew (Mishel & Epstein, 1990). Initial work on a Swedish version of the MUIS provides support for the cultural equivalence of the uncertainty concept (Hallberg & Erlandsson, 1991; Mishel, 1991), although questions remain regarding the consistency of the definition of uncertainty in the Swedish language and culture (Mishel, 1991, 1997).

Uncertainty Stress Scale

Hilton (1994) developed the Uncertainty Stress Scale (USS), which is intended to measure uncertainty, the stress occurring from that uncertainty, and the degree to which uncertainty is perceived as threatening or positive or both. The first part of the measure (60 items) asks respondents to rate their degree of uncertainty about their health condition and their coping with that uncertainty using a 5-point scale. Respondents are given the option of indicating whether the item is applicable or not applicable. The second part of the questionnaire asks respondents to rate their degree of stress related to each of the uncertainty items on a 3-point scale. The third part uses visual analog scales to measure global uncertainty, global stress, global threat, and perceptions of positive feelings arising from the uncertain state. A subscale score for each section can be obtained by summing the responses for each section.

The USS has undergone several revisions, and the author expects additional reduction of items to create a more streamlined version (Hilton, 1994). Factor analysis yielded two factors: (a) indefiniteness and lack of clarity about the present and future state of the disorder and (b) being unsettled or having doubts about coping. Internal consistency reliabilities for the factors are .96 and .94, respectively. Construct validity of the USS has been reported (Hilton, 1994). Clauson (1996) adapted the USS to create a high-risk pregnancy version.

Appraisal of Uncertainty Scale

The Appraisal of Uncertainty Scale is a 15-item questionnaire derived from a scale designed to assess coping responses (Folkman, 1982; Lazarus & Folkman, 1984). Each item represents an emotional state, such as sad, fearful, and hopeful. Respondents rate the degree to which they feel each emotion in response to the uncertainty perceived using a 6-point Likert scale ranging from "not at all" (1) to "a great deal" (6). Eight items comprise the Danger Appraisal subscale, and seven items comprise the Opportunity Appraisal subscale. Coefficient alphas range from .76 (opportunity) to .87 (danger) (Mishel & Sorenson, 1991). Table 22.1 provides a summary of selected studies that have used one or more of the questionnaires described.

➤ RESEARCH RELATED TO UNCERTAINTY IN ILLNESS

Mishel's uncertainty in illness theory related to acute (Mishel, 1981, 1988) and chronic (Mishel, 1990) illness remains the sole nursing theory specifically addressing uncertainty in illness. Linkages between concepts can be supported through direct testing of the linkages or by explaining study findings in light of existing conceptualizations (Mishel, 1997). The direct testing of linkages provides for the greatest precision because the

(text continued on page 526)

TABLE 22.1 Selected Measures for the Phenomenon of Uncertainty

Measure	Reference and Population	Reliability and Validity[a]
Appraisal of Uncertainty Scale	Mishel, Padilla, Grant, and Sorenson (1991); Adults: 100 women receiving treatment for gynecological cancer	.82 (danger), .76 (opportunity); CV-HT
	Mishel and Sorenson (1991); Adults: 131 women receiving treatment for gynecological cancer	.87 (danger), .82 (opportunity); CV-HT
	Padilla, Mishel, and Grant (1992); Adults: 100 women receiving treatment for newly diagnosed gynecological cancer	.82 (danger), .76 (opportunity); CV-HT
	Wineman, Durand, and Steiner (1994); Adults: 433 (multiple sclerosis [MS]) and 257 (spinal cord injury [SCI])	.88 for danger (MS), .86 for danger (SCI); .80 for opportunity (MS), .83 for opportunity (SCI); CV-HT
Mishel Uncertainty in Illness (MUIS)	Ellett and Young (1997); Adolescents: 105 (68 with inflammatory bowel disease, 20 with irritable bowel syndrome, and 17 healthy)	.84-.89; CV-HT
	Galloway and Graydon (1996); Adults: 40 cancer patients following surgical resection of colon cancer	.80 (total scale), .53 (complexity); alpha for ambiguity factor not reported; CV-HT
	Germino et al. (1998); Adults: 403 (201 men with prostate cancer and their family caregivers)	Coefficient alphas > .70 (specific Cronbach's alpha coefficients not reported); CV-HT
	Mast (1998); Adults: 109 women with breast cancer (58 Stage I, 50 Stage II, and 1 Stage III)	.90 (total score); CV-HT
	McCain, Zeller, Cella, Urbanski, and Novak (1996); Adults: 45 men with HIV disease	.83 (total score); CV-HT
	Mishel (1981); Adults: 134 medical, 51 rule-out, and 68 surgical patients	.91 (total scale); construct validity (known groups)
	Mishel (1984); Adults: 100 hospitalized medical patients from a Veterans Administration hospital	.89 (multiattributed ambiguity), .72 (unpredictability); CV-HT
	Mishel et al. (1991); Adults: 100 women receiving treatment for gynecological cancer	.91 (total scale); CV-HT
	Mishel and Sorenson (1991); Adults: 131 women receiving treatment for gynecological cancer	.90 (total scale); CV-HT
	Moser, Clements, Brecht, and Weiner (1993); Adults: 94 systemic sclerosis patients	.84 (total scale); CV-HT
	Northouse, Dorris, and Charron-Moore (1995); Adults: 155 (81 women with a first recurrence of breast cancer and 74 husbands)	.90 (patients); CV-HT
	Northouse, Jeffs, Cracchiolo-Caraway, Lampman, and Dorris (1995); Adults: 300 women awaiting a breast biopsy and their spouses (265)	.80 (patients); CV-HT

(continued)

TABLE 22.1 Continued

Measure	Reference and Population	Reliability and Validity[a]
	Padilla et al. (1992); Adults: 100 women receiving treatment for newly diagnosed gynecological cancer	.91 (total scale); data from current study support a three-factor structure: ambiguity about illness-wellness state (α = .88), lack of information/complexity of events information (α = .83), unpredictability of illness/treatment outcomes (α = .72); CV-HT
	Redeker (1992); Adults: 129 nonemergency first-time coronary artery bypass surgery (CABS) patients	One-week post-CABS α = .84 (ambiguity) and .75 (complexity); 6-week post-CABS α = .89 (ambiguity) and .78 (complexity); CV-HT
	Sheer and Cline (1995); Adults: 56 clinic cardiac patients	.80 and .89 for clinic pre- and postvisits, respectively; CV-HT
	Steele, Tripp, Kotchick, Summers, and Forehand (1997); Adults and children: 65 families (father, mother, and one child at least 7 years of age) in which the father had hemophilia	Alphas for father and mother data not reported; α = .83 for child sample; CV-HT
	White and Frasure-Smith (1995); Adults: male angioplasty (22) and bypass (25) patients at 1 and 3 months after treatment	.82; CV-HT
	Wineman (1990); Adults: 38 men and 80 women with MS	.82; CV-HT
	Wineman et al. (1994); Adults: 433 (MS) and 257 (SCI)	.84 (MS) and .89 (SCI); CV-HT
	Wineman, Schwetz, Goodkin, and Rudick (1996); Adults: 59 patients with progressive MS	.74; CV-HT
	Wong and Bramwell (1992); Adults: 25 mastectomy patients	Predischarge α = .91 (total scale), .87 (ambiguity), .82 (complexity); postdischarge α = .86 (total scale), .71 (ambiguity), .77 (complexity); CV-HT
Uncertainty in Illness Scale-Community Form (MUIS-C)	Bennett (1993); Adults: myocardial infarction (81: 65 men and 16 women)	.88 (ambiguity); CV-HT
	Braden (1990b); Adults: 396 patients with rheumatoid arthritis or arthritis-related conditions	.86; CV-HT
	Deane and Degner (1998); Adults: 70 women undergoing breast biopsy	.85; CV-HT
	Hilton (1989); Adults: 227 nonhospitalized women diagnosed with breast cancer	.87; CV-HT
	Janson-Bjerklie, Ferketich, and Benner (1993); Adults: 95 adults diagnosed with asthma and reversible airway obstruction	.70; CV-HT

TABLE 22.1 Continued

	Landis (1996); Adults: 94 community-based adults with a medical diagnosis of diabetes mellitus (Type I or II)	.92; CV-HT
	Lemaire and Lenz (1995); Adults: 177 women attending an educational program on menopause	.90; CV-HT
	O'Brien, Wineman, and Nealon (1995); Adults: 61 individuals with MS and their spousal caregivers	.86 (spouses); CV-HT
	Wineman, O'Brien, Nealon, and Kaskel (1993); Adults: 61 married couples with one member having MS	.85 (MS), .86 (well spouse); CV-HT
Parent/Child Perception of Uncertainty in Illness Scale	Miles, Funk, and Kasper (1992); Adults: 23 couples with premature infants hospitalized in neonatal intensive care	.83 (ambiguity), .79 (lack of clarity), .57 (lack of information), .70 (unpredictability)
	Mishel (1983b); Adults: 272 parents of hospitalized children (126 medical, 96 surgical, and 50 diagnostic)	.91 (total), .87 (multiattributed), .81 (lack of clarity), .73 (lack of information), .72 (unpredictability); construct validity (factor analysis, known groups, and CV-HT)
	Northouse, Dorris, et al. (1995); Adults: 155 (81 women with a first recurrence of breast cancer and 74 husbands)	.89 (husbands); CV-HT
	Northouse, Jeffs, et al. (1995); Adults: 300 women awaiting a breast biopsy and their spouses (265)	.80 (spouses)
	Northouse, Laten, and Reddy (1995); Adults: 81 women with recurrent breast cancer and 74 spouses	.89 (spouses)
	Sterken (1996); Adults: 31 fathers (child's biological father, stepfather, or male guardian) who had a child treated (or currently treated) for cancer	.87 (total), .84 (multiattributed ambiguity), .83 (lack of clarity), .31 (lack of information), .59 (unpredictability); CV-HT
	Yarcheski (1988); Adults: 32 parents (1 parent of each of 32 adolescents with cystic fibrosis)	.87
Uncertainty Stress Scale (USS)	Hilton (1994); Adults: 481 cancer; 31 awaiting breast biopsy; 68 cardiac; 27 vascular; 202 renal; 121 heart valve	.96 (Factor I: indefiniteness/lack of clarity), .94 (Factor II: unsettled/doubts); content validity (content experts); construct validation (factor analysis, multidimensional scaling, convergence [$r = .69$] with MUIS; CV-HT)
USS (high-risk pregnancy version)	Clauson (1996); Adults: 58 hospitalized high-risk pregnancy antepartum women	.96

a. Reliability coefficients refer to internal consistency alphas. CV-HT indicates that study results support the construct validity of the measure through hypothesis testing. The hypothesis is either directly posed in the study or can be inferred based on the literature review or the framework that guided the study or both.

researcher can ensure, at the outset of the study, that concepts are operationalized and other parameters are established in accordance with the theory to be tested. When the theory has not driven the proposal development decisions, the "fit" between the findings and the existing conceptualization referenced is likely to be less adequate.

On the basis of a review of the literature, 61 articles were found that used the MUIS, an adaptation (e.g., PPUS), or parts of the instrument. The majority of studies using the MUIS, however, were not based on any of Mishel's (1981, 1988, 1990) conceptualizations. Some studies tested an investigator-developed framework, and others were atheoretical with linkages to Mishel's (1981, 1988, 1990) conceptualizations made in light of the findings.

Studies of illness uncertainty can be divided into eight categories by type of illness (acute, chronic), person experiencing uncertainty (patient or family member), and developmental age of person (child or adult). Because Mishel's (1981, 1988) original conceptualizations were related to the acutely ill adult, most of the research is in this area. Studies to evaluate uncertainty in the chronically ill adult and in family members were stimulated when the MUIS was adapted for these populations. The evaluation of uncertainty in children and adolescents (Ellett & Young, 1997; Steele, Tripp, Kotchick, Summers, & Forehand, 1997), either as the patients or as family members, is minimal. In keeping with the original model (Mishel, 1981, 1988), this review of the literature on uncertainty in illness focuses on acute illness in adults and uses the major concepts of the model (Mishel, 1988) as the organizing force. Next, research on uncertainty related to chronic illness in adults, children and adolescents, and family members is discussed.

Acute Illness in Adults

Mast (1995) evaluated the literature on adult uncertainty in both acute and chronic illness, whereas Mishel (1997) focused on uncertainty in acute illness, including the adult patient and the family member of an acutely ill adult or child. The purpose of this discussion is to highlight the consistencies and inconsistencies related to findings on uncertainty in acute illness and Mishel's model (1988).

Stimuli Frame

Stimuli frame (characteristics of the stimulus as perceived by the individual) is proposed to be an antecedent of uncertainty, but interpretation of findings is difficult because the majority of studies in illness uncertainty did not directly test the linkage between stimuli frame and uncertainty. Mishel and Braden (1988) tested the linkage directly in women with gynecological cancer and found that symptom pattern predicted ambiguity but not complexity, whereas event familiarity predicted complexity but not ambiguity.

Diagnostic specificity may be considered an aspect of stimuli frame. Uncertainty is expected to be higher prior to diagnostic specificity when symptoms are present but a diagnosis is absent or before all diagnostic information is complete (Mishel, 1988). Overall, studies supported a linkage between diagnostic specificity and uncertainty (Fillion et al., 1996; Mishel, 1981; Northouse, Jeffs, Cracchiolo-Caraway, Lampman, & Dorris, 1995).

Cognitive Capacity

Cognitive capacity (the ability to process information) is proposed to influence uncertainty indirectly through stimuli frame. No studies in the illness uncertainty literature were found that directly tested this linkage. Severity of illness may be considered an indirect measure of cognitive capacity because severity of illness and its intensive treatment, such as the experience of pain and the use of pain medication, may influence an individual's capacity to perceive and interpret stimuli.

The majority of studies indicate a positive relationship between illness severity and uncertainty, but the findings are not conclusive (Mishel, 1997). The approaches used to assess severity of illness are varied and range from recurrence of illness (Hilton, 1994) and objective pathological indices (Staples & Jeffrey, 1997) to self-report measures of symptom distress (Christman, 1990) and functional status (Christman et al., 1988; Staples & Jeffrey, 1997). Some consistency of measuring illness severity is sorely needed. Moreover, clarification of relationships among the concepts of cognitive capacity, stimuli frame, and uncertainty requires studies that directly measure cognitive capacity.

Structure Providers

Structure providers (available resources) are proposed to influence uncertainty directly and indirectly by providing assistance in interpretation of the stimuli frame (Mishel, 1988). The literature provides greater support for the structure providers of credible authority and social support and less support for education (Mishel, 1997).

Several studies (Bennett, 1993; Davis, 1990; Mishel & Braden, 1987, 1988; White & Frasure-Smith, 1995) support an inverse relationship between social support and uncertainty across diverse populations, such as cardiac (Bennett, 1993; Davis, 1990; White & Frasure-Smith, 1995), gynecological cancer (Mishel & Braden, 1987, 1988), and trauma and postsurgical (Davis, 1990) patients. Although increased social support has been linked to less uncertainty, Mast (1995) notes that little is known about how social support ameliorates uncertainty and how unsupportive relationships may heighten the patient's uncertainty.

Credible authority was also associated with decreased uncertainty (Mishel & Braden, 1988; Molleman, Pruyn, & van Knippenberg, 1986), but the indirect path through symptom pattern was not supported in a sample of gynecological cancer patients (Mishel & Braden, 1988). In a study of 56 cardiac patients, illness uncertainty was lower in patients who perceived they had received adequate information from a credible health care provider (Sheer & Cline, 1995). Uncertainty was not decreased, however, in newly diagnosed diabetic patients when a provider-centered style of communication discouraged patients from seeking answers to their questions (Mason, 1985).

Findings related to education are inconsistent. Some studies found an inverse relationship between education and uncertainty (Christman et al., 1988; Hilton, 1994; Mishel, Hostetter, King, & Graham, 1984), whereas other studies found the opposite (Galloway & Graydon 1996; Mishel, 1984; Wong & Bramwell, 1992). There is evidence that the influence of education and social support on uncertainty may change over time (Christman et al., 1988; Mishel & Braden, 1987). Therefore, research is needed to determine the influence of structure providers across the illness process. Through the process of cognitive appraisal, the person judges the event to be a threat or an opportunity, and this in turn influences the type of coping to be used (Mishel, 1988). Although Mishel's (1988) model highlights the importance of cognitive appraisal to coping and adaptation, few model-based studies were found that sought to investigate variables influencing the cognitive appraisals of danger and opportunity. The majority of studies focused on the relationships between uncertainty or mastery and cognitive appraisals.

Appraisal

High levels of uncertainty were associated with threat of cancer recurrence in acute and chronic breast cancer survivors (Hilton, 1989), danger in women receiving treatment for gynecological cancer (Mishel, Padilla, Grant, & Sorenson, 1991; Mishel & Sorenson, 1991), and less hope in cancer patients receiving radiotherapy (Christman, 1990). There is evidence, however, that the relationship between uncertainty and cognitive appraisal is mediated by mastery (Mishel et al., 1991;

Mishel & Sorenson, 1991)—that is, the person's perception of personal resources to manage potential stressors.

Mishel (1995) identified several concepts, such as optimism (Mishel et al., 1984), sense of personal control (Braden, 1990a), and learned resourcefulness (Braden, 1990a), that may serve as other potential mediators related to inference in cognitive appraisal. Research is needed to identify other variables that may mediate between uncertainty and cognitive appraisal and to test interventions that incorporate strategies related to cognitive appraisals for promotion of healthy adaptation.

In Mishel's (1988) model, cognitive appraisal mediates uncertainty and coping. Several studies (Mishel et al., 1991; Mishel & Sorenson, 1991) of uncertainty in gynecological oncology patients support this relationship, with uncertainty appraised as a danger predicting emotion-focused coping and uncertainty appraised as an opportunity predicting problem-focused coping.

Coping

Most investigations of uncertainty and coping have examined this linkage directly rather than indirectly through appraisals of danger and opportunity. Testing of direct relationships indicated that uncertainty was associated with coping that is focused on controlling emotional distress (Mast, 1995; Mishel, 1997). Inconsistencies in the testing of direct relationships were noted, however, when subjects were studied over time (Christman et al., 1988; Mishel, 1997; Redeker, 1992).

Few studies have examined uncertainty and coping during the course of an acute illness using a repeated measures design. Also, it remains unclear how the type of acute illness, such as myocardial infarction, and previous illness experiences influence the relationship among uncertainty, coping, and adaptation. Moreover, the conceptualization and measurement of the coping variable may influence results. New measures of coping are needed that incorporate strategies relevant to

reducing the stress of uncertainty (Mishel, 1997). Qualitative studies that investigate coping with uncertainty across types of illness and over time are needed to generate items for inclusion in coping scales and to determine if there is sufficient variation in responses to warrant the tailoring of coping scales to specific clinical populations similar to Mishel's (1983a) tailoring of uncertainty scales.

Mishel (1988) proposed that coping mediates the relationship between appraisal and adaptation. In a study of 131 women receiving treatment for gynecological cancer, Mishel and Sorenson (1991) found little support for coping strategies as mediators between emotional distress and appraisals of danger or opportunity. Only two coping strategies, wishful thinking and focus on the positive, were found to mediate between danger or opportunity appraisals and emotional distress, and the mediation effect for each was small. A replication testing of the mediation effect of coping in a more heterogeneous sample of women also found limited support (Mishel et al., 1991).

Adaptation

Most studies have not tested coping as a mediator between uncertainty and adaptation but rather the direct relationship between uncertainty and adaptation. Moreover, adaptation has been operationalized in various ways, such as anxiety, emotional distress, quality of life, health, recovery, and adjustment (Mast, 1995; Mishel, 1988, 1997). In general, research has demonstrated a relationship between uncertainty and poorer psychosocial outcomes. Uncertainty has been linked to anxiety, depression, and emotional distress as well as to poorer psychosocial adjustment and quality of life in a variety of populations, such as in breast biopsy (Northouse, Jeffs, et al., 1995), breast cancer (Wong & Bramwell, 1992), cardiac (Bennett, 1993; Christman et al., 1988; Webster & Christman, 1988), gynecological cancer (Mishel & Braden, 1987; Mishel & Sorenson, 1991; Mishel et al., 1984; Padilla, Mishel, & Grant, 1992), and hysterectomy patients (Warrington & Gottlieb, 1987). Similar results were found in studies of adults with chronic illness, such as patients with arthritis (Braden, 1990b), diabetes (Landis, 1996), and spinal cord injury and multiple sclerosis (Wineman, Durand, & Steiner, 1994; Wineman, Schwetz, Goodkin, & Rudick, 1996).

In her review article, Mast (1995) posed the question of whether uncertainty inevitably produces negative patient outcomes and concluded that studies of adaptation to long-term uncertainty, such as in chronic illness, may demonstrate the phenomenon of positive reappraisal that Mishel (1990) hypothesized in her theory reconceptualization. There is evidence in the research literature that the degree and type of uncertainty may change over time, leading to the phenomenon of positive reappraisal (Hilton, 1988; Nyhlin, 1990).

Chronic Illness in Adults

There is a growing body of research related to uncertainty in chronic illness across a wide variety of populations, ranging from patients with abdominal aortic aneurysm (Patterson & Faux, 1993) and AIDS and HIV (Barroso, 1997; Gaskins & Brown, 1992; McCain & Cella, 1995; Regan-Kubinski & Sharts-Hopko, 1995; Sharts-Hopko, Regan-Kubinski, Lincoln, & Heverly, 1996; Weitz, 1989) to patients with stroke (Häggström, Axelsson, & Norberg, 1994) and ulcerative colitis (Dudley-Brown, 1996). Approximately half of the studies reviewed used a qualitative approach with phenomenological or grounded theory designs predominating.

Antecedents to Uncertainty

Several studies examined severity of illness as an antecedent to uncertainty. Uncertainty was positively correlated with severity of illness as measured by repeated surgeries in peripheral vascular disease (Ronayne, 1989) and perceptions of illness severity in rheumatoid arthritic (Braden, 1990a, 1990b) and asthmatic patients (Janson-Bjerklie, Ferke-

tich, & Benner, 1993). Mast (1998), however, found no relationship between uncertainty and disease state in breast cancer survivors. Hawthorne and Hixon (1994) found that diminished functional status was associated with uncertainty in heart failure patients and noted that patients grouped by functional status had different illness trajectories, supporting the importance of assessing severity of illness in chronicity.

Other studies have investigated the structure provider variables of education and social support as antecedents to uncertainty in chronic illness. Studies reviewed generally found an inverse relationship between education and uncertainty in persons who had been diagnosed with breast cancer (Mast, 1998), multiple sclerosis (Wineman et al., 1996), and abdominal aortic aneurysm (Patterson & Faux, 1993), extending the linkage proposed by Mishel (1988) to chronic illness. Although there was no significant difference in uncertainty between multiple sclerosis patients who agreed to participate in a clinical trial and those who refused, acceptors reported a higher educational mean (Armer, McDermott, & Schiffer, 1996).

Social Support

Uncertainty was positively correlated with perceptions of unsupportiveness or dissatisfaction with social support in 118 adults diagnosed with multiple sclerosis (Wineman, 1990). Moreover, unsupportiveness was related to purpose in life through the variable of uncertainty. Although there was a dearth of quantitative studies investigating social support and uncertainty in chronicity, social support was an important theme in many qualitative studies (Lugton, 1997; Nelson, 1996; Regan-Kublinski & Sharts-Hopko, 1995; Thibodeau & MacRae, 1997).

Similar to Mishel's (1990) description of environmental supports needed to promote a person's new and fragile life, breast cancer survivors used supportive persons to nourish their changing identities (Lugton, 1997), as did long-term survivors of AIDS, who renegotiated interpersonal relationships to maintain their reconstructed lives within the context of HIV (Barroso, 1997). For diabetic patients, searching for support, advice, and information was important in coming to terms with the uncertainty caused by the disease and the inadequacy of the health care system (Nyhlin, 1990). The "doctor-centered" style of communication used by health professionals, however, was not helpful to diabetics as they attempted to resolve their uncertainty (Mason, 1985).

Appraisal

Uncertainty was positively correlated with the appraisal of danger in persons with asthma (Janson-Bjerklie et al., 1993) and rheumatoid arthritis (Bailey & Nielsen, 1993). Ambiguity was moderately correlated with an appraisal of danger in persons with abdominal aortic aneurysm, although there was no relationship between total uncertainty scores and appraisals of danger or opportunity (Patterson & Faux, 1993). The sample size was small ($N = 27$), however, and subjects experienced many other chronic illnesses, such as arthritis, in addition to the chronic aneurysm. For both multiple sclerosis and spinal cord injury patients, danger appraisals yielded more emotion-focused coping, whereas opportunity appraisals yielded more problem-focused coping (Wineman et al., 1994). Choice of coping strategies did not explain emotional well-being once selected demographic and disability-related variables were controlled, possibly due to the coping instrument's deficiency in defining the coping dimensions important to that clinical population (Wineman et al., 1994).

Outcomes of Coping With Uncertainty

Uncertainty was associated with poorer psychosocial adjustment (Moser, Clements, Brecht, & Weiner, 1993; Mullins et al., 1995), more depression (Wineman, 1990) and psychological distress (Landis, 1996; McCain &

Cella, 1995; Wineman et al., 1996), poorer quality of life (Hawthorne & Hixon, 1994), and a lower sense of purpose in life (Wineman, 1990). Mishel's (1990) reformulation, however, allowed for growth rather than merely stability and equilibrium. The concept of growth is more clearly reflected in the qualitative studies in chronicity.

Selder (1989) proposed a life transition theory that describes how people who experience a disruption of their reality reorganize or reconstruct the existing one to create new meaning and resolve uncertainty. The idea of the process of transition was found in several qualitative studies that were reviewed. For example, breast cancer survivors learned new ways of being in the world and of putting uncertainty into life's perspective (Nelson, 1996). Cancer survivors spoke of the preciousness of life (Hilton, 1988) and changes in beliefs, values, goals, and roles that may serve as a positive experience (Halldórsdóttir & Hamrin, 1996; Hilton, 1988).

Confronting a life-threatening illness caused breast cancer survivors to think about metaphysical issues, such as the nature and meaning of life and the universe (Thibodeau & MacRae, 1997). Reappraising life and creating positive meanings were reflected in the interviews of diabetic patients facing long-term complications (Nyhlin, 1990). Women who survived a cardiac event redefined their priorities and focused on those activities that provided them with meaning and purpose (Fleury, Kimbrell, & Kruszewski, 1995).

Some studies have sought to understand uncertainty in chronicity by sampling subjects with a wide range of time since diagnosis—as much as a 53-year time span (Landis, 1996)—by collecting data cross-sectionally at only one point in time or at several points within a brief time period. Type and characteristics of uncertainty, however, may change over time. To develop an understanding of how uncertainty, appraisal, coping, and well-being can change over time and to determine what factors facilitate or deter such changes, longitudinal studies are needed to track persons from their initial diagnosis. Mixed designs, employing both quantitative and qualitative strategies, can be used to test hypothesized linkages while exploring factors less understood, such as identification of coping strategies relevant to the clinical population at each phase of the chronicity process. Finally, studies are needed to clarify how illnesses reflecting different levels of threat to life, such as arthritis versus AIDS, influence uncertainty and the process of transition in chronic illness.

Children and Adolescents

Most studies of ill children and adolescents have focused on uncertainty in the parent and not the child. Few studies were found that focused on uncertainty from the ill child's perspective.

Haase and Rostad (1994) used a phenomenological approach to explore the children's perspective of experiencing the completion of cancer treatment in seven children ages 5 to 18 years. Whereas parents' fear of recurrence focused on the child's diminished chance of survival, children's fear of recurrence focused more on having to reexperience the side effects of chemotherapy. For children, talking about their fear of recurrence was associated with a belief that their cancer would return. This study indicates the influence of the developmental stage on perceptions of and coping with uncertainty.

The MUIS was used to assess uncertainty in adolescents with cystic fibrosis, whereas the PPUS was used to assess uncertainty in parents (Yarcheski, 1988). On the basis of the results, Yarcheski postulated that some of the items on the total MUIS and PPUS may be extraneous to the concerns of adolescents with cystic fibrosis and their parents. It is also possible, however, that the MUIS and PPUS did not adequately capture the uncertainty concerns of the adolescents and their parents. Collectively, the two studies indicate the need for tailoring the measurement of uncertainty to the developmental stage and illness-related concerns of the respondent.

Family Members

Thirty-seven articles were reviewed related to studies of uncertainty in family members; the majority (20) described qualitative studies. Almost half (16) reported on studies of parents of ill children (Cohen, 1993, 1995; Cohen & Martinson, 1988; Sparacino et al., 1997), whereas 10 articles reported on spouses of ill adults (Dickerson, 1998; O'Brien, Wineman, & Nealon, 1995; Stetz, 1989). The remaining articles reported on studies of multiple family members or did not clarify whether other family members in addition to spouses were investigated (Brown & Powell-Cope, 1991; Jamerson et al., 1996; Malone, 1997).

Parents

Miles, Funk, and Kasper (1992) used the PPUS to study uncertainty in parents of preterm infants. Results indicated that the highest level of uncertainty was in the area of unpredictability, with mothers reporting higher levels of unpredictability than fathers. Uncertainty about the effects of prematurity on their child's development was also found in a qualitative study of parents attending a neonatal intensive care unit follow-up clinic, indicating a need for the provision of more developmental and parenting information (Hussey-Gardner, Wachtel, & Viscardi, 1998).

Grounded theory was used to explore the dimensions of uncertainty of parents whose children were hospitalized in an intensive care unit (Turner, Tomlinson, & Harbaugh, 1990). The results were similar to those found in the PPUS; uncertainty related to the family system and the parent-child role, however, extended Mishel's work (Turner et al., 1990).

Uncertainty or mastering uncertainty was a central theme of several qualitative studies related to parents of chronically ill children

(MacDonald, 1995, 1996; Sparacino et al., 1997). The use of hope or optimism (Siegl & Morse, 1994; Sterken, 1996) and creating meaning and purpose (Siegl & Morse, 1994) as coping strategies reflects Selder's (1989) proposal of a life transition that disrupts reality and requires creation of a new meaning and resolution of uncertainty.

Spouses

A major theme of spouses whose partners had suffered a myocardial infarction was "crushing uncertainty" (Theobald, 1997). Spouses had greater uncertainty about the illness than did cardiac (Staples & Jeffrey, 1997) and recurrent breast cancer patients (Northouse, Laten, & Reddy, 1995). Uncertainty predicted emotional distress in women experiencing recurrent breast cancer and their spouses (Northouse, Dorris, & Charron-Moore, 1995), in individuals with multiple sclerosis (MS) and their spouses (Wineman, O'Brien, Nealon, & Kaskel, 1993), and in women awaiting a breast biopsy but not in their respective spouses (Northouse, Jeffs, et al., 1995). Although illness uncertainty was an essential factoı in determining family satisfaction for the MS spouse, the congruence between each partner's perception of uncertainty was the crucial factor in determining family satisfaction for the well spouse (Wineman et al., 1993). Collectively, research in this area demonstrates the importance of investigating uncertainty in the spouse and the need to expand and test Mishel's acute (1988) and chronic (1990) illness models to incorporate the spouse and the influence of each partner's uncertainty on the well-being and growth of the other.

Other Family Members

The remaining research either studied multiple family members or did not clarify whether other family members in addition to spouses were investigated. In general, when studies investigated multiple family members

results were reported as family findings rather than by specific relationship.

The relative's illness and negotiating the health care system served as sources of uncertainty (Jamerson et al., 1996). Adult siblings often felt left out of the decision-making process and perceived that they had not received enough basic information about their relative's illness, suggesting information may not be uniformly communicated throughout the family. Family members of patients with heart transplantation (Mishel & Murdaugh, 1987), childhood cancer (Clarke-Steffen, 1997), and AIDS experienced "transitions through uncertainty" (Brown & Powell-Cope, 1991). Collectively, these studies indicate the importance of extending and testing life transition theory (Selder, 1989) in family members of those with chronic illness. Moreover, these findings indicate the importance of studying uncertainty in the family to determine how uncertainty in each of its members influences the well-being of the others.

➤ HEALTH-RELATED UNCERTAINTY

Although Mishel's (1981, 1988, 1990) conceptualizations have spawned a large body of research on uncertainty in illness, some investigators have extended the study of uncertainty beyond acute and chronic illness. An in-depth discussion of the theoretical and research literature in this area is beyond the scope of this chapter. Literature in this domain, however, bears mentioning to appreciate the breadth of and opportunities for research related to uncertainty.

Life Transitions and Events

Uncertainty has been studied in relation to normal life transitions, such as in pregnancy (Patterson, Freese, & Goldenberg, 1986), menopause (Lemaire & Lenz, 1995), infant adoption (Lobar & Phillips, 1996), and after natural disasters (Coffman, 1996). The majority of the studies reviewed used a qualitative design in which uncertainty emerged as a key concept. Models related to uncertainty in normal life transitions and following natural (or man-made) disasters are needed so that systematic research in these areas can be conducted.

Genetic Testing

As the revolution in molecular biology and genetics continues, genetic testing for various diseases is likely to become more available. Healthy persons with a family history of a potentially inheritable disease may experience substantial stress because of uncertainty about their risk for developing the disease. For diseases caused by inherited defects, such as Huntington's disease, testing is likely to produce different benefits and costs than those for diseases with multiple causes, such as breast cancer (Baum, Friedman, & Zakowski, 1997). Whereas genetic testing for Huntington's disease may decrease risk uncertainty, a positive result for the gene is likely to cause emotional distress. Cast in stress theory, Baum and associates (1997) presented a model that predicts long-term stress in genetic testing when risk uncertainty is minimally reduced, when testing results suggest a high risk or are at odds with preventive actions already taken, and when people lack the resources for coping with a high-risk result. As the use of genetic testing continues to increase, testing of this model and development of other models related to anticipation and consequences of genetic testing should prove to be fruitful areas for nursing research.

Dispositional Intolerance of Uncertainty

Whereas Mishel focuses on uncertainty in illness, several researchers, primarily from the discipline of psychology, have focused on various personality traits related to an individual's intolerance of uncertain situations (Freeston, Rhéaume, Letarte, Dugas, & La-

douceur, 1994; Krohne, 1993; Sorrentino & Short, 1986). Those who are habitually intolerant of uncertainty are likely to employ consistent vigilant behaviors by directing attention to threat-relevant information so as to avoid surprises and decrease uncertainty (Krohne, 1993). If individuals are simultaneously intolerant of emotional arousal (anxiety), however, vigilance will serve to heighten their anxiety. The end result is less effective coping characterized by fluctuations between vigilance to decrease uncertainty and avoidance to decrease anxiety. Research is needed to determine how intolerance of uncertainty and emotional arousal influences cognitive appraisal of uncertainty in illness and subsequent coping.

➤ IMPLICATIONS OF UNCERTAINTY FOR THEORY, RESEARCH, AND PRACTICE

Theory and Research

A review of the nursing literature indicates high interest in the concept of uncertainty in illness. The majority of quantitative studies have been atheoretical with reference to one of Mishel's (1981, 1988, 1990) conceptualizations made in hindsight. An understanding of the strengths and needed revisions of the current conceptualizations (Mishel, 1988, 1990) is unlikely to occur until more research is conducted in which the relevant conceptualization (acute and chronic) drives proposal development decisions.

Most studies referencing one of Mishel's (1981, 1988, 1990) conceptualizations have investigated uncertainty in ill adults. Few studies (Yarcheski, 1988) have investigated uncertainty in illness in acutely and chronically ill children and adolescents, even though developmental stage may influence perceptions of and coping with uncertainty (Haase & Rostad, 1994). Research is needed in this area and is likely to necessitate the development of different methods and measures for the assessment of uncertainty relevant to acute and chronic illness in youth. Moreover, most quantitative studies on uncertainty have used a cross-sectional design. Longitudinal studies are needed to determine how uncertainty, appraisal, coping, and adaptation and growth are related, how these relationships change over the course of acute and chronic illnesses, and what facilitates or deters healthy movement.

In addition to the need for the development of methods and measures for assessment of uncertainty in youth, Mast (1995) questioned whether the MUIS adequately measures the concept of uncertainty experienced in chronic illness because it was originally developed to assess uncertainty in acute illness. Moreover, Mishel (1997) recommended that new measures of coping are needed to incorporate strategies specific to stress reduction in uncertainty.

Most of the studies reviewed that examined illness uncertainty in family members used qualitative methods. Quantitative studies were primarily atheoretical, with results interpreted using Mishel's (1981, 1988, 1990) conceptualizations. There is evidence that uncertainty in the ill person and that in the family member are interrelated (Steele et al., 1997), with issues and problems related to the family system being a source of concern for parents of ill children (Turner et al., 1990). Collectively, research in this area points to the need for determining the unique dimensions of and relationships between uncertainty in the ill person and family member given the specific characteristics of and demands made by the illness. As research in this area progresses, it is likely that the current uncertainty conceptualizations (Mishel, 1988, 1990), which were developed with respect to ill adults, will be modified to incorporate antecedent to and consequences of uncertainty in family members.

Mishel (1997) noted that the role of personality dispositions as predictors of uncertainty or mediators between uncertainty and cognitive appraisal is limited, with some support for the mediating role of mastery. No research was found, however, that examined the relationship between uncertainty and the personality variable of intolerance for uncertainty. It is likely that dispositional intolerance for uncertainty will influence perceptions of illness uncertainty and cognitive appraisals, and this bears investigation. In addition, research (Germino et al., 1998) indicates that ethnicity influenced the relationship between uncertainty and coping. Therefore, Mast's (1995) observation that the majority of studies have examined uncertainty in Caucasian, middle-class samples indicates the need for research on uncertainty in diverse cultural populations.

Practice

Although few studies were found that investigated interventions related to illness uncertainty, most found uncertainty decreased following intervention (Braden, 1991, 1992; Hawthorne & Hixon, 1994). For example, the Self-Help Intervention Project (SHIP) for women receiving breast cancer treatment uses interventions for uncertainty management based on five goals: (a) reinforcement of opportunity appraisals; (b) promotion of elements related to cognitive structure, such as provision of information; (c) reduction of inappropriate or incorrect certainty associated with negative outcomes; (d) regulation of emotional response; and (e) promotion of personal control and probabilistic thinking (Braden, Mishel, & Longman, 1998). Although the extent to which weekly telephone interventions from the nurse contributed to a decrease in uncertainty is unclear, the study serves as a good beginning for determining the effectiveness of uncertainty interventions. Mishel (1997) concluded that the most effective interventions were educational in nature, providing information and skill building related to management of uncertainty.

Uncertainty is not necessarily detrimental (Mishel, 1988, 1990). On the basis of a literature review related to uncertainty, Wurzbach (1992) developed a guide to assess the client's degree of uncertainty and proposed interventions for use when certainty and uncertainty are deemed to be detrimental. Strategies for certainty and uncertainty are similar to strategies found in the SHIP (Braden et al., 1998) and include (a) cognitive reappraisal, (b) information provision, and (c) personal control strategies (Wurzbach, 1992). As descriptive studies further delineate the type, degree, and health consequences of uncertainty experienced throughout the illness experience, interventions can be developed and tested to target effective resolution of detrimental uncertainty (or certainty).

➤ CONCLUSION

Although the focus of this chapter was on illness-related uncertainty in ill persons and their families, it should be noted that some research has focused on uncertainty in the nurse. Studies have investigated decision making (Baumann, Deber, & Thompson, 1991), moral uncertainty about withholding or withdrawing artificial nutrition and hydration (Wurzbach, 1995, 1996), and risk uncertainty in working with AIDS patients (Reutter & Northcott, 1993). The most systematic research found, however, was in the area of perceived environmental uncertainty.

Attempts to control increasing health care costs have led to changes in the delivery of care, the availability of health care resources, and the acuity level of the patient population (Salyer, 1995). To determine how these changes influence nursing's job performance, Salyer (1995, 1996) proposed and tested a four-stage model that identified characteristics of the environment and of the nurse predicted to influence nursing performance. A key concept of the model was perceived environmental uncertainty, which was operationalized by the 11-item Perceived Environmental Uncertainty in Hospitals Scale and defined as the perception of uncertainty resulting from the need for information and the complexity, dynamism, and environmental dominance of the organization (Salyer, 1995, 1996). Research on the model is limited, and support is

mixed, ranging from partial (Salyer, 1995, 1996) to minimal (Callahan, Young-Cureton, Zalar, & Wahl, 1997).

Allred and associates (Allred, Hoffman, Fox, & Michel, 1994; Allred, Michel, et al., 1994) also investigated perceived environmental uncertainty through their Perceived Environmental Uncertainty Questionnaire (PEUQ) designed to measure the "degree of complexity, change, unpredictability, and uncertainty associated with the information, resources, or relationship factors identified as most important to providing patient care" (Allred et al., 1995, pp. 130-131). For a complete description of the four-part questionnaire with results of psychometric testing, consult articles by Allred and associates (Allred, Hoffman, et al., 1994; Allred, Michel, et al., 1994). The PEUQ identified three distinct nursing practice environments characterized by increasing levels of complexity, change, unpredictability, and uncertainty (Allred, Michel, et al., 1994). With the capacity to differentiate nursing practice environments, this questionnaire provides an opportunity for designing and testing practice models to facilitate effective and efficient nursing practice outcomes.

In conclusion, the nursing literature is replete with references to uncertainty, with most sources referring to uncertainty in acute and chronic illness. There is also a systematic and growing body of research related to perceived environmental uncertainty and efficient quality of care, however. Opportunities for research on uncertainty abound, whether the researcher is interested in focusing on the patient and family or on the nursing practice environment.

➤ REFERENCES

Allred, C. A., Arford, P. H., Michel, Y., Veitch, J. S., Dring, R., & Carter, V. (1995). Case management: The relationship between structure & environment. *Nursing Economics, 13,* 32-51.

Allred, C. A., Hoffman, S. E., Fox, D. H., & Michel, Y. (1994). A measure of perceived environmental uncertainty in hospitals. *Western Journal of Nursing Research, 16*(2), 169-182.

Allred, C. A., Michel, Y., Arford, P. H., Carter, V., Veitch, J. S., Dring, R., Beason, S., Hiott, B. J., & Finch, N. J. (1994). Environmental uncertainty: Implications for practice model design. *Nursing Economics, 12*(6), 318-326.

Armer, J. M., McDermott, M. P., & Schiffer, R. B. (1996). Psychological characteristics of MS patients: Determining differences based upon participation in a therapy regimen. *Rehabilitation Nursing Research, 5*(3), 102-112.

Babrow, A. S., Kasch, C. R., & Ford, L. A. (1998). The many meanings of uncertainty in illness: Toward a systematic accounting. *Health Communication, 10,* 1-23.

Bailey, J. M., & Nielsen, B. I. (1993). Uncertainty and appraisal of uncertainty in women with rheumatoid arthritis. *Orthopaedic Nursing, 12*(3), 63-67.

Barroso, J. (1997). Social support and long-term survivors of AIDS. *Western Journal of Nursing Research, 19,* 554-582.

Baum, A., Friedman, A. L., & Zakowski, S. G. (1997). Stress and genetic testing for disease risk. *Health Psychology, 16,* 8-19.

Baumann, A. O., Deber, R. B., & Thompson, G. G. (1991). Overconfidence among physicians and nurses: The "micro-certainty, macro-uncertainty" phenomenon. *Social Science and Medicine, 12,* 167-174.

Bennett, S. J. (1993). Relationships among selected antecedent variables and coping effectiveness in postmyocardial infarction patients. *Research in Nursing & Health, 16,* 131-139.

Braden, C. J. (1990a). Learned self-help response to chronic illness experience: A test of three alternative learning theories. *Scholarly Inquiry for Nursing Practice, 4,* 23-41.

Braden, C. J. (1990b). A test of the self-help model: Learned response to chronic illness experience. *Nursing Research, 39,* 42-47.

Braden, C. J. (1991). Patterns of change over time in learned response to chronic illness among participants in a systemic lupus erythematosus self-help course. *Arthritis Care and Research, 4,* 158-167.

Braden, C. J. (1992). Description of learned response to chronic illness: Depressed versus nondepressed self-help class participants. *Public Health Nursing, 9,* 103-108.

Braden, C. J., Mishel, M. H., & Longman, A. J. (1998). Self-help intervention project: Women receiving breast cancer treatment. *Cancer Practice, 6*(2), 87-98.

Brown, M. A., & Powell-Cope, G. M. (1991). AIDS family caregiving: Transitions through uncertainty. *Nursing Research, 40,* 338-345.

Callahan, P., Young-Cureton, G., Zalar, M., & Wahl, S. (1997). Relationship between tolerance/intolerance of ambiguity and perceived environmental uncertainty in hospitals. *Journal of Psychosocial Nursing & Mental Health Services, 35*(11), 39-44.

Christman, N. J. (1990). Uncertainty and adjustment during radiotherapy. *Nursing Research, 39,* 17-20, 47.

Christman, N. J., McConnell, E. A., Pfeiffer, C., Webster, K. K., Schmitt, M., & Ries, J. (1988). Uncertainty, coping, and distress following myocardial infarction: Transition from hospital to home. *Research in Nursing & Health, 11,* 71-82.

Clarke-Steffen, L. (1997). Reconstructing reality: Family strategies for managing childhood cancer. *Journal of Pediatric Nursing, 12*(5), 278-287.

Clauson, M. I. (1996). Uncertainty and stress in women hospitalized with high-risk pregnancy. *Clinical Nursing Research, 5*(3), 309-325.

Coffman, S. (1996). Parents' struggles to rebuild family life after hurricane Andrew. *Issues in Mental Health Nursing, 17,* 353-367.

Cohen, M. H. (1993). The unknown and the unknowable—Managing sustained uncertainty. *Western Journal of Nursing Research, 15,* 77-96.

Cohen, M. H. (1995). The stages of the prediagnostic period in chronic, life-threatening childhood illness: A process analysis. *Research in Nursing & Health, 18,* 39-48.

Cohen, M. H., & Martinson, I. M. (1988). Chronic uncertainty: Its effect on parental appraisal of a child's health. *Journal of Pediatric Nursing, 3*(2), 89-96.

Davis, L. L. (1990). Illness uncertainty, social support, and stress in recovering individuals and family care givers. *Applied Nursing Research, 3*(2), 69-71.

Deane, K. A., & Degner, L. F. (1998). Information needs, uncertainty, and anxiety in women who had a breast biopsy with benign outcome. *Cancer Nursing, 21,* 117-126.

Dickerson, S. S. (1998). Cardiac spouses' help-seeking experiences. *Clinical Nursing Research, 7,* 6-28.

Dudley-Brown, S. (1996). Living with ulcerative colitis. *Gastroenterology Nursing, 19*(2), 60-64.

Ellett, M. L., & Young, R. J. (1997). Development of the Vulnerability Scale. *Gastroenterology Nursing, 20*(3), 82-86.

Fillion, L., Lemyre, L., Mandeville, R., & Piché, R. (1996). Cognitive appraisal, stress state, and cellular immunity responses before and after diagnosis of breast tumor. *International Journal of Rehabilitation and Health, 2*(3), 169-187.

Fleury, J., Kimbrell, C., & Kruszewski, M. A. (1995). Life after a cardiac event: Women's experience in healing. *Heart & Lung, 24*(6), 474-482.

Folkman, S. (1982). An approach to the measurement of coping. *Journal of Occupational Behavior, 3,* 56-107.

Freeston, M. H., Rhéaume, J., Letarte, H., Dugas, M. J., & Ladouceur, R. (1994). Why do people worry? *Personality and Individual Differences, 17,* 791-802.

Galloway, S. C., & Graydon, J. E. (1996). Uncertainty, symptom distress, and information needs after surgery for cancer of the colon. *Cancer Nursing, 19,* 112-117.

Gaskins, S., & Brown, K. (1992). Responses among individuals with human immunodeficiency virus infection. *Applied Nursing Research, 5,* 111-121.

Germino, B. B., Mishel, M. H., Belyea, M., Harris, L., Ware, A., & Mohler, J. (1998). Uncertainty in prostate cancer: Ethnic and family patterns. *Cancer Practice, 6*(2), 107-113.

Haase, J. E., & Rostad, M. (1994). Experiences of completing cancer therapy: Children's perspectives. *Oncology Nursing Forum, 21*(9), 1483-1494.

Häggström, T., Axelsson, K., & Norberg, A. (1994). The experience of living with stroke sequelae illuminated by means of stories and metaphors. *Qualitative Health Research, 4*(3), 321-337.

Hallberg, L. R.-M., & Erlandsson, S. I.-M. (1991). Validation of the Swedish version of the Mishel Uncertainty in Illness Scale. *Scholarly Inquiry for Nursing Practice: An International Journal, 5,* 57-67.

Halldórsdóttir, S., & Hamrin, E. (1996). Experiencing existential changes: The lived experience of having cancer. *Cancer Nursing, 19,* 29-36.

Hawthorne, M. H., & Hixon, M. E. (1994). Functional status, mood disturbance and quality of life in patients with heart failure. *Progress in Cardiovascular Nursing, 9,* 22-32.

Hilton, B. A. (1988). The phenomenon of uncertainty in women with breast cancer. *Issues in Mental Health Nursing, 9,* 217-238.

Hilton, B. A. (1989). The relationship of uncertainty, control, commitment, and threat of recurrence to coping strategies used by women diagnosed with breast cancer. *Journal of Behavioral Medicine, 12,* 39-54.

Hilton, B. A. (1994). The Uncertainty Stress Scale: Its development and psychometric properties. *Canadian Journal of Nursing Research, 26*(3), 15-30.

Hussey-Gardner, B. T., Wachtel, R. C., & Viscardi, R. M. (1998). Parent perceptions of an NICU follow-up clinic. *Neonatal Network, 17,* 33-39.

Jamerson, P. A., Scheibmeier, M., Bott, M. J., Crighton, F., Hinton, R. H., & Cobb, A. K. (1996). The experiences of families with a relative in the intensive care unit. *Heart & Lung, 25,* 467-474.

Janson-Bjerklie, S., Ferketich, S., & Benner, P. (1993). Predicting the outcomes of living with asthma. *Research in Nursing & Health, 16,* 241-250.

Johnson, J. E., Fieler, V. K., Jones, L. S., Wlasowicz, G. S., & Mitchell, M. L. (1997). *Self-regulation theory: Applying theory to your practice.* Pittsburgh, PA: Oncology Nursing Press.

Krohne, H. W. (1993). Vigilance and cognitive avoidance as concepts in coping research. In H. W. Krohne (Ed.), *Attention and avoidance: Strategies in coping with aversiveness* (pp. 19-50). Seattle: Hogrefe & Huber.

Landis, B. J. (1996). Uncertainty, spiritual well-being, and psychosocial adjustment to chronic illness. *Issues in Mental Health Nursing, 17,* 217-231.

Lazarus, R. S. (1974). Psychological stress and coping in adaptation and illness. *International Journal of Psychiatry in Medicine, 5,* 321-333.

Lazarus, R. S., & Folkman, S. (1984). *Stress, appraisal, and coping.* New York: Springer.

Lemaire, G. S., & Lenz, E. R. (1995). Perceived uncertainty about menopause in women attending an educational program. *International Journal of Nursing Studies, 32,* 39-48.

Leventhal, H., Diefenbach, M., & Leventhal, E. A. (1992). Illness cognition: Using common sense to understand treatment adherence and affect cognition interactions. *Cognitive Therapy and Research, 16,* 143-163.

Lobar, S. L., & Phillips, S. (1996). Parents who utilize private infant adoption: An ethnographic analysis. *Issues in Comprehensive Pediatric Nursing, 19,* 65-76.

Lugton, J. (1997). The nature of social support as experienced by women treated for breast cancer. *Journal of Advanced Nursing, 25,* 1184-1191.

MacDonald, H. (1995). Chronic renal disease: The mother's experience. *Pediatric Nursing, 21*(6), 503-507, 574.

MacDonald, H. (1996). Mastering uncertainty: Mothering the child with asthma. *Pediatric Nursing, 22,* 55-59.

Malone, J. A. (1997). Family adaptation: Adult sons with long-term physical or mental illnesses. *Issues in Mental Health Nursing, 18,* 351-363.

Mason, C. (1985). The production and effects of uncertainty with special reference to diabetes mellitus. *Social Science and Medicine, 21,* 1329-1334.

Mast, M. E. (1995). Adult uncertainty in illness: A critical review of research. *Scholarly Inquiry for Nursing Practice: An International Journal, 9,* 3-24.

Mast, M. E. (1998). Correlates of fatigue in survivors of breast cancer. *Cancer Nursing, 21,* 136-142.

McCain, N. L., & Cella, D. F. (1995). Correlates of stress in HIV disease. *Western Journal of Nursing Research, 17*(2), 141-155.

McCain, N. L., Zeller, J. M., Cella, D. F., Urbanski, P. A., & Novak, R. M. (1996). The influence of stress management training in HIV disease. *Nursing Research, 45*(4), 246-253.

Miles, M. S., Funk, S. G., & Kasper, M. A. (1992). The stress response of mothers and fathers of preterm infants. *Research in Nursing & Health, 15,* 261-269.

Mishel, M. H. (1981). The measurement of uncertainty in illness. *Nursing Research, 30,* 258-263.

Mishel, M. H. (1983a). Adjusting the fit: Development of uncertainty scales for specific clinical populations. *Western Journal of Nursing Research, 5*(4), 355-370.

Mishel, M. H. (1983b). Parents' perception of uncertainty concerning their hospitalized child. *Nursing Research, 32,* 324-330.

Mishel, M. H. (1984). Perceived uncertainty and stress in illness. *Research in Nursing and Health, 7,* 163-171.

Mishel, M. H. (1988). Uncertainty in illness. *Image: Journal of Nursing Scholarship, 20*(4), 225-232.

Mishel, M. H. (1990). Reconceptualization of the Uncertainty in Illness theory. *Image: Journal of Nursing Scholarship, 22*(4), 256-262.

Mishel, M. H. (1991). Response to "Validation of the Swedish version of the Mishel Uncertainty in Illness Scale." *Scholarly Inquiry for Nursing Practice: An International Journal, 5,* 67-70.

Mishel, M. H. (1995). Response to "Adult uncertainty in illness: A critical review of research." *Scholarly Inquiry for Nursing Practice: An International Journal, 9,* 25-29.

Mishel, M. H. (1997). Uncertainty in acute illness. *Annual Review of Nursing Research, 15,* 57-80.

Mishel, M. H., & Braden, C. J. (1987). Uncertainty: A mediator between support and adjustment. *Western Journal of Nursing Research, 9,* 43-57.

Mishel, M. H., & Braden, C. J. (1988). Finding meaning: Antecedents of uncertainty in illness. *Nursing Research, 37*(2), 98-103, 127.

Mishel, M. H., & Epstein, D. (1990). *Uncertainty in Illness Scales manual.* Available from M. H. Mishel, University of North Carolina at Chapel Hill, School of Nursing, CB #7140 Carrington Hall, Chapel Hill, NC 27599-7140.

Mishel, M. H., Hostetter, T., King, B., & Graham, V. (1984). Predictors of psychosocial adjustment in patients newly diagnosed with gynecological cancer. *Cancer Nursing, 7,* 291-299.

Mishel, M. H., & Murdaugh, C. L. (1987). Family experiences with heart transplantation: Redesigning the dream. *Nursing Research, 36,* 332-338.

Mishel, M. H., Padilla, G., Grant, M., & Sorenson, D. S. (1991). Uncertainty in Illness theory: A replication of the mediating effects of mastery and coping. *Nursing Research, 40,* 236-240.

Mishel, M. H., & Sorenson, D. S. (1991). Uncertainty in gynecological cancer: A test of the mediating functions of mastery and coping. *Nursing Research, 40,* 167-171.

Molleman, E., Pruyn, J., & van Knippenberg, A. (1986). Social comparison processes among cancer patients. *British Journal of Social Psychology, 25,* 1-13.

Moos, R. H., & Tsu, V. D. (1977). The crisis of physical illness: An overview. In R. H. Moos (Ed.), *Coping with physical illness.* New York: Plenum.

Moser, D. K., Clements, P. J., Brecht, M. L., & Weiner, S. R. (1993). Predictors of psychosocial adjustment in systemic sclerosis: The influence of formal educa-

tion level, functional ability, hardiness, uncertainty, and social support. *Arthritis & Rheumatism, 10,* 1398-1405.

Mullins, L. L., Chaney, J. M., Hartman, V. L., Albin, K., Miles, B., & Roberson, S. (1995). Cognitive and affective features of postpolio syndrome: Illness uncertainty, attributional style, and adaptation. *International Journal of Rehabilitation and Health, 1*(4), 211-222.

Nelson, J. P. (1996). Struggling to gain meaning: Living with the uncertainty of breast cancer. *Advances in Nursing Science, 18*(3), 59-76.

Northouse, L. L., Dorris, G., & Charron-Moore, C. (1995). Factors affecting couples' adjustment to recurrent breast cancer. *Social Science and Medicine, 41,* 69-76.

Northouse, L. L., Jeffs, M., Cracchiolo-Caraway, A., Lampman, L., & Dorris, G. (1995). Emotional distress reported by women and husbands prior to a breast biopsy. *Nursing Research, 44*(4), 196-201.

Northouse, L. L., Laten, D., & Reddy, P. (1995). Adjustment of women and their husbands to recurrent breast cancer. *Research in Nursing & Health, 18,* 515-524.

Norton, R. W. (1975). Measurement of ambiguity tolerance. *Journal of Personality Assessment, 39,* 607-619.

Nyhlin, K. T. (1990). Diabetic patients facing long-term complications: Coping with uncertainty. *Journal of Advanced Nursing, 15,* 1021-1029.

O'Brien, R. A., Wineman, N. M., & Nealon, N. R. (1995). Correlates of the caregiving process in multiple sclerosis. *Scholarly Inquiry for Nursing Practice: An International Journal, 9*(4), 323-338.

Padilla, G. V., Mishel, M. H., & Grant, M. M. (1992). Uncertainty, appraisal and quality of life. *Quality of Life Research, 1,* 155-165.

Patterson, C., & Faux, S. A. (1993). Uncertainty, and appraisal in patients diagnosed with abdominal aortic aneurysms. *Canadian Journal of Cardiovascular Nursing, 4,* 4-10.

Patterson, E. T., Freese, M. P., & Goldenberg, R. L. (1986). Reducing uncertainty: Self-diagnosis of pregnancy. *Image, 18*(3), 105-109.

Pool, R. (1989). Chaos theory: How big an advance? *Science, 245,* 26-28.

Redeker, N. S. (1992). The relationship between uncertainty and coping after coronary bypass surgery. *Western Journal of Nursing Research, 14,* 48-61.

Regan-Kubinski, M. J., & Sharts-Hopko, N. (1995). Illness cognition of HIV-infected mothers. *Issues in Mental Health Nursing, 16,* 327-344.

Reutter, L. I., & Northcott, H. C. (1993). Making risk meaningful: Developing caring relationships with AIDS patients. *Journal of Advanced Nursing, 18,* 1377-1385.

Ronayne, R. (1989). Uncertainty in peripheral vascular disease. *Canadian Journal of Cardiovascular Nursing, 1*(2), 26-30.

Salyer, J. (1995). Environmental turbulence: Impact on nurse practitioner. *Journal of Nursing Administration, 25*(4), 12-20.

Salyer, J. (1996). Development and psychometric evaluation of an instrument to measure staff nurses' perception of uncertainty in the hospital environment. *Journal of Nursing Management, 4,* 33-48.

Selder, F. (1989). Life transition theory: The resolution of uncertainty. *Nursing & Health Care, 10,* 437-451.

Sharts-Hopko, N. C., Regan-Kubinski, M. J., Lincoln, P. S., & Heverly, M. A. (1996). Problem-focused coping in HIV-infested mothers in relation to self-efficacy, uncertainty, social support, and psychological distress. *Image, 28*(2), 107-111.

Sheer, V. C., & Cline, R. J. (1995). Testing a model of perceived information adequacy and uncertainty reduction in physician-patient interactions. *Journal of Applied Communication Research, 23,* 44-59.

Siegl, D., & Morse, J. M. (1994). Tolerating reality: The experience of parents of HIV positive sons. *Social Science Medicine, 38*(7), 959-971.

Sorrentino, R. M., & Short, J. C. (1986). Uncertainty, motivation, and cognition. In R. M. Sorrentino & E. T. Higgins (Eds.), *The handbook of motivation and cognition: Foundations of social behavior* (pp. 379-403). New York: Guilford.

Sparacino, P. S. A., Tong, E. M., Messias, D. K. H., Foote, D., Chesla, C. A., & Gillis, C. L. (1997). The dilemmas of parents of adolescents and young adults with congenital heart disease. *Heart & Lung, 26*(3), 187-194.

Staples, P., & Jeffrey, J. (1997). Quality of life, hope, and uncertainty of cardiac patients and their spouses before coronary artery bypass surgery. *Canadian Journal of Cardiovascular Nursing, 8,* 7-16.

Steele, R. G., Tripp, G., Kotchick, B. A., Summers, P., & Forehand, R. (1997). Family members' uncertainty about parental chronic illness: The relationship of hemophilia and HIV infection to child functioning. *Journal of Pediatric Psychology, 22,* 577-591.

Sterken, D. J. (1996). Uncertainty and coping in fathers of children with children. *Journal of Pediatric Oncology Nursing, 13*(2), 81-88.

Stetz, K. M. (1989). The relationship among background characteristics, purpose in life, and caregiving demands on perceived health of spouse caregivers. *Scholarly Inquiry for Nursing Practice: An International Journal, 3*(2), 133-153.

Theobald, K. (1997). The experience of spouses whose partners have suffered a myocardial infarction: A phenomenological study. *Journal of Advanced Nursing, 26,* 595-601.

Thibodeau, J., & MacRae, J. (1997). Breast cancer survival: A phenomenological inquiry. *Advances in Nursing Science, 19*(4), 65-74.

Turner, M. A., Tomlinson, P. S., & Harbaugh, B. L. (1990). Parental uncertainty in critical care hospitalization of children. *Maternal/Child Nursing Journal, 19,* 45-62.

Warrington, K., & Gottlieb, L. (1987). Uncertainty and anxiety of hysterectomy patients during hospitalization. *Nursing Papers/Perspectives in Nursing, 19,* 59-73.

Webster, K. K., & Christman, N. J. (1988). Perceived uncertainty and coping post myocardial infarction. *Western Journal of Nursing Research, 10*(4), 384-400.

Weitz, R. (1989). Uncertainty and the lives of persons with AIDS. *Journal of Health and Social Behavior, 30,* 270-281.

White, R. E., & Frasure-Smith, N. (1995). Uncertainty and psychologic stress after coronary angioplasty and coronary bypass surgery. *Heart & Lung, 24,* 19-27.

Wineman, N. M. (1990). Adaptation to multiple sclerosis: The role of social support, functional disability, and perceived uncertainty. *Nursing Research, 39*(5), 294-299.

Wineman, N. M., Durand, E. J., & Steiner, R. P. (1994). A comparative analysis of coping behaviors in persons with multiple sclerosis or a spinal cord injury. *Research in Nursing & Health, 17,* 185-194.

Wineman, N. M., O'Brien, R. A., Nealon, N. R., & Kaskel, B. (1993). Congruence of uncertainty between individuals with multiple sclerosis and their spouses. *Journal of Neuroscience Nursing, 25*(6), 356-361.

Wineman, N. M., Schwetz, K. M., Goodkin, D. E., & Rudick, R. A. (1996). Relationships among illness uncertainty, stress, coping, and emotional well-being at entry into a clinical drug trial. *Applied Nursing Research, 9*(2), 53-60.

Wong, C. A., & Bramwell, L. (1992). Uncertainty and anxiety after mastectomy for breast cancer. *Cancer Nursing, 15,* 363-371.

Wurzbach, M. E. (1992). Assessment and intervention for certainty and uncertainty. *Nursing Forum, 27*(2), 29-35.

Wurzbach, M. E. (1995). Long-term care nurses' moral convictions. *Journal of Advanced Nursing, 21,* 1059-1064.

Wurzbach, M. E. (1996). Long-term care nurses' ethical convictions about tube feeding. *Western Journal of Nursing Research, 18,* 63-76.

Wyler, R. S. (1974). *Cognitive organization and change: An information processing approach.* Hillsdale, NJ: Lawrence Erlbaum.

Yarcheski, A. (1988). Uncertainty in illness and the future. *Western Journal of Nursing Research, 10*(4), 401-413.

Yoshida, K. (1997). Uncertainty in the lives of people with spinal cord injury and rheumatoid arthritis. *Canadian Journal of Rehabilitation, 10,* 5-14.

PART VI

Future Directions

CHAPTER 23

Stress, Coping, Health, and Nursing

The Future

Brenda L. Lyon and Virginia Hill Rice

It is widely accepted that stress is a common experience in modern society that can affect a person's health. What is it that we do not understand about the relationship between stress and health and how is this understanding important to nursing? The purpose of this chapter is twofold: (a) to propose a conceptual model that is a holistic representation of what we currently understand about the relationship between stress, coping, and health and (b) to identify future directions for nursing theory, research, and practice in relation to stress, coping, and health. The task of grasping current knowledge as a whole is a challenge. As is clear from the preceding chapters, there is still much work to be done in the development of conceptual, measurement, and methodological guidelines to help us to consistently evaluate the role of stress-related factors on health from a nursing perspective. Not only is "stress" defined and operationalized differ-

ently, but also on a "grand" theory scale our conceptualization and measurement of health varies greatly. Nonetheless, there are some repeatedly supported dynamics among the stress-related variables and health outcomes that can be summarized here.

First, it is clear that stress-related variables are components of complex transactions among genetic, psychological, and environmental factors that affect how a person is feeling and doing as well as the body's ability to prevent or overcome disease. Currently, the theoretical framework proposed by Richard Lazarus and colleagues holds considerable promise in explaining on a grand and, with some relationships, a midrange level the dynamics between stress and health. Figure 23.1 is a conceptual model of the stress-related variables and health outcome relationships proposed in Chapters 1 through 22. The model incorporates the major variables in Lazarus's (1966) and Lazarus and Folkman's

543

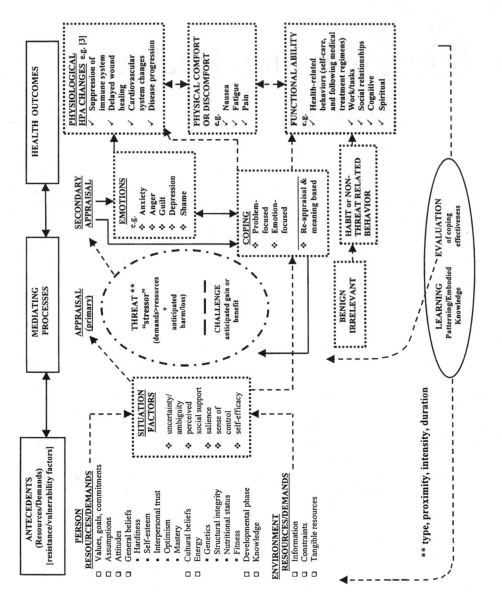

Figure 23.1. A Conceptual Model of Stress-Related Factors and Health Outcomes

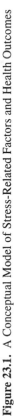

(1984) theory of stress and coping. Our portrayal is not meant to be linear but rather nonrecursive in nature, with some simultaneous occurrences and multiple feedback loops. In addition, "midrange" relationships that are empirically supported are represented by solid lines among the variables. Those that rely heavily on theoretical proposition with some but not necessarily adequate empirical support are depicted with dashed lines. It is interesting to note that many of the dashed lines are the result of the fact that it is infrequent for "appraisals" to be measured in stress, coping, and health research.

The antecedent variables in the model include person, environmental, and situational variables. The importance of all these variables lies in the possibility that they play a role in making a person resistant or vulnerable to stress experiences. Person variables include individual goals, values, commitments, attitudes, general beliefs (e.g., self-esteem, hardiness, optimism, and interpersonal trust), cultural beliefs, energy resources (e.g., genetic makeup, structural integrity of the body, nutritional status, and fitness), and knowledge. Environmental variables include available information (accuracy and clarity), constraints (social and material), and tangible resources (e.g., money, housing, and transportation). Situational factors arise from transactions between a person and his or her environment and include, but are not limited to, uncertainty, perceived social support, salience, sense of control, and self-efficacy.

There is some evidence that antecedent variables influence how a person appraises the meaning of a situation and therefore the resultant judgment of whether the situation presents a threat or challenge or is benign/positive or irrelevant. As discussed in Chapter 13, values, beliefs (general and cultural), and attitudes affect the meaning that a person derives from a given situation. Chapters 10 and 19 presented evidence that having information, in the form of sensory information, increases one's sense of personal control, thereby influencing appraisals of health care events. This in turn influences the emotions experienced.

Specifically, if a patient who desires information about what to anticipate during a medical procedure receives that information, then the patient appraises the situation as less threatening and experiences less anxiety than those who receive no information or information that only describes the medical "mechanics" of the procedure.

The important role that social support plays in affecting health-related outcomes is highlighted in Chapter 14. How social support influences health outcomes, however, is unclear. Although there is research that purports to demonstrate a direct effect of social support on health outcomes, this relationship may be spurious because "threat" tends not to be measured. It is not clear whether social support acts as a coping resource, a mediator, or a moderator of stress. It is possible that the experience of desired and satisfying social support influences the individual's primary and secondary appraisals a priori, thereby acting as a resistance resource that reduces threat appraisals and enhances coping potential.

As discussed in Chapter 21, self-efficacy is a variable that influences the initiation and maintenance of behavior, including coping effort. Behavior is proposed to be a function of the subjective value of an outcome, the subjective probability that a particular behavior or coping effort will achieve the valued outcome in a specific situation, and the individual's efficacy expectations in relation to performance. Efficacy expectations can be assessed on three dimensions (magnitude, strength, and generality) and influenced by four sources of efficacy information (mastery, vicarious experience, verbal persuasion, and physiological arousal). Many systematic reviews have supported the relationship between level of personal self-efficacy and performance of health behaviors. These are important findings to guide nursing practice as it seeks to enhance the health performance and coping of its patients and clients.

As is clear in Chapter 22, uncertainty, as a situational factor, can either increase or decrease the intensity of perceived threat depending on how a person views a situation.

There is evidence that uncertainty is positively correlated with appraisal of danger, but it is not known what factors lead a person to appraise a similar situation as nonthreatening or as a challenge. This is a classic example of viewing the glass as "half full" instead of "half empty." There is evidence that the relationship between uncertainty and cognitive appraisal of a situation is mediated by mastery, although it is not clear what variables may either moderate uncertainty or mediate between uncertainty and appraisal. Research has demonstrated a positive relationship between uncertainty and poorer psychosocial outcomes, such as anxiety, depression, psychosocial adjustment, and quality of life. It is not clear, however, what pathway or what variables may either moderate or mediate the relationship between uncertainty and psychosocial outcomes. It was also pointed out in Chapter 22 that situational factors interact with each other. For example, the presence of social support decreases perceived uncertainty in some situations.

As explained by Lazarus in Chapter 9, the appraisal of threat triggers a secondary appraisal that not only influences what stress emotion is experienced but also influences what determines coping responses. The affect of appraised threat on emotion and coping seemingly occurs simultaneously through secondary appraisal. There is considerable evidence that this proposition is valid given that researchers, as discussed in Chapters 9 and 10, often find it difficult to determine which comes first, the emotion(s) or the coping effort. Lazarus also purposes that secondary appraisal contributes to the meaning of the situation through three basic judgments: blame or credit, coping potential, and future expectations. He emphasizes the role that values, goals, belief systems, and personal resources play not only in influencing primary appraisal but also in determining the particular emotion experienced through a secondary appraisal that connects the relational meaning of the situation to how the person feels and acts.

As discussed in Chapters 2, 7, and 9, stress emotions and coping responses both influence physiological changes primarily thought to occur through the hypothalamic-pituitary-adrenal axis. In addition, there is substantial evidence, as summarized in Chapters 3 and 4, that chronic elevations in cortisol, glucocorticoids, catecholamines, and the neuromediators of norepinephrine and epinephrine have been linked to the development of disease, including coronary artery disease, hypertension, cancer, and various infectious diseases. Also, there is marked support for the proposition that elevation in these hormones and the neuromediators depresses the immune system, a factor most likely involved in the development of many illnesses.

The outcome variables of most of the research have been delimited by a focus on disease or proposed physiological correlates. Despite the absence of focus on the effect of stress-related variables on symptoms, a body of theoretical work proposes relationships between physiological correlates and selected symptoms, such as sympathetic-mediated contraction of muscles contributing to the experience of tension headaches and migraine headaches. As noted in Chapters 7 and 10, numerous intervention studies have demonstrated the beneficial effects of relaxation, cognitive interventions, therapeutic touch, sensory stimulation, back rubs and massage, guided imagery, meditation, and behavior modification on the experience of irritable bowel syndrome, temporal mandibular pain, tension and migraine headaches, anxiety, pain, sleep, nausea, and heart rate. It is interesting to note that, except for sleep, there has been a dearth of research on how stress affects functional ability, including self-care decisions and self-care behaviors.

The Acute Myocardial Infarction (AMI) Coping Model described in Chapter 16 begins to explain the relationship between knowledge of symptoms and the decision to seek care, but there is still very little consideration of what role emotions and situational or social constraints play in symptom interpretation and care-seeking behavior. Symptoms are conceptualized in the AMI model as "demands" that tax a person's resources and trigger coping responses proposed to occur in four phases: (a) symptom recognition, which includes formulation of a hypothesis about the meaning of the symptom and possible coping strategies; (b) covert construction of an action plan with the intent of restoring equilibrium; (c) overt behavior that implements the action plan (if the overt behavior does not restore equilibrium, then the process is recursive); and (d) assessment and consummation.

Many of the linkages among the variables demonstrate that how we think affects how we feel and function and vice versa. Stress-related variables help us to consider how our perceptions can trigger negative or positive emotions and how emotions affect autonomic and endocrine influences throughout the body. How a person is feeling and doing is not separate from his or her thoughts or emotions (see Chapters 9 and 10, this volume). Appraisal of threat appears to involve a simultaneous activation of biological and psychological system changes. Appraisal of threat is accompanied by a systemic arousal produced by the sympathetic nervous system and the hypothalamic-pituitary-adrenocortical axis (HPA). At the same time, depending on the meaning of the situation, stress emotions are triggered along with coping efforts that may in turn alter the physiological response.

It is striking that despite all the research conducted to date, very little has examined the relationship between stress-related variables and subjective health outcomes, including somatic discomfort (e.g., nausea, fatigue, and pain) and functional ability. In particular, because of nursing's concern about comfort and physical performance, it is surprising that nurse researchers have not focused on the effects of appraised threat, stress emotions, and coping responses on somatic symptoms or functional problems. It is even more surprising when one considers the increasing evidence of a high incidence of stress-related illnesses (including but not limited to somatoform disorders) as noted in Chapters 1 and 7.

Nursing can make a major contribution toward enhancing the experience of wellness and well-being, even in the presence of disease and illness, and therefore achieve a decrease in health care costs. The development of nursing interventions to help patients alter stress-related factors to enhance somatic comfort (physical and emotional) and functional ability is essential and should be a priority for the nursing research agenda.

➤ FUTURE DIRECTIONS FOR NURSING THEORY, RESEARCH, AND PRACTICE

Nursing's concern centers on the human experience of "illness" and "wellness." As noted in Chapters 1 and 13, human beings can experience wellness or illness in the presence or absence of disease. More important, there is sufficient reason, both research-based and anecdotal-based, to propose that middle-range stress-related phenomena, such as stress appraisals, stress emotions, and coping, influence the subjective experience of illness—in other words, how one is feeling and doing. Therefore, it is proposed here that a scientific goal for nursing is the identification of transaction patterns between stress-related variables that predict susceptibility or vulnerability to illness experiences and that predict resilience to stress and enhanced wellness experiences. Specifically, what patterns predict the experience of somatic discomforts, including stress emotions and physical discomforts and declines in functional ability below capability level, or what patterns predict somatic comfort and functional ability at or near capability level? To achieve this goal, we must (a) focus on the development of midrange theories regarding the linkages or patterns among variables (there are many midrange and situation-specific relationships embedded but not explicated in Figure 23.1); (b) develop clear conceptual and operational definitions of the constructs; (c) develop new or use existing methodologies that allow us to capture recursive, and sometimes simultaneous, changes in variables; and (d) use analysis techniques that adequately capture the nature of the relationships or influences that we are proposing. It is also important that nurse researchers develop focused programs of research that will help explicate patterns of variables that contribute to the experience of illness or wellness over time.

Midrange theories of stress-related variables include addressing the following questions: What factors contribute to a person being stress resistant or vulnerable? For example, do low self-esteem, lack of hardiness, and a pessimistic outlook place a person "at risk" for a stress-related illness in situations in which demands chronically exceed resources? Furthermore, do self-originated demands, such as expecting oneself to measure up to an "ideal" or holding onto unrealistic expectations of others, contribute to stress appraisals and, concomitantly, the stress emotions of guilt and anger? What pattern of variables predicts a threat appraisal over a challenge appraisal? Is the "hardy" person who has high self-esteem with a high degree of mastery, social support, and an optimistic disposition more likely to experience demanding or taxing situations as positively toned challenges? How are coping strategies learned? That is, are coping efforts learned through modeling, information, trial and error, or some other method? How do people determine if their coping responses are effective? Are the primary questions considered in determining coping effectiveness the following: (a) was the purpose accomplished; and

(b) did it not cost too much? Are there other factors? How are self-care behaviors and coping responses similar or different? Which person and environment factors, in addition to stress emotions and coping, are most likely to lead to specific physical discomforts or functional ability problems?

It is clear that our understanding of how stress-related variables affect health is evolving. However, there is tremendous promise for nursing research, theory, and practice in the area of stress, coping, and health. As we enter the second millennium, the role that nursing can play in helping people experience wellness, even in the presence of disease, or to not experience illness in the absence of disease will become increasingly important to policymakers and payers of health care services. It is imperative that nursing research efforts not only clearly document the variables or relationships among the variables that are affected by health outcome interventions but also document the cost-benefit ratio of the outcomes achieved through stress-related interventions.

➤ REFERENCES

Lazarus, R. (1966). *Psychological stress and the coping process.* New York: McGraw-Hill.

Lazarus, R., & Folkman, S. (1984). *Stress, appraisal, and coping.* New York: Springer.

Author Index

Subject Index

About the Contributors

Angelo A. Alonzo, PhD, is Associate Professor of Sociology at The Ohio State University. His research and scholarly activities have focused on examining cardiac delay behavior. He has served as a research sociologist with the National Heart, Lung and Blood Institute of the National Institutes of Health. He is currently a consultant to the National Heart Attack Alert Program.

Jane H. Backer, DNS, RN, is Associate Professor at Indiana University School of Nursing. Her research program is focused on stress, coping, and health outcomes of persons with chronic illness, particularly Parkinson's disease. She has published in a variety of journals. She teaches stress and coping content to graduate nursing students.

Tamilyn Bakas, DNS, RN, is Assistant Professor at Indiana University School of Nursing. Her research has focused on family caregivers of both stroke survivors and lung cancer patients using a model derived from Lazarus and colleagues' theory of stress and coping. She has developed an instrument titled the Bakas Caregiving Outcomes Scale. She coauthored a publication in *Geriatric Nursing* regarding effective caregiving approaches for patients with Alzheimer's disease.

Cecilia R. Barron, PhD, RN, CS, is Associate Professor of Nursing at the University of Nebraska Medical Center (UNMC) and Faculty Associate at the UNMC/Eppley Cancer Center. She is certified as a clinical specialist by the American Nurses' Credentialing Center in both child and adolescent and adult psychiatric nursing. Her research in the area of stress, coping, and health has been published in various research and clinical nursing journals. She is currently investigating the intermediate phase of breast cancer survivorship, including the uncertainty that occurs from the cancer diagnosis and treatment.

Susan J. Bennett, DNS, RN, is Professor at Indiana University School of Nursing. Her research program focuses on stress, coping, and quality of life in persons with cardiovascular disorders. She has published in a variety of journals, including *Nursing Research* and *Heart and Lung.*

Judith A. Cohen, RN, PhD, is Associate Professor of Nursing at The University of Vermont. Her expertise and research interests are focused in the areas of adult health, nursing theory, caring science, qualitative research methods, and health policy.

Rosanna DeMarco, PhD, RN, ACRN, is Assistant Professor and Director of Undergraduate Programs at Northeastern University, Bouve College of Health Sciences, School of Nursing. Her research interests began through an application of family theory, specifically the Framework of Systemic Organization, with staff nurses in acute care settings. Extension of her dissertation findings have yielded her research in nursing systems (administration and management) as well as client groups, specifically women living with HIV/AIDS, and lay homecare caregivers. She is also an active public policy advocate serving in an elected position on the Congress of Health Policy and Legislation of the Massachusetts Nurses Association and the Committee to Defend and Improve Health Care in Boston.

Marilyn Ford-Gilboe, RN, PhD, is Associate Professor in the School of Nursing at the University of Western Ontario. She holds a career scientist award provided jointly by the Medical Research Council of Canada and the National Health Research Development Program, Health Canada. With Dr. Helene Berman and others, she is developing the Family Health Promotion Research Program at the University of Western Ontario. Her research focuses on understanding family health promotion processes of single mothers and their children. She holds several national research grants that support both quantitative and qualitative projects in this area, including those focused on testing and refining the Developmental Health Model.

Marie-Luise Friedemann, RN, PhD, is Professor/Research Coordinator in Nursing at Florida International University. Her specialties are families and mental health. She is known for her Framework of Systemic Organization, a nursing theory for working with families. Her family assessment instrument (the Assessment of Strategies in Families-Effectiveness) is used in nursing and was also translated and tested in Mexico and Finland. Her research includes studies on family stress and unemployment, substance abuse, and the involvement of families in nursing homes.

Erika Friedmann, PhD, is Professor and Chairperson of the Department of Health and Nutrition Sciences at Brooklyn College of the City University of New York. Her research interests focus on the interaction of social, psychological, behavioral, and physiological factors as contributors to health and to cardiovascular health in particular. She is author of more than 50 research articles. She is coauthor (with S. A. Thomas and T. Eddy) of a chapter in *Companion Animals and Us: Exploring the Relationships Between People and Pets* (in press), a chapter (with S. A. Thomas) in *Companion Animals in Human Health* (1998), and an article (with S. A. Thomas, F. Wimbush, and E. Schron) in *American Journal of Critical Care* (1997).

Marlene Hanson Frost, RN, PhD, is Professional Associate in Research in the Mayo Clinic Women's Program. Her research interests include adjustment to cancer diagnosis, treatment, and survival as well as to being at increased risk for cancer. She has published on the topics of satisfaction and adjustment to prophylactic mastectomy, perceived familial risk for cancer, adjustment of women to breast cancer at various stages of the disease process, quality of life with recurrent breast cancer, and stressors associated with breast cancer health outcomes.

Martha E. Horsburgh, PhD, is Professor and Director of the School of Nursing, University of Windsor. Her research interests include adult coping with chronic illness. Results of her work are recorded in a variety of peer-reviewed journals and have been presented both nationally and internationally.

Richard S. Lazarus, PhD, is Professor Emeritus at the University of California, Berkeley. His research interests include projective methods, individual differences in perception, and perceptual defense but have mainly focused on psychological stress, emotions, and coping. He is author or coauthor of more than 200 scientific articles and 20 books, including *Psychological Stress and the Coping Process* (1966), which is considered a classic; *Stress, Appraisal, and Coping* (with S. Folkman) (1984); *Emotion and Adaptation* (1991); *Passion and Reason* (with B. Lazarus) (1994); and *Stress and Emotion: A New Synthesis* (1999).

Brenda L. Lyon, DNS, RN, FAAN, is Associate Professor of Adult Health at Indiana University School of Nursing and a clinical nurse specialist with a private practice in the diagnosis and treatment of stress-related physical illness. She is cofounder of the Midwest Nursing Research Society's Stress & Coping Research Section and served as its first chairperson from 1983 to 1985. She is author of several critical reviews of stress and coping nursing research and coeditor of the Sigma Theta Tau International monograph, *Stress and Coping: State of the Science and Implications for Nursing Theory, Research, and Practice* (1993). She is also author of several Glaxo-Wellcome monographs and videos focused on helping nurses manage stress and helping health care providers help patients who have chronic, life-threatening diseases. Her research focus has been on strategies to help patients with HIV and AIDS and patients with breast cancer manage stressful experiences. She is a fellow in the American Academy of Nursing.

Carol L. Macnee, PhD, is Associate Professor in the Department of Family/Community Nursing at East Tennessee State University and codirector of a nurse-managed clinic for homeless and indigent. Her research interests include examining the process of smoking cessation and other health behavior change from a stress and coping framework and examining outcomes of nursing care with homeless and indigent clients.

Herbert L. Mathews, PhD, is Professor of Microbiology and Immunology in the Stritch School of Medicine, Loyola University of Chicago. His research interest is the analysis of the cellular and molecular mechanisms that underlie the protective immune response to infectious agents and to cancer. Recently, his work has focused on the analysis of the immunological deficits of at-risk patients within a contextual framework of psychoneuroimmunology.

Susan McCabe, EdD, is Assistant Professor of Nursing in the Department of Professional Roles and Mental Health Nursing at East Tennessee State University and Director of Behavioral Health Care in a nurse-managed clinic for homeless and indigent. Her research interests include outcomes of advanced practice psychiatric nursing and the process of care with homeless and indigent clients.

Hamilton I. McCubbin, PhD, is Professor in the Department of Child and Family Studies and Director of the Endowed Center for Excellence in Family Studies and the Institute for the Study of Families at the University of Wisconsin-Madison. He has contributed to the advancement of family science theory and research methods through his 17 authored or coedited books and more than 100 journal articles and chapters on family stress, coping, and resiliency. He and colleagues have developed and tested more than 36 family measures that are used worldwide and have been translated into seven languages.

Marilyn A. McCubbin, RN, PhD, FAAN, is Professor at the University of Wisconsin-Madison School of Nursing, Fellow with the Center for Family Studies and the University of Wisconsin Comprehensive Cancer Center, and Nursing Core Discipline Chief with the Pediatric Pulmonary Center at the University of Wisconsin-Madison. She is coauthor (with H. I. McCubbin) of the Resiliency Model of Family Stress, Adjustment, and Adaptation and has also developed instruments to measure aspects of family functioning, such as family hardiness, family problem-solving communication, and parental coping with a child's chronic illness.

Margot L. Nelson, RN, PhD, is Associate Professor of Nursing and coordinator of the master's in nursing program at Augustana College. Her research has focused on psychoneuroimmunology and stress and coping experiences, particularly for people with HIV and AIDS. Her teaching and nursing practice emphasis is on adult health, chronic health conditions, and nursing research. Recent publications focus on the advocacy role of nurses and design of an education-practice model responding to care of underserved populations.

Patricia K. Pierce, DNS, RN, is Assistant Professor at Indiana University-South Bend School of Nursing. She has more than 30 years of experience in practice and nursing education and has taught graduate nursing courses for the past 8 years, including Stress and Coping and Nursing Research. Her clinical focus is adult health, especially coping with chronic illnesses.

Carol Mattson Porth is Professor Emeritus at the University of Wisconsin-Milwaukee School of Nursing. She teaches courses in pathophysiology and pharmacology. Her area of research expertise focuses on autonomic control of blood pressure and cardiovascular function in humans. She is author of *Pathophysiology: Concepts of Altered Health* (5th ed., 1998).

Edith D. Hunt Raleigh, PhD, RN, is Dean of Graduate Studies and Professor of Nursing at Madonna University. Her research and teaching interests focus on coping and hopefulness in chronic physical conditions. She is on the editorial board of the *Journal of Nursing Measurement.*

Nancy R. Reynolds, PhD, RN, CNP, is Assistant Professor of Nursing at The Ohio State University College of Nursing. Her research and scholarly activities have focused on examining mechanisms of and strategies for enhancing adaptation to chronic illness. Her work has been guided by a stress and coping framework, principally self-regulation theory. Her current research is focused on HIV symptoms and adherence behavior.

Virginia Hill Rice, PHD, RN, CS, FAAN, is Professor of Nursing at the Wayne State University College of Nursing and Professor of Oncology at the Wayne State University College of Medicine and the Karmonos Cancer Institute. She holds a doctorate in social psychology and is a certified medical-surgical clinical nurse specialist. She has a long history of funded research and numerous publications and presentations in the field of stress, coping, and health. She received the Nightingale Award for Excellence in Nursing Research, the Midwest Nursing Research Society's Stress and Coping Research Section's Advancement of Science Award, and the MNRS Distinguished Contributor to Nursing Research in the Midwest Award. She is a fellow in the American Academy of Nursing.

JoAnn B. Ruiz-Bueno, PhD, ARNP/CNM, is Director of the Family Nurse Practitioner Program at the University of Cincinnati. She is a certified nurse-midwife.

Nancy A. Ryan-Wenger, PhD, RN, CPNP, is Professor and Chair of the Department of Community, Parent-Child and Psychiatric Nursing. Her research and other scholarly work are in the area of stress, coping, and health in children. She developed the Schoolagers' Coping Strategies Inventory to measure children's frequency and effectiveness of coping behavior.

Vicki W. Sharrer, MS, RN, CPNP, is Associate Professor in Nursing at Ohio University. She teaches pediatric nursing and practices as a pediatric nurse practitioner. She has conducted and participated in several research projects related to stress and coping in school-age children.

Debra Siela, DNSc, RN, CCNS, CS, CCRN, RRT, is Assistant Professor in the School of Nursing at Ball State University. She conducts research in the areas of chronic obstructive pulmonary disease (COPD), self-efficacy, and ventilator weaning. She has a particular interest in gender differences related to symptom interpretation and management. She is currently completing her dissertation at Rush University that examines gender differences in self-efficacy, dyspnea, and functional performance in COPD patients.

Sue Ann Thomas, RN, CSP, PhD, FAAN, is Professor of Nursing at Georgetown University School of Nursing. She is a clinical specialist in psychiatric nursing and a family therapist. Her research interests are in holistic cardiovascular health. She is author of more than 50 research articles. She is coauthor (with E. Friedmann and T. Eddy) of a chapter in *Companion Animals and Us: Exploring the Relationships Between People and Pets* (in press), a chapter (with E. Friedmann) in *Companion Animals in Human Health* (1998), and an article (with E. Friedmann, F. Wimbush, and E. Schron) in *American Journal of Critical Care* (1997).

Patricia W. Underwood, PhD, RN, is Director for Research and Faculty Development at the Kirkhof School of Nursing, Grand Valley State University. She has conducted several studies examining stress, coping, and social support within the context of childbirth, developed a scale to measure perceived satisfaction with received social support, and coauthored (with Joanne Ruiz-Bueno; 1999)

a synthesis of nursing research for the years 1991 to 1995 that examined coping resources.

Lorraine M. Welch, RN, EdD, is Associate Professor of Nursing at The University of Vermont. She has taught psychosocial concepts and psychiatric mental health nursing as well as educational concepts to undergraduate and graduate students. Her research interest is in transformative experiences for students and faculty in nursing education. She is also studying caregiver-client experiences as they cope with degenerative neurological disease.

Joan Stehle Werner, RN, DNS, is Professor of Adult Health Nursing at the University of Wisconsin-Eau Claire. Her research has focused on occupational stress and health in various populations of health care providers and on stress and quality of care in long-term care. She has authored and coauthored several chapters and articles on stress, coping, and related topics. Her educational research and writing are in the area of clinical reasoning. Her areas of teaching expertise are nursing practice in adult health, human responses, research, and chronic mental illness.

Jill M. White, PhD, is Assistant Professor in the School of Nursing at the University of Wisconsin-Milwaukee. Her areas of research expertise focus on the use of music therapy to improve cardiac autonomic function after myocardial infarction and women's experiences with myocardial infarction. She has authored multiple articles and book chapters in these and related areas.

Ann W. Wieseke, DNS, RN, is Associate Professor in the School of Nursing at Ball State University. She conducts research in the areas of health care economics, maternal depression, and self-efficacy. She is currently completing work related to maternal depression. Several articles have been published reporting the works of her research.

Frances B. Wimbush, PhD, is a faculty member and Program Director in the Acute Care Nurse Practitioner Program at Wayne State University. Teaching and research interests include the role of stress in the development of disease states, especially as related to cardiovascular disease.

Linda Witek-Janusek, RN, PhD, is a physiologist and Professor of Nursing at the Marcella Niehoff School of Nursing, Loyola University of Chicago. Her program of research is aimed at understanding the relationship among stress, neuroendocrine activation, and the immune response in vulnerable populations. She is directing studies aimed at understanding the stress-immune response in women at risk for breast cancer and in individuals with HIV. She is also investigating the immunobiology of infant antifungal defense mechanisms.

Christine A. Wynd, PhD, RN, CNAA, is Professor in Nursing at the University of Akron. She teaches research methods and conducts research in the area of health promotion and smoking cessation. She uses a stress-coping model as the framework for much of her research.